Primary Health Care in the Making

Edited by
Ulrich Laaser   Raoul Senault   Herbert Viefhues

With 87 Figures and 175 Tables

Springer-Verlag
Berlin Heidelberg New York Tokyo

Priv.-Doz. Dr. med. Ulrich Laaser
Deutsches Institut zur Bekämpfung
des hohen Blutdruckes
Postfach 10 14 09
D-6900 Heidelberg 1

Professor Dr. Raoul Senault
Centre de Medecine Preventive
F-54501 Vandoeuvre-lès-Nancy Cédex

Professor Dr. med. Herbert Viefhues
Universitätsstraße 150
D-4630 Bochum 1

Library of Congress Cataloging in Publication Data
International Congress of Preventive and Social Medicine (10th : 1983 : Heidelberg, Germany) Primary health care in the making. Bibliography: p. Includes index.
1. Community health services-Congresses. 2. Medicine, Preventive-Congresses. 3. Social medicine-Congresses. 4. Health education-Congresses. I. Laaser, U. (Ulrich), 1941 –. II. Senault, R. III. Viefhues, Herbert. IV. Deutsche Gesellschaft für Sozialmedizin. V. Deutsches Institut zur Bekämpfung des Hohen Blutdruckes. VI. Title.
RA422.I63 1983 362.1 84-24050

ISBN-13: 978-3-642-69979-5 e-ISBN-13: 978-3-642-69977-1
DOI: 10.1007/978-3-642-69977-1

Softcover reprint of the hardcover 1st edition 1985

Graphischer Betrieb, Würzburg.
2119/3140-543210

Preface

Since the historical conference held in Alma Ata in 1978, it has been possible to observe a reorientation of the medical profession. More and more, issues of health enter the stage and curative medicine is not just loosing ground but some interest. 'How effective is health education?' and 'Whose task is primary prevention?' are questions which stimulate great concern and public debate. It seems also to be the first time since the last decades of the 19th century that the social dimension of health receives adequate consideration. Thus the recent publication of the so-called Black Report on *Inequalities in Health* (Penguin 1982) led to a heated discussion in Great Britain, certainly of relevance to many other countries. The 6 years since 1978 are much too short a time to proceed far towards 'Health for All', as the slogan of the World Health Organization puts it, but the concepts are spelled out, vaguely but convincing to many of us. It is the right time to discuss first experiences and to move from philosophy to empirical work. This work – as it relates to the process evolving since Alma Ata – is characterized by participation, cooperation and prevention:

Participation, because 'disease' concerns only the individual patient, his or her family and immediate social environment, while 'health' concerns everyone and should involve everyone. It is a task of the whole of society rather than the domaine of a single profession or party.

Cooperation, because the promotion of health must take place in daily life, subject to many influences and guided by goals and desires often unrelated to a medical preception of health and disease. Therefore a better mutual understanding between the medical and especially the social professions is of utmost importance.

Prevention, because some time during life health is succeeded by disease and whatever we as physicians can do to prevent premature morbidity and death, we are obliged to do it. The main motive for a preventive orientation of the medical profession is not the doubtful economic benefit possibly accruing from the retardation of chronic disease, it is simply an ethical one. For this reason prevention became a major focus in general medicine irrespective of the varying types of health care systems.

To bring good medical care close to the people is the essence of primary health care, and nowadays this includes preventive medicine, equal cooperation with other professions and participation of the patient in the diagnostic and therapeutic decision making. Still at the beginning of its modern development, primary health care takes as many forms as there are countries and identified deficiencies in the traditional delivery of health care. *Primary Health Care In The Making* is based on the proceedings of the Xth International Congress of Preventive and Social Medicine with the theme preventive and social aspects of primary health care. It was the first congress of its kind to be held in the Federal Republic of Germany and is a highlight in the history of the German Society of Social Medicine. The contributions mirror the differing stages of development throughout the world and for several countries provide a detailed insight into and description of their health problems and resources. This information has not always been easily accessible, like from many countries in the third world. Therefore, we have given special attention to the presentation of their data and experience. There are fascinating similarities between attempted solutions in developing as well as in developed societies, e.g. with regard to the increasing role of medical assistant personal.

However, primary prevention relates to the general, healthy population and in so far to daily lifestyles and habits, i.e. it reaches out beyond the organized health care system. The more 'primordial' prevention is, the more it has to rely on lay involvement and participation because there are no other ethical ways of inducing motivation for lifestyle change. This is where modern education for health through competence comes in, where mutual aid or self-help and self-organization as new social developments become relevant for the promotion of health. Promotion of health does not only relate to the system of health care, but depends on many other conditions which influence the quality of life. In this approach epidemiology acquires a new social dimension: we have to measure the state of well-being, of functioning, and of coping efficiency of the individual, family, and community. We are not only asking for a healthy mind in a healthy body, but a healthy person in a healthy society; we must build up a real epidemiology of health (G. A. Canaperia).

Heidelberg, December 1984

H. Viefhues R. Senault U. Laaser

Contents

Part I
The Physician and Primary Health Care 1

A. Changing Mentality in Medical Training

B. Paccagnella
Changing Mentality in Medical Education 3

R. Senault and J. P. Deschamps
Medical Education: Proposals for the Future 11

E. Musil
Education in Social Medicine 14

J. Gofin, N. Mainemer, and S. L. Kark
Community Health in Primary Care – A Workshop on Community-Oriented Primary Care 17

R. Rothenberg, V. R. Coleman, and P. Zabetakis
Seminars in Clinical Preventive Medicine 22

T. D. Dublin
The Migration of Physicians to the United States – A Study of Candidates for ECFMG Certification, 1969–1982 25

B. Primary Health Care by the Physician and Allied Personnel

B. Kosanke
Cooperation Between Different Professions and Lay Personnel 31

F. Holldack-Heckmann
The Group Medical Practice – A Prospect for Doctors and Patients? . 34

U. Hoffmann
Division of Tasks and Cooperation: Learning Processes in Inter-professional Group Practices 38

B. Meifort and H. Paulini
Legal, Institutional and Educational Conditions for Interdisciplinary Teamwork Between Allied Health Professions 42

A. Geiger
Social Work in Health Care Services 46

A. A. Talbot, P. Curtis, L. MacLaren, A. F. Sanchez, and R. Bissonette
Telephone Medicine: A Training Need in a Technological Society . . 49

F. Fontana and A. Orsini
Family Counselling Services in the Veneto Region of Italy:
Structural and Functional Aspects 60

C. Brühne-Scharlau and F. W. Schwartz
Health Counselling – A Pilot Programme 67

G. Wendt
Primary Prevention by the General Practitioner? 70

H. Noack
Medical and Psychosocial Problems in Primary Care 74

H. E. Kerek-Bodden, P. Kramer, E. Schach, and F. W. Schwartz
Mental Health Problems in the Offices of General Practitioners
and Internists 80

M. Heydthausen and F. Koch
Diagnostic Language in Primary Health Care – A Structural and
Semantic Analysis of Diagnoses on Health Service Medical Cards . . 86

H.-D. Klimm
Early Detection of Disorders of Peripheral Circulation in General
Practice: A Model for a Research Project of the German Society
for General Medicine 90

R. Laessle and R. Ellmann
Effects of the Social Situation on Health and Utilization of Medical Care
Services: Results from the Munich Follow-up Study 95

R. Ellmann and R. Laessle
Social Class and Utilization of Primary Medical Care Services:
Class-Specific Patterns of Utilization Behaviour in the Munich
Follow-up Study 100

M. Patel
Choice of Best or Cheapest Drugs: A Note on Regulating Drug Supplies 105

W. Koenig, U. Keil, J. Stieber, A. Döring, S. J. Pöppl, and M. Mraz
Epidemiology of Digitalis Use – Results from a Random Sample
of the Munich Population 109

Part II
Special Groups for Primary Health Care 117

A. Maternal and Child Care

M. Nikolić, M. Gec, G. Nikolić, and G. Sbutega
Some Relevant Ecological Factors and Their Influence on Pregnancy . 119

M. Gec, M. Nikolić, V. Sulovic, and G. Sbutega
Some Maternal and Social Factors in Relation to the Birth Weight of Infants . . . 122

M. H. Schmidt and G. Esser
The Diagnosis of "Minimal Brain Dysfunction" – Implications for Social Medicine . . . 125

B. Childhood and Adolescence

L. Neradović, D. Plećaš, and M. Havelka
Physical Fitness of Obese Children and Its Relationship to Age, Sex and Nutritional Intake . . . 128

B. Legetić, M. Planojević, V. Grujić, and J. Pisarev
Knowledge, Habits and Standpoints of Novi Sad Adolescents in Relation to Cardiovascular Diseases and Possibilities of Their Prevention as Part of a Comprehensive Community Cardiovascular Control Programme . 132

U. Laaser and P. Allhoff
Review of the Results and Recommendations of the Cologne Study . . 135

S. G. Gerberich, M. Hays, J. S. Mandel, R. W. Gibson, and C. J. Van der Heide
Analysis of Suicides in Adolescents and Young Adults: Implications for Prevention . . . 137

D. Repovš
"Health Education" – A New Subject in the Secondary Schools of SR Slovenia, SFR Yugoslavia . . . 146

R. Fehr and E. O. Krasemann
Some Results of the "Schülerstudie Gesundheitserziehung Hamburg" 150

H. Hildebrandt
An Ecological Concept of Health Promotion in Child and Youth Work – Projekt Gesundheit/Bund Deutscher Pfadfinder . . . 156

P. Franzkowiak
Growing Up into the 1980s: An Ecological Framework for Health Promotion for Youth . . . 161

C. The Occupational Setting

W. Maschewsky
Industrial Jobs and Coronary Heart Disease . . . 167

M. T. Tenconi, A. Taccola, C. Mercuri, G. B. Gotti, M. R. Spina, and G. Bellotti
Coronary Prone Behaviour Related to Occupational Stress in a Sample of Male Workers . . . 170

I. Weber and J. Siegrist
Work Stressors and Coronary Risk: Two Perspectives . . . 175

K. Undeutsch and C. Halhuber
Some Aspects of the Return to Work After Myocardial Infarction . . 179

W. Huber, E. Marquard, and W. K. Schreiber
Vocational Rehabilitation in Hypertension and Renal Diseases . . . 183

S. Poser, P. Denecke, H. Friedrich, and R. Schipper
Occupational Performance of Patients with Multiple Sclerosis 188

S. Koifman, V. L. G. Blank, and J. A. M. Souza
Mortality and Accidents in the Electrical Industry 192

J. S. Vobecky, J. Vobecky, and D. Shapcott
Nutritional Habits and Their Relation to Health in the Occupational Environment 197

U. Canaris and J. Töppich
Alcohol in the Working Environment 205

D. Environmental Risks

J. van Reek
Air Pollution and Health Indicators: Regional Findings for the Netherlands 209

P. Lercher and W. W. Kofler
Possibilities and Limits of Data Drawn from the "Gesundenuntersuchung" for an Epidemiological Study of the Connection Between Air Quality and Chronic Bronchitis 215

W. Jedrychowski, M. Krzyzanowski, and B. Wojtyniak
Biological Effect of the Air Quality Measured at the Population Level . 223

E. The Chronically Ill

U. Gerhardt
Family Rehabilitation in Chronic Illness 227

B. Luban-Plozza
Family Psychology and "Family Confrontation" 230

G. Mall
Who Treats the Chronically Ill: The General Practitioner or the Internist? 235

A. Füller
Compliance – A "Risk Factor" for Chronic Diseases? 240

J. Ananijević-Pandey and H. Vlajinac
Non-fatal Myocardial Infarction in Women Under 50 Years of Age, with Reference to Oral Contraceptive Use in Belgrade 244

M. Arndt, D. Rühland, R. Keferstein, and W. Pircher
Rehabilitation After Surgery for Chronic Vascular Disease: Goal and Reality 249

J. Resch
Multiple Sclerosis and Geophysical Factors 252

J. Kunow
Chronic Mental Illness: Social Factors and Rehabilitation Outcomes . 256

G. Krüger, H. Biehl, B. Krumm, and C. Schubart
Longitudinal Pattern of Aftercare in a Cohort of Recent Onset Schizophrenics 261

H. D. Brenner, W. Böker, K. Andres, and W. G. Stramke
Efforts at Compensation with Regard to Basic Disorders Among Schizophrenics 267

L. von Ferber, H. J. Jesdinsky, A. Schröer, and H. J. Trampisch
Identification of Specific Patterns of Work Incapacity Related to Chronic Illness: Analysis of Data Gathered by the Health Insurance Funds in Western Germany 274

F. Migrants in Germany

A. Geiger and F. Hamburger
Migration and Health 281

C. Schöning-Kalender
Sickness in the Process of Migration 284

I. Theilen
Illness and Health of Turkish "Citizens" in West Germany as Seen Against the Background of Their Personal Life Narratives 288

H. Mergerian and W. Bommer
Studies on Social Hygienic Problems Appertaining to Foreign Children and Their Families in the Federal Republic of Germany 294

M. Akkent, G. Franger, and N. Gültepe
The Living Conditions and Education of Turkish Infants in the Federal Republic of Germany: Report on a Model Project in Nürnberg 297

F. Poustka
Are New Counselling and Psychotherpeutic Patterns Necessary for Children of Foreign Employees (Guest-workers)? Results of an Epidemiological Study 300

J. Korporal, J. A. Marmor, and A. Zink
Migration and Health – Thoughts on Past and Current Research . . . 304

Part III
Health Education in Primary Health Care 311

A. Education for Health through Participation

T. Fülöp
Health for All by the Year 2000: A Challenge for the Education of Health Personnel 313

J. McEwen
Primary Health Care: The Challenge of Participation 320

E. A. Sand
The Promotion of Health Through Changes in Life-style:
Epidemiological, Psychosocial and Ethical Aspects 326

K. Orth-Gomér, B.-M. Wallin, and A.-L. Undén
Social Support and Coronary Risk Factors 330

B. Learning from the Third World Experience

R. P. Bernard and S. Sastrawinata
Maternal and Perinatal Death in Indonesian University Obstetrics:
Risk Display for Selected Social and Biological Determinants 335

C.-L. Chen, Y.-M. Chang, C.-C. Lin, and J.-Y. Lin
Maternal Transmission of Hepatitis B and Its Prevention 352

L. V. Adekunle and O. S. Oduntan
Psychosocial Factors in Childhood Diseases in Nigeria:
A Preliminary Study 356

V. B. Saxena
Primary Health Care and Feasibility of Yaws Eradication in India . . 370

G. Lachenmann
Human Resources for Primary Health Care in Developing Countries . 377

T. D. Wilson, L. M. Irwig, and L. D. Saunders
Evaluation of Polyclinic Services Run by Primary Health Care (PHC)
Nurses in Soweto 381

W. Bichmann
Primary Health Care – A New Strategy? Lessons to Learn
from Community Participation 386

C. Modification of at Risk Behaviours

B. Mausner and D. Brandspiegel
The Relation of Pattern of Support for Smoking and Achievement
Motive in Young Women 391

M. F. Schuntermann
On the Effectiveness of Smoking Cessation Treatment Methods . . . 394

V. Milošević
Cigarette Smoking, COHb Level and Physical Fitness 398

F. Schmidt
Reduction of Cigarette Consumption as the Most Important Task
of Preventive Medicine and Health Policy 402

E. Poetter, L. P. Krall, K. Huth, F. W. Schmahl
A New Approach to Diet Counseling of Overweight Patients and Diabetics . . . 408

I. Cleres-Kaiser
Adiposity – A Challenge to the General Practitioner in Therapy and Prevention . . . 416

Part IV
Cooperative Prevention Programmes in Primary Health Care . . . 419

A. The Control of Elevated Blood Pressure in the Community

1. Presuppositions for Community-Wide Blood Pressure Control . . . 421

D. Ganten
High Blood Pressure Control in the Community . . . 421

W.-P. Tseng
Epidemiological Study of Hypertension and Stroke in Taiwan . . . 424

M. Maiwald
Home Blood Pressure Measurement – A Useful Tool in the Management of High Blood Pressure? . . . 428

V. R. Coleman
An Education Program for Instruction in Self Blood Pressure Measurement . . . 434

P. Strazzullo, F. Contaldo, F. P. Cappuccio, A. Fischetti, P. R. A. Soda, A. De Leo, C. Iovine, and M. Mancini
Serum Insulin and Glucose Tolerance in Obese Patients with or Without Associated Arterial Hypertension . . . 436

P. S. Sever
The Treatment of High Blood Pressure: Non-Pharmacological and Pharmacological Measures . . . 442

J. Menard, G. Chatellier, and P. Corvol
What Can Be Learnt from the Results of the High Blood Pressure Trials? . . . 451

U. Härtel, U. Kail, V. Cairns, A. Döring, and J. Stieber
Medical Care Utilization and Self-Reported Health of Hypertensives: Results of the Munich Blood Pressure Study . . . 456

2. Blood Pressure Control Programmes and Their Effectiveness . . . 464

W. T. Friedwald
The American National High Blood Pressure Education Program . . . 464

B. Ravnikar, N. Erzen, P. Jezersek, J. Turk, and D. Zrimsek
Epidemiological Situation of Cardiovascular Diseases in Slovenia and Possibilities for Prevention and Control . . . 468

D. S. Silverberg, L. Baltuch, Y. Hermoni, and P. Eyal
Application of Epidemiology in Primary Health Care – Treatment of Hypertension . . . 472

W. Höbel, J. Stieber, P. Potthoff, and R. Thurmayr
Severity Rating of Hypertension as a Measure of Individual Rehabilitation Effects . . . 477

H. Wenzel und U. Laaser
Cost-Effectiveness of Treating Hypertensives in the Federal Republic of Germany: A Model Analysis . . . 483

B. Community Health Promotion by Lay Involvement

G. De Backer, M. Dramaix, M. Kornitzer, F. Kittel, and K. Vuylsteek
Social Differences in the Long-Term Effects of Health Education in Reducing Coronary Risk . . . 488

D. S. Thelle, O. H. Førde, and E. Arnesen
The Tromsø Heart Study: The Effect of Dietary Intervention in Hyperlipaemic Men – 5-Year Follow-up . . . 495

A. Füller and R. Pitsch
Health Committees – A Way to Consumer Participation in Health Care Systems . . . 500

F. Haux
A Model for Co-ordinated and Integrated Lifelong Health Security . . . 505

R. Rodale
Community Prevention: The Program of the People's Medical Society . . . 509

P. Lemke and F. Pfirrmann
The Role of Health Insurance Companies in Primary Prevention . . . 512

K. Becker and B. Laugsch
Health Work in a Working-Class District of Mannheim . . . 516

S. Panico, R. Landolfi, and L. Minelli
Health Promotion in A Large Citty . . . 521

U. Laaser
Lay Involvement in the Primary Prevention of Cardiovascular Disease: The Rhein-Neckar Community Study (GRN) . . . 524

Subject Index . . . 541

List of Contributors

L. V. Adekunle
Department of Preventive and Social Medicine, College of Medicine, University of Ibadan, Ibadan, Nigeria

M. Akkent
Institut für Tropenhygiene, Im Neuenheimer Feld 324, 6900 Heidelberg, Federal Republic of Germany

P. Allhoff
Arbeitsgruppe für Interdisziplinäre Gesundheitsforschung, Postfach 45 01 09, 5000 Köln 91, Federal Republic of Germany

J. Ananijević-Pandey
Institute of Social Medicine Statistics and Health Research, School of Medicine, University of Belgrade, Dr. Subotića 15, 11000 Belgrade, Yugoslavia

K. Andres
Psychiatrische Universitätsklinik Bern, Bollingenstrasse 111, 3072 Bern, Switzerland

M. Arndt
Chirurgische Universitäts-Klinik, Jungeblodtplatz 1, 4400 Münster, Federal Republic of Germany

E. Arnesen
Institute of Community Medicine, University of Tromsø, Postboks 417, 9010 Tromsø, Norway

G. De Backer
National Found for Scientific Research, Bruxelles, Belgium

L. Baltuch
Hypertension Control, Medical and Nursing Division of Kupat Holim of the Histadrut, Health Insurance Institut of the General Federation of Labor, Tel-Aviv, Isreal

K. Becker
Gemeindestudie Rhein-Neckar, Deutsches Institut zur Bekämpfung des hohen Blutdruckes, Postfach 10 14 09, 6900 Heidelberg 1, Federal Republic of Germany

G. Bellotti
Clinica Neuropatologiea, Via Palestro 1, 27100 Pavia, Italy

R. P. Bernard
International Federation for Family Health, 22 Ave. Riant Parc, 1209 Geneva, Switzerland

W. Bichmann
Institut für Tropenhygiene und Öffentliches Gesundheitswesen am Südasien-Institut der Universität Heidelberg, Im Neuenheimer Feld 324, 6900 Heidelberg, Federal Republic of Germany

H. Biehl
Zentralinstitut für Seelische Gesundheit, Postfach 59 70, 6800 Mannheim 1, Federal Republic of Germany

R. Bissonette
Medicus mundi International, Mozartstrasse 9, 5100 Aachen, Federal Republic of Germany

V. L. G. Blank
Public Health Department of C.C.S. Universidade Federal de Santa Catarina, Campus Universitário-Florianopolis, CEP 88000, Brazil

W. Böker
Psychiatrische Universitätsklinik Bern, Bolligenstrasse 111, 3072 Bern, Switzerland

W. Bommer
Institut für Allgemeine Hygiene und Tropenhygiene, Georg-August-Universität, Windausweg 2, 3400 Göttingen, Federal Republic of Germany

D. Brandspiegel
Beaver College, Glenside, PA 19038, USA

H. D. Brenner
Psychiatrische Universitätsklinik Bern, Bolligenstrasse 111, 3072 Bern, Switzerland

C. Brühne-Scharlau
Zentralinstitut für die kassenärztliche Versorgung in der Bundesrepublik Deutschland, Haedenkampstrasse 5, 5000 Köln 41, Federal Republic of Germany

V. Cairns
MEDIS-Institut für Medizinische Informatik und Systemforschung der Gesellschaft für Strahlen- und Umweltforschung, Ingolstädter Landstrasse 1, 8042 München-Neuherberg, Federal Republic of Germany

U. Canaris
Bundeszentrale für gesundheitliche Aufklärung, Ostmerheimer Strasse 200, 5000 Köln 91, Federal Republic of Germany

F. P. Cappuccio
Institute of Internal Medicins and Metabolic Disease, Center for Ateriosclerosis, 2nd Medical School, University of Naples, Naples, Italy

Y.-M. Chang
National Taiwan University Hospital, Taiwan, Republic of China

G. Chatellier
Inserm U36, 17, rue du Fer-à-Moulin, 75005 Paris, France

C.-L. Chen
Taipei Municipal Women and Children Hospital, Taipei/Taiwan, Republic of China

I. Cleres-Kaiser
Fedderbach 4, 5108 Monschau-Kalterherberg, Federal Republic of Germany

V. R. Coleman
New York State Department of Health, New Rochelle Regional Office, 145 Huguenot Street – 5th Floor, New Rochelle, NY 10801, USA

F. Contaldo
Institut of Internal Medicine and Metabolic Disease, Center for Arteriosclerosis, 2nd Medical School, University of Naples, Naples, Italy

P. Corvol
Inserm U36, 17, rue du Fer-á-Moulin, 75005 Paris, France

P. Curtis
Medicus mundi International, Mozartstrasse 9, 5100 Aachen, Federal Republic of Germany

P. Denecke
Klinik und Poliklinik für Neurologie, Georg-August-Universität Göttingen, Robert-Koch-Strasse 40, 3400 Göttingen, Federal Republic of Germany

J.-P. Deschamps
Centre de Médecine, Préventive, 2, Avenue du Doyen J. Parisot, 54500 Vandoeuvre-lès-Nancy, France

A. Döring
MEDIS-Institut für Medizinische Informatik und Systemforschung der Gesellschaft für Strahlen- und Umweltforschung, Ingolstädter Landstrasse 1, 8042 München-Neuherberg, Federal Republic of Germany

M. Dramaix
Laboratoire d'Epidémiologie et de Médecine Sociale, Université Libre de Bruxelles, Bruxelles, Belgium

T. D. Dublin
2938 Garfield Street, N.W., Washington, DC 20008, USA

R. Ellmann
Max-Planck-Institut für Psychiatrie, Kraepelinstrasse 10, 8000 München 40, Federal Republic of Germany

N. Eržen
Public Health Institute of SR Slovenia, Ljubljana, Trubarjeva 2, Yugoslavia

G. Esser
Zentralinstitut für Seelische Gesundheit, Kinder- und Jugendpsychiatrische Klinik, Postfach 59 70, 6800 Mannheim 1, Federal Republic of Germany

P. Eyal
Hypertension Control, Medical and Nursing Division of Kupat Holim of the Histadrut, Health Insurance Institute of the General Federation of Labor, Tel-Aviv, Israel

R. Fehr
Gesundheitsbehörde Hamburg, Abt. 65, Gesundheitsvorsorge und -fürsorge, Seewartenstrasse 7, 2000 Hamburg, Federal Republic of Germany

L. von Ferber
Medizinische Statistik und Biomathematik, Medizinische Einrichtungen der Universität Düsseldorf, Moorenstrasse 5, 4000 Düsseldorf 1, Federal Republic of Germany

A. Fischetti
Institute of Internal Medicine and Metabolic Disease, Center for Arteriosclerosis, 2nd Medical School, University of Naples, Naples, Italy

F. Fontana
Institute of Hygiene, University of Padua, Via Loredan 18, 35100 Padova, Italy

O. H. Førde
Institute of Community Medicine, University of Tromsø, Postboks 417, 9010 Tromsø, Norway

G. Franger
Institut für Tropenhygiene, Im Neuenheimer Feld 324, 6900 Heidelberg, Federal Republic of Germany

P. Franzkowiak
Forschungsgruppe Jugend und Gesundheit, Kaiserstrasse 63, 6900 Heidelberg, Federal Republic of Germany

W. T. Friedewald
National Heart, Lung, and Blood Institute, National Institutes of Health, Federal Building, Room 212, Bethesda, MD 20205, USA

H. Friedrich
Abteilung für Medizinsoziologie, Humboldtallee 1 d, 3400 Göttingen, Federal Republic of Germany

A. Füller
Deutsches Institut zur Bekämpfung des hohen Blutdruckes, Postfach 10 14 09, 6900 Heidelberg 1, Federal Republic of Germany

T. Fülöp
Division of Manpower Developement, World Health Organization, 1211 Geneva 27, Switzerland

D. Ganten
Deutsches Institut zur Bekämpfung des hohen Blutdruckes, Postfach 10 14 09, 6900 Heidelberg 1, Federal Republic of Germany

M. Gec
Institute of Hygiene and Medical Ecology, School of Medicine, University of Belgrad, Dr. Subotiĉa 5, 11000 Belgrade, Yugoslavia

A. Geiger
WIAD, Godesberger Allee 54, 5300 Bonn 2, Federal Republic of Germany

S. G. Gerberich
School of Public Health, University of Minnesota, Institute for Athletic Medicine, Minneapolis, MN 55455, USA

U. Gerhardt
Medizinisches Zentrum für Psychosomatische Medizin, Abt. Medizinische Soziologie, Klinik der Justus-Liebig-Universität Giessen, Friedrichstrasse 24, 6300 Giessen, Federal Republic of Germany

R. W. Gibson
School of Medicine, University of Minnesota, Duluth, MN 55455, USA

J. Gofin
Department of Social Medicine, Hadassah Medical Organization and the Hebrew University, School of Public Health and Community Medicine, Jerusalem, Israel

G. B. Gotti
Centro per le malattie cardiovascolari professionali, Dipartimento di Medicina Preventiva, Occupazionale e di Comunità – Sezione di Medicina del Lavoro, Via Boezio, 27100 Pavia, Italy

V. Grujiĉ
Institut za zdravstvenu zaštitu, Bulevar Revolucije 91, 21000 Novi Sad, Yugoslavia

N. Gültepe
Institut für Tropenhygiene, Im Neuenheimer Feld 324, 6900 Heidelberg, Federal Republic of Germany

U. Härtel
MEDIS-Institut für medizinische Informatik und Systemforschung der Gesellschaft für Strahlen- und Umweltforschung, Ingolstädter Landstrasse 1, 8042 München-Neuherberg, Federal Republic of Germany

C. Halhuber
Innere Medizin, Kardiologie und Sportmedizin, Abteilung 1, Herz-Kreislauf-Klinik, 5920 Bad Berleburg, Federal Republic of Germany

F. Hamburger
Pädagogisches Institut der Universität Mainz, Postfach 3980, 6500 Mainz, Federal Republic of Germany

F. Haux
AOK-Kurklinik Pfaffenberg, Innere Medizin, Pfaffenbergstrasse 6, 3423 Bad Sachsa, Federal Republic of Germany

M. Havelka
Institute for Hygiene and Medical Ecology, School of Medicine, University of Belgrade, Dr. Subotiča 5, 11000 Belgrade, Yugoslavia

M. Hays
School of Public Health, University of Minnesota, Minneapolis, MN 55455, USA

C. J. Van der Heide
Children's Health Center, Minneapolis, MN 55455, USA

A. Hermoni
Hypertension Control, Medical and Nursing Division of Kupat Holim of the Histadrut, Health Insurance Institute of the General Federation of Labor, Tel-Aviv, Israel

M. Heydthausen
Institut für Medizinische Soziologie, Universität Düsseldorf, Universitätsstrasse 1, 4000 Düsseldorf, Federal Republic of Germany

H. Hildebrandt
c/o Hesselmann, Lutterothstrasse 3, 2000 Hamburg 20, Federal Republic of Germany

W. Höbel
MEDIS-Institut für Medizinische Informatik und Systemforschung der Gesellschaft für Strahlen- und Umweltforschung, Ingolstädter Landstrasse 1, 8042 München-Neuherberg, Federal Republic of Germany

U. Hoffmann
Sonderforschungsbereich 101, Hohenzollernstrasse 81, 8000 München 40, Federal Republic of Germany

F. Holldack-Heckmann
Pfeufferstrasse 33, 8000 München 70, Federal Republic of Germany

W. Huber
Rehabilitationsklinik Heidelberg, Bonhoefferstrasse, 6900 Heidelberg 1, Federal Republic of Germany

K. Huth
Diakonissen-Krankenhaus, 6000 Frankfurt, Federal Republic of Germany

C. Iovine
Institute of Internal Medicine and Metabolic Disease, Center for Arteriosclerosis, 2nd Medical School, University of Naples, Naples, Italy

L. M. Irwig
Medical Research Council and the University of the Witwaterstrand, York Road, Darktown, 2193 Johannesburg, South Africa

W. Jedrychowski
Department of Epidemiology, Institute of Social Medicine, Medical School, Kopernika 7, Kraków, Poland

H. J. Jesdinsky
Medizinische Statistik und Biomathematik, Medizinische Einrichtungen der Universität Düsseldorf, Moorenstrasse 5, 4000 Düsseldorf 1, Federal Republic of Germany

P. Jezenšek
University Clinical Center, Ljubljana, Trubarjeva 2, Yugoslavia

S. L. Kark
Department of Social Medicine, Hadassah Medical Organization and Hebrew University, School of Public Health and Community Medicine, Jerusalem, Israel

R. Keferstein
Chirurgische Universitätsklinik, Jungeblodtplatz 1, 4000 Münster, Federal Republic of Germany

U. Keil
MEDIS-Institut für Medizinische Informatik und Systemforschung der Gesellschaft für Strahlen- und Umweltforschung, Ingolstädter Landstrasse 1, 8042 München-Neuherberg, Federal Republic of Germany

H. E. Kerek-Bodden
Zentralinstitut für die kassenärztliche Versorgung, Haedenkampstrasse 5, 5000 Köln 41, Federal Republic of Germany

F. Kittel
Laboratoire d'Epidémiologie et de Médecine Sociale, Université Libre de Bruxelles, Bruxelles, Belgium

H.-D. Klimm
Abteilung für Allgemeinmedizin, Universität Heidelberg, Friedrichstrasse 81 a, 7554 Kuppenheim, Federal Republic of Germany

F. Koch
Institut für Medizinische Soziologie, Universität Düsseldorf, Universitätsstrasse 1, 4000 Düsseldorf, Federal Republic of Germany

W. Koenig
MEDIS-Institut für Medizinische Informatik und Systemforschung der Gesellschaft für Strahlen- und Umweltforschung, Ingolstädter Landstrasse 1, 8042 München-Neuherberg, Federal Republic of Germany

W. W. Kofler
Department of Social Medicine at the University of Innsbruck, Adamgasse 1, 6020 Innsbruck, Austria

S. Koifman
Department of Epidemiology, National School of Public Health, Rio de Janeiro, Brazil

M. Kornitzer
Laboratoire d'Epidémiologie et de Médecine Sociale, Université Libre de Bruxelles, Bruxelles, Belgium

J. Korporal
Fachhochschule für Sozialarbeit und Sozialpädagogik Berlin, Karl-Schrader-Strasse 6, 1000 Berlin 30, Federal Republic of Germany

B. Kosanke
Zentralinstitut für die kassenärztliche Versorgung, Haedenkampstrasse 5, 5000 Köln 41, Federal Republic of Germany

L. P. Krall
Joslin Diabetes Center and Harvard Medical School, Boston, USA

P. Kramer
Zentralinstitut für die kassenärztliche Versorgung, Haedenkampstrasse 5, 5000 Köln 41, Federal Republic of Germany

E. O. Krasemann
Gesundheitsbehörde Hamburg, Abteilung 65, Gesundheitsvorsorge und -fürsorge, Seewartenstrasse 7, Federal Republic of Germany

G. Krüger
Zentralinstitut für Seelische Gesundheit, Postfach 5970, 6800 Mannheim 1, Federal Republic of Germany

B. Krumm
Zentralinstitut für Seelische Gesundheit, Postfach 5970, 6800 Mannheim 1, Federal Republic of Germany

M. Krzyzanowski
Department of Epidemiology, Institute of Social Medicine, Medical School, 7 Kopernika Street, Kraków, Poland

J. Kunow
Psychiatrisches Landeskrankenhaus Weinsberg, 7102 Weinsberg/Weissenhof, Federal Republic of Germany

U. Laaser
Deutsches Institut zur Bekämpfung des hohen Blutdruckes, Postfach 10 14 09, 6900 Heidelberg 1
Federal Republic of Germany

G. Lachenmann
German Development Institute, Fraunhoferstrasse 33–36, 1000 Berlin 10, Federal Republic of Germany

R. Laessle
Max-Planck-Institut für Psychiatrie, Kraepelinstrasse 10, 8000 München 40, Federal Republic of Germany

R. Landolfi
Servizio di Epidemiologia, Ecologia ed Educazione Sanitaria, USL 39 Napoli, Piazza Ettore Vitale 66, 80100 Napoli, Italy

B. Laugsch
Deutsches Institut zur Bekämpfung des hohen Blutdruckes, Postfach 10 14 09, 6900 Heidelberg 1, Federal Republic of Germany

B. Legetić
Dispanzer KVB-dom zdravlja "Novi Sad", Bulevav Avnoj-a 77, 21000 Novi Sad, Yugoslavia

P. Lemke
Deutsches Institut zur Bekämpfung des hohen Blutdruckes, Postfach 10 14 09, Federal Republic of Germany

A. de Leo
Institute of Internal Medicine and Metabolic Disease, Center for Arteriosclerosis, 2nd Medical School, University of Naples, Naples, Italy

P. Lercher
Department of Social Medicine at the University of Innsbruck, Adamgasse 1, 6020 Innsbruck, Austria

C.-C. Lin
National Taiwan University Hospital, Taipei, Taiwan, Republic of China

J.-Y. Lin
National Taiwan University Hospital, Taipei, Taiwan, Republic of China

B. Luban-Plozza
Piazza Fontana Pedrazzini, 6600 Locarno, Switzerland

J. McEwen
Academic Department of Community Medicine, King's College, School of Medicine and Dentistry, Denmark Hill, London SE5 8RX, United Kingdom

L. MacLaren
Medicus mundi International, Mozartstrasse 9, 5100 Aachen, Federal Republic of Germany

N. Mainemer
Department of Social Medicine, Hadassah Medical Organization and the Hebrew University School of Public Health and Community Medicine, Jerusalem, Israel

M. Maiwald
Forschungsgruppe Stress, Medizinische Universitätsklinik Heidelberg, Alte Bergheimer Strasse 5, 6900 Heidelberg, Federal Republic of Germany

G. Mall
Krankenhaus St. Trudpert, Innere Abteilung, Wolfsbergallee 50, 7530 Pforzheim, Federal Republic of Germany

M. Mancini
Institute of Internal Medicine and Metabolic Disease, Center for Arteriosclerosis, 2nd Medical School, University of Naples, Naples, Italy

J. S. Mandel
School of Public Health, University of Minnesota, Minneapolis, MN 55455, USA

J. A. Marmor
Department of Anthropology, The University of Conneticut, RFD'2 Daleville School Road, West Wellington, CT 06279, USA

E. Marquard
Rehabilitationsklinik Heidelberg, Bonhoefferstrasse, 6900 Heidelberg 1, Federal Republic of Germany

W. Maschewsky
Fachhochschule Hamburg, Fachbereich Sozialpädagogik, Saarlandstrasse 30, 2000 Hamburg 60, Federal Republic of Germany

B. Mausner
Department of Psychology, Beaver Bollege, Glenside, PA, 19038, USA

B. Meifort
Bundesinstitut für Berufsbildung, Fehrbelliner Platz 3, 1000 Berlin 31, Federal Republic of Germany

J. Menard
Inserm U36, 17, rue du Fer-à-Moulin, 75005 Paris, France

C. Mercuri
Dipartimento di Medicina Preventiva, Occupazionale e di Comunità-Sezione, Via Forlanini 1, 27100 Pavia, Italy

H. Mergerian
Institut für Allgemeine Hygiene und Tropenhygiene, Georg-August-Universität, Windausweg 2, 3400 Göttingen, Federal Republic of Germany

V. Milošević
Institute of Hygiene and Medical Ecology, School of Medicine, University of Belgrade, Dr. Subotića, 11000 Belgrade, Yugoslavia

L. Minelli
Istituto di Igiene, Università di Perugia, Via del Giochetto, 06100 Perugia, Italy

W. Mraz
Institut für Klinische Chemie, Klinikum Großhadern, Universität München, Marchioninistrasse 15, 8000 München 70, Federal Republic of Germany

E. Musil
Mariahilferstrasse 177, 1150 Wien, Austria

L. Neradović
Institute of Hygiene and Medical Ecology, School of Medicine, University of Belgrade, Dr. Subotića 5, 11000 Belgrade, Yugoslavia

G. Nikolić
Paediatric Surgery Clinic, University of Belgrade, Tiršova 10, 11000 Belgrade, Yugoslavia

M. Nikolić
Institute for Hygiene and Medical Ecology, School of Medicine, University of Belgrade, Dr. Subotića 5, 11000 Belgrade, Yugoslavia

H. Noack
Institut für Sozial- und Präventivmedizin, Universität Bern, Finkenhubelweg 11, 3012 Bern, Switzerland

O. S. Oduntan
Department of Preventive and Social Medicine, College of Medicine, University of Ibadan, Ibadan, Nigeria

A. Orsini
Institute of Hygiene, University of Padua, Via Loredan 18, 35100 Padova, Italy

K. Orth-Gomér
National Institute for Psychosocial Factors and Health, Box 60210, 10401 Stockholm, Sweden

B. Paccagnella
Università degli Studi di Padova, Instituto di Igiene, Via Loredan 18, 35100 Padova, Italy

S. Panico
Istituto di Medicina interna e Malattie Dismetaboliche, Clinica Medica 2, 2 Facoltà di Medicina, Università di Napoli, Via Pansini 5, 80131 Napoli, Italy

M. Patel
Department of Community Medicine, University of Manchester, Stopford Building, Oxford Road, Manchester 1113 9PT, Great Britain

H. Paulini
Bundesinstitut für Berufsbildung, Fehrbelliner Platz 3, 1000 Berlin 31, Federal Republic of Germany

F. Pfirrmann
Deutsches Institut zur Bekämpfung des hohen Blutdruckes, Postfach 10 14 09, 6900 Heidelberg 1, Federal Republic of Germany

W. Pircher
Chirurgische Universitätsklinik, Jungeboldtplatz 1, 4400 Münster, Federal Republic of Germany

J. Pisarev
Institut za zdravstvenu zaštitu, Bulevar Revoluije 91, 21000 Novi Sad, Yugoslavia

R. Pitsch
Deutsches Institut zur Bekämpfung des hohen Blutdruckes, Postfach 10 14 09, 6900 Heidelberg 1, Federal Republic of Germany

M. Planojević
Dom zdravlja, "Novi Sad", Bulevar Avnoj-a 75, 21000 Novi Sad, Yugoslavia

D. Plećas
Institute for Hygiene and Medical Ecology, School of Medicine, University of Belgrade, Dr. Subotića 5, 11000 Belgrade, Yugoslavia

S. J. Pöppl
Forschungszentrum GSF, MEDIS-Institut, Ingolstädter Landstrasse 1, 8042 München-Neuherberg, Federal Republic of Germany

E. Poetter
Institut für Arbeits- und Sozialmedizin, Wilhelmstrasse 27, 7400 Tübingen, Federal Republic of Germany

S. Poser
Klinik und Poliklinik für Neurologie, Georg-August-Universität Göttingen, Robert-Koch-Strasse 40, 3400 Göttingen, Federal Republic of Germany

P. Potthoff
MEDIS-Institut der Gesellschaft für Strahlen- und Umweltforschung, Ingolstädter Landstrasse 1, 8042 München-Neuherberg, Federal Republic of Germany

F. Poustka
Zentralinstitut für Seelische Gesundheit, Kinder- und Jugendpsychiatrische Klinik, Postfach 59 70, 6800 Mannheim 1, Federal Republic of Germany

B. Ravnikar
Public Health Institute of SR Slovenia, Ljubljana, Trubarjeva 2, Yugoslavia

J. van Reek
Department of Medical Sociology, University of Limburg, Tongersestraat 53, 6200 MD Maastricht, The Netherlands

D. Repovš
Social Medicine, Institute of Public Health for SR Slovenia, P.O. Box 260, 61001 Ljubljana, Yugoslavia

J. Resch
Robert-Koch-Strasse 52, 6836 Oftersheim, Federal Republic of Germany

R. Rodale
People's Medical Society, 33 E. Minor Street, Emmaus, PA 18049, USA

R. Rothenberg
Bureau of Chronic Disease Prevention, New York State Department of Health Corning Tower, Empire State Plaza, Albany, NY 12237, USA

D. Rühland
Chirurgische Universitäts-Klinik, Jungeboldtplatz 1, 4400 Münster, Federal Republic of Germany

A. F. Sanchez
Medicus mundi International, Mozartstrasse 9, 5100 Aachen, Federal Republic of Germany

E. A. Sand
Ecole de Santé Publique, Université Libre de Bruxelles, Campus Erasme 590/5, 1070 Bruxelles, Belgium

S. Sastrawinata
International Federation for Family Health (IFFH), 1200 Genève, Switzerland

L. D. Saunders
Medical Research Council and the University of the Witwaterstrand, York Road, Darktown, 2193 Johannesburg, South Africa

V. B. Saxena
Department of Preventive and Social Medicine, Pt. JNM. Medical College, Raipur, Madhya Pradesh, India

G. Sbutega
Institute for Hygiene and Medical Ecology, School of Medicine, University of Belgrade, Dr. Subotiča 5, 11000 Belgrade, Yugoslavia

E. Schach
Universität Dortmund, Postfach 50 05 00, 4600 Dortmund 50, Federal Republic of Germany

R. Schipper
Multiple Sklerose, Informations- und Beratungsstelle, Gosslerstrasse 10 e, Göttingen, Federal Republic of Germany

F. W. Schmahl
Institut für Arbeits- und Sozialmedizin, Wilhelmstrasse 27, 7400 Tübingen, Federal Republic of Germany

F. Schmidt
Forschungsstelle für Präventive Onkologie, Klinische Fakultät Mannheim, Universität Heidelberg, Maybachstr. 14–16, 6800 Mannheim 1, Federal Republic of Germany

M. H. Schmidt
Zentralinstitut für Seelische Gesundheit, Kinder- und Jugendpsychiatrische Klinik, Postfach 59 70, 6800 Mannheim, Federal Republic of Germany

C. Schöning-Kalender
Heinrich-Hertz-Strasse 2, 6800 Mannheim 24, Federal Republic of Germany

W. K. Schreiber
Rehabilitationsklinik Heidelberg, Bonhoefferstrasse, 6900 Heidelberg, Federal Republic of Germany

A. Schrör
Institut für Medizinische Soziologie, Medizinische Einrichtungen der Universität Düsseldorf, Moorenstrasse 5, 4000 Düsseldorf 1, Federal Republic of Germany

C. Schubart
Zentralinstitut für Seelische Gesundheit, Postfach 59 70, 6800 Mannheim 1, Federal Republic of Germany

M. F. Schuntermann
Verband Deutscher Rentenversicherungsträger, Eysseneckstrasse 55, 6000 Frankfurt 1, Federal Republic of Germany

F. W. Schwartz
Zentralinstitut für die kassenärztliche Versorgung in der Bundesrepublik Deutschland, Haedenkampstrasse 5, 5000 Köln 41, Federal Republic of Germany

R. Senault
Centre de Médicine Préventive, 2, Avenue du Doyen J. Parisot, 54500 Vandoeuvre-lès-Nancy, France

P. S. Sever
Department of Clinical Pharmacology, St. Mary's Hospital Medical School, Northfolk Place, London, W2, IPG, United Kingdom

D. Shapcott
Department of Pediatrics, Faculty of Medicine, University of Sherbrooke, Sherbrooke, Quebec, Canada

J. Siegrist
Medizinische Soziologie, Fachbereich Humanmedizin, Universität Marburg, Bunsenstrasse 2, Federal Republic of Germany

D. S. Silverberg
Hypertension Control, Medical and Nursing Division of Kupat Holim of the Histradut, Health Insurance Institute of the General Federation of Labor, 62908 Tel-Aviv, P.O. Box 16250, Israel

P. R. A. Soda
Institute of Internal Medicine and Metabolic Disease, Center for Arteriosclerosis, 2nd Medical School, University of Naples, Naples, Italy

J. A. M. Souza
National School of Public Health, Av. Leopoldo, Bulhoes 1480, 8. andar, Rio de Janeiro, CEP 21041, Brazil

M. R. Spina
Dipartimento di Medicina Preventiva, Occupazionale e di Comunità-Sezione di Igiene, Via Forlanini 1, 27100 Pavia, Italy

J. Stieber
MEDIS-Institut für Medizinische Informatik und Systemforschung der Gesellschaft für Strahlen- und Umweltforschung, Ingolstädter Landstrasse 1, 8042 München-Neuherberg, Federal Republic of Germany

W. G. Stramke
Arbeitsgruppe für Evaluative Forschung, Zentralinstitut für Seelische Gesundheit, Postfach 59 70, 6800 Mannheim 1, Federal Republic of Germany

P. Strazzullo
Istituto di Medicina Interna e Malattie Dismetaboliche II Facoltà di Medicina e Chirurgia, Università di Napoli, Via Pansini 5, 80131 Napoli, Italy

V. Sulovic
Institute of Hygiene and Medical Ecology, School of Medicine, University of Belgrad, Dr. Subotića 5, 11000 Belgrade, Yugoslavia

A. Taccola
Centro per le malattie cardiovascolari professionali, Dipartimento di Medicina Preventiva, Occupazionale e di Comunità-Sezione di Medicina del Lavoro, Via Boezio, 26100 Pavia, Italy

A. A. Talbot
Medicus mundi International, Mozartstrasse 9, 5100 Aachen, Federal Republic of Germany

M. T. Tenconi
Dispartimento di Medicina Preventiva, Occopazionale e di Comunità-Sezione di Igiene, Via Forlanini 1, 27100 Pavia, Italy

I. Theilen
Scheffelweg 11, 6901 Wiesenbach, Federal Republic of Germany

D. S. Thelle
Institute of Community Medicine, University of Tromsø, Postboks 417, 9010 Tromsø, Norway

R. Thurmayr
Institut für Medizinische Statistik und Epidemiologie, Sternwartstrasse 2, 8000 München 80, Federal Republic of Germany

J. Töppich
Bundeszentrale für gesundheitliche Aufklärung, Ostmerheimer Strasse 200, 5000 Köln 91, Federal Republic of Germany

H. J. Trampisch
Medizinische Statistik und Biomathematik, Medizinische Einrichtungen der Universität Düsseldorf, Moorenstrasse 5, 4000 Düsseldorf 1, Federal Republic of Germany

W.-P. Tseng
Department of Medicine, National Taiwan University Hospital, 1 Chang-te Street, Taipei, Taiwan, Republic of China

J. Turk
University Clinical Center Ljubljana, Trubarjeva 2, Ljubljana, Yugoslavia

A.-L. Undèn
National Institut for Psychosocial Factors and Health, Box 60210, 10401 Stockholm, Sweden

K. Undeutsch
Herz-Kreislauf-Klinik, Innere Medizin, Arbeitsmedizin und Sportmedizin, Abteilung II, 5920 Bad Berleburg, Federal Republic of Germany

H. Vlajinac
Institut of Epidemiology, School of Medicine, University of Belgrade, Višegradska 26, 11000 Belgrade, Yugoslavia

J. Vobecky
Department of Community Health, Faculty of Medicine, University of Sherbrooke, Sherbrooke, Quebec, Canada

J. S. Vobecky
Human Nutrition Research Center, Faculty of Medicine, University of Sherbrooke, Quebec, Canada

K. Vuylsteek
Department of Hygiene and Social Medicine, State University Ghent, Bruxelles, Belgium

B.-M. Wallin
National Institute for Psychosocial Factors and Health, Box 60210, 10401 Stockholm, Sweden

I. Weber
Medizinische Soziologie, Fachbereich Humanmedizin, Universität Marburg, Bunsenstrasse 2, 3550 Marburg, Federal Republic of Germany

G. Wendt
Deutsches Institut zur Bekämpfung des hohen Blutdruckes, Postfach 10 14 09, 6900 Heidelberg, Federal Republic of Germany

H. Wenzel
Friedrichstrasse 61, 7750 Konstanz, Federal Republic of Germany

T. D. Wilson
Medical Research Council and the University of the Witwaterstrand, York Road, Darktown, 2193 Johannesburg, South Africa

B. Wojtyniak
Department of Epidemiology, Institute of Social Medicine, Medical School, 7 Kopernika Street, Krakòw, Poland

P. Zabetakis
Lenox Hill Hospital, 100 East 77 Street, New York, NY 10021, USA

A. Zink
Fachhochschule für Sozialarbeit und Sozialpädagogik Berlin, Karl-Schrader Strasse 6, 1000 Berlin 30, Federal Republic of Germany

D. Zrimšek
Primary Institution, Skofja Loka, Trubarjeva 2, Yugoslavia

Xth International Congress of Preventive
and Social Medicine
Heidelberg-Mannheim 1983

Under the auspices of
The International Federation of Hygiene, Preventive Medicine
and Social Medicine

in official relations with
The World Health Organization

in co-operation with
The European Association of Social Medicine
The German Society for Social Medicine
The Society for Social Hygiene, Baden-Württemberg

under the patronage of
The President of the Federal Republic of Germany

was organized by
The German Society for Social Medicine

in co-operation with
The German Institute for High Blood Pressure Research

and supported by
Bundesministerium für Jugend, Familie und Gesundheit
Ministerium für Arbeit, Gesundheit und Sozialordnung,
Baden-Württemberg
Deutsche Forschungsgemeinschaft
Bayer AG
Paul Martini Stiftung
Zentralinstitut für die kassenärztliche Versorgung

with contributions from
Boehringer Mannheim GmbH
Byk Gulden GmbH
Gödecke AG
Klöckner AG
Koch AG
Mack KG
Sanol Schwarz GmbH

Part I

The Physician and Primary Health Care

A. Changing Mentality in Medical Training

Changing Mentality in Medical Education

B. Paccagnella

Introduction

During the 1950s many of the university teachers in the European faculties of medicine began to realize that the time had come when teaching had to be changed, but it was not very clear what could be changed and the reason why it should be changed. Consequently WHO organized seminars and workshops in many European countries, such as those in Hamburg, Madrid, San Remo and Copenhagen, to discuss the various subjects connected with medical pedagogy.

At the same time in some universities study groups were formed (United Kingdom, Sweden, Holland, U.S.A., Canada etc.) to plan a new methodology for the school of medicine. Scientific associations were developed for the same purpose, and more publications became available on the subject.

In brief, the analysis of the pedagogic problems showed a need to introduce different methods involving workshops in place of the traditional ex cathedra lectures that provided the undergraduates with only a passive knowledge of the subject. This method was used for centuries in the universities, but today undergraduates consider it outdated and completely unsatisfactory.

At the same time, analysis of the pedagogic problems revealed that the curricula in the medical schools were addressed to forming a type of doctor who knew a great deal about somatic medicine (anatomy, physiology, pathology, and medical and surgical treatment) but almost nothing as far as mental health was concerned (this topic was discussed only during the lectures in neuropsychiatry); moreover, no or only inadequate consideration was being given to the social problems and the social factors associated with human health.

It was evident that the university curriculum for the education of a present-day doctor was not sufficiently in tune with the new concept of health considered valid by all the countries of the world since 1946. It was inadequate for the development and organization of public health services for the modern world.

The above-mentioned new concept regards health as the physical, mental and social well-being of the individual. Hence psychosocial factors and their influence on health have to be taken into consideration in the training of all those who will be involved in the health of human beings. At the same time, the new types of disease that have developed in the industrialized countries (as revealed by epidemiological studies) as well as the increase in psychosomatic and be-

Primary Health Care in the Making
Ed. by U. Laaser, R. Senault, H. Viefhues

havioural disorders and the new environmental health problems (dramatically pointed out by an increasing incidence of intoxications) confirmed the necessity of bringing the formative curriculum into line with present-day needs. The already qualified doctor was not in a position to meet these needs as his training had concerned practically only physical medical aspects rather than combined psychophysical and social aspects.

Just as during the past three decades it was not easy to make changes and many justified doubts were expressed, today the future changes in health problems and the optimal development of health services based on primary health care as laid down by the Alma Ata Declaration can only be speculated upon. Consequently caution must be exercised in facing the social difficulties of this age.

The Eras of Medical Science

In reflecting on the changing mentality in medical education, I think it is useful to dwell on the identification and the comparative analysis of the stages or recent eras in medical science as suggested by McGavran quoted by [1], Barton [1] and Bryant [2]. McGavran pointed out four important eras in medical history between the middle of the last century and the middle of this one, i.e. between 1850 and 1950. These were (a) the *"empirical era"* up to the middle of the last century, when emphasis was placed on empirical diagnosis and treatment of symptoms; (b) the *"basic science era"* during the second half of the last century, which was bacteria or infectious disease centred, the emphasis being on diagnosis and treatment of disease; (c) the *"clinical science era"* during the first half of this century, which was patient centred, placing emphasis on diagnosis and treatment of the individual; and (d) the *"public health science era"* from the middle of this century onwards, which is community centred and places emphasis on diagnosis and treatment of the community. According to McGavran (quoted by [1]) the fourth stage began after the introduction of antibiotics and insecticides, when the great problems of environmental health arose in the industrialized countries and the correlation between health and the biophysical and social environment was brought to light by epidemiological studies.

Barton in 1979 [1] proposed McGavran's classification again and developed it by prophesying developments up to the year 2000. He recognized a new era after the Alma Ata Declaration (1978) and called it the "political health science era". This new era was to be based on a medical approach taking into account the entire population, "the total body politic", in a global process for health promotion and protection.

A careful reading of Table 1 is sufficient to enable one to understand the essential elements of the changes that have occurred in medical science since the middle of the last century and of those that will be seen in the near future. What is so striking is the rapidity of the evolution. If we take into consideration the elements shown in Table 1, i.e. the purpose and philosophy of medical

Table 1. Development of medical science up to the year 2000 [1]

	Empirical health era	Basic science era	Clinical science era	Public health science era	Political health science era
	1850	1900	1950	1975	2000
Purpose and philosophy	Symptom centred	Bacteria or Disease	Patient centred	Community centred	People centred
	Empirical diagnosis and treatment of symptoms	Diagnosis and treatment of disease	Diagnosis and treatment of the individual	Diagnosis and treatment of the community	Diagnosis and treatment of total body politic
Education	Lectures Authoritarian instruction	Laboratory instruction	Clinical instruction Bedside teaching	Clinical public health instruction Community-side teaching	Social experience learning Social and economic understanding Managerial acumen Political psychology and process Country health programming
Research	Historical	Basic Laboratory Development of new tools	Clinical development of clinical techniques	Community Development of community Measurements and criteria Planning techniques	Social and economic development Subjective indices for quality of life Intersectorial activity process Network process
Behavioural science	Unknown	Not needed Individual activity	Ancillary Social sciences – an adjunct to medicine Speciality group necessary	Integrated Social sciences Sophisticated skills Co-equal with public health science Interdisciplinary team	Interrelated Social, health, economic and political sciences Intersectorial team

science, the prevailing form of education, the direction of research and the relationship with the behavioural and social sciences, I think that nearly all those who have graduated in medicine, even in recent years, direct their attention to the patient-centred clinical era. The hospital bed still remains a reference point, a symbol! However, scientific research, the relationship with the social, economic and behavioural sciences, and many teaching experiments already reveal new characteristics typical of the future era. In fact, the political health science era has already commenced.

According to Barton [1] this era involves the whole community, that is the whole political body responsible for the running of the health services together with social, political and economic sciences and other sectors such as agriculture, industry, transport and town planning, in an intersectorial relationship for health care. This does not mean that by the year 2000 health services will be available for everybody on the basis of the principle of social equity; rather we will all be involved in improving health care [6]. Recently Bryant [2] studied the evolution of and the interaction between the three main components of health care, i.e. the health services, health manpower and the universities, in the clinical science era and in the era of social and preventive medicine, which corresponds to the one McGavran (quoted by [1]) called the public health science era. In addition, he forecast the evolution of a health-for-all era in accordance with the global programme of the World Health Organization (corresponding to the era of political health science of Barton [1]).

The roles of the three components in health care have been detailed by Bryant [2] in Table 2, where the following lines of evolution can be identified:

1. The services that in the clinical science era were addressed to the individual and later to the community in a selective way are foreseen as being addressed to the whole population through the development of the political science era.
2. During the clinical science era health manpower comprised doctors assisted by nurses and auxiliaries. Later it was made up of two large categories of workers – the doctors and the nurses/auxiliaries – each with an independent role – and there is now the prospect of three large categories of health workers, i.e. "community health workers", doctors and nurses/auxiliaries.
3. The Universities, which had always interested themselves in research and education as well as clinical duties, later took up the causes and prevention of diseases related to the community and will in future direct their attention to the study and teaching of health for the entire population. This entails an extension of research into new fields of interest such as analysis of the different needs of the population, epidemiological analysis, the study of information systems and methodologies for the programming as well as the management of the health service network. The university will also have to take into consideration evaluation of the service, that is, they must analyse its utilization, costs and measures of effectiveness.

The changes that occurred from era to era, traced in mere detail here, were determined by cultural, socio-economic, technological and political changes

Table 2. Evolving roles of health services, health manpower and universities [2]

	Health services	Health manpower	Universities
Clinical era	Focus of care:	Levels of care:	Predominant emphases:
Coverage: individuals Manpower: one tier Emphases: clinical	Hospitals Health centres	• Doctor assisted by nurse, auxiliaries	Service: clinical Research: Basic and clinical Education: clinical
Preventive and social medicine era	Focus of care	Levels of care:	Predominant emphases:
Coverage: selective in communities Manpower: two tiers Emphases: clinical Preventive: social	Hospitals Health centres Selected communities Components of PHC: nutrition immunizations environmental control	• Doctor • Nurse/auxiliary	Service: clinical and community Research: basic; clinical; community-related causes of disease, prevention and control; assessment of effectiveness Education: clinical; concepts of prevention, social relationships; roles of team in PHC
Health for all era	Focus of care:	Levels of care:	Predominant emphases:
Coverage: universal, with effective services Manpower: three tiers Emphases: Clinical preventive social managerial + development	Defined population Total coverage Network of facilities PHC to communities Community participation	• Doctor • Nurse/auxiliary • Community health worker	Service: Comprehensive care to defined population Research: basic; clinical; health services, including epidemiology, coverage, utilization, costs, measures of effectiveness, management, evaluation; relationship with development Education: clinical; prevention; competencies for universal coverage with effective services; roles of team, especially leadership; development

and also by the changes in disease patterns and by the inability of the available therapy to cure the new types of disease. As many diseases cannot be cured, preventive medicine has come into its own. In addition, the evolution in medical care has been determined by the change of opinion regarding the role of the doctor, by the incredible importance attached to the medical alternatives (homeopathy, acupuncture etc.) and by the new concept of self-care, the community interesting itself in health and not leaving everything to the doctors.

The Impact on the Faculties of Medicine

We must admit that the changes that have taken place during the last three decades in the concept of health have hit the faculties of medicine in striking ways. In fact, the gradual evolution from "medical services" to "health services" involves great structural and functional change. Important changes in health manpower must be made; this is especially true of those people who do not work in the hospital, and the alterations must be both in their professional attitude and in their practical ability and knowledge concerning the roles allotted to them. Study of the new professional profiles is necessary so as to identify the needs of the profession, and base the new educational curricula on these needs. However, in my opinion very few faculties are ready to co-operate in re-orienting the curricula to produce doctors who will fit into the new era based on primary health care.

New methodology should be used as well as active educational methods, thereby integrating with the health services outside the hospital. Scientific research in line with primary health care should be carried out, and there should be interaction with other faculties and with sectors of the social and economic services. Environmental conditions need to be created which are compatible with the health of the people and which promote a more healthy life-style. We can say that passing from the clinical science era to subsequent eras has certainly caused disturbing problems and has thereby changed many theories inside the faculties of medicine. However, the more important changes have not yet been made and so the rapidity of social evolution is striking in comparison to the adjustments made by many medical schools to face the needs of the community.

Professional Attitudes

Even though the above-mentioned eras have occurred almost everywhere, it is well-known that different countries have found varying solutions to health problems; in fact, there are great differences in the organization of health and social services. At the same time the changes of mentality regarding medical education can vary vastly in relation to culture, tradition and social characteristics as well as economic and political ones. Thus generalization is imprudent and dangerous.

During the last 3 years in Italy the organization of the health services has changed greatly. A National Health Service was introduced in 1978, and obviously this service can meet the needs of the people not only by giving assistance to everybody but, above all, by providing efficacious and pertinent service, that is, by providing an efficient health service. The Italian National Health Service was based on the following principles:

1. The prevention of disease and health promotion
2. Giving a total coverage to health by integrating and collaborating with the various services in question
3. Centralizing the services at a local and regional level through the setting up of local units of health and social services in such a way that the community can take part in the running of the service.

At present, primary health care in Italy is organized on a district basis; in these districts the local health units are subdivided so that multidisciplinary teams are available to communities of about 10 000 – 12 000 people.

Study of the functions attributed to doctors under the present national and regional Italian sanitary law shows a very different professional profile from the traditional one of the general practitioner whose function was to diagnose and cure disease either at home or in the surgery. In fact, the new doctor must participate in different ways in the National Health Service programme and in the organization and co-ordination of the district team he belongs to. He must carry out preventive medicine, not only performing immunization against infectious diseases but also instituting precautions against toxicological risks and taking responsibility for the health education of the population. This, according to the law, is his first duty because he must promote the awareness of the community regarding their health. Not only that, the physician must diagnose, cure and rehabilitate patients as well as collaborate in assisting invalids and patients with chronic degenerative diseases.

As the reader can see, this is a professional profile that has a community basis and requires a very different mentality from that of the clinical science era doctor. Therefore it is absolutely essential that the traditional curriculum of the medical school be changed. The scientific contribution made by medical research during the last 3 years is of fundamental importance in respect of medical teaching. It has been of great help in enabling us to better understand that the doctor must have diverse attributes: (a) adequate knowledge, (b) practical ability, and (c) an appropriate attitude to his work. These fundamental components are necessary in different ways according to what the doctor is called upon to do. The person who draws up a curriculum must bear this in mind, as the three components cannot be divided in as much as they are interdependent in their action. It appears that the third component (attitude) is of major importance because of the fact that the new doctor must fully understand the community approach. The altered mentality consists chiefly in the doctor regarding health problems as having a community dimension, in contrast to the individual dimension emphasized during the clinical science era.

"The commitment is to convince the General Practitioner to think in terms of health and pathological needs of the population, asking himself on the efficacy of his own work which is to improve the quality of the assistance given and to reduce the waste of resources" [3]. Besides a change in the attitude of doctors, multidisciplinary teamwork is indispensable in developing primary health care, contrasting with the monodisciplinary work typical of curative medicine.

In conclusion, there is no doubt that a change in mentality must be supported by adequate knowledge and vice versa. However, it seems opportune to give particular attention to professional *attitudes* in drawing up new curricula; we must not limit ourselves to considering only the knowledge and practical abilities that new doctors should have.

References

1. Barton WL (1979) Alma Ata: signpost to a new health era. World Health, July:10 – 15
2. Bryant JH (1983) Health care, health manpower and universities. An historical and future perspective. WHO Consultation 11 – 14 April 1983 (Working document)
3. Evans JR (1981) Measurement and management in medicine and health services. Rockefeller foundation, New York
4. Paccagnella B (1981) La ricerca epidemiologica nel Servizio Sanitario Nazionale. Proceedings of the Congress on statistics and epidemiological research, Bressanone. CLEUP, Padova
5. Paccagnella B (to be published) La dimensione comunitaria della medicina e il medico di comunità. Fed Med 8
6. Rossi-Espagnet A (1982) La salute per tutti e tutti per la salute. Proceedings of the 56th National Congress of the Italian Association Medici Condotti, Acireale, 19 – 24 Sept, 1982

Medical Education: Proposals for the Future

R. Senault and J. P. Deschamps

In his report Professor Paccagnella claims that it was back in the 1950s that we became aware of the need to modify medical education. Teaching methods based on ex cathedra lectures allowed no active participation by the students, and this old university practice became completely outdated. It also became obvious that this traditional education produced a particular type of doctor – treating physical but not psychological problems, and not relating to the individual as a complete person and even less to a social group. In short, he was not the kind of doctor who could relate to an individual as a member of a social group.

However, the new concept of health, as the World Health Organisation defined it, called for doctors to play a wider role. At the same time the evolution of health problems towards a more psychosomatic and behavioural pathology confirmed the urgent need for reform.

Quoting from several works written in the last three decades, Professor Paccagnella recalls how medicine has evolved from an empirical era (prior to the 19th century) to a clinical era (during the first half of this century). This was followed by the public health era, where the emphasis was on the community rather than the individual. We are at present approaching a new era, the political health science era, where the emphasis is on entire populations. Professor Paccagnella points out that medical education remains in the clinical era, symbolised by the fact that the hospital bed is still its basic point of reference.

I would myself like to stress the gap which exists in almost all of our countries between

- the importance attributed by national or international officials to giving priority to primary health care, preventive medicine, individual and community participation in health care, the problems involved in considering health policy as one element of a whole within the socioeconomic system, and the fact that doctors form only *one* group of the health workers with whom they work; and
- the fact that curricula are persistently based on acquiring biological and pathological knowledge, taking none of the above "priorities" into account.

My observation may seem harsh. I know there are remarkable examples of updated teaching in schools of medicine both in industrialised countries and in the Third World. Dr. F. M. Katz and Dr. T. Fulop have made an excellent pre-

Primary Health Care in the Making
Ed. by U. Laaser, R. Senault, H. Viefhues

sentation of these examples at the World Health Organisation, revealing a significant evolution in both the content and form of a certain number of curricula offered in universities. However, our purpose is not to delight in successes, but rather to try to discuss together solutions to the remaining problems. And I am afraid that these examples are still exceptions, pilot schemes which the majority of medical schools do not take up. In the latter, education is still extremely conventional despite small improvements here and there, such as devoting a few extra hours to teaching community health, epidemiology or medical economics, or replacing lectures with work done in small groups.

As yet in our universities I have not felt the wave of reform required to educate doctors for the year 2000 according to the health needs they, along with others, will have to satisfy, and the social and economic context in which they will practise medicine. The improvements made up until now are few and far between, and what we need to consider are not the exceptions, but rather the bulk remaining.

Analysing the causes of such a situation would be a lengthy process. However, they no doubt lie in those areas whose understanding requires a sociological approach. It is not easy to understand why medicine makes such advances with the techniques it devises or employs, yet remains so conservative in using these innovations to improve the health of the population. In France, for example, it is paradoxical that a doctor's work has undergone a complete change in a matter of decades, but that the medical profession refuses to consider – even on a trial basis – assuming forms of medical practice other than those exercised a hundred years ago. It is deplorable that medical schools continue to educate doctors well-informed in 20th century technology, but prepared only to practise 19th century medicine.

There are many faults in need of correction, such as:

- attempts to maintain authority within the university network and the medical profession;
- research into the most lucrative forms of medical practice;
- the fear associated with abandoning a position as a technician/magician for the more difficult role of technician/instructor;
- the inability to master the application of increasingly sophisticated technologies.

However, the first stage must be to change mentalities *via* medical education.

It is too often said that medical students should be taught the *techniques* of medicine, and that they will learn the rest from experience during the first few years of their work as professionals. This is not so, however, since today the techniques of medicine constitute, above all, this "rest". A doctor will never be a biologist, chemist, electronics expert or whatever. He will, however, need to know how to work alongside these professionals, and more important than that even, to know how to listen to, communicate and analyse a group situation, solve problems, manage, present dossiers, train workers and evaluate his own work. The professionals he will have to be able to work with include:

1. health experts, colleagues rather than inferiors (nurses, community health workers); and
2. experts in psychology, social anthropology, sociology, economics etc.

He will also be required to work with the community and its political, union and associative representatives, and to establish new relations with the population as a whole, based on conversation and knowledge sharing. If this were possible, and if medical education could train doctors for it, then the Alma Ata Declaration would stand more chance of success.

In practice we have to persist in introducing reforms in medical education in our countries. Of the important and realistic objectives, I propose the following points for discussion:

1. It is both necessary and possible to give a modified training to future lecturers in medical faculties, since they are at present insufficiently prepared for their teaching role and lack an overall view of health problems outside the limits of their own particular fields.
2. It is both necessary and possible to bring medical students *out* of the hospitals.
3. It is both necessary and possible to accept that doctors in the "Health for All in the Year 2000" era cannot be expected to know everything about medicine, that they must not receive a vulgar, simplified, piecemeal sort of universal medical education, but rather that they should be capable, above all, of solving problems, making decisions and advisedly using the skills of technicians from all disciplines.
4. It is both necessary and possible to educate, to some extent at least, various professionals in the health service (doctors, nurses, midwives etc.) so that team-work need not be a painful discovery on leaving university, but rather a work method already experienced during the course of study.

Education in Social Medicine

E. Musil

Institutes for Social Medicine and Occupational Health have been established in many countries since the end of the Second World War, and knowledge concerning the psychology of learning and didactics has also improved. One of the most important innovations is the realisation that not only cognitive experience is essential; rather the affective or emotional dimensions must also be kept in mind. Research into these problems has been conducted by the European Association for Medical Education, the World Health Organization, the World Medical Association and some universities.

The inadequacy of medical education in our time lies not in the lack of academic sociology but in the deficiency of contact between theory and practical application. Additional study of sociology does not improve the situation, but within the study of social medicine, education in sociology should be as comprehensive as is necessary for medical practice. Knowledge of medical psychology and psychosomatics is of great advantage inasmuch as a physician is thereby enabled to understand the patient's psychosocial problems.

During a symposium on medical sociology in Vienna in 1982 88% of the students claimed that the practical education during the medical curriculum is unsatisfactory. The author's inquiries among 650 physicians of every age and specialty have yielded the same result. Considering the present situation at the universities, it seems curious that the above-mentioned panel of students pleaded for an increasing number of students in general. The "Bundesärztekammer", in contrast, warns against a greater number of students due to a significant lack of education and opportunities in hospitals and institutes.

At the same symposium, a great number of students expressed the opinion that they are not essentially interested in mathematical and statistical medicine. No doubt the theoretical sciences are of great value for education in connection with practical examples. Theory is absolutely necessary as a basis for application. Consequently theoretical knowledge of symptoms, syndromes and statistical material enables the physician to reach a diagnosis after computing the reports.

Bershewa Experiment

In 1975, at the Ben-Gurion University in Bershewa in the Negev region of Israel, a didactic experiment was undertaken, especially with regard to basic

Primary Health Care in the Making
Ed. by U. Laaser, R. Senault, H. Viefhues

medicine and family medicine. The dean is also health director of the region. Not only medical doctors (including general practitioners) but also nurses and administrators teach at the university. Since their inception, the courses have always been highly esteemed. The curriculum lasts 6 years and covers prophylaxis, rehabilitation, ecology and social problems pertaining to in- and/or outpatients. There is no specific university building, because education is performed in a variety of settings, e.g. in laboratories, in hospitals and in the homes of patients.

Maastricht Experiment

An experiment was started in 1972 in Maastricht, Holland, wereby practice and theory are taught together from the beginning of the course. In the course, which lasts 6 years, no particular branches of medicine are taught; rather the whole human being is always considered. The courses are not performed in large lecture theatres but with small groups of students who develop their knowledge by gaining experience step by step. As theoretical lectures are not included in the curriculum, anatomy, physiology, histology, social factors etc. are taught upon the basis of the topical diseases of the patient under consideration. The student also has to work in general practice. The examinations are set not only by professors but also by general practioners and interns of the hospital.

Such a system has not been realised in Europe but shows interesting possibilities for development. Special courses on industrial medicine would not be necessary because the normal education covers all the social and vocational problems.

There are three aspects of teaching:

1. *Cognitive,* i.e. conveying facts so that they are learned and internalised.
2. *Affective or emotional.* Many faculties have tried to experiment in this area, especially as regards topics like relation between physician and patient, medical ethics and health education. In the future there should be more emphasis on the affective aspect of teaching.
3. *Sensorimotoric,* i.e. conveying skill and working knowledge with regard to operations, giving injections, percussion etc.

In 1970 the regional bureau for Europe of the WHO worked out standards with regards to how lecturers in universities should be prepared. It was recommended that discussion groups with lecturers and students be set up to consider how education, seminars and examinations should be arranged.

At every clinic and every institute there should be at least one member of staff who is responsible for pedagogic matters. He should organize workshops on problems and should make proposals on how to arrange lectures. In addition he should ensure that the results of discussions are disseminated.

At the beginning of every semester an analysis of the content of lectures should be carried out. The aim of the lectures should be to enable the students to become qualified physicians in respect of a specific population in a specific area, and this should be reflected in their content.

Discussions, questionnaires and interim tests indicate the level of the students' knowledge. Such examinations should be performed in a manner which motivates the student to learn with avid pleasure. Techniques for learning vary according to the individual, and every student has to search for a satisfactory method. The use of aids, such as minicomputers, video recorders and simulators, is admissable. Books and articles should be printed with impressive headings; chapters should be well arranged so that information is readily accessible and there should be sufficient illustrations. As lectures in lecture theatres do not seem to be the best method of instruction, smaller groups offering students the possibility to pose questions if anything is unclear are to be preferred. The Socratic method, when the instructor guides the student with regard to questions, is advantageous. The teacher should place himself in the student's place in this endeavour.

Exercises, Courses and Seminars

The most important practical exercise in social medicine for the student is to observe and report on a family with social difficulties and ailments. Such a report and the proposals regarding solutions should be discussed in groups under the guidance of the teacher. There should also be excursions and discussions in relation to the following topics:

Health offices
The orphanages handicapped
Courts for working people
Sports medicine
School children
Preventive medicine etc.

Role play should be performed with control by a video recorder to establish the student's faults in treating a patient and talking to him.

For practical exercises in statistics, specific health problems or ailments should be analysed and proposals for their solution or treatment made accordingly.

References

Grundy F, Mackintosh JM (1957) The teaching of hygiene and public health in Europe. WHO Monogr Ser 34
Stuart-Harris C (1972) Medicine today and the role of science in medical education. University of Sheffield, University of Southampton
Musil E (1977) Einführung in die Sozialmedizin. Facultas, Vienna
Cole RB, Engel CE (1975) Planning a course of continuing education for general practice. British Medical Association, London
Zwell ME, Zabarenko L (1974) Training for family practice. University of Pittsburgh 1970
Winter E (1974) Epidemiologie, WEB, Berlin

Community Health in Primary Care – A Workshop on Community-Oriented Primary Care

J. Gofin, N. Mainemer, and S. L. Kark

The Hadassah Community Health Center at Kiryat Yovel in Western Jerusalem has been exploring various ways to develop a comprehensive approach to the provision of primary health care in the community. The basic features of the practice we have developed are: a focus on the health of the community as a whole and on its subgroups when appraising needs, planning and providing services and evaluating their effects, and this is done in the framework of a care. This is done in the framework of a practice providing primary clinical care for individuals and families in the community, with special attention to continuity of care. This integration of some aspects of community medicine with primary health care in the community has been referred to as "community-oriented primary care" (COPC) [1].

The Health Center is the teaching and research center of the Hebrew University-Hadassah School of Public Health and Community Medicine and it has been used to provide field experience and operational research in the practice of community health care. The School conducts two Master of Public Health courses, one for Israelies and the other for International students, both of which include a workshop on community-oriented primary care.

The workshop on Community-Oriented Primary Care

The objectives of the Workshop are:

1. To study COPC as it is carried out by the Community Health Center at Kiryat Yovel, Jerusalem
2. To apply the principles and strategies of COPC as illustrated at the Hadassah Community Health Center, to specific communities in students' countries of origin

This report is concerned with the workshop for the 66 international students who have participated in the most recent ones in 1981 and 1982. The students were from different professional backgrounds, mainly physicians, but also nurses, dentists, social workers, behavioral scientists, biologists, and sanitarians. The group included students from countries in Latin America and Asia with a limited number from Africa, Western Europe, and North America. Many of

Primary Health Care in the Making
Ed. by U. Laaser, R. Senault, H. Viefhues

them are in key positions in their countries in the areas of public health administration and primary health care; others are teachers in the field of public health and community medicine.

The workshop extends over a trimester of ten weeks, with two full days per week assigned for this purpose. The total number of hours is 160, but students arrange informal work-group sessions beyond these times.

Before the commencement of the workshop, a manual is prepared for the use of both students and staff as a guide to the program. It contains a brief outline of the general principles of COPC and a description of the Community Health Center's main activities and programs. It also includes a bibliography for each section of the workshop.

The general arrangement of the workshop is as follows:

1. Prior to leaving their countries, the students receive a letter requesting them to bring basic health information on the community in which they work or on a community which they know.
2. The information is discussed before the commencement of the workshop in three or four preparatory sessions, thereby providing the opportunity to assess the quality of the data and to exchange information about the students' different communities.
   This provides the basis for the selection of the most appropiate communities.
3. The first two weeks are devoted to an introduction to COPC at the Health Center in Jerusalem and includes discussion of the meaning and scope of COPC, together with observations on the main activities related to the care of individuals and families while, simultaneously learning the organization of COPC at the Health Center. As part of learning the functions of the Health Center, the role of different staff members are studied through interviews with many of them, as well as by accompanying them as they go about their daily activities.
4. Observation and study of at least one of the various community health programs which have been developed in the primary care practice of the Health Center. This usually extends over a period of four weeks. For this purpose the class is divided into two groups of about twelve to fifteen students each, for the study of the following: I. Programs focussed on maternal and child health, e.g., "PROD" (promotion of the growth and development of infants and children) and the "28-day program" (health surveillance and care through pregnancy and its outcome up to the 28th day after birth) [1, 2], and II. Programs focussed on the health of adult population, such as the community program for the control of risk factors for cardiovascular diseases [1–4].
   The teaching of the programs is carried out by the program directors together with other members of the staff and of the community.
5. Following the more detailed study of at least one community health program, the seventh week of the workshop is dedicated to a further review by the workshop central team, with the total student group, emphasizing some of the basic features of COPC as developed in the Health Center: a) uses of epidemiology in COPC, b) the composition of the health team, and c) community involvement.

6. The students' study communities. For the main assigment in the workshop, the students are expected to apply the principles and methods used in the COPC of the Health Center to various communities in their countries of origin. They are requested to present a plan of a community-focussed health program, to be developed in the primary care setting of their community. During the first seven weeks of the workshop, a weekly session is devoted to consideration of applicability to their own communities of the principles of COPC. Then the students spend the last three weeks completing their assignments on these communities, at the end of which they present their reports to a joined student staff session.
7. The students' work-groups. The class is divided into groups of three to six students working on developing COPC programs for each selected community. They are advised by specially appointed tutors.

Each group selects one health-related condition or a health problem on which a community program is later formulated. The criteria considered for the selection of one among several health conditions are: prevalence and severity of the condition, the extent of community concern, and the practical possibilities of dealing with the problem by existing primary health care service in that particular community.

Some examples of the health conditions selected are: tuberculosis (in an urban community), infant mortality (in a rural area), hypertension (in an urban community), gastroenteritis and malnutrition (in small rural villages), family planning (in several differing communities), and teenage pregnancy (in a large city community).

The Development of COPC by the Students' Work-Groups

The development of the COPC requires a process involving several components [5, 6] which are illustrated to the students by the community health programs at the Kiryat Yovel Health Center. Their community health program plan and presentation are expected to be executed along the same lines:

Preliminary steps. This includes the uses of the available information on the population, the existing health services and the health status in the community as the basis for deciding on priorities and selection of the health condition that needs further investigation and action.

Community diagnosis. This implies diagnosis of the state of health of the community as a whole in relation to the specific condition chosen and its determinants.

Planning of intervention. Based on the knowledge gathered through the preliminary steps and the community diagnosis, the students need to formulate the general and the specific objectives of the intervention program, the description of the programs activities, the design of records, the training and role definition of the health workers, allocation of the resources, a system of health surveillance, and evaluation of programs.

Implementation and surveillance of health. The actual implementation can not be done in the classroom, but methods can be formulated for the surveillance of the community's health and monitoring of health activities.

Evaluation includes the measurement of the performance of the activities and evaluation of outcome (effectiveness), efficiency, and community satisfaction.

Evaluation of the Workshop

The students are evaluated on their participation during their various studies of the Health Center programs. This is done by the health team demonstrating each of the programs and by the tutors in the student work-group. The presentations are assessed as a group performance in which each student's contribution is taken into consideration.

The students were requested to evaluate the workshop through various weekly sessions and its conclusion. This was done by completing a questionnaire and by informal discussion with members of the central team. Their comments related to the structure, organization, content, teaching methods, tutors, reading assignments, and function of the student groups.

When students were asked whether they would apply the principles learned in this workshop seminar to their future work, the majority of them responded positively. They stated that the application might be in developing new community health programs or assessing existing programs, teaching medical students, nursing students, physicians and other health workers as well as research and conducting community health surveys.

Discussion

The services provided by the Community Health Center at Kiryat Yovel are particularly appropriate for the teaching base of the workshop. The Health Center's role in the development of COPC was recognized in a conference that was organized by the Institute of Medicine of the National Academy of Sciences in the United States in 1982, to discuss ways of extending the practice of COPC in the United States. The Center's experience was the basis for discussion at the conference [6, 7].

The workshop demonstrates a combination of community-oriented care perspective through the use of epidemiology in primary health care. We believe that this approach will encourage more health workers to have experience similar to those provided by this workshop, thus giving the scientific support that is needed to strengthen the quality of care at primary local level.

The workshop is a learning experience that contributes to a community orientation of primary health care, and in this way to WHO [8] aim of "primary health care for all people". The workshop context offers the students an opportunity for both observing COPC and considering the problems involved in planning a similar approach in their own communities. The community approach and use of epidemiology in the practice demands knowledge and a change in attitude to the scope of medical pratice and health care in the community. This is one of the main challenges of this particular workshop.

References

1. Kark SL (1981) The practice of community oriented primary health care. Appleton Century-Crofts, New York
2. Kark SL (1974) Epidemiology and community medicine. Appleton Century Crofts, New York
3. Kark SL, Kark E, Hopp C, Abramson JH, Epstein LM, Ronen I (1976) The control of hypertension, atherosclerotic diseases and diabetes in a family practice. JR Coll Gen Pract 26:157–169
4. Abramson JH, Gofin R, Hopp C, Gofin J, Donchin M, Habib J (1981) Evaluation of a community program for the control of cardiovascular risk factors: the CHAD program in Jerusalem: Isr J Med Sci 17:201–222
5. Kark SL, Abramson JH (1981) Community focussed health care. Isr J Med Sci 17:65–70
6. Abramson JH, Kark SL (1983) Community oriented primary care: meaning and scope. In: Connor E, Mullan F (eds) Community oriented primary care: new directions for health services delivery. National Academy Press, Washington, D.C.
7. Mullan F (1982) Community oriented primary care: an agenda for the 80's. New Eng J Med 307:1076–1078
8. World Health Organisation (1978) Report of the international conference on primary health care, Alma-Ata, USSR. WHO, Geneva

Seminars in Clinical Preventive Medicine

R. Rothenberg, V. R. Coleman, and P. Zabetakis

Background

In January, 1982, the New York State Legislature created a Heart and Hypertension Institute in the Department of Health. Its mandate was to develop further the program for screening, detection, and follow-up of hypertension, to conduct research in the field of cardiovascular epidemiology, and to promote programs of professional education and training for physicians, nurses, pharmacists, and persons in the health professions for the prevention of heart disease.

Rationale

Our initial efforts, called "Seminars in Clinical Preventive Medicine", have been targeted to practicing physicians. Several perceptions underlie this rationale: First, illness is part of a whole spectrum of causes and effects. The individual arrives where he is for a variety of reasons. Often, the patient–physician encounter is the earliest, and perhaps the only, opportunity for intervention. Despite the rising interest in risk alteration, it is an opportunity for health promotion that is frequently missed.

Second, the physician is in a unique position to put the weight and force of community prestige behind such an effort. In turn, adoption of a preventive approach by the physician (i.e., recognizable concern for the maintenance of health) is likely to add to that prestige. From the viewpoint of strategy for social change, it is important to attempt to involve the recognized leadership as quickly as possible.

Third, physicians have traditionally approached health from the perspective of treating disease. It is, of course, entirely appropriate that recognition and management of disease states should be a primary focus of the practitioner.

In 1900 the ten leading causes of death in the United States were dominated by communicable and infectious diseases, but in 1975 the ten leading causes were chronic disease and trauma for which some preventive measures are available. However, little background information on risk or organized procedures for intervention are imparted during medical training. Physicians have in general not been offered the clinical and behavioral tools required for treating risk.

Primary Health Care in the Making
Ed. by U. Laaser, R. Senault, H. Viefhues

Curriculum

With this perspective, we designed a curriculum around the following questions: What is the current state of our health and what puts us at risk for premature disease and death? What do current trends portend for the future health status of our society? What action should the practitioner take, and what tools are available for such action?

The planning process included creation of an Advisory Board of experts in preventive medicine, chronic disease, and cancer to provide consultation, program review, and, in some instances, direct technical input. The final product, however, was developed as a combined effort of the Bureau of Chronic Disease Prevention of the New York State Department of Health. The final format selected was a 1-day intensive session for physicians, providing six credit hours of Continuing Medical Education. The subject matter focused on the epidemiologic basis, tools, and strategies for risk intervention in the areas of hypertension, nutrition, exercise, smoking, stress, diabetes, and cancer (Table 1).

Table 1. Tools for clinical intervention

Hypertension	Joint National Committee guidelines and statistics for New York State for diagnoses and management
Poor nutrition	Regimens for fat reduction, sodium reduction, and weight reduction, healthful diets, and review of fad diets. Plus some suggestions the physician could give for modifying patient's diet behavior
Smoking	Methods of smoking cessation and mortality statistics
Diabetes	Guide for diagnoses and management. Guidelines for patient education for prevention of five major complications
Sedentary lifestyle	Graded exercise prescriptions
Cancer	Plan for systematic screening with a timetable for early detection procedures
Stress	Stress management techniques reviewed

Educational Techniques

A variety of educational methodologies are used during the presentation, including audiovisuals, lectures, discussions, and participatory exercises. The sessions are conducted by two physicians – an epidemiologist and a practitioner – who begin the day by administering a Health Risk Appraisal. This questionnaire elicits a standard data base concerning health history, lifestyle, and medical conditions. It is identical to the one that physicians are encouraged to use in their practice, and is processed on site using a portable terminal. At the end of the day, each participant receives his/her personal printout identifying actual age, appraised age and achievable age. A summary of current risks and the modifications that the individual can make to obtain the achievable age are also provided. A video-cassette is then shown of a "typical" physician–patient interview wherein the opportunities for health risk intervention are handled in a disorganized way. The object lesson, for the end of the day, is the greater ease with which risk may be approached using the organization of the Health Risk Appraisal.

The Migration of Physicians to the United States – A Study of Candidates for ECFMG Certification, 1969–1982

T. D. Dublin

Since World War II, the United States has been a major recipient – as opposed to donor – of medical manpower. Physicians, and also nurses, have been seeking opportunities there for advanced professional training as well as for career practice. Prior to World War I and continuing to a substantial degree until World War II, the prevailing migratory pattern of physicians was away from the United States rather than to it. At that time many American physicians aspiring to positions of eminence within their profession, whether in teaching, research, or practice, sought to extend their educational experience with graduate training obtained in the leading medical centers of Europe.

The more recent flow of physicians *to* the United States gained impetus from the post-war Good Neighbor policies typified by the Fulbright Educational Exchange Act of 1946. This legislation and subsequent amendments to the Immigration and Nationality Act removed or reduced longstanding barriers to migration of foreign nationals to the United States and encouraged the flow of physicians as "exchange visitors" for graduate training in the medical specialties in American hospitals. It was assumed that a limited period of advanced training would aid these visiting physicians to prepare themselves for a higher level of professional practice in their own countries. Only with the enactment of Medicare and Medicaid legislation in the mid-1960s and the subsequent recognition of a severe shortage of young physicians to fill hospital staff positions, were restrictions on length of stay relaxed and actual inducements offered to these visiting physicians to remain permanently in the States.

In 1976, however, the United States Congress, in enacting Public Law 94–484, determined that a shortage of physicians no longer existed. That legislation reinstituted barriers both to the entry of foreign national physicians, even on a temporary basis, and to the conversion of a visitor visa to one permitting permanent residence. New regulations now require foreign-trained physicians, whether temporary visitors or permanent residents, to demonstrate that they meet the same standards of professional competence as those expected of graduates of domestic (and Canadian) medical schools.

An additional major source of inflow of graduates of foreign medical schools has arisen as a result of the substantial increase in the number of United States citizens going abroad to obtain their undergraduate medical education. These individuals whose homes and families remain within the United States intend to return to the States to complete their graduate medical training and to

Primary Health Care in the Making
Ed. by U. Laaser, R. Senault, H. Viefhues

enter career practice there. This trend has developed despite a remarkable expansion both in the number of United States medical schools and the number of students enrolled during the past decade. Because our concerns focus on the entry of all graduates of foreign medical schools into the mainstream of graduate training and medical practice in the United States we must perforce include this group of American citizens in our present evaluations. A more detailed review of the antecedents of the present study has previously been published [1].

The magnitude of the flow of foreign medical school graduates (FMGs) to the United States in recent years, as compared with the total number of United States-trained physicians, is reflected in tabulations prepared annually by the American Medical Association from its comprehensive Physician Masterfile [2–4]. In 1959, when the first comprehensive enumeration was made of the sources of medical education of all physicians in the United States, the 20 575 FMGs identified constituted 8.5% of the total supply. Eleven years later, in 1970, the number had increased to 63 391 (19.0% of the total). As of 1 January 1982, 110 542 FMGs were listed in that roster and constituted 22.8% of the total. Thus, during the past 22 years there have been net additions of 90 000 foreign medical graduates to the overall supply of physicians in the United States, more than a fourfold increase in number, and an average annual increase of more than 4000[1].

Since 1957, the Educational Commission for Foreign Medical Graduates (ECFMG), created by a consortium of nongovernmental professional associations concerned with medical education and standards of medical practice within the United States, has been assigned responsibility for the evaluation of the educational credentials and other professional qualifications of the graduates of foreign medical schools who seek entry to an accredited program of graduate medical education in this country. In addition, each of the 54 medical licensure jurisdictions in the United States now stipulates that FMGs applying for licensure to practice must hold ECFMG certification or have completed 1 or more years of residency training in an accredited program in the United States.

The year 1982 marked the completion of 25 years of the Commission's operations. Its 50th semiannual test of the medical knowledge of applicants against standards of performance established by graduates of domestic medical schools on similar examinations was offered in July of that year in 147 examination centers, 40 located within the United States and the balance, 107, abroad. During this 25-year period, more than 300 000 individual candidates applied for ECFMG certification and have taken over 561 000 separate ECFMG examinations. The testing procedures include an assessment of each applicant's ability to comprehend and utilize the English language.

Since 1977, the ECFMG has also been responsible for the administration of the Visa Qualifying Examination (VQE), an additional test of medical knowl-

[1] In 1959, 5421 of the 20 575 FMGs identified, or 2.2% of the total physician supply, were graduates of Canadian schools; the corresponding figures in 1970 were 6174 or 1.8% and in 1982, 7780 and 1.6% respectively. This subgroup of FMGs is often merged with graduates of medical schools in the United States as the procedures for accreditation of institutions providing medical education in Canada are identical with those employed in the United States

edge, and during these past 6 years a total of 30 559 examinations of this type have been given, some to candidates who had previously taken one or more ECFMG examinations and some to others with no prior ECFMG examination experience. This recent Federal legislation requires that FMGs seeking graduate clinical training or wishing to perform services as a physician in the United States must achieve a passing score on that examination before becoming eligible to enter the country either on a temporary visitor or permanent resident visa. ECFMG certification continues as a prerequisite for the appointment of an FMG to an accredited training program. To reduce the confusion created by a seemingly duplicative examination needed for the granting of a visa to enter the United States, a passing score on the VQE is now accepted as meeting the medical knowledge requirements for ECFMG certification.

The Commission is now conducting a large-scale study involving the compilation and correlation of extensive data from multiple sources on more than 200 000 graduates of medical schools located outside of the United States and Canada who have taken at least an initial ECFMG certifying examination during the 14-year period, 1969 – 1982. This population, representing approximately two out of three of all of the candidates who have ever applied to the ECFMG for examination and certification, has been selected because of the completeness and accuracy of the detailed, computerized records now available on their demographic, educational, and other professional characteristics and qualifications. In addition, these data provide a starting point for a long-term follow-up study of graduates of foreign medical schools who have gained entry to the health care system in the United States. Briefly stated the objectives of the studies now in progress are:

1. To characterize the graduates of foreign medical schools who have applied for ECFMG certification and have taken an initial ECFMG examination (and possibly subsequent examinations) during the 14-year period 1 January 1969 through 31 December 1982
2. To characterize those candidates who have met the examination and other requirements for ECFMG certification and to assess the extent to which success or failure in achieving that objective is determined by such factors as country of origin, medical school attended, other elements of educational background, and English language competence
3. To identify those FMGs who, after achieving ECFMG certification, have actually come to the United States and have received graduate clinical training in a medical specialty in an accredited hospital residency program and compare that training experience with the training received by graduates of United States and Canadian medical schools
4. To identify and characterize those ECFMG certified physicians who, following the completion of their training in the United States, have returned to their countries of origin compared with ECFMG certified physicians who have remained to practice their profession in the United States
5. To identify and characterize the United States nationals who have received their undergraduate medical education at foreign medical schools and who have applied for ECFMG certification as a means of reentry into the mainstream of American medical practice, and to evaluate the factors that may

be influencing United States nationals to choose to attend medical schools abroad

The first two phases of this study, concerned with the identification and characterization of the study cohort of 205 542 candidates for ECFMG certification, have now been completed and a full presentation of the findings to date is being prepared for publication.

The Study Population

In this limited presentation, it is possible only to list some of the important demographic and other characteristics of the study population. These include, for example, year of application for certification, age and sex, the 155 nationalities represented, the 109 countries where they received their medical education in 955 different medical schools, their native language (English or other), language of instruction in medical school, the year of graduation, the interval between completion of medical school education and initial ECFMG examination, and the site of the examination center where they took their initial ECFMG examination. These are being taken into account in analyses now in progress bearing upon the success or failure of candidates on their initial or subsequent ECFMG examinations. They will also be considered, individually and in combination, in our efforts to identify those factors that may influence candidates who, having successfully achieved ECFMG certification, elect to seek graduate training in hospitals in the United States, factors that may determine the direction and course of their entire professional careers.

Recently, the ECFMG has announced that beginning with the examination to be offered in July 1984, its test of medical knowledge will more closely approximate the assessment of knowledge of the basic medical sciences and clinical subjects covered in Parts I and II of the National Board of Medical Examiners, examinations taken by a large majority of the students attending medical schools in the United States. This new test will include a larger number of questions than has the examination given by the ECFMG in the past and will require 2 days rather than 1 to complete. Also, it is anticipated that this revision in screening procedures will obviate the need for a separate Visa Qualifying Examination and that ECFMG certification based on the new examination will meet the special visa requirements of the United States government for physicians wishing to enter the United States for graduate training or for practice. These developments also underscore the timeliness of the studies now in progress.

Discussion

What are the ultimate objectives of the studies briefly outlined in the above presentation? There is, of course, a justifiable purpose served in summarizing and evaluating the unique experience of the Educational Commission for Foreign Medical Graduates over the first 25 years of its existence. During that period it has employed the best techniques available to validate the educational credentials of graduates of foreign medical schools who seek opportunities for further professional training in the United States and to assure that those physicians satisfying its criteria for certification will benefit from such training, while at the same time conforming to the standards of practice and patient care in the United States. It is reasonable to anticipate that the ECFMG and its sponsoring educational and professional bodies will utilize the findings of these analyses in developing their own policies and plans for the future. However, the objectives of these studies extend beyond that goal.

There are sound bases for the prediction that large numbers of physicians trained in many countries around the world, some of them in various stages of economic and social development and sorely in need of additional medical manpower, will wish to come to the United States and to other of the so-called developed nations for such advanced professional training as may not yet be available to them in their homelands. How many of them will have the opportunity to do so? How many could and would benefit by such an educational experience? How many might be diverted from the intended purposes of such training programs, choosing to become emigrees rather than migrant physicians seeking to enhance their professional competence, contributing thereby to progress in medical care in their homelands? It is possible that the analyses now in progress may establish that present mechanisms and procedures – in which the individual physician develops his own plans and negotiates his own arrangements, often at considerable distance from a prospective training site – may not be, in fact, as beneficial to the physicians and the countries concerned as our conventional wisdom has dictated. It is also possible that past and present experience, supported by documentation derived from analyses in progress and others contemplated for the immediate future, will point the way to more systematic approaches involving the cooperative sharing of responsibilities for both planning and operations by institutions, organizations, and governmental agencies in both 'donor' and 'recipient' countries.

Viewed in the perspective of the general theme of this Congress – Preventive and Social Aspects of Primary Care – it may by appropriate to ask whether the analytic data to be derived from these follow-up studies of ECFMG candidates will provide support for the continuation of hospital residency programs in highly specialized tertiary care institutions as the predominant if not the sole mechanism for the provision of high-quality graduate educational experience for exchange visitor physicians, as well as for graduates of foreign medical schools who expect to enter career practice in the United States. There is reason to believe that these studies will supply important data in support of alternative programs and a broader range of educational opportunities that could prove both attractive and beneficial to graduates of both foreign and domestic medical schools.

In the conceptual framework established earlier in this century by Professors Grotjahn, Sand, and Ryle as well as by other pioneers in the discipline of social medicine, it is essential that medical education and the deployment of health manpower, whether on an intranational or on an international scale, be considered in the context of their social as well as their technological parameters. It is hoped that the forthcoming data from the studies briefly described in this presentation will prove useful in the promotion of such objectives.

Summary

The background, objectives, and current status of a major epidemiological study of 205 542 graduates of medical schools located outside of the United States and Canada who, during the 14-year period 1969–1982 have taken at least an inital ECFMG examination of their medical knowledge and English language competence have been briefly outlined. These examinations have been taken in order to gain ECFMG certification, which, since 1961, has been a prerequisite for appointment to accredited programs of graduate training in the medical specialties in hospitals in the United States. Such certification is also a requisite for licensure to practice medicine within the United States for all graduates of foreign medical schools. The data being analyzed indicate the marked diversity in the demographic characteristics and the educational background of the candidates included in the study population. This presentation also suggests some of the ways that data from these studies may assist in coping more effectively with the educational and social forces underlying the election of large numbers of graudates of foreign medical schools to migrate to the United States as well as to other countries.

Acknowledgment. The author wishes to express his appreciation of the invaluable assistance provided by the staff of the ECFMG and of Vector Systems in the preparation of this presentation. Special acknowledgment is made to Ray L. Casterline, MD, Vice President and Chief Operating Officer, ECFMG; B. S. Bloom, PhD, and Robert S. Knorr, MPH, of the Department of Research Medicine, University of Pennsylvania; and to Mr. Leo Genovese, Vector Systems Corporation.

References

1. Dublin TD (1981) The changing role of the foreign medical graduate in the practice of medicine in the US. Educational Commission for Foreign Medical Graduates, Philadelphia
2. Stewart WH, Pennell MY (1961) Medical school alumni. Public Health Service Publication no 263, Washington, DC, Health manpower source book, sect 11
3. Distribution of physicians in the US 1971 (1972) American Medical Association, Chicago
4. Physician characteristics and distribution in the US 1982. (1983) American Medical Association, Chicago

B. *Primary Health Care by the Physician and Allied Personnel*

Cooperation Between Different Professions and Lay Personnel

B. Kosanke

One of the pet ideas of the 1970s was more cost-effective care by means of greater co-operation. We admire the multidisciplinary group practices in the United States and the health centres in the Netherlands and the United Kingdom, and it is difficult to understand why the Federal Republic of Germany should not be able to keep up with these countries. In fact we have only small two-doctor partnerships and widespread sharing of expensive technical equipment; there is little patient-oriented teamwork.

In this paper I shall first give some reasons for this relative lack of co-operation in German public health care, and then call into question some of the team initiatives in the 1970s. Thirdly, I shall describe the more promising starting point of recent developments towards co-operation between physicians, welfare and lay personnel. Finally, I shall analyse the chances of these new initiatives having a good cost-benefit ratio.

Why can we not keep up either with U.S. group practices or with the Dutch health centre movement? Is the German physician a sort of monomaniac entrepreneur, lacking the well-known Anglo-saxon spirit of teamwork?

Man acts and reacts because of severe necessity or very strong incentives (as Oscar Wilde said: "I can resist everything except temptation"), or because desired benefits are easily obtained. The starting point of the U.S. group practices was mere necessity. American surgeons offer out-patient care four times more often than do surgeons in Germany, and anaesthetists do so 35 times more often. Both the surgeon and the anaesthetist absolutely need easily available support from those engaged in other disciplines.

Another reason for the lack of teamwork in Germany is that we have a two times higher ratio of general practitioners. Their best offer is confidentiality, personal understanding, which does not necessarily dovetail with teamwork. A third reason is that German physicians who are fond of co-operation simply work in a hospital. The ratio of such physicians to others is one and a half times higher than in the United States.

The preconditions for teamwork in Germany are therefore directly inverse to those in the United States. Concerning the Dutch health centres, we had neither the strong incentives nor the facilities of well organized first-line social services such as the Cross organizations in the Netherlands.

During the 1970s many young physicians in Germany were fascinated by the concept of the health centre because it was largely in line with the new para-

Primary Health Care in the Making
Ed. by U. Laaser, R. Senault, H. Viefhues

digm of medical care, i.e. priority of prevention, and treatment of chronic and psychosomatic diseases. Some physicians imported the health centre concept, but quickly got into trouble, in part because of incompatibility with the established health system.

Sectors of the public health administration and trade unions also issued plans, programmes and models of teamwork. The catchwords were integration, centralization and intersectorial co-operation. Paperwork proliferated; expert assessments were ordered, but ideas were seldom implemented. Judging by a bird's eyeview today, I think that a strong necessity for co-operation has not really been demonstrated. There was much lip service to the idea and even more strategies. Operational research was often a committed rather than a sceptical supporter of greater co-operation, piling up a host of data with no evidence at all, and seldom proving greater cost-effectiveness of co-operation on the full scale of intervening variables. Most of this research ended with the refrain that further research was needed.

Today, however, we are observing new initiatives that have a more promising starting point because they answer an obvious need in respect of a co-ordinated set of different services for the care of severely handicapped patients, e.g. retarded children, cancer patients, the elderly, the mentally ill, alcoholics, drug addicts and other fringe groups. All of these groups need close co-operation between three different services: medical treatment, rehabilitation services, and support of daily activities. Specialized medical care alone will never permit full reintegration of the handicapped into daily life. Rather it must be supported by rehabilitation services, and neither can be successfully applied if there is no help in respect of daily needs and activities.

Up to now, such patients have mostly been cared for in hospitals and other institutions, which thwarts re-integration into social life owing to the side-effects of hospitalization. In fact, ambulatory care that keeps the patient within his social environment is the most direct way to optimal reintegration. The problem here is to organize the necessarily permanent and comprehensive set of services between service providers who, by tradition, operate in quite different institutions.

Some doctors have coped with this difficulty. They work in a team providing the medical treatment and the necessary co-ordination of the rehabilitation services. The latter services are offered by welfare personnel team members – together with the family, the neighbours or self-help groups, i.e. lay care that renders daily life outside of hospitals and other institutional care units possible.

This makes a big difference to the health centres mentioned above: they are not reacting to an idea, but to the need of well-defined target groups. They do not offer a wide range of medico-psycho-social services; rather they specialize in only one target group. This is more appropriate to our health system. The Central Research Institute in Cologne is doing operational research on these models. The criteria of effective care for these handicapped patient groups are quite clear-cut. They are:

- The frequency of prevented hospitalization
- The frequency of longer periods of well-being and shorter episodes of relapse

- A less disturbed pursuit of daily life and a better acceptance of the patient within his social surroundings.

This evaluation will need only limited data collection. Other problems under observation are the feasibility of patient-oriented co-operation in different types of organization, the development of quality standards and indicators of need.

Two major problems will need a long-term policy: financing and the motivation of a sufficient number of care providers to guarantee a network of services that covers a given area.

Man reacts through necessity or strong incentives. Handicapped patients badly need permanent and comprehensive, i.e. co-operative, services allowing them to stay within their accustomed social surroundings. The service providers will not necessarily react to this need. But the chances are not too bad: the increasing number of young physicians in primary health care will not have the money to compete with the very high standard of technical equipment and qualification we have already got in primary care. They must look for other ways of competing. There are not many, but teamwork with welfare and lay personnel is one of them.

The Group Medical Practice – A Prospect for Doctors and Patients?

F. Holldack-Heckmann

In the Federal Republic of Germany the term 'group medical practice' encompasses quite different types of co-operation:

– the 'Apparategemeinschaft', also known as 'partielle Praxisgemeinschaft',
– the 'Praxisgemeinschaft' and
– the 'Gemeinschaftspraxis'.

In recent years these types of practice have become increasingly important. Their number has more than doubled since 1978. According to the NAV, in 1982 there were 1054 'Apparategemeinschaften' (consisting of 20 352 doctors) and 6960 doctors had joined together in 3380 'Gemeinschaftspraxen'. Unfortunately, for the 'Praxisgemeinschaft' there are only the records from 1977/78, showing 128 practices with 268 doctors.

Let me describe the different forms of practice in detail:

The 'Apparategemeinschaft'

'Apparategemeinschaften' are formed by doctors of similar or different specialization in order to share equipment for diagnostic or therapeutic purposes. Each doctor has full responsibility for the treatment of his own patients and for bills on his own behalf to the 'Kassenärztlichen Vereinigungen' (physicians' billing organizations). That is, the partners carry on their own practices completely independent of each other and are also spatially separated. The co-operation primarily concerns certain medicotechnical services but also makes possible the common procurement of medical supplies.

The reason for this form of co-operation lies without doubt in the development of highly sophisticated and expensive technical apparatus. These instruments make possible an improvement and a rationalization of diagnosis. Their acquisition and upkeep would be uneconomic, if not impossible, for a single private doctor. The 'Ärztliche Apparategemeinschaft Lemgo' can be given as an example of a highly efficient form of such rationalized medicotechnical services. The members of this 'Apparategemeinschaft' are very heterogeneous and very unusual for the Federal Republic of Germany: private

Primary Health Care in the Making
Ed. by U. Laaser, R. Senault, H. Viefhues

doctors, hospitals and 'Vertrauensärztliche Dienststellen' of the LVA. The most important advantages of this co-operation, accruing from its size, are:

- Automation and data processing
- Rationalization of the chemical tests, with a reduction in costs and an increase in quality
- Employment of highly qualified personnel
- Unification of excat laboratory standards for a larger area with the consequence that the strict division between ambulatory and hospital medical care no longer exists, at least as far as some aspects of diagnosis are concerned
- It helps to relieve private doctors of problems with staff and with regulations concerning quality control and it improves patient care in rural regions. Unnecessary hospital stays can be prevented, while the medical records are available in case of hospital admittance.
- Great gaps in knowledge between hospital doctors and their colleagues in private practice can be prevented by discussions about the patients' records and regular seminars

The 'Praxisgemeinschaft'

The co-operation between doctors of similar or different specialization in a 'Praxisgemeinschaft' consists in the common use of practice rooms and equipment, but also in the common employment of personnel. The treatment of the patients, however, is done separately and the doctors also bill their services with the 'Kassenärztliche Vereinigung' independently of each other.

A wide range of forms of co-operation can be found which bear the name 'Praxisgemeinschaft'. Sometimes it differs from the 'partielle Praxisgemeinschaft' only by virtue of its spatial proximity; sometimes it resembles the 'Gemeinschaftspraxis', whose members co-operate so intensely that separate billing with 'Kassenärztlichen Vereinigungen' and the formal assignment of patients takes place only for legal reasons. So far the 'Gemeinschaftspraxis' with doctors of different specialization has not been permitted.

It is characteristic of the 'Praxisgemeinschaft' that forms of co-operation are not limited to common medical technical facilities with the necessary accompanying personnel, but that there is also an extension of co-operation into the area of office organization, such as a common entrance, waiting room, staff room, office etc.

Close proximity and the use of the above-mentioned increases in efficiency make possible not only a more economic organization of the practice and the procurement and upkeep of high-quality technical facilities, but also colleague consultation, mutual further education, discussions about mutual patients, and decisions as to vacations and emergency duty. These factors do improve the quality of the individual doctor's services as well, as improving his working conditions.

The 'Gemeinschaftspraxis'

The third form of co-operation between private doctors, the 'Gemeinschaftspraxis', is the most all-encompassing. It comprises not only common office space, facilities and mutual employment of personnel, but also the common use of patients' records and common charging of performed services to the 'Kassenärztliche Vereinigungen'. The 'Gemeinschaftspraxis' can be considered as a form of 'collective private property' which includes not only practice equipment but also the collective disposal of the practice income. Thus, this form of co-operation stands in complete contrast to the individual – one could say – 'archiac' single practice which prevails in the Federal Republic of Germany.

This might have been an important reason for the prohibition of the 'Gemeinschaftspraxis' before 1965; the duty to register was first introduced in 1968. However, the mutual practice of doctors of different specialities, the so-called interdisciplinary group practice, has been forbidden up to the latest decision of the Bundessozialgericht.

Even though group practices consisting of more than two persons are considered to be the most advanced form of co-operation, they are hardly found in the Federal Republic of Germany today. Below I shall try to demonstrate the advantages they offer.

Basically, there is hardly any doubt that the medical group practice offers more advanced possibilities of diagnosis and therapy in comparision with the isolated service of the individual doctor. The necessity for close medical co-operation is the consequence of the increasing specialization of medical service and the development of medical technology. However, the necessity for close co-operation results also from the shift within the spectrum of diseases to be treated; in former times infectious diseases were the centre of medical concern, but nowadays (after having successfully stemmed epidemics) special attention has to be paid to chronic diseases. Furthermore, the high percentage of diseases caused by unsolved psychological problems and social living conditions shows a need for co-operation between doctors and professional groups such as psychotherapists, psychologists and social workers as well as lawyers. I would like to refer in this context to Hoffmann et al. [2], who analysed in particular new models of psychosocial services.

Another point can be derived from problems of medical care in the suburbs and rural areas. A practice equipped with modern facilities which offers the opportunity for co-operation might attract the young hospital doctor to settle in areas of insufficient supply, because working conditions there (i.e. regular duty hours, free time for further education) resemble to a greater extent the conditions in hospitals than those in individual practices. Also, the tendency to shift from 'curing' to 'preventive' medicine, with increasing demands on working hours and practice equipment, encourages co-operation.

Results from early research into group medical practice proved that the equipment in group medical practice was superior to that in comparable individual practices. Furthermore, the number of cases per doctor was less in group medical practice, i.e. there was more time for the individual patient and for further education [1, 3]. Our study of a three-member partnership primarily revealed the possibility of division of labour within a single medical sector as well as between different sectors.

There are also several other sociopsychological considerations which call for co-operation between doctors in the form of group medical practices. Furthermore, an improvement in the ambulant sector radiates into other sectors of health services, as I showed in my doctoral thesis.

References

1. Amon T (1984) Gemeinschaftspraxen in der Bundesrepublik Deutschland. KV Niedersachsen, Hannover
2. Hoffmann U, et al. (1982) Gruppenpraxis und Gesundheitszentrum. Campus, Frankfurt
3. Wolff M (1973) Die Gruppenpraxis. Institut für Freie Berufe, Nürnberg

Division of Tasks and Cooperation: Learning Processes in Inter-professional Group Practices

U. Hoffmann

Introduction

In the last few years much of the discussion about primary health care has centred on health personnel and their activities. Considerable emphasis has been placed upon the importance of teamwork. While some progress has been made in inter-professional co-operation and in training for inter-professional teamwork, progress in general in this area has been very disappointing. Finding ways of working together and communicating across occupational boundaries has turned out to be more difficult than anticipated. In contrast to the growing number of medical group practices, inter-professional group practices (including different categories of health personnel as well as non-medical professionals) to date account for less than 1% of practices in the Federal Republic of Germany.

Explicit and unconscious aims in co-operation as well as promotive and hindering factors have been the focus of a study of eight group practices, undertaken by the Sonderforschungsbereich 101 at the University of Munich in 1980 and 1981 [1]. In this paper it is my intention to present some of the findings of this study.

I begin by reviewing the underlying concept of group practice initiatives. I shall secondly describe two different forms of inter-professional group practice and then outline some of the major difficulties encountered in the actual process of inter-professional co-operation.

The Underlying Concept of Group Practice Initiatives

In contrast to the medical concept of disease, a *'holistic' approach,* embracing a number of aspects relevant to an individual's well-being, is fundamental to all group practice initiatives. Holistic assumptions suggest that the health of an individual involves varied dimensions including the interaction between social, emotional and environmental factors and physical illness. Besides medical treatment, the idea of *'comprehensiveness'* further requires co-operation with social workers and psychologists. The appropriate pattern of common contributions by the personnel involved may be classified as a *pattern of merged con-*

Primary Health Care in the Making
Ed. by U. Laaser, R. Senault, H. Viefhues

tributions, meaning co-operation in a feed-back process with common discussions and common planning of treatment [2, p. 22]. Formal or informal regulations regarding decision making and *participation of all members* of the group are presumed to be a necessary precondition of this concept. Obviously this touches upon the crucial issue of hierarchy. Hierarchy and the distribution of income are closely intertwined. It follows that the pooling and redistribution of income, too, require formal or informal regulation.

Two Generations of Group Practice Initiatives

Starting from these principles in the mid- and late-1970s *four health centres* were established in the Federal Republic and West Berlin, all of which included general practitioners, specialists in various fields, i.e. specialists for internal diseases, surgeons, gynaecologists, orthopaedists etc., receptionists, nurses, technical assistants, physiotherapists, occupational therapists, dieticians, psychologists and social workers. The health personnel sometimes amounting to 100, the health centres have been stricken by increased bureaucracy, the contributions of the personnel tending to be parallel or additive rather than merged. In some cases they have eventually split up into single practices. The health centres have certainly failed to cope with the problem of hierarchy, last but not least due to the fact that the doctors had raised high loans to finance extensive technical facilities. Because it was they who had brought the money in, participation of other health personnel was repressed in a number of cases. Particularly in times of financial pressure they were elbowed out.

In contrast to the previous concept of big health centres, *a second generation* of group practice initiatives came into existence in the late-1970s and early-1980s based on a more general orientation. In practical terms, all of them included general practitioners, no specialists, and a limited number of other professionals, in each case in a distinct combination. The limitation of the group size to between 7 and 15 members is considered a necessary condition for achieving a high level of co-operation. The low level of technical facilities may foster positive effects concerning the equitable sharing of power and benefits.

Difficulties Encountered in the Process of Co-operation

Given the limits and constraints arising from present financing principles, making health teams work raises plenty of challenges in the actual process of work itself. Don't expect me to list the exact duties of each category of health personnel. Instead, let me outline some of the difficulties encountered in *identifying* appropriate tasks and finding ways of working together across occupational boundaries.

The tasks of the same category of health personnel differ to some extent among the different group practices, and the *division of tasks* is in fact subject to an ongoing process of change. This has given rise to the following problems.

Whereas doctors are expected to be competent in the area of medical treatment and are thus provided with a well defined task, the professional roles of other personnel apparently lack coherence. It is because of this lack of definition that different professions to some extent perform overlapping services which, of course, is not bad in itself. Yet at the same time this undermines the self-confidence of the personnel involved and imposes constant difficulties in focusing on distinct fields of activity.

The alternation of theoretical and concrete work, of teamwork and individual effort, is significant to inter-professional group practices. Periodic meetings provide scope for feedback, common discussions and common planning of treatment. Just to mention some such meetings, there may be regular weekly team discussions, working groups on specific topics, Balint groups, case discussions etc. *The timing and harmonizing of different occupational perspectives,* however, is rendered difficult by irritations. Often there is no congruence between the professionals' expectations of each other.

Let me give an example. Doctors usually favour a pattern of additive contributions based on distinct and well defined tasks and competences. Thus a doctor may say: "I expect a social worker to handle problems he or she is more apt at than I am according to my area of activity." A social worker may put emphasis on a broader concept of merged co-operation. "Co-operation means an intensive effort towards mutual interchange. The knowledge and experience of both doctor and social worker meet and lead to a new, enlarged perception of the patient in respect of whom the new perspective will be proved, developed and altered."

Diffuse areas of activities and different frames of reference particularly affect the co-operation between doctors, social workers and psychologists, thus threatening to impair the possible extent of multidisciplinary professional contributions in the *psychosocial* field.

Other categories of health personnel have been faced with quite the opposite problem: tasks that are too well defined. This certainly is the case with *receptionists* but the problem affects other professionals as well. Patronizing attitudes on the part of doctors are commonly associated with the belief that the appropriate role of receptionists is to help reduce *their* workload and help in performing *their* functions. This has set limits to enlarging the receptionists' area of work. They still have to make do with the donkey work, their jobs lacking the prerequisites of self-fulfilment and personal growth, factors which, in their turn, probably contribute most to a high degree of teamwork motivation. Co-operating with self-help groups which have been established in a number of group practices may be a means of enhancing receptionists' work.

Conclusion

Interprofessional co-operation in primary health care still occurs in unsatisfactory circumstances with respect to training and funds. Co-operation has not yet been given a real chance. A crucial issue in making health teams work is time – time to understand and develop the tasks of different professionals in a patient and ongoing process of experimentation against the background of mutual sharing and support.

The real issue, however, centres on whether or not the medical establishment will accept inter-professional co-operation as a positive development rather than resisting the sharing of power and resources.

References

1. Hoffmann U, Schubert I, Tatschmurat C, Zettel O (1982) Gruppenpraxis und Gesundheitszentrum. Campus, Frankfurt
2. Westrin CG (1983) Organisation and management of primary health care from a medical perspective. Report of a European Seminar on Research in Primary Health Care, October 1982. Available from European Centre for Social Welfare Training and Research, Vienna (Eurosocial Reports no 21, pp 15–21)

Legal, Institutional and Educational Conditions for Interdisciplinary Teamwork Between Allied Health Professions

B. Meifort and H. Paulini

This paper is based on results of the research project "Consequences for the allied health professions of developments in health services" conducted by the Federal Institute of Vocational Education. The points of interest in this context refer only to the paramedical professions, which are to be interpreted as registered health professions.

The legal, institutional and educational conditions of teamwork in primary health care (aimed at patient-oriented care) will be discussed below. Some consequences for vocational training with reference to co-operation will then be derived from this discussion.

Legal Conditions

Trends in educational policy are towards isolated structured professions in the field of the allied health professions rather than towards comprehensive basic qualifications and specialization during further education. In the Federal Republic of Germany these trends are visible in both state and federal policy. The allied health professions belong to a *separate field of the vocational educational system.* Legally they are based on special vocational laws, the general vocational education act applying only to medical (as well as dental) assistants. Therefore the splitting of the professions is legally guaranteed.

There exist *a large number of different professions* working in the same or in a similar area (cf. Table 1): 18 professions are based on federal regulations and 16 on state regulations. Each of them involves only a few special qualifications and tasks which could make these professions genuine. Furthermore, only the *professional titles* are protected by law, not the profiles of professional activity. Qualified activities can be taken over at any time by members of any other profession. For instance, the physicians' assistants take over professional tasks from medical technical assistants or medical technicians. In this way the higher qualified professions can be dislocated by low level professions without the staff having learned the necessary skills and without them being paid equally.

Besides the absence of a legal definition of professional tasks, the *denomination* of the allied health professions as "assisting" or "helping" professions gives a good impression of the restricted possibilities of their professional ac-

Primary Health Care in the Making
Ed. by U. Laaser, R. Senault, H. Viefhues

Table 1. Survey: The professional field in health care – a selection

	Training time (years)	Sort of regulation[a]
Primary health care professions		
Medical assistants	2	FR
Dental assistants	2–3	FR
Veterinary assistants	2–3	FR
Diagnostic-technical health professions		
Medical laboratory technician	2	FR
X-ray technician	2	FR
Veterinary laboratory technician	2	FR
Cytology assistant	1–2	SR
Pharmacy technician	2½	FR
Nursing professions		
Registered nurse	3	FR
Pediatric registered nurse	3	FR
Licensed practical nurse	1	FR
Midwife	3	FR
Midwifes aide	½	FR
Dietetics assistant	2	FR
Nursing-home nurse	2–3	SR
Rehabilitation professions		
Masseur	1	FR
Masseur/medical bath attendant	2½	FR
Physical therapist	2	FR
Ergotherapist	3	FR
Mental health nurse	3–4	SR
Speech therapist	3	FR
Orthoptist	2–2½	SR
Neuro-otologic assistant	3	SR

[a] SR, state regulation; FR, federal regulation

tivities. This situation is based on our Constitution, the Basic Law, and is one reason for the dominant position of physicians. Last but not least, from the point of view of vocational education, there is no permeability between professions, even when they are in the same professional field.

To summarize: The legal limits of co-operation are based on the separation of professions, on the absence of legally defined tasks, on the lack of permeability between professions and on the limited definition of those professions as "helpers".

Institutional Conditions

In primary health care the tasks of prevention, care, rehabilitation and social counselling are linked. Corresponding to these activities, the multifunctional professional structure of these areas shows the necessity of co-operation.

Case studies in primary health care centres have revealed somewhat improved health care as well as the introduction of co-operation. For example, in these centres the medical (and dental) assistants have a broader range of activities: thus they carry out new tasks in health counselling and health education, like the counselling of pregnant women, dietetic counselling or hygiene counselling. These experiences have to be evaluated and their transferability to other institutions ascertained.

The vocational training in the allied health professions is primarily carried out in hospitals. Because of the rigid separation between in-patient hospital-care and ambulant health care in West Germany, primary health care work as an increasing future professional activity has not been paid enough attention in educational policy up till now.

In summary, the institutional conditions for teamwork show signs of improving, but limits to this tendency are also evident, as in the educational organization.

Curricular Conditions

Starting from the hypothesis that there must be a similar fundamental content in every vocational training field, which could be taught similarly in every profession in that field, we analysed the contents of the subjects on the curricula of selected allied health professions and compared them. Those subjects of vocational education which are similar in content in all professional areas of health care are:

- Professional and legal basics
- Basics in psychosocial sciences (sociology, psychology, pedagogics)
- Basics in medical/biological sciences (anatomy, physiology)

Concerning the subject "Professional and Legal Basics", something all members of the health professions have in common is the *occupational field orientation.* Vocational education in the health field should inform students about the problems, structures and tasks of the health care system in general, and about the functions and limitations of different professions. But in reality, especially in primary health care professions, "professional and legal basics" are normally taught on a strictly functional basis (i.e. with reference only to the profession concerned).

Concerning the "Basics in Psychosocial Sciences", something all members of the health professions have in common is a *patient orientation.* So, for example, psychosocial knowledge and capabilities could be offered similarly, in all allied health professions, which would undeniably be an important basis for co-operation and a more developed patient orientation. But, as we found out, the curricula are – when they exist at all in this subject – strictly functional too. Hence there is a specific kind of psychology for physical and speech therapists, a specific kind of pedagogics for mental health nurses etc. In primary health care professions these subjects are not taught at all during vocational training.

Concerning the "Basics in Medical/Biological Sciences" something all members of the health professions have in common is an orientation towards the *organic structure* and the function of the human body. In vocational education for the primary health care professions, this subject is treated only superficially. In the rehabilitation professions it is related to the tasks of single professions. Only the nursing professions offer a relatively broad curriculum on this subject.

Consequences for Vocational Training with Reference to Teamwork

From this brief analysis the following consequences can be derived:

1. It will be necessary to establish new working patterns, i.e. there should be comprehensive planning of the use of labour:
   - Implementing integrated social and health care stations with a multi-functional professional structure of staff.
   - Professionally and hierarchically separated tasks, such as those in physical therapy and nursing, should be reunited.
   - New tasks such as psychosocial care should be integrated into 24- hour health care; this should not, however, lead to the development of a new specialization.

   This comprehensive professional planning is the basis for a patient-oriented and comprehensive curriculum in the vocational training for the allied health professions.
2. In vocational training a broad and transfunctional basic education should be developed; specific functional subjects should be taught later.
3. Practical experiences in the primary health care system should be integrated into the vocational training for all allied health professions.
4. To achieve equality in interdisciplinary teamwork the field of professional activities should be legally guaranteed. Only knowledge and consciousness of a defined, independent area of competence will enable all members of the allied health professions to co-operate on an equal basis. Therefore a high level of qualifications is necessary, a level that ensures all employees to be able to fulfil their tasks with a certain professional self-sufficiency.

Social Work in Health Care Services

A. Geiger

The limits of health services in the Federal Republic are becoming apparent. The enormous increase in chronic illnesses (heart and circulatory illnesses, cancer etc.) and the rising costs in the health sector document the situation in a health care – or perhaps one should say "illness care" – service which sees its main task in the treatment of illnesses which cannot be cured by medical therapy alone.

Curative medicine, aimed at the individual patient, is limited in its abilities with regard to structural problems, risk factors and pressures relevant to health. This is because social structures and prerequisites making health possible in the first place are, for the most part, generated in a political, work and learning context outside of the medical field. The processes leading to acute or chronic illness and the results of such illness necessitate, in addition to medical intervention, a growing number of preventive and rehabilitative measures. This, however, implies a direct contact to the individual's professional and personal surroundings, which is hardly possible in our current medical health system.

The social worker, a "social expert", is, thanks to his training, experience and personal professional ethic, able to establish both physical and social contact with the individual in question. His integration into the medical health team therefore implies an expansion of the spectrum of intervention in the therapeutic sector and, above all, an increasing recognition of preventive and rehabilitative goals. This means, generally speaking, a concrete formulation of fields of focus in areas in which social workers have long been employed (for example, work in hospitals), but at the same time a description of possibilities in the ambulatory areas which calls, above all, for implementation of rehabilitative and preventive measures (consulting services, "non-specific health services").

Politically or structurally influenced hindrances to integration set limits to the current conditions for social work. On the one hand, they limit an increase or specialization in the employment of social workers (for example, in group practices, ambulatory clinics, health departments etc.), and on the other hand the first steps towards positive co-operation which have been taken by medical personnel and social workers (for example in psychiatric work) do not become apparent.

Concerning the direct co-operation between medical and non-medical personnel, and particularly social workers, three levels can be described:

Primary Health Care in the Making
Ed. by U. Laaser, R. Senault, H. Viefhues

1. Areas in which the co-operation or teamwork has made considerable progress. For example, the area of psychiatric care and the general fields of social work which have been most strongly influenced by the trend towards psychosocial counselling.
2. Areas in which, for reasons relating to the low status of social workers, social work has been seen as identical to traditional charity work and thus has often been misused, e.g. by the health departments, which often make exaggerated use of their role as employers in order to uphold traditional notions of the roles of those involved and which, for reasons of social and medical deficits, demand a segmentation of health care services and thus limit or hinder the work of the social worker.
3. Areas in which the contacts between medical and social personnel is relatively rare. For example, the social services in hospital, where, due to an overload of administrative work, the social worker is not able to carry out his real tasks in psychosocial counselling; here intensive co-operation between the medical and paramedical personnel is indeed necessary.

The current training of social workers results in an action competency that is specifically social based; a specialization in the field of health services, however, is missing. This can be traced to the developments at the *"Fachhochschulen"* in the early 1970s, where the compensatory and emancipatory goal-orientation of the training diametrically contradicted the medical personnel's concept of training. One expression of this relationship can be seen in the fact that medical personnel with a specialty in the social area have been employed at Fachhochschulen only in the last few years and that various Fachhochschulen even today do not offer satisfactory instruction in the field of social medicine.

This was the starting point for the introduction of a major field of study in "social work in the health services" as part of the basic curriculum for social work at the Fachhochschule BS/WF. It is directed at the following three goals, which correspond to the above-mentioned areas:

1. Qualified training for areas in which social workers have already been employed (health departments, in-patient institutions etc.), including, of course, a more concrete formulation of the tasks.
2. Training for expanding fields in the ambulatory area (counselling services, Pro Familia, drug counselling etc.).
3. Training which takes into consideration the structural changes in the medical field (health centres etc.).

Following a two-semester course of basic studies, during which basic aspects of social work are taught and two practical courses are completed in health institutions, the major focus of the course of study, concerning health care, begins with third semester. One of the chief components of the newly established study programme is training in the form of projects which cover the fields of

- psychiatry
- help to the handicapped
- work with acutely and chronically ill patients

- social work in terms of preventive medicine in industry
- non-school health education

In addition to a general trend towards project-oriented training in the study of social work, project-based work during the training in the health field is to be recommended
- to achieve a concrete formulation of the areas of employment,
- to test innovative methods in areas which are new to social work, and
- to accustom the students to being able to work as a team.

The experimental phase of the pilot project, financed by the Federal and State Commission for Educational Planning and Support of Research and directed at developing such a curriculum, has proved that the main fields of employment for its graduates will be, in addition to the traditional psychiatric areas,
- public health services,
- the ambulatory and preventive area, and
- the curative area.

In public health the necessity has become apparent for a more concrete formulation or, in part, a shift of accent concerning the main areas of employment (for example in the social-psychiatric area).

The health department, traditionally unpopular among social workers, has become much more attractive due to the close co-operation with various institutions and the job descriptions which could thus be formulated. It must be added that health-related aspects were discovered in other branches of public administration (for example, the social welfare agency) and these institutions thus have become more relevant for graduates in their practical work.

Potential employers are therefore various institutions and counselling services in the public domain. Health work in the ambulatory or preventive area means, with reference to the WHO's definition of health, intervention from a rehabilitative or primarily preventive point of view. Of course, counselling, for example in areas of social problems, is not to be neglected. A neighbourhood or public orientation is most effective in this work, to achieve the highest possible measure of activity (for example in the area of health education). Close co-operation with the ambulatory medical services is necessary. First steps in this direction, for example the employment of a social worker as a "communication channel for socio-therapeutic help" vis-à-vis the medical doctor, have been very successful. Employers here would be the health insurance companies, the public health services, health centres and the ambulatory medical care system in general.

The curative area aims at work with the acutely and chronically ill (for example, hospital social services), and here a closer job description should stress the psychosocial care of the patients rather than administrative activities. Experience in the work in the pilot project has shown that, on the basis of such job descriptions of the specific competence of social workers, the co-operation with the medical and paramedical personnel improved considerably and was much more effective.

Telephone Medicine: A Training Need in a Technological Society

A. A. Talbot, P. Curtis, L. MacLaren, A. F. Sanchez, and R. Bissonette

In the past decade, increasing attention has been given to the telephone as a means of patient access to health care and physician management of medical problems [1 – 10]. Telephone contacts involving medical intervention have been estimated to form 10% – 15% of all patient encounters in the United States [11]. This proportion is even greater among primary care physicians, such as pediatricians, internists, and family physicians, who may spend 20% or more of their practice time in telephone conversations with patients. With few exceptions, however, past research on telephone encounters has described single practice profiles without comparative data from comparable sites over an adequate sampling period [12 – 15].

This paper describes the profile of after hours telephone encounters and tests the relationship between practice context, problem content, and management, and physician-patient interaction in three US family practice residency programs. The data support the thesis that systematic training in telephone medicine should be an integral facet of residency experience in family medicine and primary care [16 – 18].

Materials and Methods

The data collected for this study were compiled in 1978 – 79 as part of the After Hours Call Survey of the Department of Family Medicine of the University of North Carolina at Chapel Hill. The After Hours Call Survey, conducted over five consecutive years from 1976 through 1981, was designed to develop materials and methods that could be implemented easily and processed reliably in family medicine and allied health training programs.

Research Sites

The first research site included in the present study was the original location of the study, the Family Practice Center of the University of North Carolina at Chapel Hill (i.e., UNC-CH). As shown in Table 1, Chapel Hill is a community of approximately 50 000, located in the eastern piedmont, at one corner of the

Primary Health Care in the Making
Ed. by U. Laaser, R. Senault, H. Viefhues

Table 1. A comparison of after hours telephone calls to three US family practice residencies: practice profiles

	Chapel Hill	Charlotte	Buffalo
Demography			
Social milieus	University town	Metropolis	Urban core
Population	50 000	350 000	475 000
Crime rate	8 400	22 900	25 200
Adjacent hospital size	645 beds	830 beds	320 beds
Familiy practice center			
Clinic Visits during study	13 000	11 000	17 000
% Medicaid*	5	10	50
% black*	25	33	60
Number of residents studied	18	12	32
*% after hours coverage**			
2nd year residents	17	49	26
3rd year residents	67	51	30
After hours coverage period			
Weekdays	17:00–8:00	16:30–8:00	17:00–8:00
Weekends	17:00–8:00 (Fri) (Mon)	16:30–8:00 (Fri) (Mon)	17:00–8:00 (Fri) (Mon)
Method used to triage after hours calls	Answering service	Hospital exchange	Hospital exchange

metropolitan area of Raleigh-Durham called the Research Triangle, an area that includes a population of 450 000. To the south, west, and north, Chapel Hill is surrounded by rolling woodland hills, fringe suburbs, numerous small towns, and farms which host some of the most important dairy farming industry in the state. The rural, pastoral influence of the area on the quality of life is revealed in the crime rate (of nearby Raleigh), which is only about one-third that of the more urban research sites. While most of the 8000 active patients from 2500 families, who made about 12 000 visits per year during the 1978–79 study period, are drawn from the immediate Chapel Hill community and Orange County, some patients also come from several surrounding counties. For the most part, the Family Practice Center serves a predominately white (75%), middle class group in which over 70% of the population have attended college. The middle class character of the practice population is also reflected in the fact that only 5% of the UNC-CH Family Practice Center patient population have payment supports through Medicaid. During the 1978–79 study year, 18 residents participated in the call schedule as well as several faculty attendings, postgraduate fellows, and community physicians. At UNC-CH, residents take call from late afternoon (5:30 p.m.) until the next morning when the clinic opens (8:00 a.m.) or for a 24-hour period at the weekend. Patients contact the practice through an answering service, but the responding physicians might take the call from the hospital, emergency room, family practice center, or their own home.

The second research site was the Family Practice Center of the Charlotte Memorial Hospital and Medical Center (i.e., CMH), a residency program from the same general geographic region as Chapel Hill, but located in a much more densely urbanized area. The Charlotte residency program is located in North Carolina's second largest metropolitan area and is situated at the southern end of a geographic corridor through central North Carolina that contains a majority of the state's population, wealth, and industry and has come to be known as the Piedmont Crescent. The Family Practice Center at CMH is located adjacent to an 830-bed regional hospital near the heart of downtown Charlotte. As shown in Table 2, the Charlotte Family Practice Center provides care for approximately 2400 families who recorded nearly 11 000 encounters per year. The proportions of black (33%) and Medicaid (10%) patients as well as the structure of the daily on-call period at the Charlotte residency program are fairly similar to Chapel Hill. Because of the month-long, on-call rotation schedule at Charlotte, however, only 12 of the 18 residents took calls during the study year: Also, the residents at Charlotte often covered services at CMH, and consequently took calls outside the medical complex less frequently than did residents at

Table 2. Patient profiles, diagnosis and management: a comparison of after hours telephone calls to three US family practice residencies

	Chapel Hill	Charlotte	Buffalo
After hours telephone calls			
After hours telephone calls during study year	1350	1108	432
Rate/100 clinic visits*	112.5	100.7	25.4
*Patient profile %**			
Caller = Pt	49	44	64
0–18	29	41	31
56+	8	7	23
Males	35	33	22
Blacks	24	25	44
*Dxs %**			
Infectious	18	11	11
Respiratory	15	12	12
Digestive	9	12	11
Pregnancy	3	5	6
Psychosocial	4	6	17
*Rxs for (tracers[a]) %**			
Drugs prescribed	16	39	25
Advice/counsel	82	28	63
None	2	29	10
*Follow-up (tracers) %**			
Pt should call again, if needed	33	22	50
Pt should make appointment at FPC	33	29	13
None	29	33	19

* $P < 0.01$

[a] Tracer Dxs = acute URI, viral syndrome, anxiety, cystitis, fever, abdominal pain

Chapel Hill. Researchers at Charlotte recorded only telephone calls after hours during the study period; hence, the comparative analysis in this paper is limited to this common data base in the three research sites.

The third study site was the Deaconess Hospital Family Practice Center, an affiliate of the State University of New York at Buffalo (i.e., SUNYAB). Located at the eastern end of Lake Erie, Buffalo is an industrial, predominately blue-collar metropolitan center that is popularly known as America's coldest city because of its inclement weather. As a research site, Buffalo provided a sharp regional contrast with the North Carolina residency programs and also allowed a comparison of family practice center patient care in locations of contrasting urban size. The Deaconess Hospital Family Practice Center is located downtown in the Buffalo urban core. Consequently, although the Buffalo metropolitan area has a predominantly white population, the Deaconess Family Practice Center serves a black catchment area (60%) with a sizable proportion of older, Medicaid patients (50%). The residency at Deaconess Hospital is the largest of the three research sites; 32 residents are trained at this program. The Deaconess Center has an active practice population of over 11 000 patients from 5200 families who presented over 17 000 office encounters during the study year. The Deaconess Family Practice Center was not used at all for patient visits after hours. Residents took call only when on duty, usually in the emergency room. All telephone encounters that required immediate follow-up were seen in the Deaconess Hospital Emergency Room.

Data Collection

Procedures for the survey were developed so that following each patient encounter, the responding physician completed a two-part, cheque-sized, adhesive data card designed to become part of the medical record. The data card and collection process [11] included: type of encounter (e.g., phone), relationship of caller to patient (e.g., mother), sex and race of patient, time of call, regular family doctor, presenting symptoms, subsequent diagnoses, treatment and follow-up plan, and signature of the responding physician. On a second part of the card, the responding physician made several ratings for each call, including: the patient's motive for calling (e.g., necessary, unnecessary), social problem involvement of the patient's problem (e.g., none, major), as well as the physician's subjective reaction to the encounter (e.g., anger = strong negative, satisfaction = strong positive) and attempts to reassure the patient (e.g., Likert scale, 0 = none, 5 = special effort).

All after hours telephone calls to the Charlotte Memorial Hospital Family Practice Center and Deaconess Hospital Family Practice Center at Buffalo during the study period were recorded on the data sticker, coded on site, then forwarded to Chapel Hill for data processing. Generally, missing information and other data errors were minimal. Information from Charlotte Memorial and Buffalo Deaconess was compared with the After Hours Survey data from the Family Practice Center of the University of North Carolina at Chapel Hill for that year.

Results

Call Rate

As shown in Table 2, a number of differences emerge when the after hours telephone practices of the three residencies are compared. During the study year, 432 telephone encounters were recorded at Buffalo, equivalent to 2.5% of the total practice at the Deaconess Family Practice Center. This proportion is notably less ($P < .01$) than the rate recorded at either North Carolina residency. Information of 1108 after hours telephone encounters was recorded during the study year at Charlotte, or 10% of all patient contacts. This proportion was very similar to the number recorded at Chapel Hill during the study year (11.5%).

Patient Profile

The data suggest systematic differences between the residencies in terms of the patients who telephone for care at night. The pattern suggests differences in the family component of the practices ($P < .01$). During the study year, Buffalo recorded the highest proportion of calls from patients themselves (64%), while Charlotte (44%) recorded the fewest. Conversely, Charlotte recorded the highest proportion of calls from a parent or spouse (46%), while Buffalo recorded the fewest (30%) from these family members. The family profile of telephone encounters at Chapel Hill resembled the pattern at Charlotte more than Buffalo.

The residencies also differed in the age, sex, and race profiles of the after hours telephone practices ($P < .01$). It is consistent with the family profiles that Charlotte recorded the most calls for patients under 18 (41%) and Buffalo had the highest proportion of calls from the older segment of the practice (23%). The proportion of calls from older patients at Chapel Hill (8%) was similar to Charlotte (7%), but the percentage of pediatric calls (29%) was more similar to Buffalo (31%). The proportion of males calling at Chapel Hill (35%) was quite similar to Charlotte (33%) and both were notably higher than the proportion recorded at Buffalo (22%). The percentage of calls from black patients at Chapel Hill (24%) and Charlotte (26%) was similar and notably less than the number recorded at Buffalo (44%). Yet, in proportion to the number of regular clinic encounters at the family practice centers, the number of after hours telephone calls from blacks at Charlotte and Buffalo was less than at Chapel Hill.

Diagnoses

Infectious, respiratory, general, and digestive problems were among the most common ICHPPC-2 diagnoses in each data set [19]. Cardiac, vascular, allergic-metabolic-endocrine-nutritional disorders, neoplasms, prophylactic, blood, prenatal care and congenital genetic diagnoses formed less than 10% of the telephone diagnoses at each residency. Nevertheless, systematic differences emerge between the programs. For example, Charlotte and Buffalo recorded fewer infectious and respiratory diagnoses, but significantly more digestive and pregnancy problems than Chapel Hill ($P < .01$). The North Carolina practices, however, counted fewer psychosocial problems and more general problems, accidents/poisons, and eye and ear problems than Buffalo. The biggest difference between the three programs was the proportion of telephone encounters involving a psychosocial diagnosis at Buffalo (17%), a proportion notably greater than at Charlotte (6%) or Chapel Hill (4%).

Problem Management and Follow-up

A comparison of the ten most frequent and six selected tracer diagnoses (tracer Dxs = acute URI, viral syndrome, anxiety, cystitis, fever, abdominal pain) showed that the management of problems ($P < .01$), as well as follow-up styles ($P < .01$), differed consistently among the programs. On similar sets of problems, residents at Charlotte prescribed medication (39%) more often and reported less counseling (28%) than other sites. Conversely, residents at Chapel Hill reported giving counseling to patients (82%) much more often than prescriptions (6%). Buffalo residents prescribed more medication (25%) than those at Chapel Hill, but counseled patients more often (63%) than recorded at Charlotte. Also, Charlotte residents were more likely to report no therapy given (29%) than residents at the other sites. The most common follow-up strategy at Buffalo was to have the patient call later (50%). At Charlotte and Chapel Hill, residents were more likely to have patients make a regular clinic appointment or to record no follow-up.

Physician Response to After Hours Telephone Calls

Following the completion of after hours encounters, the on-call physician rated these patient contacts on several dimensions including: probable reason the patient called, social problem aspects of the presenting complaint(s), necessity of the call, physician's personal reaction to the encounter, and the extent to which the patient was offered reassurance. Table 3 shows that these ratings varied systematically among the residency programs. Some of these differences are due to the variation in diagnostic profiles and management styles. Yet, patterns emerge which are not easily correlated with these differences.

About two-thirds of all after hours telephone encounters were estimated by the physician to be due to a physical problem. The proportion of calls estimated by the physician to be due to emotion-based problems was fairly similar at Chapel Hill (21%) and Charlotte (24%), but significantly less than at Buffalo (35%) ($P < .01$). This proportion is consistent with the high number of psychosocial diagnoses reported by Buffalo family practice residents. In addition, 26% of the after hours telephone contacts at Buffalo were estimated to have a major social problem component, while the proportion of cases at Chapel Hill (7%) and Charlotte (5%) was much lower ($P < .01$). At Chapel Hill (11%) and Char-

Table 3. Physician response(s): a comparison of after hours telephone calls to three US family practice residencies

	Chapel Hill	Charlotte	Buffalo
*MD ratings of calls (%)**			
Presenting problem is: organic based	68	65	62
emotion based	21	24	35
Problem has major social component	7	5	26
Call was unnecessary	20	11	32
Call produced anger frustration	10	9	20
Attempt to reassure patient: none	18	42	14
special	48	12	28
MDs' personal reaction to encounter predicts[a]			
Attempt to reassure Pt	+	+	+
Estimate of necessity of call	+	+	+
Estimate of social problem component	–	–	–
MDs' estimate of the necessity of call predicts[a]			
Estimate of Pt's motive for calling	–	–	–

* $P<0.01$

[a] Signs indicate direction of significant ($P<0.01$) regression coefficient

lotte (11%), approximately one in ten calls was for prescription refills or lab test results. The proportion of these calls at Buffalo (4%) was remarkably less ($P < .01$) and consistent with the Deaconess Hospital Emergency Room policy which fiercely discouraged patients from calling after hours for administrative requests.

The proportion of calls estimated to be necessary was higher in Charlotte (24%) and Buffalo (23%) compared with Chapel Hill (18%). Charlotte reported fewer (11%) and Buffalo reported more (32%) unnecessary calls than residents at Chapel Hill (18%). In general, estimates of the necessity of calls at Chapel Hill approximated a statistically normal distribution, while the distribution at Charlotte was weighted toward necessity, and the proportions at Buffalo were heavy at both extremes ($P < .01$).

The comparison of physician reaction also produced a crossover pattern. Physicians at Buffalo reported more anger and frustration (20%) than those at Charlotte (9%) and Chapel Hill (9%). Physicians at Charlotte reported neutrality (56%) most often in response to the after hours telephone encounters. At Chapel Hill (63%) and Buffalo (54%) the most common response was interest and satisfaction. The data indicate, then, sharp and unique differences in the modal emotional response of physicians at the three sites, with the most extreme differences emerging at Buffalo ($P < .01$).

The reported attempts to reassure patients also produced modal differences, and these are consistent with the distribution of emotional responses of physicians studied. Residents at Chapel Hill reported giving the greatest amount of reassurance. Nearly half (48%) of the requests for care led to a special effort by the physician to reassure the patient. At Charlotte, where the greatest proportion of neutral reactions to encounters was reported, the highest proportion of encounters where no reassurance was offered (42%) was recorded. At Buffalo, where after hours telephone calls were most likely to be rated as unnecessary and produce anger or frustration in the responding physician, most efforts to reassure patients (58%) were reported to be low ($P < .01$).

In sum, after hours telephone calls at Buffalo were assessed more often as due to emotion-based problems with major social problem components, as unnecessary, and as engendering anger or frustration in the responding physician. In contrast, residents at Chapel Hill reported giving more reassurance to patients and deriving more interest or satisfaction from encounters. Charlotte residents, who reported the most neutral reactions, also recorded the most calls where no reassurance was offered.

Physician Response: Path Analysis

A multiple regression analysis of the relationship between variables in the response patterns of physicians showed several consistent tendencies ($P < .01$) [20–23]. In each data set, the physician's emotional response and estimate of the necessity of the call were central to other assessments. As shown in Table 3, the provider's emotional reaction was consistently and positively associated with the amount of reported reassurance and the estimated necessity of the call, and negatively associated with diagnoses of emotion-based problems. Interestingly, however, physician reactions did not seem to be associated directly with patient motives for seeking care by phone. The estimated necessity of a telephone call was not correlated with the amount of reassurance reportedly given. Finally, the associations between the social problem component of a call and the amount of reassurance reported were related only inconsistently.

Implications

The data indicate that telephone medicine, at least as practiced in this sample of family medicine residency programs, is not a simple phenomenon. The findings reinforce earlier assertions concerning the wide disparity between the routines of telephone care delivery, the knowledge base attendant to this phase of medicine, and the development of training programs to evaluate and enhance its effectiveness [16–18]. The comparative analysis reported above illustrates many of the subtleties characterizing after hours telephone medical practice and testifies to the systematic variation in resident experience in this phase of training.

The analysis suggests that the morbidity profiles of after hours telephone encounters at these three residency programs may be more similar than practice demography and styles of problem management. This similarity may explain, in part, why past concerns about telephone medicine typically have been limited to administrative issues: who should take call; how often; what kind of answering service; which problems should be seen immediately, followed with a later clinic visit, or ignored? The similarities among the residencies disguise substantive differences in the fundamental character of on-call practices and the uneven practice experience of residents in this phase of training.

The study shows substantial variation in methods used to manage similar problems. These differences are most striking in the patterns of counseling and prescriptions. The management styles exhibited by residents in response to after hours telephone calls may reflect philosophies and practice styles of their faculty or other particular attitudes in their training ethos.

The analysis suggests a multivariate understanding of telephone medicine. Teachers of family medicine need to assimilate some background about the local practice population base, the methods and context used by patients to access care, practice styles of relevant mentors, and provider attitudes towards after hours care.

To some degree, the data reflect different expectations or traditions in primary medical care. At Buffalo, for example, the family practice residency is surrounded by a population conditioned toward episodic, impersonal care. Social context and history create considerable dissonance between the shared definitions of patients and providers concerning access to after hours care. This mismatch in expectations has been a persistent impediment to the application of concepts like continuity of care. Similarly, the clear resemblance between the two North Carolina programs is partly due to the legacy of their design and development in a similar political geography. In this light, the similarities of the North Carolina programs in structure and patient demography is not too surprising.

It seems clear that the structural and characterological aspects of a residency program exert a pervasive influence on the experience of residents with after hours telephone medicine during their training years. We would argue that family practice residencies should develop specific training programs for telephone medicine. This may require:

A Conceptual Pivot: Patient contact by telephone should be formalized as a conceptual phase of medical care delivery. Telephone medicine can no longer be relegated to the status of an ad hoc consequence of a high technology society. Indeed, in this phase of patient contact, the medium does seem to be the message. The message is that the telephone has fundamentally expanded patient access to, and experience with, primary medical care and the approach of providers needs to be rethought [24].

A Quality Control Pivot: Training programs should monitor the delivery of telephone medicine in their practice(s). The exact details of such arrangements depend necessarily upon local resources and interest. The general requisites, however, should allow educators routinely to describe the parameters of their telephone practice and to organize them for feedback to individual trainees. The authors have developed one technique to accomplish this goal that may serve as a useful guide in the development of telephone medicine training tools [25].

A Training Pivot. This training should include *orientation* toward the age- sex morbidity, epidemiology, demography, occupational environment, and psychosocial aspects of practice. Residents should be made aware of the rationale for on-call arrangements and of how their experience will aid in attaining the educational goals of the program as well as the administrative arrangements of after hours coverage. *Simulations and protocols* should be used to illustrate principles and problems of telephone encounters in the training experience of residents. Simulations are especially helpful in providing examples of the range of common problems and unusual conditions which ave evoked the anger or frustration of providers in past encounters. Simulated encounters can be used quite effectively in group or individual sessions with either professional staff or office personnel. Simulations are especially helpful in developing understandings of patient requests for care, in eliciting personal and interactional facets of treatment by telephone, for examining rationales of problem management, and in facilitating a broad range of administrative and interpersonal skills. Eventually, standard protocols for telephone encounters may be designed to facilitate training and to insure uniform minimums of care. Training programs should provide *regular feedback* to individual residents concerning their personal telephone practice. One example of this information which was developed at the University of North Carolina Family Practice Center at Chapel Hill for computerized printouts is available from the senior authors. Feedback can include morbidity profiles, demographic summaries, styles of problem management, and a comparative analysis of tracer diagnoses with typical resident experience in the training program.

References

1. Cooper CR, Toshioka SS, Greenlick MR (1971) Determinants of medical care utilization. The use of the telephone for reporting symptoms. J Health Soc Behav 12:155–162
2. Greenlick MR, Freeborn DK (1973) Determinants of medical care utilization: The role of the telephone in total medical care. Med Care 2:121
3. Westbury RC (1974) The electric speaking practice. Can Fam Phys 20:69
4. Nickerson HJ, Biechler L, Witte F (1975) How dependable is diagnosis and management of earache by telephone? Clin Pediatr 14:920–924
5. Hall DW (1976) The off-duty arrangements of general practitioners in four European countries. J Coll Gen Pract 26:19
6. Perrin EC, Goodman HC (1978) Telephone management of acute pediatric illness. N Engl J Med 298:130–135
7. Rosenblatt RA (1978) On-call in a family practice residency: Implications for patient care and residency training. J Fam Pract 6:327–331
8. Hoffman BD, Merritt K (1978) Analysis of after-hours calls and visits in a family practice. J Fam Pract 7:1185
9. Heagerty MC (1978) From home calls to telephone calls. Am J Public Health 1:14
10. Katz HP, Pozen J, Mushun AJ (1978) Quality assessment of a telephone care system utilizing non-physician personnel. Am J Public Health 1:31
11. Curtis P, Talbot AA (1979) The after-hours call in family practice. J Fam Pract 9:901–909
12. Spencer DC, Daugird AJ (1981) After hours health care in family practice. Fam Med 8:7–10
13. Brown SB, Eberle BJ (1974) Use of the telephone by pediatric house staff: A technique for pediatric care not taught. J Pediatr 84:117
14. Talbot AA, Mangum JR (1980) The structure of physician response to the after hours call in a family practice residency program. Fam Med Rev 1:72–90

15. Mayer TR, Solberg L, Seifert M, Cole P (1983) After-hours telephone calls in private family practice. J Fam Pract 2:327–332
16. Curtis P, Talbot AA (1980) After-hours calls: A forgotten item of education in family practice. Med Teach 2:245–247
17. Curtis P, Talbot AA (1980) After-hours call: An aspect of primary care education. J Med Educ 55:55–57
18. Curtis P, Talbot AA (1981) The telephone in primary care. J Comm Health 6:194–203
19. International classification of health problems in primary care, Version 2. Oxford University Press, New York
20. Blalock HM (1972) Multiple and partial correlation. In: Blalock HM (ed) Social statistics, 2nd edn. McGraw-Hill, New York
21. Boyle RP (1970) Path analysis and ordinal data. Am J Soc 75:461–480
22. Lyons M (1971) Techniques for using ordinal measures in regression and path analysis. In: Costner HL (ed) Sociological methodology. Jossey-Bass, San Francisco
23. Goodman LA (1972) A modified multiple regression approach to the analysis of dichotomous variables. Am Sociol Rev 37:28–46
24. de Sola Pool I (ed) (1981) The social impact of the telephone. MIT Press, Cambridge, MA
25. Evens S, Baer C, Smart A, Berolzheimer N (with Slatt L, Curtis P) (1982) Telephone skills for medical office personnel. Health Sciences Consortium, Chapel Hill, NC

Family Counselling Services in the Veneto Region of Italy: Structural and Functional Aspects

F. Fontana and A. Orsini

Objective and Methods

The objective of this study was to assess through an ad hoc survey, the situation of family counselling services (FCS) in the Veneto region a few years after their institution. Data about (a) organizational aspects of FCSs and (b) the numbers, qualifications and professional functions of the staff members were collected by questionnaires. On the other hand, data on the demands of the population and the job descriptions of the staff's activities were the result of several workshops directly involving the manpower of FCSs.

General Picture

Family counselling services were instituted by a State law in 1975 as an initial step in the health care system reform that was comprehensively carried out in 1978 by an act of Parliament (law no. 833) laying the foundation of the National Health Service (NHS).

The NHS is organized at three main levels:

- *National level,* with legislative and general planning tasks.
- *Regional level.* At this level there is the implementation of the national laws, planning and administrative control of the local health units (LHUs) within the regional area.
- *Local level.* Management of services and provision of care are carried out at this level through the LHUs. The population covered by each LHU ranges from 50 000 to 200 000.

FCSs act within the LHU and are a component of the primary health care system, aiming to achieve the integration between social and medical aspects, with particular emphasis on prevention. The Veneto region, with a population of 4 351 313 and an area of 18 378 km² is divided into 35 LHUs.

Primary Health Care in the Making
Ed. by U. Laaser, R. Senault, H. Viefhues

Structural Organization

In the whole region there are 101 FCSs, 91 of which are directly administered by LHUs. Private FCSs are officially recognized by regional administration only if they satisfy specific standards.

The catchment area of each FCS includes 5000 – 100 000 people (45 000 on average).

FCS Staffing

FCS is an autonomous working unit whose staff includes at least a psychologist, a gynaecologist and a social worker. When the need arises, the staff may include other health workers such as: nurses, midwives, educational advisers and legal advisers.

An innovative concept has been introduced into FCS work, i.e. the individual cases are dealt with by the whole staff working as a team so that the care and the operational guidelines are divided amongst the different specialists.

The activities of the FCSs are planned according to the guidelines laid down by a steering committee of the LHU. The practical work is mainly concerned with psychological, pedagogic, social and legal advice and assistance, referring to personal and interpersonal problems arising from family and pregnancy. Furthermore, antenatal care is also provided and advice offered on contraception and problems associated with sexuality and sterility. In this context, genetic counselling is given in order to prevent hereditary diseases and to ensure early diagnosis of pregnancies at risk. Birth control advice and assistance in the termination of unwanted pregnancies are also part of the activities of the FCSs. Information and education through the diffusion of scientific and psychosocial information on sexuality, pregnancy and family problems in general are also functions carried out by the FCS's team. In addition, FCS staff deal with problems of minors (e.g. adoption, marriage of minors) in co-operation with legal bodies collecting and furnishing information on families and their social background. Furthermore, the FCS staffs are expected to improve their professional knowledge, skills and attitudes through update activities and continuing education.

Depending on the case concerned, the team may co-operate with other services, directly working with them or sending the patient(s) to them. Table 1 shows the different possibilities of co-operation between FCS and other services.

The total number of professionals working at FCSs in the Veneto region is 456, 368 of whom work in public services and 88 in private ones. The job description of each member of the staff, made up from the list of their specific functions, can be summarized as follows:

Psychologist:
- Provision of information
- Health education
- Counselling

Table 1. Possibilities of co-operation between FCSs and other services

Services \ Demands	Family planning	Sterilization	Antenatal classes	Care in pregnancy	Advice for parents of newborn children	Puberty	Adolescence	Menopausal problems	Male menopause	Problems of the elderly	Diseases of the urino-genital tract	Prevention of breast and uterus cancers	Adoption
Family counselling services	+	+	+	+		+	+	+	+		+	+	+
General practitioner	+	+	+	+		+	+	+	+	+	+	+	
Paediatrician					+								
Worker in the health district						+	+			+			
Polyclinic	+	+		+	+	+		+	+		+	+	
Hospital		+	+	+	+			+			+	+	
Mental health services													
Drug addiction services													
Occupational med. services													
Public health services													
Health education office													
Mother and child health services					+								
Voluntary organizations										+			
Regional specialist services											+		
Local authority										+			
Provinces													
Courts													+
Schools						+							
Parishes													
Trade unions													
Job centre													

							+								+	+			+	+	Sexual problems
							+								+	+			+	+	Genetic counselling
															+	+			+	+	Abortion
																	+			+	Personal problems of couples
																	+			+	Problems between parents and children
				+		+		+	+								+	+		+	Problems of young people and minors
			+						+					+			+	+	+	+	Developmental problems
				+		+								+			+			+	Juvenile delinquency
																			+	+	Problems related to hysterectomy and mastectomy
				+																+	Separation and divorce
																	+			+	Legal advice on employment and the family
		+				+											+			+	Unmarried mothers
		+																		+	Preparation for marriage
+	+																				Unemployment counselling
						+															Housing problems
+						+															Economic support
			+																+	+	Sexual education
			+						+								+			+	Information and advice on pedagogic aspects
								+									+			+	Difficulties of socialization and communication

	–	Psychological intervention
	–	Programming of the activities of FCS
Gynaecologist:	–	Provision of information
	–	Health education
	–	Counselling
	–	Treatment
Social worker:	–	Provision of information
	–	Health education
	–	Promotion of the FCS activities
	–	Contacts with other services on the territory
	–	Co-operation with legal bodies
	–	Co-ordination among the members of the staff
Nurse:	–	Provision of information[1]
	–	Health education[1]
	–	Supporting the gynaecologist
Midwife:	–	Provision of information
	–	Health education
	–	Counselling
	–	Assistance of pregnant women

Demands of the Users on the FCS

The most frequently expressed needs are listed in Table 2. They are divided into different categories, according to their characteristics. It has to be stressed that several needs brought to the FCS are outside its institutional framework; some of these cases are nevertheless taken on. Examples of such demands are: requests for flats and jobs, help in cases of drug addiction, financial support, psychological support for physically and mentally handicapped people and care for the elderly.

Conclusion

The most relevant feature of the FCS is its comprehensive nature: the need to approach family problems in a multidisciplinary way is clearly seen; thus the contribution of professionals on the staff with different cultural backgrounds makes it possible to solve problems that are not considered as simply medical, or psychological or social. It has to be underlined that these services have been planned mostly for preventive purposes.

---

[1] Especially on knowledge of the human body, contraception, pregnancy and childbirth, diet in pregnancy etc.

Table 2. The needs expressed most frequently to the FCSs

Biological needs	Psychological needs	Sociocultural needs	Economic needs	Educational needs
Family planning	Problems of couples	Adoption of children	Economic support in cases of separation	Sex education
Care of pregnant women and puerperas	Problems between parents and children	Problems of living together	Requests for abortion due to economic needs	Family planning
Menopause problems	Psychological care for sexual problems	Difficulties of inter-personal relationships		Relationships between parents and children
Genetic counselling	Psychological care for abortion	Support of socialization and development in childhood		Health education
Documents requested for abortion	Psychological care in pregnancy	Separation and divorce		Information and advice on educational aspects
Prevention of cancer of the breast and genital organs	Family planning	Unmarried mothers		Assignment of children to other relatives
Information and treatment for sexual problems	Adaption of children	Sexuality		Prevention of cancer of the breast and genital organs
Treatment of diseases of male genital organs	Male and female meno-pausal problems	Family planning		
Antenatal care	Genetic problems	Antenatal care		
Problems of puberty and adolescence	Antenatal classes	Abortion		
The male menopause	Psychological problems of puerperium	Puberty		
	Pubertal problems	Problems linked to the presence of old people in families		
	Developmental problems	Social problems related to mastectomy, hyster-ectomy and sterilization		
	Abnormal behaviour of adolescents	Legal advice on family and working mothers' rights		
	Difficulties of sociali-zation and communi-cation	Social support for families in cases of juvenile delin-quency		
	Psychological problems related to mastectomy, hysterectomy and sterili-zation	Menopause		

References

1. Busnelli E (1979) Identità professionale ed equipe interdisciplinare. UI Congresso Naz. Ucipem, Salsomaggiore
2. Donati P (1981) Consultorio familiare, salute e sistema socio-sanitario: quale prevenzione? VII Congresso Naz. Ucipem, Senigallia
3. Paccagnella B (1979) Il consultorio familiare come servizio inserito nella comunità locale. VI Congresso Naz. Ucipem, Salsomaggiore
4. Saraceno C (1980) Modelli di famiglia; da: Ritratto di famiglia degli anni '80. Laterza, Bari Rome
5. Legge Nazionale 23 December 1978 no 833 "Istituzione del Servizio Sanitario Nazionale"
6. Legge Nazionale 29 July 1975 no 405 "Istituzione dei Consultori Familiari"
7. Legge Regionale Veneta 25 March 1977 no 28 "Disciplina dei Consultori Familiari"
8. Legge Regionale Veneta 7 March 1980 no 13 "Organizzazione dell'Unità Sanitaria Locale"
9. Legge Nazionale 22 May 1978 no 194 "Norme per la tutela sociale della maternità e sull'interruzione volontaria della gravidanza"
10. Circolare Regionale Veneta 15 June 1977 no 37

Health Counselling – A Pilot Programme

C. Brühne-Scharlau and F. W. Schwartz

Health counselling by practising physicians is a pilot programme for preventive counselling. It is directed to persons who are still healthy but may be exposing themselves to risk factors such as smoking, overweight, lack of physical exercise and stress. Target groups are 30- to 50 year-old insurees covered by any of six sickness funds. They are chosen by random sampling and invited to participate by their insurance company. This pilot programme began in February 1982 and lasted until June 1983. The regions studied are covered by two State Associations of Doctors Admitted to Health Insurance Practice (Kassenärztliche Vereinigungen): Hamburg, a city district, and Pfalz, a rural district.

The pilot programme was designed to meet the need for individual preventive care. The motto of the programme is 'Help people to help themselves'. Three gratis preventive consultations are offered.

Practising physicians primarily are not responsible for patients who are not yet ill. Under the law, health insurance covers only therapeutic services. Until now the only exceptions have been for prenatal care, child preventive health care and cancer check-ups. Thus our pilot programme for the first time allows physicians to charge for extensive preventive counselling at contractually established rates.

The first of the three health counselling consultations consists of a medical history, a physical examination (without ECG and extensive laboratory testing) and a very thorough interview about behaviour which endangers health. The emphasis in the doctor–patient discussion following the interview is placed on realistic changes which could be made in everyday life in the most direct manner possible. The basic consideration is that general advice like "don't smoke so much" or "do get more exercise" is not very successful. The problem is not what to do but how to do it. Therefore the physicians support their patients in finding possible areas for change in everyday life.

Most initial consultations last for an hour or even more. At the end of the session the doctor and patient fix a date for the next health counselling session – if there are risk factors and the patient is interested in continuing the consultation. The results of the counselling session are recorded in a booklet received by the insuree. A copy (without the patient's name, of course) is used for the evaluation.

External support is possible: If it becomes evident in the course of the consultation that the patient needs and asks for extra support beyond the health

Primary Health Care in the Making
Ed. by U. Laaser, R. Senault, H. Viefhues

counselling, the doctor can refer the patient to local bodies which organize weight reduction courses, jogging groups, anti-smoking seminars, relaxation training etc. We have encouraged local bodies to offer appropriate courses. Physicians are kept informed about the local availability of such support programmes.

Our pilot programme is not an epidemiological experimental study but rather an open field study and feasibility study. Although scientific evaluation has not been completed we can roughly answer the following questions:

1. Do physicians accept the supplemental educational programme and the underlying concept of health counselling?
2. Are the insurees interested in the offer of health counselling?
3. Is health counselling feasible under the given conditions?

With regard to the first question: In both regions 170 general practitioners and internists took part (the number was limited). They were obliged to undergo an initial supplemental education programme on health counselling methods. The evaluation of the questionnaires showed that the majority of the participating physicians accepted the programme as a whole.

One of the main effects within the doctors' learning process was a somewhat modified appreciation of the physicians' role: one which helps the patient take advantage of opportunities to help himself. The health counselling plan allows the physicians to take considerable time for the consultation and accordingly corresponds better to the classical image of the physician and to a more intensive doctor–patient relationship. It is worth mentioning that one side-effect reveals the influence of the programme: in the course of the training 27% of the physicians reduced their own risk factors.

As to the second question: The interest shown by insurees in this new oppurtunity has been promising: The participation rate for the first health counselling session remains at about 20%. Until now about 10 000 insurees have participated. About half of them fixed a date for a second counselling session. For those who did not continue, three reasons are documented: about half of them do not have any risk factor; 9% are not entitled to participate because of a chronic illness; 13% do not have any further interest.

Thus, keeping in mind the third question ("Is health counselling feasible?"), the results promise a positive answer as to the acceptability of the programme to both the insurees and the physicians. Nevertheless, the various single factors have to be isolated and focussed concerning their transferability.

So, although the answers to the above questions tend to be affirmative, the answer to the main question remains: "Did the insurees change their behaviour towards a more healthy life-style because of the health counselling?" i.e. whether the health counselling will be effective in the long run. Hence, the scientific study will have to determine the type as well as the duration of modifications in behaviour. For this purpose, questionnaires have been sent out and personal interviews conducted. The evaluation of these data is in progress, and results will be available later this year.

References

1. Bengel J, Koch U (1983) Erwartungen und Erfahrungen der an der Fortbildung teilnehmenden Ärzte. Freiburg
2. Breslow L, Enstrom JE (1980) Persistence of health habits and their relationship to mortality. Prev Med 9:469–483
3. Brühne C, Heuser MR, Koch H (1983) Erster Zwischenbericht zum Modellversuch 'Gesundheitsberatung durch Ärzte'. Hamburger Ärztebl 11:381–383
4. Department of Health and Social Security (1982) Prevention and health: avoiding heart attacks. London
5. Ettlinger PRA, Freeman GK (1981) General practice compliance study: is it worth being a personal doctor? Br Med J 282:1192–1194
6. Fischer N (1983) Ärztliche Gesundheitsberatung als Hilfe zur Selbsthilfe. In: Bundesvereinigung für Gesundheitserziehung (ed) Gesundheit für alle – Aufgabe für jeden. Bonn, pp 173–177
7. Harris DM, Guten S (1979) Health-protective behavior: an exploratory study. J Health Soc Behav 20:17–29
8. Hochbaum GM (1971) Measurements of effectiveness of health education activities. J Health Educ 14:54–59
9. Russel MHH, et al. (1979) Effect of general practitioners advice against smoking. Br Med J 2:231–235
10. Schwartz FW (1980) Prävention im System der gesetzlichen Krankenversicherung. Thesen und Empfehlungen. Zentralinstitut für die kassenärztliche Versorgung, Cologne (Wissenschaftliche Reihe, vol 19)
11. Steptoe A (1981) Psychological factors in cardiovascular disorders. London
12. Wissenschaftliches Institut der Ortskrankenkassen (ed) (1979) Gesundheitspolitisch relevante Herz- und Kreislauferkrankungen. WIdO, Bonn (WIdO-Materialien, vol 7)
13. Zentralinstitut für die kassenärztliche Versorgung (ed) (1977) Herz-Kreislauf-Vorsorgeprogramme in der Bundesrepublik Deutschland. ZI, Cologne (Tagungsberichte, vol 1)
14. Zielke M, Brühne C (1983) Ergebnisse und Schlußfolgerungen aus den Kursleiter-Interviews zum Fortbildungsprogramm. ZI-Berichte, Cologne

Primary Prevention by the General Practitioner?

G. Wendt

Frequently, prevention is considered to be the sole responsibility of physicians; as a matter of fact, all problems related to health or sickness are more or less thoughtlessly passed on to the doctor. This procedure is problematic in the Federal Republic of Germany because little practical experience in the field of prevention is available there. Remarkable exceptions are the model of Community Prevention at Eberbach/Wiesloch and the pilot study "Health Advice and Health Promotion" under the auspices of the AOK (General Local Sickness Insurance Scheme) in the district of Mettmann. As these studies represent the experience of several years, only the most important results will be summed up here.

Considering the fact that the prevention of modern diseases caused by civilization makes intervention in the everyday life of the population necessary, measures taken in Eberbach and Wiesloch aim "at the free initiative of the population – supported by the community administration – in using the conditions provided at their place of residence to promote health and prevent diseases" [7, p. 81].

If a doctor wishes to become active in the field of primary prevention he leaves – metaphorically speaking – his practice. In the latest publication of the initiators of the model Community Prevention, the expectation is expressed that the conventional roles of doctor and patient should be changed, and the following example is given: "The physicians who generally used to wait for their patients or to be called by them must change their position in the case of the prevention of cardiovascular disease." So-called *established communities*, e.g. "kindergarten, schools, factories and associations" are named as venues for activities in the field of primary prevention [2, p. 81]. *The local working groups for preventive health care within communities* – clearing offices for eventual activities – are composed mainly of lay personnel; physicians are included only as advisors [2, p. 82].

Although this model does not include the general practice as a suitable venue for primary preventive activities, health advice (e.g. as a part of primary prevention) has been given at the general practitioner's office in various models of health insurance – with doubtful results, as we now know. Less than 50% of the physicians invited and only 3.6% of the patients entitled participated in the pilot study *Health Advice and Health Promotion* [8, pp. 4–7].

Primary Health Care in the Making
Ed. by U. Laaser, R. Senault, H. Viefhues

The question must be raised as to whether a general medical practice, with its typical, hard to modify general conditions, is the right place for preventive activities. Instead of giving ready answers, some results of research will be presented.

Frequency in Making Use of Medical Services

Contacts with physicians are episodic, frequent and continuous visits occurring only as a consequence of continued illness and old age. A large number of people – greatly underestimated – *never or hardly ever visit a doctor.* In case of an inquiry by Infratest, 15% of the adult inhabitants of the Federal Republic of Germany stated that they had not visited a doctor for more than a year (Infratest 1979, Das Ärztebild in der Gesellschaft, unpublished manuscript). Among young people – the age group mainly addressed by preventive measures – an even higher percentage must be assumed. Just recently, these facts have been confirmed by an extensive inquire [5, p. 159].

Time Available

The normal (meaning frequent) consultation of a physician *leaves* – even in the presence of good-will – *no time* for primary prevention by the doctor. An average consultation time of 5.7 min is mentioned in the literature [3, p. 18]. It may be doubted whether the routine of a general medical practice, directed at diagnosis and therapy, represents a suitable framework for health education. Primary prevention by physicians on the whole could take place only rarely. Actually each patient has little time to communicate with the physician (Table 1), so that there are few chances to discuss the risk situations at work, within the home and in neighbourhood [1].

Table 1. Length of conversation during consultations with general practitioners [1]

Conversation between doctor and patient in a general practice	First consultation	Advice given to chronic patients
Average length of diagnosis-oriented part of conversation	3.2 min	0.5 min
Average length of the part of conversation dominated by patient	0.8 min	0.1 min
Average length of the part of conversation dominated by doctor	2.4 min	0.4 min
Number of patients	$n=78$	$n=92$

Consequences of Deficiencies of the Medical Service

One further problem is the diverse density of medical practices in cities and urban districts. We can say that in rural districts, outskirts of cities and workers' quarters we find fewer physicians, so the inhabitants have to accept long periods of waiting and shorter consultations [10]. This brings about discrimination against exactly those social groups which – as is known from various inquiries – show a certain reserve towards all preventive measures as a consequence of their working and living conditions. With reference to the so-called preventive health checks, a medical service paid by health insurance schemes, it has been proved for some time that: "Only 30% to 40% of the population regularly make use of this offer and that members of the upper and middle class do so significantly more often than members of the lower classes" [9, p. 116]. Preventive measures taken by physicians therefore would result, willy-nilly, in social selection and would be a serious disadvantage for a population especially endangered with regard to health.

Language of the Physician – Language of the Patient

In concluding I would like to point to the results of research in a largely unknown branch of science, sociolinguistics, which might be relevant in this connection. Exactly analysing communications pertaining to diagnosis and therapy, Ferber [4] discovered that the use of a *different idiomatic language* greatly impedes the conversation of the physician and patient with regard to finding ways together of changing unhealthy living conditions and behaviour (Table 2). Health education and information serving primary prevention aimed at the elimination of unhealthy living conditions should, therefore, rather be undertaken by lay persons belonging to the same social sphere, i.e. colleagues.

Altogether, judging from the cited results of research, primary prevention by *general practitioners at their office* should be looked upon rather sceptically. On the other hand, the recently established *Working Groups for Health Education* [6] and the *Community Health Panels* initiated by the German Cardiovascular Prevention Study (Deutsche Herz-Kreislauf-Präventionsstudie 1983), both of which include the engaged co-operation of physicians, would seem to

Table 2. Idiomatic differences in the language used by patients, general practitioners and clinicians [4]

The socially idiomatic language of the		
... patient	... general practitioner	... clinician
is modelled by his		
... environment	... therapeutic community	... scientific community
and therefore is		
... experience-oriented	... action-oriented	... science-oriented

offer great promise in achieving results in this so important field. A condition for their success, however, is that they succeed in obtaining the necessary cooperation of physicians and interested lay persons.

References

1. Ahrens S (1976) Erste Ergebnisse einer Untersuchung über die Arzt-Patient-Interaktion in der Allgemeinpraxis – Teil I und Teil II. Prakt Arzt 3/4:403–410, 703–709
2. Buchholz L, et al. (1983) Interventive Erfahrungen im Eberbach-Wiesloch-Projekt. In: Nüssel E, Lamm G (eds) Prävention im Gemeinderahmen. Zuckschwerdt, Munich Bern Vienna
3. Eberlein R (1974) Der Zeitbedarf in der ärztlichen Allgemeinpraxis. In: Brandlmeier P (ed) Die Allgemeinpraxis. Springer, Berlin Heidelberg New York
4. Ferber L von (1979) Sozialdialekte in der Medizin – Das Sprachverhalten von Laien, Praktikern und Wissenschaftlern. In: Böhme G, Engelhard M von (eds) Entfremdete Wissenschaft. Suhrkamp, Frankfurt
5. Gesellschaft für Strahlen- und Umweltforschung (ed) (1983) Jahresbericht 1982. Munich
6. Ministerium für Arbeit, Gesundheit und Sozialordnung (1982) Erlaß vom 30. August 1982
7. Nüssel E (1981) Ärztliche Aufgaben in der Prävention. In: Troschke J von, Stößel U (eds) Möglichkeiten und Grenzen ärztlicher Gesundheitsberatung. Gesomed, Freiburg
8. Rege J, Burkhardt T, Modellversuch "Gesundheitsberatung und Gesundheitsförderung": Erste Ergebnisse. Munich (IFT-Berichte, vol 25)
9. Schmädel D (1975) Schichtenspezifische Unterschiede im Gesundheits- und Krankheitsverhalten der Bevölkerung der Bundesrepublik Deutschland. In: Ritter-Röhr D (ed) Der Arzt, sein Patient und die Gesellschaft. Suhrkamp, Frankfurt
10. Wendt G (1983) Disparitäten der ärztlichen Versorgung in Großstädten der BRD. Medical dissertation, University of Göttingen

Medical and Psychosocial Problems in Primary Care *

H. Noack

Questions and Methods

This contribution addresses two questions: (1) What views do primary care doctors hold about the health problems of their patients. (2) To what extent do these views correspond with the diagnostic classifications they apply to the problems presented by their patients. Preliminary answers were sought within the context of a study which investigated the reasons of adult patients for seeking primary medical care, and of their expectations of it [H. J. Schaufelberger, B. Cloetta, H. Noack, U. Berner, S. Altbisser (1983) Der Patient in der ambulanten ärztlichen Versorgung, unpublished research report]. This study was undertaken in a medical out-patient department and in the private practices of ten internists and nine general practitioners. Private practitioners had been selected on the basis of a mail questionnaire sent to all internists and general practitioners in a particular urban area in the German-speaking part of Switzerland.

Data collection included a 1-hour interview with 259 patients (40.3% in the out-patient department, 33.2% in the internists' and 26.6% in the general practitioners' offices). Doctors were asked to record for each of these patients, among other things, the reason for visiting a doctor and his diagnosis or classification of the problem presented, using a patient record form derived from the form employed in the U.S. Ambulatory Medical Survey [2]. Finally, a semi-standardised interview was conducted with 26 of the 30 doctors participating in the study (11 junior physicians in the out-patient department, nine internists and six general practitioners). The results reported here were collected with the patient record form and the semi-standardised interviews of doctors. Suitable categories of medical and non-medical problems were developed in a content analysis of the interview protocols.

* Supported by Schweizerischer Nationalfonds, Nationales Forschungsprogramm Nr. 8, Gesuch Nr. 4.393-0.80.08 (Project directors: Prof. U. C. Dubach, Universität Basel; Prof. H. G. Pauli, Universität Bern)

Primary Health Care in the Making
Ed. by U. Laaser, R. Senault, H. Viefhues

Results

Reasons for Visit

In order to discuss the doctors' diagnoses or problem classifications as well as their views about the medical and non-medical problems of their patients in a somewhat broader context, the reasons for visiting a primary care institution were investigated. The most frequently registered reasons for visit were: symptoms of the musculoskeletal system, symptoms of the digestive system, general symptoms, symptoms of the respiratory system, symptoms of the nervous system (excluding sense organs) and a request for a medical examination and for preventive measures (Fig. 1, right side).

These results were compared with results obtained with very similar methods from far bigger samples in the U.S. and in the Federal Republic of Germany [5]. The distribution of symptoms found in the Swiss study tends to resemble the results of the West German study more closely than the results of the U.S. National Ambulatory Medical Survey (Fig. 1).

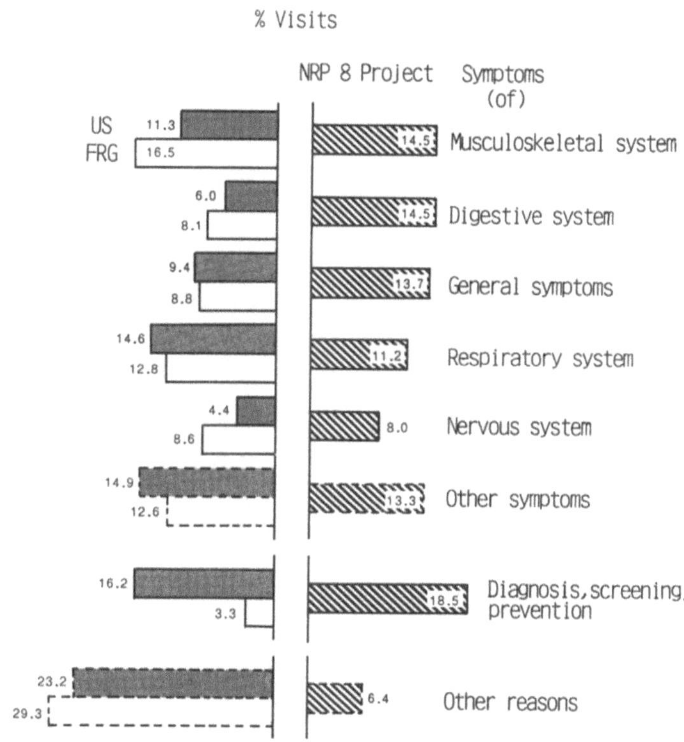

Fig. 1. Reasons for visit of primary care institutions in the Swiss NRP 8 Project ($n = 249$), in the U.S. Ambulatory Medical Survey ($n = 229\,919$) and in a survey in the Federal Republic of Germany ($n = 13\,488$)

Diagnoses and Other Problem Classifications

The most frequently recorded principal or main diagnoses and problem classification were: diseases or disorders of the musculoskeletal system and connective tissues, of the circulatory system, the respiratory system, the digestive system, symptoms and ill-defined conditions, mental and psychological disorders and endocrine, nutritional and metabolic diseases (Fig. 2, right side). Except for mental and psychological disorders and for diseases of the circulatory system, the rank order of these diagnostic classifications corresponds to the rank order of the reasons for visit described previously.

Because of the well-known phenomenon of multiple morbidity in primary care [4], principal diagnoses do, however, provide an incomplete picture. Thus, the mean of the number of diagnoses or problem classifications recorded by the doctors in this study was 2.3. If all diagnoses and problem classifications are taken into account (Fig. 2, left side) psychological or mental disorders, diseases of the circulatory system and endocrine, nutritional and metabolic disorders tend to be more frequent.

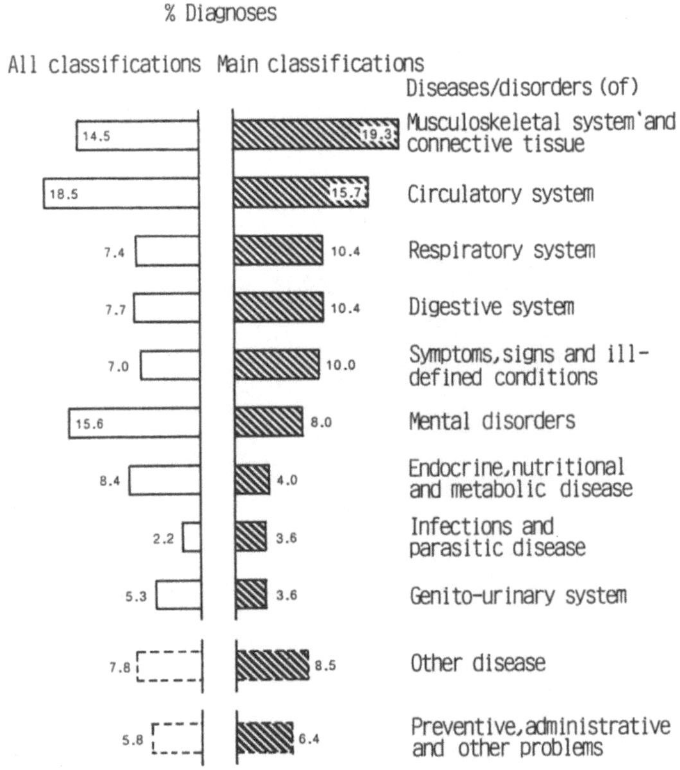

Fig. 2. Diagnostic classifications in primary care ($n = 249$ patients) according to the International Classification of Health Problems in Primary Care [6]

Frequently Reported Medical and Psychosocial Problems

In order to give a preliminary account of the doctors' views of their patients' health problems, they were asked in the final interview: "When you consider the diseases, complaints or requests of your patients, which of these have been particularly frequent in your own practice/in the out-patient department?" As shown in Table 1, over three-quarters of the doctors reported psychosomatic diseases or symptoms as frequently perceived health problems in primary care; two-thirds reported problems referable to the circulatory system; roughly two-fifths reported generalized or specific pain, and psychological or mental problems; and close to one-third reported complaints referable to the digestive system. In one of the doctor's own words: "These are psychosomatic complaints or disturbances of function. ... It can be multiple somatic complaints or symptoms referable to an organ which are related to some psychosocial conflict. On the whole I would say: approximately 50% to 70% are psychosomatic disorders. ... What I have in mind frequently are, for example, heart pain or heart complaints; ... in women frequently an abnormal feeling in the genitourinary region, and these women may have a specific history, for instance, of hysterectomy. ... Perhaps in males disturbances of the musculoskeletal system are more frequent; ... and abdominal disturbances, including irritability of the colon, certainly are the most frequent complaints, and – in addition – headache" (0105).

Frequently Reported Non-medical Problems

Another related question on the physician interview was: "Quite often one can read or is told that some patients seeking medical help do in fact suffer from a problem or request help of a non-medical nature. ... Could you estimate the proportion of such patients (in your own practice/in the out-patient department)?" Of the 21 doctors who replied to this question, ten felt that the proportion of such non-medical problems tended to be rather small (not big, smaller than 30%) and eight felt that it was rather big (largest part, bigger than 30%), whereas three seemed to find the delineation of medical problems implied by this question difficult.

All doctors were asked a further question: "What sort of non-medical problems do you have in mind, for example?" About two-thirds of the doctors interviewed mentioned problems of social relationships in the marriage or family, roughly one-half reported problems related to job or occupation, over two-fifths psychosomatic disorders and almost one-third psychological problems and social conflicts or psychosocial strain (Table 2). To quote two of the doctors interviewed: "Yes, very frequently problems of social relations ... within the family. Furthermore, excessive demands of the job; to use a rather worn-out expression: the stress of the work-place ..., a feeling of insufficiency in private as well as in professional life ..." (0200) "... Then there are these various stresses and pressures from outside: financial as well as status problems. ... There are also many people who simply want some advice as to what they should do; for example, whether they should enter further education or training ..." (5900).

Table 1. Frequently reported medical problems

Type of problem	Number of doctors[a]
1. Psychosomatic diseases or symptoms, including those accompanying somatic illness; disturbance of body functions such as nervous heart condition or nervous stomach	20
2. Diseases of or symptoms referable to cardiovascular system, e.g. abnormal heartbeat, status following ischaemic heart disease, hypertension	18
3. Generalized pain and pain referable to a specific body system such as headache, chest pain, abdominal pain	11
4. Psychological or mental disorders or symptoms, e.g. depression, anxiety, nervousness, insomnia	10
5. Disease of or symptoms referable to the digestive system, e.g. diarrhoea, constipation or irritable bowel syndrome	8
6. Endocrine and metabolic disorders or symptoms referable to such conditions, e.g. diabetes, hyperthyroidism, overweight	6
7. Upper respiratory infection, flu, common cold, cough, bronchitis	6
8. Rheumatic disorders such as arthritis, arthrosis or symptoms referable to rheumatism	4
– All other diseases or symptoms referable to other body systems, e.g. general symptoms such as tiredness, exhaustion	16
– Request for check-up, medical examination or health certificate; concern about health or symptoms	11

[a] Of 26 doctors replying to the interview question (11 junior doctors in medical out-patient department, 9 internists, 6 general practitioners)

Table 2. Frequently reported non-medical problems

Type of problem/comment	Number of doctors[a]
1. Marriage problem, conflict with partner or within family, including educational problems with children or school problems	17
2. Occupational or job problem including conflicts with collaborators, work pressure or strain, unemployment	13
3. Psychosomatic diseases or symptoms including complaints or disturbance of body functions referable to sustained tension	11
4. Psychological or psychiatric problem such as anxiety, depression, death and dying; problems related to self-concept, drug use	8
5. Social conflict or psychosocial strain, e.g. those referable to social environment of neighbourhood, housing, social status, income	8
– Other non-medical problems referable to daily life, personal development, education and training, health certificate	10
– Each of these problems also reflects a medical problem; however not in a traditional sense	9
– Medical and non-medical or psychosocial problems are interdependent and cannot be seperated from each other	6

[a] Of 25 doctors replying to the interview question (11 junior doctors in medical out-patient department, 8 internists, 6 general practitioners)

Overall, 23 of the 25 doctors who replied to this question reported psychosocial and social problems and 16 out of 25 referred to psychosomatic and psychological problems. The junior doctors of the medical out-patient department did not differ from their almost 20-year-older colleagues in private practice with regard to the frequency of reporting either psychosocial and social or psychosomatic and psychological problems. Most doctors interviewed seemed to consider a delineation of medical and non-medical problems difficult if not meaningless.

Conclusions

The exploratory nature of this study permits only tentative answers to the questions stated at the beginning of this paper: (1) Doctors in different primary care institutions tend to interpret a larger proportion of the problems presented by their patients as psychosomatic and psychosocial problems, in addition to or along with common disorders of the major organ systems. Although primary care doctors may differ with regard to more specific aspects, many of them seem to explain the nature and the conditions of ill-health from a holistic point of view. (2) The patients' problems most frequently perceived by primary care doctors seem to resemble their diagnoses and other problem classifications only to some extent. Thus, epidemiological studies based upon clinical classifications of diseases, even classifications attempting to take the specific aspects of primary care into account [6], are likely to provide an incomplete picture of primary care morbidity.

The results reported in this paper can be discussed in the context of empirical studies of primary care in the U.K. and the U.S. [1, 3]. These studies revealed that primary care doctors differ in their views or opinions as to whether psychosocial and psychosomatic disturbances represent trivialities not worth presenting to a doctor, or rather legitimate medical problems.

References

1. Cartwright A (1967) Patients and their doctors. Routledge and Kegan Paul, London
2. Ezzati T, McLemore T (1980) The National Ambulatory Medical Survey. 1977 Summary. National Center for Health Statistics. US Department of Health, Education, and Welfare, US Government Printing Office, Washington, DC
3. Mechanic D (1978) Medical sociology. Free Press, New York, pp 389–400
4. Moehr JR, Haehn KD (eds) (1977) Verdenstudie – Strukturanalyse allgemeinmedizinischer Praxen. Deutscher Aerzteverlag, Köln-Lövenich
5. Schach E, Brecht JG, Schwartz F-W (1982) Ambulante medizinische Versorgung, Vergleich zwischen der Bundesrepublik und den USA. MMW 124:675–678
6. World Organization of National Colleges, Academies, and Academic Associations of General Practitioners/Family Physicians (WONCA) (1979) International classification of health problems in primary care, ICHPPC-2. Oxford University Press, Oxford New York Toronto

Mental Health Problems in the Offices of General Practitioners and Internists

H. E. Kerek-Bodden, P. Kramer, E. Schach, and F. W. Schwartz

Introduction: Methods and Data

The data presented constitute the first results of a survey among ambulatory care physicians in the Federal Republic of Germany (EVaS). The study was based on a sample of 969 ambulatory care physicians of almost every specialty. This physician group represents a 10% sample of doctors in an area representative of the Federal Republic of Germany with respect to variables such as distribution of physicians by specialty, population distribution by age and sex, and health insurance status. The response rate was 62%. The survey was conducted in the last 3 months of 1981 and the first 3 months of 1982. Analyses are based on office contacts by ambulatory care patients selected at random by physicians. The reporting period for physicians was 2 days.

The survey's main aim was to provide information on contacts by ambulatory care patients with their physicians or their offices by patient characteristics, reasons for contact, severity of morbidity as evaluated by patient and physician, services provided and disposition. Reasons for visit as indicated by patient and diagnoses assigned to the principal reason by the physician were coded with the Reason for Visit Classification, developed by the National Center of Health Statistics [3]. This classification scheme was transcribed into German [2] and substantially extended in the course of coding the data for this study.

Results

Contacts with General Practitioners and Internists by Patient Characteristics

This paper presents results about mental health-related patient contacts with general practitioners and internists.

The majority of contacts with general practitioners' offices are made by women (Fig. 1a). Out of 100 patient-physician contacts, 56 are by females and 44 by males. This discrepancy is even wider for internists. For this physician group we observe 61% of contacts by females and 39% of contacts by males (Fig. 1b). As expected, Fig. 1 shows that contact percentages for older persons

Primary Health Care in the Making
Ed. by U. Laaser, R. Senault, H. Viefhues

are higher than for the younger age groups. In particular, the contacts with persons beyond the age of 44 years of age are higher for internists (68.4% of total contacts) than for general practitioners (60.1% of total contacts). Furthermore, we observe great differences of contact percentages by health insurance status. While about 4% of contacts with general practitioners are by privately insured patients, this figure is about 8% for internists.

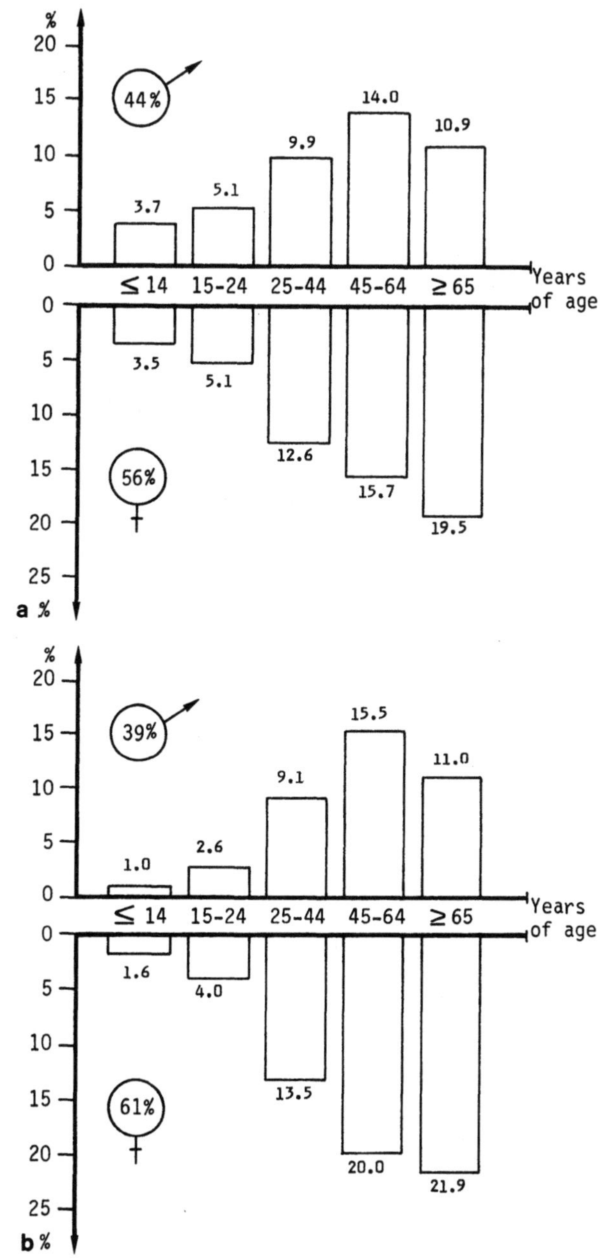

Fig. 1. **a** Contacts (in %) with general practitioners by sex and age. **b** Contacts (in %) with internists by sex and age

Mental Health Problems as Reasons for Contact

The definition of a mental health problem-related contact is as follows in terms of RVC categories: Symptoms referable to psychological or mental disorders (S100–S199), Diagnoses referable to mental disorders (D300–D349), General psychiatric or psychological examination (X130), Psychotherapy (T410), and Social problem counselling (T700–T799). About 3% of study contacts are associated with a mental health problem as the principal reason.

This order of magnitude holds true for general practitioners as well as for internists. If we take all reasons for contacts into consideration, we observe that at least one mental health reason is mentioned in 9% of contacts with general practitioners and in 8% of contacts with internists. Mental health problems by patients and physicians are mostly expressed as symptoms. While about 80% of patients' reasons are given in the form of symptoms, the corresponding physicians' statements are noted down as symptoms in 60% of the entries. This observation confirms the well-known fact that as regards reasons for patient–physician contacts in primary care related to mental health problems, a coding scheme such as the International Classification of Diseases (Der Bundesminister für Jugend, Familie und Gesundheit, 1979) is less suitable than a scheme designed to code reasons as given by the patient (e.g. the RVC).

Figure 2 compares total and mental health-related contacts with general practitioners and internists by age. As contact percentages add to 100 across age by contact category and within a physician group, we may compare the structure of total contacts and mental health-related contacts by age and physician group. Mental health-related contacts (mental health problem as principal reason) are rare for contacts by persons below the age of 15 years. Beyond that age mental health-related contact percentages increase with age approximately as total contact percentages increase. This holds true for general practitioners and internists with the exception of contacts for one age group: general practitioners report 31.6% of mental health-related contacts as being by persons aged 25–44 years, while only 22.5% of their total contacts are by persons in that age group. This difference requires further study.

Severity of Mental Health Problems as Assessed by Patients and Physicians

The severity of mental health-related contact reasons (mental health problem as principal reason) was reported by patients and physicians. This severity statement by the patient may be interpreted as an indicator of urgency. The corresponding physician's assessment is given after diagnosis, relates to the principal reason for contact given by the patient and describes the physician's evaluation of the need for treatment. Figure 3 shows mental health-related contacts with general practitioners and internists by severity as assigned by patients and physicians. As percentages add up to 100 across severity categories within patient and physician groups, we may compare contact percentages for physicians and patients for each physician group. Patients' assessment and

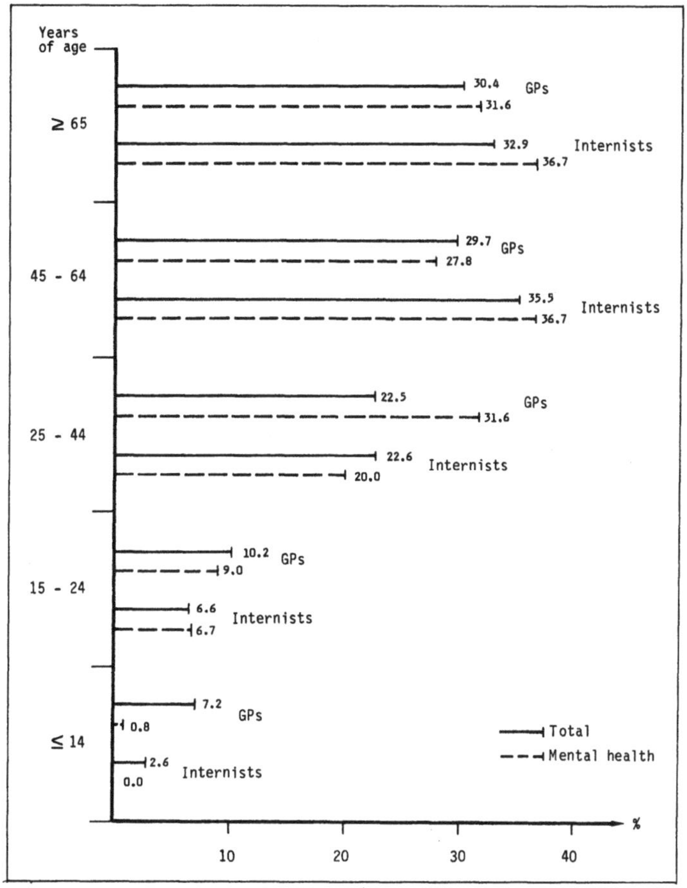

Fig. 2. Total contacts and contacts in which mental health problems are the principal reason for contact: contacts in per cent by age and physician group

physicians' assessment agree roughly, when they are compared across physician specialty. While physicians tend to classify between 39.8% (general practitioners) and 33.3% (internists) of mental health-related contacts with their offices as serious, patients do so for 51.5% (general practitioners) and 61% (internists) of contacts. In general, physicians tend to assign severity categories of a less serious nature to reasons for mental health-related contact than do patients.

Selected Services Provided for Mental Health-Related Contacts

In the framework of the study, services provided by physicians in ambulatory care are measured in broad categories only. Table 1 displays the most frequent services provided for contacts related to mental health problems. It shows that for both physician groups, prescription and medical counselling are the major

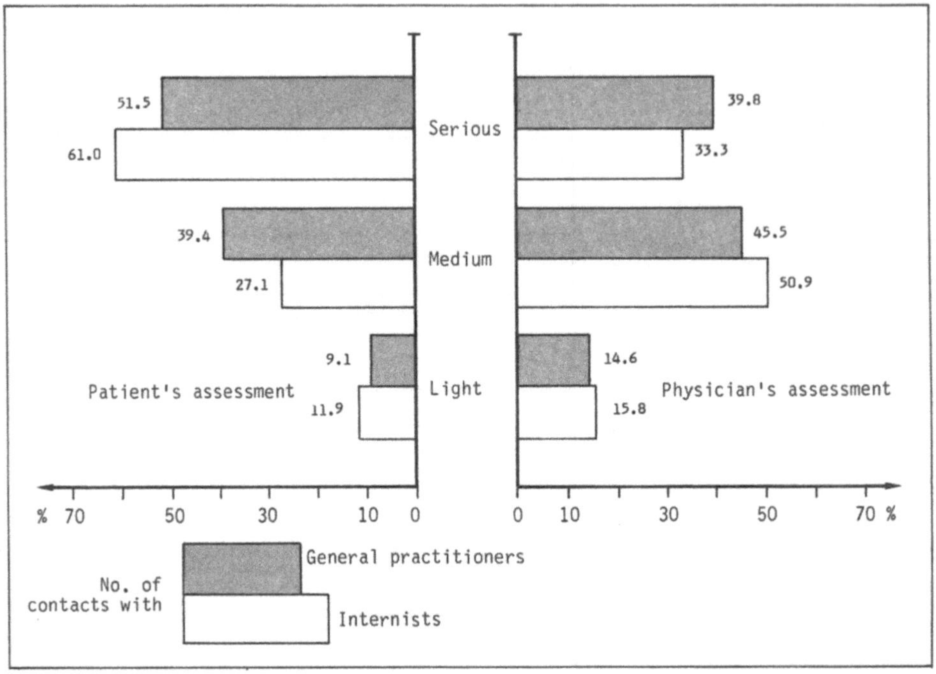

Fig. 3. Contacts (in %) by severity of mental health problem as assessed by patient and physician (contacts with mental health problem as principal reason for contact)

Table 1. Selected services provided per 100 contacts with a mental health problem as the principal reason for contact

Services provided[a]	General practitioner	Internist
Prescription	66	45
Medical counselling	62	48
Blood pressure check	43	39
Physical examination	29	31
History	20	32
Therapeutical listening	29	19
Psychotherapy	7	7

[a] Multiple services possible

therapeutic services provided to patients contacting for mental health-related reasons (principal reason). In particular, 66% of mental health-related contacts with general practitioners and 45% of such contacts with internists are associated with a prescription. A prescription only and no other services are provided for about 10% of contacts to each physician group. Medical counselling occurs in 62% of such contacts with general practitioners and in 48% of such contacts with internists. It should also be pointed out that about one-fifth or more of contacts with a mental health problem as the principal reason for contact are associated with therapeutic listening on the part of the physician. Psychotherapy occurs in 7% of such contacts for both physician groups.

Summary

The paper describes the mental health-related contacts with the offices of general practitioners and internists with respect to selected patient and contact characteristics. The percentage of contacts associated with a mental health problem as the principal reason are about 3% for both physician groups. This percentage is increased to 8% for internists and 9% for general practitioners when all contacts with at least one mental health reason are taken into consideration. This implies that three times more contacts are somehow associated with a mental health problem than contacts with a mental health problem as the principal reason for contact. The percentage of contacts with physicians is higher for the older age groups. This observation holds true for all contacts as well as for mental health-related contacts and for both physician groups. Patients and physicians frequently do not concur in their assessment of the degree of severity of the reason for contact, physicians tending to assign a less severe code to the same principal reason. The majority of mental health-related contacts are associated with prescriptions and/or medical counselling as the major forms of therapy. It turns out that general practitioners provide either or both of these services in more than 60% of their office contacts and internists in slightly less than 50% of their contacts. This may imply a difference in therapeutic procedure between the two physician groups which requires further scrutiny.

References

1. Der Bundesminister für Jugend, Familie und Gesundheit (ed) (1979) Handbuch der Internationalen Klassifikation der Krankheiten, Verletzungen und Todesursachen (ICD) 1979, 9th revision, vol I: Systematisches Verzeichnis. Consulting, Wuppertal; vol II: Alphabetisches Verzeichnis. Girardet, Wuppertal
2. Kramer P, Schach E, Schwartz FW (1982) A reason for visit classification for ambulatory care – Ein Klassifikationsschema für Kontaktanlässe in der ambulanten Versorgung. Deutsche Fassung der Reason for Classification des National Center for Health Statistics (1979). Zentralinstitut für die kassenärztliche Versorgung in der Bundesrepublik Deutschland, Cologne
3. Schneider D, Appleton L, McLemore L (1979) National Center for Health Statistics. A Reason for visit classification for ambulatory care. Data evaluation and methods research, no 78. DHEW Publ no (PHS) 79–1352, Public Health Service, Hyattsville, MA (Vital and health statistics, series 2)

Diagnostic Language in Primary Health Care – A Structural and Semantic Analysis of Diagnoses on Health Service Medical Cards

M. Heydthausen and F. Koch

Introduction

For the identification and analysis of time patterns of chronic diseases based on data which have their origin in primary health care, exact and information-retaining handling of free-text diagnoses is necessary. The problems in the area of text processing include the detection of the vocabulary and syntactic structures used and, above all, the question of whether there exists a semantic model which is generally applied when diagnostic statements are formulated.

Consequently, the subject of this paper will not be a discussion of the problem of whether there is sense in using "primary diagnoses" for any investigations. Our aim, rather, is to answer the question of whether the dataset of primary diagnosis can be technically analysed for further use, especially on an algorithmic level. The main elements of the paper are a short report on the origin of the investigated dataset, a summary of the results of grammatical analysis and the definition of a semantic model for primary diagnoses by giving a multidimensional highly structured nomenclature.

The Dataset

The dataset for these investigations consisted of about 9000 diagnostic statements which we derived from all kinds of Health Serivce Medical Cards in free text. Of course, all statements are written in German medical language. Consequently the results of the grammatical and syntactic analysis only give evidence for the German language area.

Grammatical Structures

Analysing the grammatical constructions of the diagnostic statements, we found a set of nominal phrases with a very simple structure. Most of these statements consist of just a few words. In detail: 96.9% of all phrases were composed of at most five words, with an average word length of eight characters.

Primary Health Care in the Making
Ed. by U. Laaser, R. Senault, H. Viefhues

Diagnostic statements consist mainly of nouns, perhaps supplemented by adjectives, adverbs, another noun, the genitive form of a noun or a prepositional construction. Verbs seldom occur.

Summarizing, we found that primary health care physicians use a mode of expression in diagnosis that is generally short, firm in its sense, uncomplicated and without structural redundancy.

A Semantic Model

As already stated, in analysing diagnostic statements from Health Service Medical Cards, exact and information-retaining handling of the diagnoses is necessary. Use of the ICD system for this purpose is difficult. As an alternative and even more as a basis for a semantic model for diagnosis we explain below the construction of a multi-dimensional nomenclature especially for use in social medicine and for diagnosis which has its origin in primary health care.

The Dimensions of Medical Knowledge

A diagnostic statement consists of medical terms. These terms can be divided into different items, related to the different dimensions of medical knowledge. We decided to take into account the following dimensions, which we call reference systems:

Topography (abbreviated T)
Nosology (abbreviated N)
Etiology (abbreviated E)
Modifiers (abbreviated M)

The informal definition behind these dimensions is: A certain disease (N) at a certain site (T) caused by a certain fact (E). All this or parts of it can be modified (M).

As an example, take the statement "chronic viral pneumonia", which can be divided into the following terms: T: Pneumon; N: Pneumonia; E: Virus; M: Chronic.

Simple and Complex Diagnosis

Of course, diagnostic statements can be more complicated than the previous example, in which case the preceding model does not fit. We call diagnosis that obeys the preceding model, simple diagnosis. Simple diagnosis can be combined by suitable relations to complex diagnosis. Suitable relations are temporal coincidence (*), temporal sequence (→), causal sequence (⇒) and exclusion (¬).

As an example of a complex diagnosis, take the statement "inflammation and fibrosis" which combines N: inflammation and N: fibrosis by means of temporal coincidence: (N: inflammation) * (N: fibrosis)

The Vocabularies of the Reference Systems, Independent Terms

The vocabularies of the reference systems are derived directly from the actual free-text diagnostic statements of Health Service Medical Cards. So, they represent the actual mode of expression in German medical language in the area of primary health care. The terms are related to the different reference systems in the following manner: terms are as short as possible (morphema like "itis") and terms are as long as necessary to express an independent semantic unit.

Terms obeying this definition are called independent terms. It is clear that there are different ways of defining such independent semantic units. But this is throughout a wanted effect, because the needs of defining diagnostic meaning in social medicine differ from the needs of defining meaning in, for example, pathology.

Classification Systems

Each vocabulary of a reference system can be combined with an arbitrary number of classification systems (cs). The nomenclature we use actually consists of four vocabularies, one for each reference system, and five classification systems. The two classification systems for Topography allow two methods of clustering the T-items: for each T-item we can define to which organic system it belongs and to which region of the body.

Example: independent term "vertebra" of T-vocabulary is assigned to cs "System" class "vertrabral column" and cs "Region" class "dorsum".

Representation of Medical Knowledge

The same technique of assignment can be used for representation and definition of medical knowledge. Now, any independent item of any vocabulary can be linked with any classification system whenever the meaning of the item requires. Of course, new classification systems can be generated whenever necessary to define knowledge.

The N-item "chalazion", for example, means: chronic inflammation of glandulae tarsales. Expressed by means of linking and assigning, references are set

from	N-vocabulary	chalazion
to	cs "Systems"	glandulae tarsales
	cs "Regions"	eye
	cs "N"	inflammation
	cs "M"	chronic

Semantic Patterns

The semantic structure of simple diagnosis is evident. Any simple diagnosis can be related to one of these patterns: N or TN, perhaps completed by E- or M-items. In the investigated data set more than 90% of diagnoses were simple. Analysing the complex diagnoses we found four patterns covering 80% of them (Table 1). With these few patterns we can assign a well defined semantic pattern to 98% of all diagnosis.

Table 1. Four patterns found in analysing complex diagnoses

Pattern	Meaning	Example (in German)
(T . . T) N	Disease at different sites	Gastroenteritis
N . . N	Different diseases, no explicit sites	Weit-stabsichtigkeit
(TN) N	Disease at site combined with disease	Emphysembronchitis
N → N	Temporal sequence of diseases	Postcholecystektomie-syndrom

Summary

Diagnoses on Health Service Medical Cards written in German medical language have a simple syntactic structure. Making use of the outlined semantic model, a well defined meaning can be assigned to nearly all diagnosis. Only 10% of the diagnoses were complex and highly structured. The rest were simple diagnoses. Even 80% of the complex statements can be divided into simple semantic patterns.

Early Detection of Disorders of Peripheral Circulation in General Practice: A Model for a Research Project of the German Society for General Medicine

H.-D. Klimm

Arteriosclerosis and its sequelae occupy first place in all developed countries in the western world with respect to morbidity and mortality. Even though the risk factors and risk profiles for arteriosclerosis that have been identified as a result of widespread epidemiological studies are being increasingly detected, interpreted and treated in general practice and the first signs of a change in trend can be seen, there is still a great deal of uncertainty with respect to early detection and interpretation of the precursors and early manifestations of arteriosclerosis itself. Thus the clinician generally perceives and recognises such syndromes when they have already become manifest in their classical form, i.e. when they have reached the diagnostic level in the dynamic development of the disease.

In contrast, the family doctor, who looks after 90% of all patients medically, sees the development right up to manifestation of the disease. Because he lives and acts in the same biotope, he experiences with his patients the fluctuating disorders of well-being and the always variable but consistent symptoms and symptom complexes of an illness in their individual dynamics long before the final stage of diagnosis can be reached.

He has the task and the unique chance to recognise degenerative changes in their earliest form and to be able to positively influence their fateful course. He must, however, be provided with aids that are effective, practical and economic; methods that have a balanced relationship between cost and benefit and which can be applied, without major investment in personnel or technical equipment, on a large number of people in a relatively short time.

The Deutsche Gesellschaft für Allgemeinmedizin (DEGAM: German Society for General Medicine) has developed a research programme and model for the early detection of disorders of peripheral circulation which may fulfil the criteria for prevention given above. This programme is based on the following two observations:

- A general practitioner will generally initiate and carry out specific diagnostic measures for the determination of disorders of peripheral circulation if the patient reports the typical symptoms that the practitioner has learnt during his training and postgraduate studies. In stages I and II a, however, peripheral disorders of circulation are without symptoms.
- Upon examination of 6400 apparently healthy subjects, Wittmer in Basle found stenosis or occlusion of a limb artery in 1% of the 45- to 50-year-olds

Primary Health Care in the Making
Ed. by U. Laaser, R. Senault, H. Viefhues

and in 7% of the 65- to 75-year-olds, but the people concerned did not show or report the typical symptoms of claudication.

A main aim of the research project of the DEGAM presented here for discussion will be, in addition to determining the frequency and severity of disorders of peripheral circulation, to develop a catalogue of subjective symptoms and symptom complexes that may be assigned to stages I and IIa.

It is planned to carry out the study as follows:

1. A representative selection of general practices in urban margins and rural areas throughout the Federal Republic of Germany will be studied. It is intended to include 30 practices from each of the three groups. The individual practices will be identified by consecutive numbering.
2. Selection on representatively selected weekdays in these practices of all patients aged 15 years and over who visit the practice for any reason whatsoever. The individual patients will be identified by consecutive numbering in the practice concerned.
3. Completion of a questionnaire for each patient on familial, social and medical characteristics and questioning about disorders of peripheral arterial circulation with typically recognised symptoms and recording of spontaneous reports of symptoms in the legs.
4. Measurement of the blood pressure over the radial artery bilaterally by means of cuff and stethoscope.
5. Subsequently, measurement of the blood pressure by means of ultrasonic Doppler measuring probe over the radial artery bilaterally.
6. Subsequently, measurement on both lower limbs as follows: Application of a congestive cuff with manometer at the distal end of the lower leg, placed over the posterior radial artery instead of the stethoscope–ultrasonic Doppler measuring probe.
7. To complete the examination, an exercise test in the form of a simple Ratschow's test. The patient lies down and must raise his legs at right angles for 5 min.
8. Determination of the ratio of malleolar pressure to upper arm pressure, which in healthy subjects = 1. Pressure ratios < 0.9 are pathological.
9. Evaluation of the pressure ratios found according to Heinemann as follows:

   a) With pressure values of less than 100 mmHg over the posterior radial artery, pathological conditions can be assumed.
   b) Values between 100 and 130 mmHg are in the suspect range.
      - If the pressure falls on raising the legs by more than 20%, then pathological conditions can be assumed.
      - If there is a pressure difference of more than 15 mmHg to the detriment of the lower leg pressure in comparison with the values above the radial artery, then one can assume pathological conditions.
   c) With pressure values above 130 mmHg one can assume normal flow conditions. Exception: pressure ratios of more than 15 mmHg to detriment of the lower leg pressure.

10. Attempt to subdivide according to stages using the following schedule:
    Mean absolute systolic arterial pressure at rest in normotensive patients
    - greater than 90 mmHg = ischaemia stage I
    - greater than 80 mmHg = ischaemia stage IIa
    - 50–80 mmHg = severe to moderate ischaemia stage IIb or III
    - less than 50 mmHg = ischaemia stage IV
11. Collection and recording of all known risk factors for the individual patients by means of the existing files in the individual practices.
12. Statistical analysis and attempt to objectify the correlation of subjective symptoms with the objective data on the pressure measurement.
13. Formation of patient cohorts in the age groups
    - 15–30 years
    - 30–60 years
    - 60–90 years and
    - over 90 years,

    who should be examined at regular intervals according to the same schedule in order to determine an indication of the incidence of arteriosclerosis and of disorders of peripheral circulation in particular.
14. Regular follow-up of the patients with objectively determinable disorders of peripheral circulation, to determine the effectiveness of exercise and conservative drug therapy.

An investigation is currently running in Heidelberg as a pilot project and has been carried out according to the above model. The two medical students concerned, Frl. Marianne Franze and Herr Thomas Stegmeier, have so far examined 395 patients in four general practices. The intermediate results are available. Out of a total of 395 patients, 105 were less than 40 years old and 290 older than 40 years.

In a total of 59 of these 395 patients (= 14.9%) a blood pressure difference was detected. Of the 105 patients less than 40 years old, ten (= 9.5%, five men, five women) had pathological differences in blood pressure, and of the 290 patients over 45 years old, 49 (= 16.8%, 24 men, 25 women) had pathological findings.

In the 10 patients under 40 years old who had pathological differences in pressure, such differences could be measured in three bilaterally, in four only on the right and in three only on the left.

In the 49 patients over 40 years old who had pathological differences in pressure, there were pressure differences bilaterally in 18 patients, pressure differences only on the right in 17 patients and pressure differences only on the left in 14 patients.

Perhaps the intermediate results regarding the risk profile should also be briefly mentioned. In the ten patients under 40 years old with pathological differences in pressure, three (two men and one woman) did not have any risk factors, whilst in the 49 patients over 40 years old with pathological results only four were without risk profile (three men and one woman).

Whilst many years of nicotine abuse in patients under 40 years old with pathological differences were found only in two out of the ten, in the patients over 40 years old 22 of the 49 showed many years of abuse of nicotine. One of the ten patients under 40 years old had had hypertension for several years, whereas seven of the 49 over 40 had it. One of the ten under 40 had been obese for a number of years, whereas 14 out of the 49 over 40 had suffered from obesity for many years. Diabetes was not detectable as a risk factor in the under 40-year-old patients, compared with long-term diabetes in three patients over 40. It is both striking and worthy of note that six of the ten patients under 40 years old with pathological differences in pressure had a clear family predisposition, as did 30 of the 49 patients over 40 years old. With respect to the summation of long-term risk factors, then, five of the ten patients under 40 years old with pathological results had one risk factor and two patients had two risk factors simultaneously, whilst in the 49 patients over 40 years old the following constellations were found: 10 had one risk factor, 22 had two, and 15 had three or more.

Unfortunately, data on subjective symptoms and their correlation with the individual pathological data found cannot be given as the investigation is still running and the results are not available. This is only intended to give an insight into the current investigation as a basis for discussion.

Before the DEGAM undertakes this programme it hopes that this congress will provide a critical assessment of its plan, competent aids and the support of experienced epidemiologists, workers in social medicine and angiologists. Fruitful co-operation is also hoped for, taking into account particular wishes and ideas.

Summary

Arteriosclerosis and its sequelae occupy first place in all developed countries in the western world with respect to morbidity and mortality. Even though the risk factors and risk profiles for arteriosclerosis that have been identified as a result of widespread epidemiological studies are being increasingly detected, interpreted and treated in general practice and the first signs of a change in trend can be seen, there is still a great deal of uncertainty with respect to early detection and interpretation of the precursors and early manifestations of arteriosclerosis itself. Whilst in hospital only those syndromes are seen and recognised that are present in their manifest classical form, the family doctor, who looks after 90% of all patients, sees the development of these diseases. It is his task and unique chance to be able to recognise degenerative changes in their early stages and to be able to influence their fateful course positively. The Deutsche Gesellschaft für Allgemeinmedizin (German Society for General Medicine) intends to investigate throughout the Federal Republic of Germany the early stages of disorders of peripheral circulation by means of Doppler sonographic examination and determination of the known risk factors and by the use of a questionnaire in selected practices for all patients aged 15 years and older who visit these practices. Four main topics will be considered:

1. Determination of the frequency of patients with disorders of peripheral circulation in stages I and IIa by means of Doppler sonographic exami-

nation (determination of differences in blood pressure between the upper and lower limbs).

2. Determination and recording of known risk factors in all the patients examined.
3. Determination and questioning for specific profiles of symptoms that could correspond to objectively detectable blood pressure differences in accordance with the treated circulatory disorders of stages I and IIa.
4. Formation of patient cohorts which will be followed up at regular intervals according to the same schedule to determine the incidence of disorders of peripheral circulation.

In addition to the detailed programme of the proposed research, initial results of a pilot project that has been carried out by means of this model by two medical students in four general practices in Heidelberg are presented for discussion.

Effects of the Social Situation on Health and Utilization of Medical Care Services: Results from the Munich Follow-up Study *

R. Laessle and R. Ellmann

Although numerous studies have shown that socioeconomic status (SES) is related to health and utilization behaviour, the criticism has often been made not only that results vary with method of status measurement [10, 11], but also that such results do not disclose why social class differences emerge [3, 8]. In the meantime, various researchers have attempted to find variables which could help to explain the influence of social class [2, 3, 5, 9]. A closer look at individual components of SES (e.g. income, occupation, education) can be a first step in studying this relationship. Further, it seems obvious that SES reflects only part of the individual's social situation. Other variables, such as working conditions, housing conditions, place of residence and social support, could conceivably play important intervening roles.

On the basis of our results on class-specific patterns of utilization behaviour and amount of services used (see the contribution of Ellmann and Laessle in this volume), the present paper deals with the following topics:

1. What are the effects of certain components of SES (e.g. income, education, occupation) on health and utilization measures?
2. Do other variables characterizing the individual's social situation (e.g. objective material conditions, employment status, social support) show closer relationships to utilization behaviour than SES?
3. Which variables describing the individual's social situation contribute to status-specific differences in health?

Method

The analysis is based on data from a 7-year follow-up study on a representative sample of the adult population of the Federal Republic of Germany ($n = 419$). Data collection, sample and dependent variables (health and utilization measures) are described elsewhere (Ellmann and Laessle in this volume).

Independent variables: The components of SES include education (four levels), occupation of head of household (five categories) and houshold income

* This work was supported in part by the Robert Bosch Foundation

Primary Health Care in the Making
Ed. by U. Laaser, R. Senault, H. Viefhues

(dichotomized). Other variables characterizing the individual's social situation were gathered using a semi-standardized interview schedule (Faltermaier 1982, unpublished). This measures objective restrictions and stressful conditions in a variety of areas of life, as well as the degree of dissatisfaction with these areas, based on self-report data. Each separate area (i.e. work conditions, housing conditions or leisure activities) is rated on a 4-point scale; total scores ranging from 0 to 100 are built separately for objective conditions and for dissatisfaction (higher values indicate more restrictions or greater dissatisfaction).

Two social support measures were derived: a global score (range 1–7; higher values mean less support) and a specific measure (living together with a partner vs. living alone). Other variables we considered are employment status (full-time vs. part-time or unemployed) and place of residence (rural vs. urban).

Results

Multiple regression analysis was used to estimate the relative contribution of each SES component to health and utilization behaviour, as depicted in Table 1 for our male sample. A comparison of the beta weights of the status components with regard to health measures seems to indicate that the reported class differences in health ratings can be attributed to differences in income and occupation. Although there was a significant relationship between the combined status index and health, neither of these single effects alone reached significance. Nonetheless, there is a tendency for people with lower income and lower occupation to report poorer health status.

The amount of service use (number of physician visits in the last 12 months) showed no significant relationship to the combined SES measure. In Table 1 we see that it is also unrelated to the individual status components.

The results for patterns of use are as often reported in the literature [e.g. 7]: men with less education prefer the general practitioner for medical care (beta = -0.20; $t = -2.38$, $P < 0.02$), whereas more educated men show a greater tendency to consult an internist (beta = .27; $t = 3.18$, $P < 0.02$). Controlling for place of residence did not influence these relationships.

For the women in our sample we obtained similar results regarding the health measures and amount of use.

In a stepwise multiple regression approach we examined how initial estimates of the SES–utilization relationship and the SES–health relationship change when groups of other variables describing the individual's social situation are added in the analysis [5]. As we found no significant relationship between extent of service use and SES, we were especially interested in analysing whether other variables characterizing the social situation would prove to be better predictors of utilization behaviour. Table 2 depicts the relationship between extent of services used and SES, considering the other social variables, for our male sample. Regression equation I shows that there is no linear effect of social status when controlling for age and health status. The same is true for

Table 1. Effects of the components of SES on health and utilization measures (standardized beta coefficients), men ($n = 207$)

	Income	Occupation	Education
Global health rating[a]	−0.11	−0.13	0.01
Somatic complaint list[a]	−0.08	−0.13	0.00
Number of physician visits[b]	0.04	0.02	0.05
Number of different specialists[b]	0.08	0.09	0.00
Preference for G. P.[b]	0.07	0.00	−0.20***
Preference for internist[b]	0.00	−0.14*	0.27***

* $P<0.10$; ** $P<0.05$; *** $P<0.02$
[a] Controlling for age
[b] Controlling for age and health

Table 2. Relationship between number of physician visits and SES, considering variables describing the social situation: comparison of different regression equations (standardized beta coefficients), men ($n = 207$)

Regression equation	I	II	III
Age	0.10	0.08	0.07
Health rating	0.42***	0.39***	0.41***
Somatic complaint list	0.09	0.08	0.08
SES	0.08	0.10	0.11*
Objective material conditions (total score)	–	0.13**	0.14**
Employment status	–	−0.07	−0.10
Residency	–	0.07	0.08
Degree of dissatisfaction	–	–	−0.09
Social support (global score)	–	–	0.00
Partner	–	–	0.00
Explained variance	26%	29%	29%

* $P<0.10$; ** $P<0.05$; *** $P<0.02$

the women in our sample. When adding the variables describing the objective conditions of the social situation (equation II), we found a significant effect for the total score of objective material conditions (beta = 0.13; $t = 2.01$, $P < 0.05$). This effect remains significant (beta = 0.14; $t = 2.10$, $P < 0.05$) even when considering satisfaction and support variables in equation III; i.e. high restrictions and many stressful conditions in the individual's objective situation go hand in hand with more physician visits, independent of SES.

The results for women are somewhat different insofar as satisfaction and partnership proved to be important, in addition to objective material conditions. Women living together with a partner use fewer services (beta = −0.17; $t = -2.47$, $P < 0.05$). Dissatisfied women also tended to use fewer services (beta = −0.16; $t = -1.90$; $P < 0.10$), which was contrary to our expectations.

Table 3. Relationship between health measures and SES, considering variables describing the social situation: comparison of different regression equations (standardized beta coefficients), men ($n = 207$)

Regression equation	I	II	III
Age	0.34***	0.34***	0.36***
SES	−0.18***	−0.14***	−0.14**
Objective material conditions (total score)	–	0.13*	0.08
Employment status	–	−0.11*	−0.08
Residency	–	−0.05	−0.08
Degree of dissatisfaction (total score)	–	–	0.22***
Social support (global score)	–	–	0.04
Partner	–	–	0.00
Explained variance	19%	22%	27%

* $P < 0.10$; ** $P < 0.05$; *** $P < 0.02$

Change in the relationship between SES and health (as measured by the global health rating), when adding the other variables characterizing the social situation, is shown in Table 3 for our male sample.

Regression equation II shows that the effect of SES remains significant (beta = −0.14; $t = -2.12$, $P < 0.02$), but is somewhat reduced, when introducing additional variables. Part of the variance in health status which was attributed to SES in equation I, therefore, may be due to objective material conditions (beta = 0.13; $t = 1.93$, $P < 0.10$) and employment status (beta = −0.11; $t = -1.67$, $P < 0.10$).

When adding variables measuring social support and degree of dissatisfaction in regression equation III, there is no change in the social class effect, but the effects of objective material conditions and employment status, which appeared significant initially, are reduced to non-significance. Of the newly included variables, only degree of dissatisfaction had a significant effect (beta = 0.22; $t = 2.91$, $P < 0.02$). The beta-weight indicates that it is a rather important variable: dissatisfied men give poorer health ratings. For women we obtained similar results.

Summing up the results on health, it is apparent that people with lower SES tend to give poorer health ratings, but part of status differences in health ratings can be explained by other variables. Objective material conditions do relate to health; however, individual dissatisfaction seems to play an important intervening role. It is reasonable to assume, though, that the relationship between poor health and dissatisfaction is one of mutual influence.

Our results demonstrate that it is possible to find more specific variables which could explain differences in health better than a global SES measure alone. Also, we were able to identify specific factors which relate to extent of utilization behaviour, although the global SES index itself showed no significant effects. Indeed, the amount of explained variance of extent of services used, taking all our independent variables into account (see Table 2), is 30% and much higher than in other studies [3, 6, 12]. Nevertheless, the remaining 70% suggest that the model should be expanded to include other variables which previous research has shown to be relevant, such as attitudional factors and insurance coverage [1, 4, 5].

References

1. Becker M, Haefner D, Kasl S, Kirscht J, Maiman L, Rosenstock I (1977) Selected psychosocial models and correlates of individual health-related behaviors. Med Care [Suppl] 15:27–46
2. Bush PJ, Osterweis M (1978) Pathways to medicine use. J Health Soc Behav 19:179–189
3. Coburn D, Pope CR (1974) Socioeconomic status and preventive health behavior. J Health Soc Behav 15:67–77
4. Crandall LA, Duncan RP (1981 Additional and situational factors in the use of physician services by low-income persons. J Health Soc Behav 22:64–77
5. Dutton B (1978) Explaining the low use of health services by the poor: costs, attitudes, or delivery systems? Am Sociol Rev 43:348–368
6. Kohn R, White KL (1976) The use of health services: an international collaborative study. Main report of the WHO/International collaborative study of medical care utilization. Oxford University Press, London
7. Kronenfeld J (1982) Organisation of ambulatory care by consumers. Sociol Health Illness 4:183–200
8. McKinlay J (1972) Some approaches and problems in the use of services – an overview. J Health Soc Behav 13:115–151
9. Rundall TG, Wheeler RC (1979) The effect of income on use of preventive care: an evaluation of alternative explanations. J Health Soc Behav 20:397–406
10. Schmädel D (1975) Schichtspezifische Unterschiede im Gesundheits- und Krankheitsverhalten der Bevölkerung der Bundesrepublik Deutschland. In: Ritter-Röhr D (ed) Der Arzt, sein Patient und die Gesellschaft. Suhrkamp, Frankfurt, pp 112–121
11. Steinkamp G (1980) Klassen- und schichtenanalytische Ansätze in der Sozialisationsforschung. In: Hurrelmann K, Ulich D (eds) Handbuch der Sozialisationsforschung. Beltz, Weinheim, pp 253–284
12. Wolinsky F (1978) Assessing the effects of predisposing, enabling, and illness-morbidity characteristics on health service utilization. J Health Soc Behav:384–396

Social Class and Utilization of Primary Medical Care Services: Class-Specific Patterns of Utilization Behaviour in the Munich Follow-up Study *

R. Ellmann and R. Laessle

Over the last three decades a great amount of research has been carried out dealing with the question of equity in the delivery of medical services [1, 2, 9]. Most commonly, utilization of medical services has been examined by studying volume of services utilized or entrance rates to the professional medical care system (i.e. mere presence or absence of physician contacts within a specified time period). It has, however, often been pointed out that utilization behaviour should preferably be considered to be a multidimensional concept [3, 6], and utilization research has dealt not only with the amount of services utilized but also with more specific variables such as types of services utilized, sources of care and number of affiliations with medical care providers [7, 8, 10, 14]. In studying social class differences in utilization behaviour it thus seems important to consider patterns of utilization behaviour as well as total amount of services utilized.

In the Federal Republic of Germany there has been relatively little research to date on utilization, neither regarding equity in the amount of services delivered nor regarding patterns of utilization behaviour [4, 5, 12]. This paper addresses itself to the following questions:

1. Are there differences in West Germany in the amount of services utilized in relation to socioeconomic status? More specifically, does the lower class tend to underutilize medical services?
2. Are there specific patterns of use, i.e. differences in types of services used, which can be identified as typical for a certain social class?

Method

Analyses are based on interview data collected from a representative sample (207 men and 212 women, 26–63 years old) of the adult population of West Germany. This sample was part of a larger 7-year follow-up study described elsewhere [16].

Utilization behaviour in the 12 months prior to interview was measured by the following variables: the amount of services used was measured by total

* This research was funded in part by the Robert Bosch Foundation

Primary Health Care in the Making
Ed. by U. Laaser, R. Senault, H. Viefhues

number of physician visits in the last 12 months. Preferences for certain sources of care were measured by calculating for each subject the percentage of his total physician visits in the last 12 months accounted for by a general practitioner, by an internist and by a gynaecologist. The number of different specialists consulted in 12 months, whereby the general practitioner is also counted, reflects the breadth of care, what has been referred to as "compactness of care" [14].

Two subjective health status measures were included: a global health rating (5-point scale) and the Somatic Complaint List developed by von Zerssen and Koeller [15], which measures number and severity of complaints.

The independent measure was socioeconomic status, which was measured using an index combining educational, occupational and income level. On the basis of this index the sample was divided into three classes, referred to as the upper middle class, the lower middle class and the lower class.

All analyses were carried out separately for men and for women. Results reported are based on analysis of variance, except when otherwise stated.

Results

The first question, whether there is a relationship between social class and amount of services used, should be formulated more precisely, as we are interested in the adequacy of medical services and this, of course, relates to need. We hypothesized that there would be a relationship between social class and health and this indeed proved to be the case. Figure 1 shows the relationship between social class and the Somatic Complaint List. The global health rating showed a similar significant relationship for both sexes: subjects of lower social class tend to have poorer health status.

It is thus very obvious that one must control for health status when studying class differences in the amount of medical services utilized. Therefore, all of the

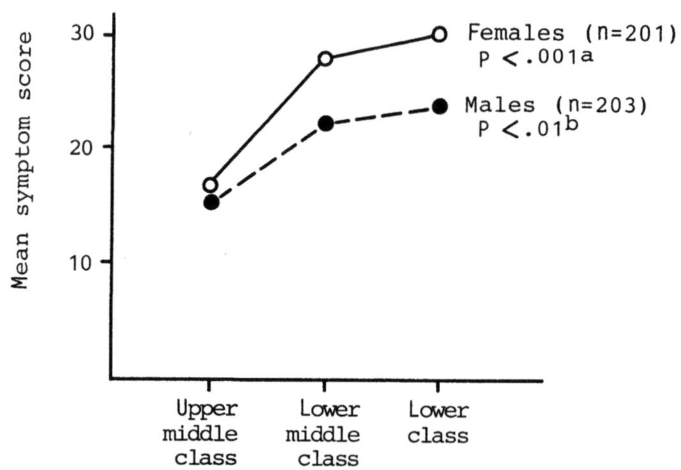

Fig. 1. Health status and social class – Somatic Complaint List. [a]ANOVA F = 8.04, [b]ANOVA F = 5.38

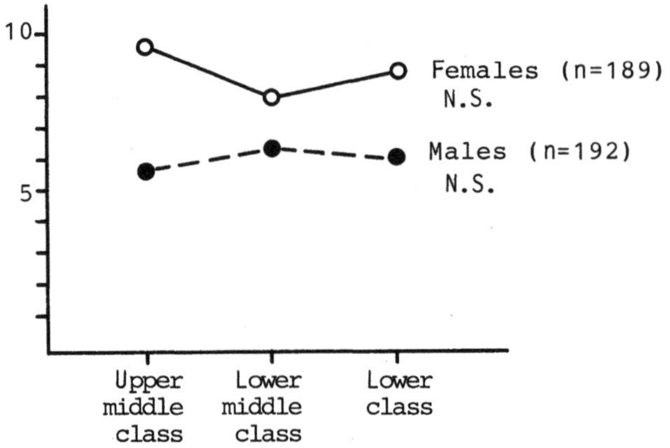

Fig. 2. Average number of visits to physician in last 12 months, adjusted for level of health (subjective rating; Somatic Complaint List)

following analyses control for age and for level of health (using both health measures) within each sex.

Figure 2 shows that there are no significant class differences in total number of physician visits. This seems to answer the first question directed towards the issue of equity in the amount of services quite clearly. Specifically, there is no evidence of underutilization by the lower class. One must naturally consider that this measure is a very rough estimate of utilization, containing no information on the specific services received or on the quality of care. In addition, controlling for levels of health by means of subjective health ratings has certain drawbacks due to probable social class differences in symptom perception [2].

We must also recognize that our lower class encompassed about 39% of our sample. It is still possible that a much smaller group representing the lower extreme of the socioeconomic status scale or subgroups not included in our sample (e.g. the aged, the homeless or foreign workers) show reduced utilization of medical services. We can only conclude at this point in our data analysis that we have found no evidence of widespread underutilization connected with lower socioeconomic status.

The second question to be examined deals with class-specific patterns of utilization. The following hypotheses are to be tested: that subjects of lower social class tend to consult fewer different doctors; and that subjects of lower social class show a preference for consulting a general practitioner, while tending to consult internists and gynaecologists less often.

Figure 3 shows that our first hypothesis could only partially be confirmed: lower class men did show a tendency to use fewer sources of care. Here we controlled not only for age and level of health but also for total number of visits to the doctor. That is, this variable reflects actual degree of the tendency to use fewer or more different sources of care, given the same number of total visits.

Results pertaining to preferences for certain sources of care, our second hypothesis, are shown in Fig. 4. The differences between lower middle class and lower class are in the direction postulated: lower class men and women show the greatest preference for the general practitioner. Lower class women also show less preference for the gynaecologist. The upper middle class, however, shows results we had not anticipated: greater preference for the general practitioner, and less preference for the gynaecologist than the lower middle class. When one compares preference for the general practitioner with preference for the gynaecologist, one sees that the values are very close for the lower middle class, suggesting that here the gynaecologist has gone farthest in taking over the role of being the primary source of care.

The differences between social classes with regard to preference for the internist were not significant using analysis of variance. Regression analysis, however, showed a linear trend ($P < 0.06$) for the men. The trend is as hypothe-

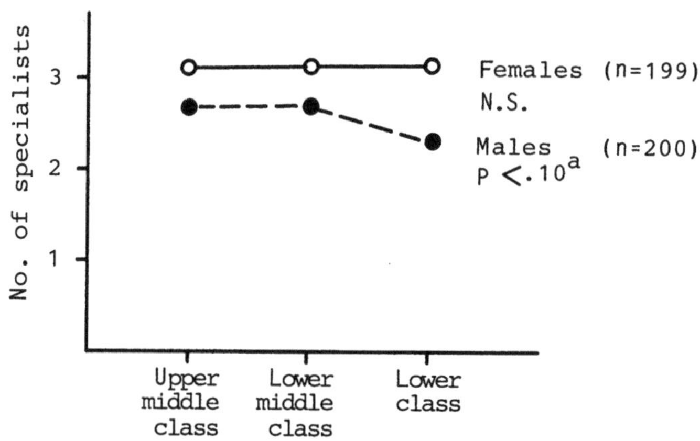

Fig. 3. Average number of specialists consulted (over 12 months), adjusted for level of health, age and total number of visits by each sex. [a]ANOVA F = 2.75

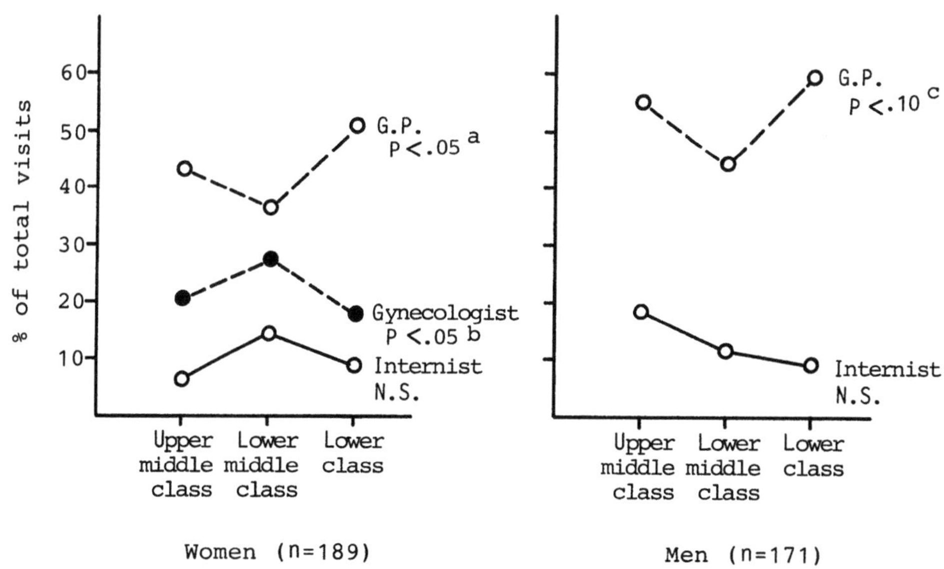

Fig. 4. Mean percent of total physician visits (over 12 months) accounted for by various specialists, adjusted for level of health and age within each sex. [a]ANOVA F = 4.03, [b]ANOVA = 3.13, [c]ANOVA = 2.72

sized, with the lowest degree of preference in the lower class and the highest degree of preference in the upper middle class.

One can conclude that it is indeed possible to identify class-specific patterns of utilization behaviour, even though the total amount of utilization, as measured by total number of physician visits, seems to show no social class differences. These results are, of course, incomplete until one has carefully examined how these patterns of utilization behaviour relate to quality of care or to health outcome. Previous research has shown that such relationships can be found between patterns of utilization behaviour and quality of care [11, 13]. Caution would be advisable in making cross-cultural generalizations, however, considering the differences in type of insurance coverage and medical training and practices between the U.S.A. and West Germany. As this issue could be of particular relevance for future social policy decisions, it would seem especially worthy of further research.

References

1. Andersen R, Aday LA (1978) Access to medical care in the U.S.: Realized and potential. Med Care 16:533–546
2. Berkanovic E, Reeder L (1974) Can money buy the appropriate use of services? Some notes on the meaning of utilization data. J Health Soc Behav 15:93–99
3. Bice T, White K (1971) Cross-national comparative research on the utilization of medical services. Med Care 9:253–271
4. Bundesminister für Arbeit und Sozialordnung (ed) (1979) Untersuchungen zur Schichtenspezifität der Inanspruchnahme medizinischer Leistungen und der Krankheitsverläufe in der sozialen Krankenversicherung, Vorstudie, Vol 1. Bundesministerium für Arbeit und Sozialordnung, Bonn
5. Geißler U (1983) Daten zur Inanspruchnahme ärztlicher Leistungen in der Bundesrepublik Deutschland. Mensch Med Ges 8:5–10
6. Hershey J, Luft H, Gianaris J (1975) Making sense out of utilization data. Med Care 13:838–854
7. Kronenfeld J (1978) Provider variables and the utilization of ambulatory care services. J Health Soc Behav 19:68–76
8. Kronenfeld J (1982) Organisation of ambulatory care by consumers. Sociol Health Illness 4:183–200
9. McKinlay J (1972) Some approaches and problems in the use of services – an overview. J Health Soc Behav 13:115–151
10. Moscovice I (1977) A method for analyzing resource use in ambulatory care settings. Med Care 15:1024–1044
11. Ross C, Duff R (1982) Returning to the doctor: The effect of client characteristics, type of practice, and experiences with care. J Health Soc Behav 23:119–131
12. Schmädel D (1975) Schichtspezifische Unterschiede im Gesundheits- und Krankheitsverhalten der Bevölkerung der Bundesrepublik Deutschland. In: Ritter-Röhr D (ed) Der Arzt, sein Patient und die Gesellschaft. Suhrkamp, Frankfurt, pp 112–121
13. Shortell S, Richardson W, LoGerfo J, Diehr P, Weaver B, Green K (1977) The relationships among dimensions of health services in two provider systems: A causal model approach. J Health Soc Behav 18:139–159
14. Solon J, Rigg R (1972) Patterns of medical care among users of hospital emergency units. Med Care 10:60–72
15. von Zerssen D, Koeller D (1976) Die Beschwerden-Listen (B-L). Beltz, Weinheim
16. Wittchen H-U, von Zerssen D, Ellmann R, Moeller H-J (1983) Der Verlauf behandelter und unbehandelter psychischer Störungen: Methodik und erste Ergebnisse. In: Kommer D, Röhrle B (eds) Gemeindepsychologische Perspektiven, vol 3. DGVT, Tübingen, pp 118–124

Choice of Best or Cheapest Drugs: A Note on Regulating Drug Supplies

M. Patel

Expenditure on health has increased so rapidly in both the developed world and in developing countries that there is now growing concern over the efficiency of resource allocation within the health sector. One aspect of this concern is shown in discussions on the regulation of the supply of prescription drugs. The range of prescription drugs available to physicians and consumers may be controlled by two types of regulatory action. One deals with the use of generic names [1], while the second deals with the prohibition of harmful or therapeutically ineffective drugs [2].

The use of generic rather than brand names for pharmaceutical products can be achieved either through the adoption of specific laws and regulations dealing with the supply of drugs, or through a revision of trade mark laws dealing with the distribution and advertising of drugs. If only generic names were used it could be expected that the cheapest of the chemically identical products would normally be chosen to fill generic prescriptions. More expensive brands would then disappear from the market.

The second type of regulatory action places restrictions on the range of chemical products permitted in national markets. This can take the form of a ban implemented by public authorities on products found to be harmful in some respect, or of a ban on products considered not therapeutically useful enough for the price charged. Both of the initiatives in these areas, that of the WHO to restrict drug lists on the basis of therapeutic utility and price of drugs, and that of the UNCTAD to negotiate import contracts in bulk under generic names, have met with mixed reactions from the medical profession. It has been argued that the quality of medical treatment would suffer if public authorities intervened in the pharmaceuticals market.

It is true that doctors must do the best for their patients, and demands to choose between prescription drugs on the basis of their relative prices can be met with a certain amount of indignation. The justification for this indignation rests on the tenet that in the absence of economic considerations the product chosen will be the clinically optimal one. It will be the best product for that patient. It is further argued that if price was considered as relevant then the product prescribed would be the best value for that patient in purely clinical terms. Thus many patients would be prescribed 'second best' or even 'third best' drugs, and the doctor could no longer be seen as doing his best for those patients. If

Primary Health Care in the Making
Ed. by U. Laaser, R. Senault, H. Viefhues

the consideration of prices results in sub-optimal treatment, it follows that doctors can improve the health of their patients more by ignoring drug prices.

This model rests on a number of naive assumptions that have been firmly exploded as well as some not so naive assumptions that are worth exploring further.

The most visible of these concerns the difference between individual and social optimality. The best situation for each individual patient would be that the doctor devoted all their time to that one patient. Doctors must see the larger picture and share time, which is scarce to them, between all their patients by terminating consultations once the marginal utility of an extra minute spent with one patient equals the marginal utility gained by spending that minute with another patient. If, as they say, time is money, then it can be seen that, in these terms, the value or cost of diagnosis is rationed between patients and doctors.

The clear difference between rationing the value of diagnosis and rationing the value of prescriptions is that, unlike time, the value of prescriptions does not appear to the individual doctor as a scarce resource. In fact the value of a prescription appears to the individual doctor as the value of time appears to the individual patient. It has the appearance of a commodity that can be consumed in greater quantities with positive benefits at no additional cost to that individual. Indeed, in neither case does the real additional cost incurred fall even on an identifiable individual.

In both cases costs are spread over a group. The patients who consume more than their 'fair share' of time ensure that other patients will be treated with less time. The doctor incurring excess expenditure in prescribing ensures that other expenditures of the health services will be budgeted for at a reduced level accordingly. Increase in pharmaceutical imports can be achieved only at the expense of other import-dependent sectors of the economy.

The above is relatively straightforward and is simply a logical extension of the model contained in the first paragraph. This continues to generate the conclusion that the drug that is best in socially cost-effective terms can be only as good as, or worse than, the drug that is best in purely clinical terms for that individual patient. In the second section we shall examine this apparently inviolable strict ranking in the light of the principle of indeterminacy. The concept of the 'optimal product in purely clinical terms' will be shown to be a concept with its own economic dimensions independent of all social and cost-effective criteria raised so far.

The choice of the best product for the patient in purely clinical terms is a choice of one or several products from a larger range of products. That knowledge of these is necessarily finite in itself makes no difference. The actual choice made for any patient is a choice based on the diagnosis and the knowledge that the doctor has of the products considered [3, 4]. To establish that a clinically optimal choice (that ignores economic considerations) is possible, it is necessary to show that the knowledge that the doctor has of the products to be chosen from is itself unbiased. To examine the assertion that a doctor's knowledge of products is unbiased we must consider the sources of such knowledge [5].

Sources of knowledge are by no means uniform in their quality. We may consider as distinct in this respect medical education, textbooks, medical indexes, articles in journals, advertisements and drug company representatives. Some of these sources will be more scientifically acceptable than others. What constitutes an acceptable source may vary somewhat between prescribers, health service institutions and countries. The acceptance of a source of information as not totally meaningless implies that the source is then endowed with some ability to influence decisions. The amount that any source will influence a prescription decision may depend on how acceptable, in scientific or clinical terms, that source is [6].

The mere discounting of sources according to their relative quality would be sufficient to ensure the clinical optimality of prescription decisions in a static framework under one condition, i.e. that the relative quality of the different sources must be known with certainty. Given that condition we may go on to investigate clinically optimal prescribing within a dynamic framework, a framework in which time passes.

We can isolate two major and distinct influences of time on clinically optimal prescribing. The first is that over time advances in medical science will result in increases in medical knowledge as a whole, and with some finite time lag, in the medical knowledge of each practitioner. The extent of this time lag will vary according to the source of information that each doctor uses to update his knowledge. Medical representatives and advertisements will be more up-to-date than medical textbooks. It must be noted that the source that is the most up-to-date may not be the most reliable or scientifically acceptable source. In any case where the ranking of sources by data and accepability is non-identical (it is not always the more reliable source that is also the most up-to-date one and thus information from that source is not always to be preferred unambiguously), the doctor must balance the date attached to a source against its reliability. (Are more doctors now turning to brand Z? Is product A the best treatment for . . .?)

The above juggling act is still a simplification of the problem facing the doctor who seeks to maintain his awareness of pharmaceutical products in such a state that he can be confident of making optimal judgements. The doctor only has a limited amount of time that can be spent keeping abreast of new developments. The amount of information that the average doctor receives through the post alone is more than he may have time to read. The amount available in specialist and medical libraries far surpasses that. Yet information in libraries is relatively inaccessible. It takes longer to obtain and is harder to digest than advertisements. Journal articles may occupy an immediate position and be more accessible than information in libraries but less available than advertisements. Thus the date and acceptability of a source of information must also be weighed against the accessibility of that source.

The last effect of time we shall consider is that effect it has on any item of knowledge. From one position in time medical education will be the major determinant of knowledge of pharmaceuticals. From another medical education may be a minor one. This result would arise even without memory decay. As the size of a field of knowledge increases, the relative size of any fixed unit decreases.

From this it is clear that prescription optimality in clinical terms is an elusive goal. The choice that is made in prescribing a product is not one in which unambiguous rankings for all products can always be made. Such rankings would imply that knowledge itself was optimal or perfect. The choice that is made is, in effect, one of choosing a suitable, rather than choosing the optimal, product. The level of indeterminancy associated with a choice is too contingent on quantitatively unassessable factors, whether consciously so or not, to meet the strict demands of absolute optimality.

It is at this point that the relevance of cost-efficiency prescribing and legislative restrictions on imports and distribution of drugs returns. No economist would suggest that a doctor should ever choose a product that is unsuitable for a patient. The suggestion has always been that the prescriber should choose the product that is most cost-efficient out of the range of products that are suitable for that patient. The contention of this essay is simply that the range of products that are suitable in this manner and that cannot be unambiguously ranked by any other means is somewhat larger than might otherwise be supposed to be the case. Public authorities basing policy on careful definitions of these ranges could improve economic cost-efficiency of overall prescribing at no cost to the individual patient in therapeutic terms.

References

1. UNCTAD Secretariat (1977) Pharmaceutical policies in Sri Lanka. Trade and Development Board, Geneva, TD/B/C6/21
2. WHO Expert Committee (1977/1979) The selection of essential drugs. WHO Tech Rep Ser 65:641
3. Julian P, Herxeimer A (1977) Doctors' anxieties in prescribing. Coll Gen Pract 27:662
4. Herxeimer A, Lionel NDW (1978) Minimum information needed by prescribers. Br Med J 2:1129–1132
5. Dadja R (1978) Drug advertising and prescribing. J R Coll Gen Pract 23:538–541
6. Yudkin J (1979) Pharmaceutical industry. World Med

Epidemiology of Digitalis Use – Results from a Random Sample of the Munich Population

W. Koenig, U. Keil, J. Stieber, A. Döring, S. J. Pöppl, and W. Mraz

Introduction

The Federal Republic of Germany (FRG) leads other industrial nations in the consumption of digitalis [5, 8]. Up to now known figures refer to the consumption data provided by pharmaceutical companies. To our knowledge, epidemiological studies on digitalis use have not yet been carried out. We therefore analysed the drug history of a random sample of the Munich population which was part of the Munich Blood Pressure Study. Furthermore, electrocardiographic findings and the serum creatinine which were available for the majority of the participants were evaluated. The goal of this analysis was the provision of data on the frequency of digitalis intake in the Munich population as well as data about prescribed dosages.

Material and Methods

The Munich Blood Pressure Study was designed as a representative cross-sectional study (MBS I 1980/81) with a follow-up study (MBS II 1981/82). The principal goal of this study was the provision of baseline data on the prevalence, awareness, treatment and control of hypertension in the population of Munich (Fig. 1) [15]. The participants were interviewed by specially trained personnel (mainly nurses) by means of a standardized questionnaire which asked about history of hypertension, attitudes and knowledge concerning hypertension, history and family history, use of medical care, life-style, socioeconomic variables and a detailed drug history. After the interview the sampled citizens underwent three blood pressure measurements and the recording of weight and height. All participants were asked to present the package or information sheet of all current medication (taken within the last 7 days) at the interview to provide reliable data.

In the Munich Blood Pressure Study II (MBS II 1981/82), a resting ECG (12 leads) was done on all participants who had given informed consent, and blood samples were drawn to measure the following parameters: total cholesterol, HDL-cholesterol, γ-GT, uric acid and serum creatinine (Scr). Besides these procedures the standardized interview and blood pressure measurements were carried out as in the preceding study (MBS I).

Primary Health Care in the Making
Ed. by U. Laaser, R. Senault, H. Viefhues

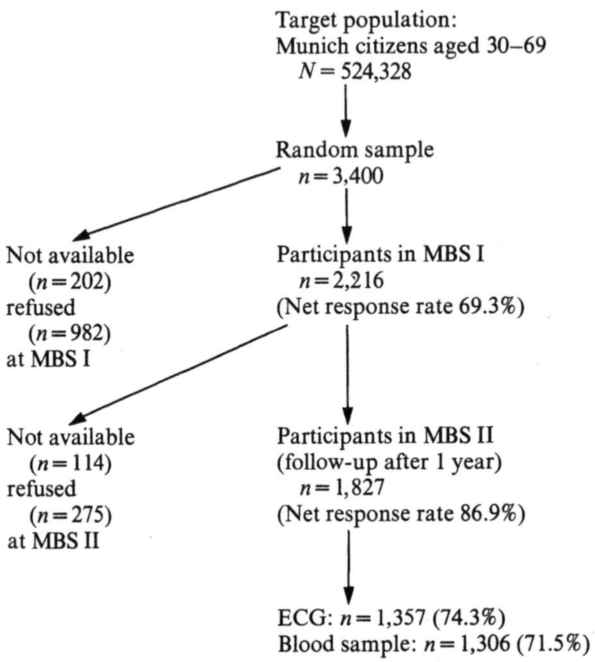

Fig. 1. Details of the Munich Blood Pressure Study (cross-sectional study with follow-up)

The following data on digitalis use refer to the MBS II, because the electrocardiogram and the results of serum creatinine analysis are needed for further interpretation. Percentages of participants taking digitalis were similar in both studies (6.9%; 95% confidence interval 5.9%–8.0%, vs 7%). The following parameters were calculated:

The creatinine clearance (Crea Cl in ml/min) according to the equation of Cockcroft and Gault [3]

$$\text{Crea Cl} = \frac{(140 - \text{age}) \times \text{weight (kg)}}{72 \times \text{Scr (mg/dl)}} \times \text{Fs},$$

where Fs means correction for sex differences (female 0.85, male 1.00).

The expected maintenance dose according to the equation of Schaumann et al. [12] is

for methyl-digoxin: $E = 0.000931 \times (150 - \text{age}) \times (1 + \text{Fs} \times 1.22/\text{Scr})$

for digoxin: $E = 0.001025 \times (150 - \text{age}) \times (1 + \text{Fs} \times 1.64/\text{Scr})$.

According to the recommendations of the authors, a minimum value of 0.9 mg/dl for serum creatinine was used. For β-acetyldigoxin and other glycosides no equations could be found in the literature. Assuming that β-acetyldigoxin has pharmacokinetic properties similar to those of digoxin [2], we used the equation for digoxin to calculate the maintenance dose of that drug. In addition, the daily prescribed dose of digitalis was recorded for each participant. Furthermore, the dosage interval was taken into account.

Results

One hundred and twenty-seven participants, i.e. 7% of the sample ($n = 1{,}827$), including 57 males and 70 females with a mean age of 61.3 years, took chemically defined glycosides. Eighty-seven (68.5%) were older than 60, and 55 (43%) were aged 65 or more. The age and sex distributions of the participants in the MBS I taking digitalis were similar. Extrapolating this percentage to the total number of German citizens aged 30–69 years (about 30 million) would mean that 2.1 million people in this age group in the FRG take digitalis. According to Schüren and Rietbrock [13] there are a total of about 4 million patients taking digitalis in the FRG. Since the glycoside consumption in people under 30 years of age can be neglected, the remaining 1.5–1.9 million would apply to the age group 70 and above. Barely 6.4 million people of this age group live in the FRG, which means that out of these about 25% are taking digitalis constantly.

Figure 2 shows the frequency distribution of the prescribed glycosides. Ninety-one percent was covered by three drugs, namely β-acetyldigoxin, β-methyldigoxin and pure digoxin. Digitoxin was taken by only two participants. Of the 127 citizens, 94% stated that they were taking their drug regularly; 6% were taking it at irregular intervals.

In 87 of the 127 participants blood samples could be drawn. Only in one case was the value of the serum creatinine above 1.2 mg/dl. The mean value for men was slightly higher than for women (1.00 ± 0.21 vs 0.84 ± 0.20 mg/dl). Calculating the creatinine clearance according to the equation of Cockcroft and Gault [3], nine participants showed a value of less than 50 ml/min; 35 had 50–80 ml/min and 22 others showed 80–100 ml/min.

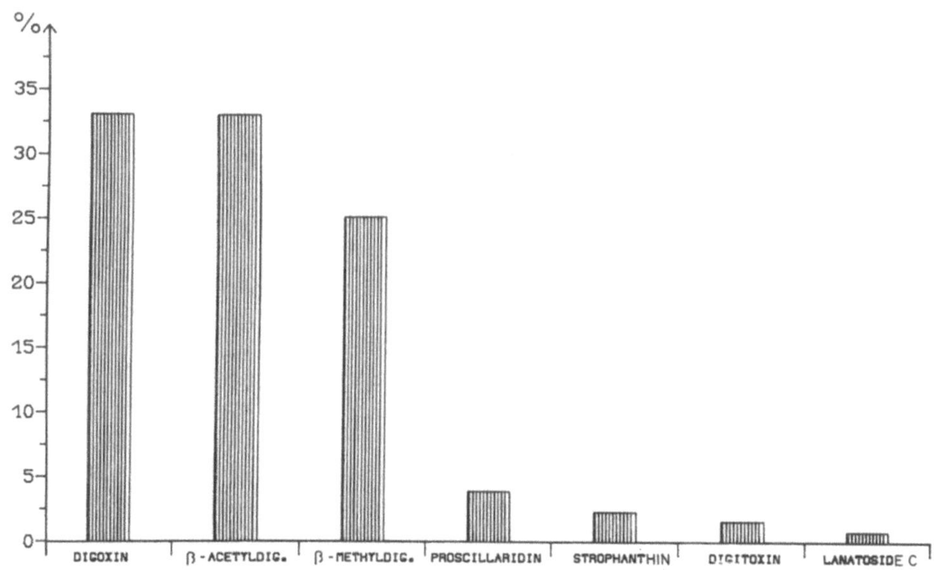

Fig. 2. Distribution of prescribed glycosides ($n = 127$). Munich Blood Pressure Study II (MBS 1981/82)

In the age group 60–69 taking digitalis ($n = 60$) and showing normal creatinine values we found 58% to have a creatinine clearance less than 80 ml/min; of these nine had less than 50 ml/min. In the group aged 70 and above the proportion of such patients should be even higher.

Calculating the expected maintenance doses for digoxin, β-acetyldigoxin, and β-methyldigoxin using the equations of Schaumann et al. [12] and comparing these data with the information of the participants regarding the prescribed daily doses of glycosides, we found that 44% were taking doses equivalent to the calculated maintenance dosage. In 29% of the cases the prescribed dose was below and in 27% above the calculated dosage (Fig. 3). These figures are in accordance with the literature [1, 7]. A difference between the two dosages was considered only when the calculated and the prescribed dosages differed by more than half a tablet (i.e. 0.05 mg). In 79 of 115 participants these data could be obtained. In a prospective study with β-methyldigoxin on 212 hospitalized patients, Isbary et al. [6] found a considerably lower intoxication rate (2.4%) after administration of a maintenance dose according to the equation of Schaumann and associates. This percentage was reported for ambulatory patients [9], whereas in hospitalized patients digitalis intoxication was seen in up to 20% [4, 9].

Figure 4 shows the different frequency distributions between the calculated and the prescribed maintenance doses. In contrast to the results of Schaumann et al. [12], the median of the calculated dose in our study differed only for β-methyldigoxin from the prescribed daily dose (0.15 mg vs 0.20 mg) and was identical for pure digoxin and β-acetyldigoxin (0.25 mg and 0.20 mg). The better coincidence of dosages can be explained by the fact that the participants in our study may not have suffered more severe forms of congestive heart failure

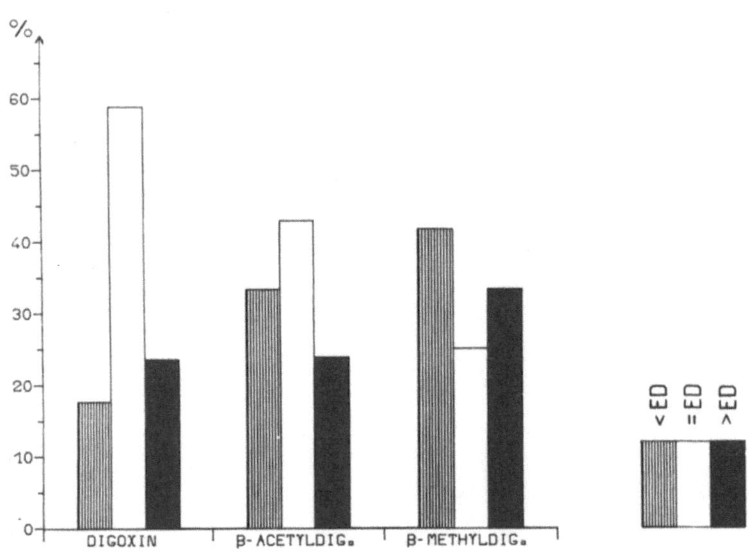

Fig. 3. Prescription patterns of the three most frequently used glycosides ($n = 79$). *ED*, calculated maintenance dose. Munich Blood Pressure Study II (MBS 1981/82)

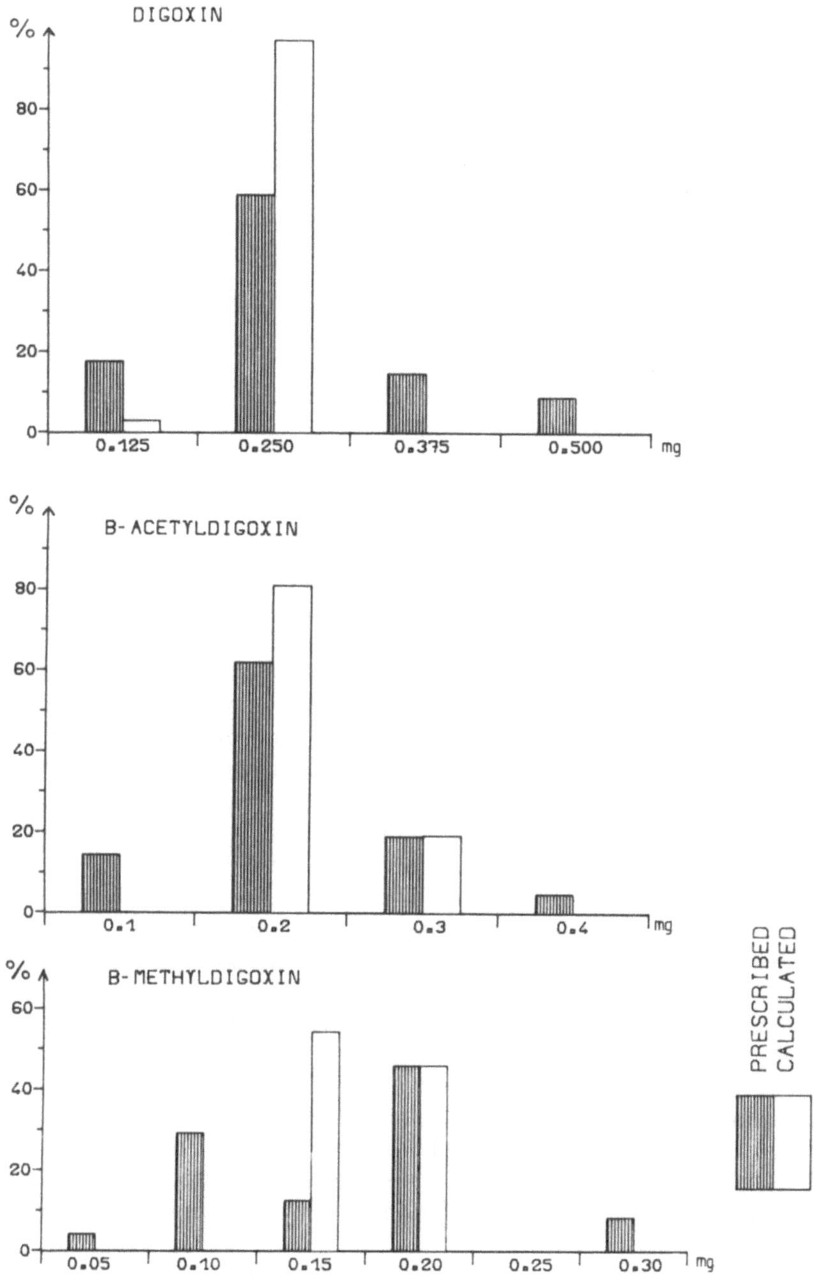

Fig. 4. Distribution of the calculated maintenance dose (Schaumann et al. [12]) and the prescribed daily glycoside dose for digoxin, β-acetyldigoxin and β-methyldigoxin ($n = 79$). Munich Blood Pressure Study II (MBS 1981/82)

Table 1. Electrocardiographic findings in 94 participants under constant digitalis medication.[a] Munich Blood Pressure Study II (MBS 1981/82)

Findings	Frequency (%)	Cases
Normal ECG	61.7	58
Sinus arrhythmia	6.4	6
Bradycardia (< 60/min)	5.3	5
Atrial fibrillation	9.6	9
I° AV block	6.4	6
Intraventricular blocks	4.3	4
ST-segment depression	23.4	22
Shortened QT interval	1.1	1
Premature contractions (SVPC + VPC)	5.3	5
Myocardial infarction	7.4	7

[a] Combinations possible

requiring higher doses. Furthermore, β-methyldigoxin obviously was prescribed in a dose of 0.15 mg much less frequently than could be expected from the distribution of the calculated maintenance dose.

Table 1 shows a synopsis of the ECG findings. In 94 of 127 participants under digitalis medication a high quality ECG tracing was recorded. More than 90% of them were in stable sinus rhythm. An abnormal recording was seen in 36 participants. Most frequently ST segment changes were found. 5.3% showed bradycardia, 6.4% I° AV blocks (which were of more than 240 ms duration in only one case) and 4.3% intraventricular blocks. In 7.4% ECG signs consistent with an old transmural myocardial infarction were detected.

Looking at the total number of prescribed drugs for the 127 participants, only seven took exclusively a glycoside. In 33 people, three drugs were prescribed and in seven eight different medications were prescribed. About 80% therefore had two or more drugs in addition to their glycoside. The intake of diuretics was found to be low at only 16%, and vasodilators were not prescribed at all.

Only 46% of the 127 participants, knew the reason for their digitalis use. In an investigation by Schwartz et al. [14] of 178 chronically ill ambulatory patients, 59% had made mistakes in taking their medications. Most frequently the drug was omitted several times. This was seen particularly in those patients who did not know the reason for their drug use and who were prescribed several drugs at the same time.

Finally the prevalence of hypertension in our sub-sample has to be mentioned. Slightly more than 20% revealed hypertensive blood values and 30% presented with borderline pressure (BP). In the Framingham study [10] hypertension preceded in 75% of patients who developed congestive heart failure over a period of 16 years and were initially free of that disease. It is suggested that controlling these patients for their high BP would lead to a reduction in the need for digitalis.

Conclusions

1. The number of about 4 million patients using digitalis as calculated from figures of medication intake appear to be accurate.
2. The large proportion of patients over 60 years of age with beginning renal impairment necessitates digitalis dosages adjusted for creatinine clearance [11].
3. A large proportion of patients do not seem to take their medication regularly.
4. Compliance could be improved if all patients knew the reason for their digitalis prescription.

References

1. Bodem G, Ochs HR, Meyer R, Baur MP (1979) Prospektive Untersuchungen zur Digitalistherapie von Patienten bei der Klinikaufnahme. Z Kardiol 68:41–49
2. Clasen R, Kemmeter H, Gilfrich HJ (1979) Biologische Verfügbarkeit von Digoxin und Beta-Acetyldigoxin nach Einmalapplikation. Dtsch Med Wochenschr 104:543–546
3. Cockcroft DW, Gault MH (1976) Prediction of creatinine clearance from serum creatinine. Nephron 16:31–41
4. Flasch H (1982) Nebenwirkungshäufigkeit bei der Digitalistherapie. Therapiewoche 32:6235–6242
5. Friebel H (1982) Arzneimittelverbrauch. Ein Vergleich der Verbrauchssituation in einigen europäischen Ländern. Dtsch Apotheker Z 15:815–818
6. Isbary J, Doering W, Roth F, König E (1983) Senkung der Intoxikationsrate durch individuelle Glykosiddosierung. Herz Kreisl 10:479–485
7. Johnston GD, McDevitt DG (1980) Epidemiology of plasma digoxin concentrations in three patient populations. Ir J Med 149:43–48
8. Larbig D (1981) Aktuelle Digitalistherapie – klinische Gesichtspunkte. Arztl Forsch 28:3–14
9. Lichey J, Schröder R, Rietbrock N (1977) Aktuelle Plasma-Digoxinkonzentration von Patienten bei Krankenhausaufnahme. Dtsch Med Wochenschr 102:1056–1060
10. McKee P, Castelli WP, McNamara PM, Kannel WB (1971) The natural history of congestive heart failure: The Framingham study. N Engl J Med 285:1441–1446
11. Rietbrock N, Alken RG (1980) Die Therapie der Herzinsuffizienz mit Digitalis. Dtsch Med Wochenschr 105:1622–1628
12. Schaumann W, Glocke M, Kaufmann B (1981) Berechnung der voraussichtlichen Erhaltungsdosen von Metildigoxin und Digoxin aus Geschlecht, Körpergewicht, Alter und Serumkreatinin. Herz Kreisl 7:349–358
13. Schüren KP, Rietbrock N (1982) Digitalisbehandlung in Deutschland. Beispiel einer unkritischen Arzneimittelverordnung. Dtsch Med Wochenschr 107:1935–1938
14. Schwartz D, Wang M, Feitz L, Goss MEW (1962) Medication errors made by elderly, chronically ill patients. Am J Public Health 52:2018–2026
15. Stieber J, Döring A, Keil U (1982) Häufigkeit, Bekanntheits- und Behandlungsgrad der Hypertonie in einer Großstadtbevölkerung. MMW 124:747–752

Part II

Special Groups for Primary Health Care

A. Maternal and Child Care

Some Relevant Ecological Factors and Their Influence on Pregnancy

M. Nikolić, M. Gec, G. Nikolić, and G. Sbutega

Introduction

Aircraft noise has been reported to have remarkable physiological effects, especially because of its level and frequency [1, 2]. Our previous investigations have shown a significant influence on the performance of mental tasks, and it was clear that the effects of the noise varied with the sex, age and emotional stability of each person examined [3]. There is evidence that noise may also be a risk factor in pregnancy. The effects of noise at the place of work are well-known [4], and our own observations under experimental conditions were remarkable in showing far more deaths among the young of guinea pigs subjected to noise stress [5, 6]. The influence of aircraft noise on the course of pregnancy and the state of newborns has been investigated by Japanese authors [7], who found changes in newborns when mothers were exposed to noise. The main task of this paper is to evaluate how great is the effect of noise on pregnancy in relation to other factors.

Methods

This study was conducted in a small suburban community, a few kilometres from Belgrade airport. Aircraft noise was measured by standard methodology in the years 1975, 1979 and 1983 [8]. This involved the use of moving apparatus (Brüel and Kjaer) which registered the noise level and made logarithmic recordings.

The 108 women who delivered babies between May 1979 and May 1982 were interviewed in their homes. Socioeconomic information was recorded, as well as some factors related to health behaviour. Conditions of life were inspected and special attention was paid to the women's attitude of the aircraft noise.

Primary Health Care in the Making
Ed. by U. Laaser, R. Senault, H. Viefhues

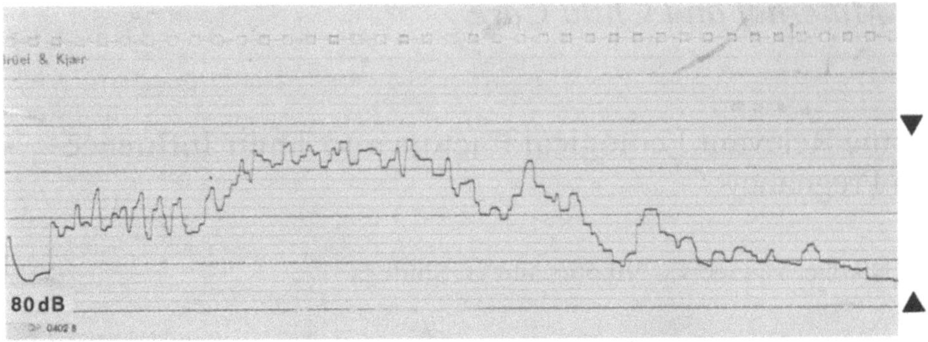

Fig. 1. Aircraft noise near to Belgrade airport

Table 1. Attitude of pregnant women to noise exposure ($n = 108$)

Attitude	%
Does not make me nervous	33
Makes me anxious	24
Makes me irritable	43
Total	100

Table 2. Harmful effects of noise on pregnant women ($n = 100$)

Effects on	%
Hearing alone	13
Nerves alone	34
Both	42
Pregnancy	7
Other	4
Total	100

Results

Estimation of the aircraft noise near to Belgrade airport showed that levels were between 80 and 103 dB in 1983 (Fig. 1). The frequency of overflights was every 5 min.

The personal reaction of pregnant women is displayed in Table 1. Thirty-six women (33.3%) said that noise did not make them nervous. Anxious behaviour was established in 46 women, and 26 said that noise made them quick-tempered. In terms of the effect of the noise on health, a majority of the women (89%) considered that noise has a bad influence on nerves and hearing. Less of them considered that pregnancy may be interfered with (Table 2). As far as personal attitudes to the noise are concerned, the outstanding feature was that 40% of the women were afraid of an aircraft crashing owing to the fact that the runway is close to their homes.

Discussion

The results of noise measurement showed that the level was above that recognized as acceptable for a community, so one would expect it to be an annoying factor. It is quite clear that the noise level around Belgrade airport did not change between 1975 and 1979 [8].

From the subjective reactions of pregnant women, one would expect objective and physiological responses and changes that could be risk factors for the course of pregnancy.

Only a prospective analysis would provide more reliable data which could estimate the influence of noise on the health of pregnant women.

Acknowledgements. This study was supported by a grant from the Republic Association of Science of the SR of Serbia.

References

1. Zondek B, Tari J (1967) Effects of auditory stimuli on reproduction. Ciba Found Study Group 26:4–7
2. Osada Y, Yoshida K, Tshunashima S, Hirokawa K, Nakamura K, Okokubo C, Haruta K (1972) Influence of sex and age on the physiological responses to intermittent noise. Bull Inst Public Health 21/1:14–19
3. Nikolić M (1976) Methodology of noise investigation in urban conditions with relation to health of population. Thesis, School of Medicine, University of Belgrade
4. Ivković C (1978) Utjecaj buke na fertilnu sposobnost žena u tekstilnoj industriji. XII GAN SLD, Zb Rad:132–136
5. Perunović M, Paunović J, Milković K (1975) Uticaj stresa bukom na trudne ženke i ponašanje štakora. Perinatalni dani, Zagreb, Zbornik:103
6. Peruzović M, Milković K (1975) Utjecaj stresa na tjek trudnoće i razvitak mladunčadi štakora. Perinatalni dani, Zagreb, Zbornik:285
7. Audo J, Hattari H (1973) Statistical studies of the effects of intense noise during human fetal life. 27/1:101–107
8. Pravica P, Nikolić M, Savićević M, Kušić S, Pjerotić Lj, Plavšić Z, Petrović N, Budisavljević M (1979) VII Kongres Prv Med, Bled, Zbornik rezimea:T_8

Some Maternal and Social Factors in Relation to the Birth Weight of Infants

M. Gec, M. Nikolić, V. Sulovic, and G. Sbutega

Introduction

This investigation was a part of a study designed to measure the impact of air craft noise on the course and outcome of pregnancy. Although there is evidence for the importance of noise as a determinant of the course and outcome of pregnancy [1, 2], it continues to be difficult to establish direct correlations under the conditions of various ecological influences.

Because newborn birth weight is often used as an indicator of the successful outcome of pregnancy, attempts are very often made to explain variability in birth weight on the basis of maternal and environmental factors [3–5]. The task of this paper was to investigate the relationship between birth weight and maternal age, years of education, cigarette smoking, gestational age and maternal body measures. Quantification of the impact of these factors on human reproductive performance is important for better planning of preventive measures.

Methods

Sample

This study, which was part of an "Aircraft noise and Pregnancy" project, was conducted in a small suburban community a few kilometres from Belgrade airport. The number of births during the previous 3 years was established (May 1979 to May 1982), and an attempt was made to contact every woman who delivered a baby during this period.

Subjects

The 107 women for whom data were available ranged in age from 17 to 43, with a mean of 24.4 ± 4.54 years. Pregnant women had 8.9 ± 3.62 years education on average. The mean number of persons in the household was 5.3 ± 2.4. Fifty-two women smoked during pregnancy and the mean number of cigarettes per day being 15.1 ± 8.43.

Primary Health Care in the Making
Ed. by U. Laaser, R. Senault, H. Viefhues

Data Collection

Subjects were interviewed in their homes. Socioeconomic information was recorded, as well as some factors concerning health behaviour. Obstetric information such as birth weight of the baby, weight at first clinic visit and delivery weight based on weight at last clinic visit before delivery was obtained from physicians' records. Weight gain was calculated. Information on smoking was obtained to determine whether the women had smoked during pregnancy and the amount smoked.

Statistical Analysis

Statistical analysis were performed using simple linear correlation tests. The significance of correlations was determined using *t*-transformation.

Results

There was a significant positive correlation ($r = 0.623$, $P < 0.01$) between birth weight of the infant and delivery weight of the mother. There was a potential correlation between birth weight and initial weight ($r = 0.209$, $P < 0.10$) and weight gain ($r = 0.207$, $P < 0.10$) (Table 1). Birth weights of the 107 infants ranged from 1.950 to 4.800 g, with a mean of 3.314 ± 591 g. Mean weight gain during pregnancy was 10.6 ± 2.51 kg.

When simple correlation tests were performed, initial weight and weight gain were highly correlated ($P < 0.05$) with delivery weight. The number of weeks of gestation was significantly and positively correlated with birth weight ($r = 0.431$, $P < 0.01$) (Table 1). From the results it is obvious that the length of gestation had positive effects on the weight gain and delivery weight also ($P < 0.05$).

Table 1. Results of simple linear correlation analysis to determine the relationship between birth weight and maternal factors

Maternal factors	Birth wt.	Age	Initial wt.	Wt. gain	Delivery wt.	Pregnancies	Weeks of gestation	No. in household	Years of education
Age	−0.02								
Initial wt.	0.21	0.25							
Wt. gain	0.21	0.19	−0.20						
Delivery wt.	0.62**	0.11	0.34*	0.27*					
Pregnancies	−0.02	−0.04	0.15	0.22	0.25				
Weeks of gestation	0.43**	−0.25	0.17	0.27*	0.33*	−0.16			
No. in household	−0.19	−0.13	−0.05	−0.07	0.13	0.44**	−0.22		
Years of education	0.03	0.02	0.01	−0.03	−0.02	−0.34*	−0.02	−0.13	
No. of cigarettes	−0.26*	0.01	−0.05	−0.16	−0.24	−0.06	−0.13	−0.18	−0.20

* $P<0.05$; ** $P<0.01$

Smoking was negatively related to birth weight ($r = -0.259$, $P < 0.05$), with a possible effect on delivery weight of the mother ($r = -0.245$, $P < 0.10$). The mean birth weight of the infants of the 52 women who reported smoking during pregnancy was 3,158 ± 528, significantly less ($P < 0.05$) than the mean birth weight of 3,408 ± 690 g for infants of women who said that they did not smoke during pregnancy. Mean weight gain during pregnancy was 10.3 ± 5.3 kg for smokers and 11.2 ± 4.9 kg for nonsmokers ($P < 0.10$). Some socioeconomic factors, as age, population residence, education were not found to be significant.

Discussion

Previous investigators have reported that mother's weight gain and prepregnant weight are the two strongest influences on birth weight [6, 7]. In this case delivery weight, which is in function of prepregnant weight and weight gain was the variable selected. That means whereas it is optimal to enter pregnancy in well nourished state, sufficient weight gain during pregnancy leading to an increased delivery weight is important to the outcome, also. In this study, delivery weight was the most consistent measure of maternal size, because initial weight was determined at various times during the first three months of pregnancy. Gestational age has been used in previous investigations [8] and was discovered to have positive relationship to birth weight.

Many studies have related smoking during pregnancy to low birth weight. Our results indicate the same relationship, though the sample was small. Rush (9) pointed out some of the effects of smoking on birth weight to a deppression in caloric intake as reflected by lower maternal weight gain. The same trend was found in this study. Smokers gained less weight, but, it was difficult to show a significant effect.

Caution must be exercised when interpreting the above results, because correlation coefficients do not necessarily indicate a causal relationship between factors. So, we can conclude that improving nutrition of the mother is important in increasing birth weight. In addition, the effect of smoking may, also, be mediated by lowered weight gain. Educational programs emphasizing the relationship between these significant variables and birth weight could be extremely valuable.

Acknowledgements. This study was supported by a grant from the Republic Association of Science of the SR of Serbia.

References

1. Osada Y, Yoshida K, Tsunashima S, Ogawa S, Hirokawa K, Nakamura K, Okokubo C, Haruta K (1972) Influence of sex and age on the physiological responses to intermittent noise. Bull Inst Public Health 21/1:14–19
2. Zondek B, Tamari J (1967) Effects of auditory stimuli on reproduction. Ciba Found Study Group 26:4–7
3. O'Sullivan JB, Gellis SS, Tenney BO (1965) Aspects of birth weight and its influencing variables. Am J Obstet Gynecol 92:1023–1026
4. Weiss W, Jackson EC (1969) Maternal factors affecting birth weight. In: Perinatal factors affecting human development. PAHO Sci Publ no 185, Washington, DC, pp 54–55
5. Lewis R, Charles M, Pathwary KM (1973) Relationship between birth weight and selected social, environmental and medical care factors. Am J Public Health 63:973–979
6. Aninger W, Bauer P (1974) Relations of infant weight, placental weight and weight and height of the mother. Arch Gynecol 217:69–83
7. Simpson JW, Lowles RW, Mitchell AC (1975) Responsibility of the obstetrician to the fetus. 2. Influence of prepregnancy weight and pregnancy weight gain on birth weight. Am J Obstet Gynecol 45/5:481–487
8. Cagini P (1977) Intrauterine growth evaluated from birth weight and duration of gestation: Relation to different risk factors. Minerva Pediatr 29:10–15
9. Rush D (1974) Examination of the relationship between birth weight, cigarette smoking during pregnancy and maternal weight gain. J Obstet Gynecol Br Commonw 81:746–752

The Diagnosis of "Minimal Brain Dysfunction" – Implications for Social Medicine*

M. H. Schmidt and G. Esser

As in other psychological-medical disciplines, efforts are being made in child psychiatry to devise a system of classifying the observed disorders according to their aetiology. Where this goal cannot be achieved, classification based on the involved organs is attempted, in order to advance from the lowest possible nosological level of merely defining symptoms or syndromes. In line with this general intention, various behavioural disorders of children (and, in particular, of school-age children) are often regarded as different aspects of a single common syndrome which is associated with functions of the central nervous system. Besides providing satisfactory frameworks for physicians involved in diagnosis and treatment, this way of classification is also welcomed by parents since it meets their frequent desire for causal explanations. Parents are in an extremely difficult situation when they are confronted with their child's symptoms and cannot be given answers as to their causes and origins. Such a lack of information often encourages them to disregard seemingly unspecific therapeutic directions – especially if more parental efforts are called for than merely supervising the application of a prescribed drug. As long as it remains unclear to what extent, by which means and even whether at all parents' reactions can influence their child's problem behaviour they have no reason to respond to the symptomatic behaviour in a specific manner. Thus, such parental non-compliance is in the final analysis based on our present inability to satisfy their understandable demand for causal explanations.

The above considerations provided the setting for our reflections on the social-medical significance of research results concerning the justification of the minimal brain dysfunction (MBD) diagnosis. Before evaluating the findings of several relevant epidemiological studies, we would like to point out that these investigations were originally expected to support the MBD concept and to underpin its implications. As shall be seen, the results are in contrast with the tested hypotheses, representing one of the rare occasions where the original assumptions are falsified.

Our results originate from an epidemiological project investigating the prevalence, dimensionality and significance of cerebral dysfunction in school-age children. Subjects studied belonged to a representative sample of 400 8-year-old children living in Mannheim. In addition, we investigated a clinical

---

* We thank our colleague Dipl.-Psych. W. Woerner for translating this paper from German

Primary Health Care in the Making
Ed. by U. Laaser, R. Senault, H. Viefhues

sample of 100 8-year-old out-patients of the child psychiatric clinic of the Zentralinstitut für Seelische Gesundheit.

For many decades, milder forms of infantile cerebral palsy have been regarded as sequelae of so-called minimal brain damage. In the early 60s, however, British child neurologists recommended that the term be discarded and replaced by minimal brain dysfunction. This suggestion represented a step backwards in the development of clinical classification, as an aetiologically oriented term was dismissed in favour of a merely organ-oriented one. Nevertheless, this conclusion seemed justified on account of the observed weakness of associations between brain damage and brain dysfunction: Confirmed brain damage without brain dysfunction was found just as frequently as functional brain disorders without demonstrable brain lesions.

In clinical practice, however, traumatic, inflammatory and toxic brain injuries continued to be connected with the term cerebral dysfunction. American and German publications (e.g., Strauss, Göllnitz, Lempp and Corboz) describing uniform psychopathological consequences after infantile minimal brain damage spread the belief in the existence of a specific syndrome. The various aspects thought to be involved included facultative neuroanatomical, neurophysiological, neuropsychological, anamnestical and developmental abnormalities, along with an obligatory behavioural cluster referred to as the infantile brain organic psychosyndrome in a narrow sense. It was generally agreed that this syndrome represented a risk factor for the development of child psychiatric disorders.

The causal nature of this model along with the high prevalence rates of the described syndrome as reported for unselected samples led to its application to various childhood disorders. The facultative status of many symptoms within the syndrome facilitated this extension of the concept. Child psychiatrists, somewhat more cautiously also child neurologists, but, above all, paediatricians and general practitioners made use of the concept and seemed to confirm the high prevalence rates of minimal brain dysfunction. On the other hand, critical voices were also raised. Several investigations questioned the uniform psychopathology, and others objected to the circular reasoning used when defining the syndrome or criticized the large variability of the reported prevalence rates, which ranged from 2% to 18%.

Although originally we had no intention of questioning the concept, our results demonstrated an extremely low extent of overlap among neurophysiological, neuropsychological and behavioural signs typically constituting the MBD diagnosis. Over 90% of the children with neurophysiological abnormalities failed to show specific skill deficiencies and vice versa. Occurrence rates of the genuine syndrome are probably as low as 1% in random samples and no higher than 4%–7% in clinical samples. The postulated association between cerebral dysfunction and psychiatric disorders was confirmed, but was confined to the correlation of psychiatric disorders and specific skill deficiencies. Behavioural patterns in the sense of a brain organic psychosyndrome may possibly be present in a small core group of children but not in the vast majority of subjects to whom the term of minimal brain dysfunction has been applied owing to undue generalization and extension of diagnostic criteria.

With respect to clinical practice, an alteration of present diagnostic strategies is inferred from our results. In the absence of performance deficiencies, neurophysiological methods can be entirely dispensed with, since neurophysiological disorders by themselves contribute little towards explaining behavioural symptoms.

When counselling parents, we are no longer able to offer them the conclusive causal model. This will presumably lead to increasing emphasis on the responsibility of other – genetically or socially determined – factors in the development of behavioural disorders. On the other hand, the dangers of stigmatization will be reduced for many children. Well-proven therapeutic methods such as psychoeducational training programmes and the application of stimulant drugs to hyperactive children will be maintained, even though the notion of cerebral alterations can no longer serve as a rationale for stimulant drug therapy. Furthermore, parent–child interactions will necessarily become more incorporated into therapeutic practice. Here, the prevention of parental guilt feelings is one point deserving serious consideration. At the same time, the stronger responsibility experienced by parents may provide a better chance to change their child-rearing behaviour. These counselling tasks cannot be left to child psychiatrists alone, but should rather be accomplished by primary health care agents such as general practitioners and school psychologists.

A newly arising problem concerns the cost settlements by health insurance bodies. Until now, the cost of educational training programmes has been met by health insurance only if underlying organic causes could be assumed. In the future, this claim will be restricted to the genuine MBD group, leaving the large number of children with learning disorders without financial support. While a certain amount of expenditure for medical diagnostics will be economized by limiting their application to this core group, the distribution of insurance liabilities with respect to psychoeducational and medical intervention will have to be reconsidered in general.

The loss of causative explanations remains unsatisfactory, not only to parents. Simpler approaches towards explaining psychological disorders having failed, research efforts must now center on the development of new, more complex models of pathogenesis. One of the areas calling for elucidation concerns the relations between hereditary factors, organic risks and parent–child interactions. Due to the extreme difficulty of assessing genetic factors with our currently available methods, future research will concentrate on the connections between organic risk factors and conditions of socialization which need to be assessed in a differentiated and detailed manner. Such an approach would also lead to the formulation of preventive psychohygienic means of improving parent–child interactions.

B. Childhood and Adolescence

Physical Fitness of Obese Children and Its Relationship to Age, Sex and Nutritional Intake

L. Neradović, D. Plećaš, and M. Havelka

Introduction

Physical activity is essential for a child's somatic and emotional health [10], but the fact is that obese children have a low level of leisure time physical activity [1, 8]. The actual level of physical activity is difficult to measure accurately [4, 13], and the measurement of physical work capacity (PWC) can be used to define the range from the obese to the non-obese children indirectly.

This study aimed to examine the relationship of fitness to other anthropometric and nutritional factors, and to measure physical fitness in obese children in the course of dietary therapy.

Materials and Methods

Forty-five obese girls and 27 obese boys from 8 to 17.4 years of age and attending primary and high schools in Belgrade were studied. Thirty normal weight girls and 20 normal weight boys of the same age were tested as a control group.

Height and weight were measured by a standard technique [11]. Obesity was defined by relative body weight (RBW) $\geq$ 120% and when the percentage of body weight as fat (BWF) was 2 SD above the mean according to age and sex [3]. RBW was calculated on the basis of the difference between the real weight and the ideal weight that a child and an adolescent should have for their height, according to the tables by Jelliffe [6]. The skinfold thickness (SFT) was measured at the right mid-biceps, triceps, subscapular and supra-iliac sites with the child standing, using John Bull calipers. From the score of the four SFT measurements, BWF was calculated using a method based on densiometric studies [3]. PWC was performed on a mechanically braked bicycle ergometer, and a standard calibration procedure was used [12].

A 4-day dietary record was kept by each child. From the dietary records analyses were made of the protein, fat, carbohydrate and food energy content using standard tables [2]. The data elements were analysed using the coefficients of correlation [7].

Primary Health Care in the Making
Ed. by U. Laaser, R. Senault, H. Viefhues

Results

The levels of PWC 150 and 170 according to age group for normal weight boys and girls are shown in Table 1 and Fig. 1. The boys' PWC was greater than that of the girls of the same age and increased rapidly from 11.5 to 17.4 years.

Table 2 and Fig. 2 show that the obese boys' PWC was greater than that of obese girls of the same age group, and, in general, PWC for obese boys and girls was significantly smaller than that for the normal weight boys and girls.

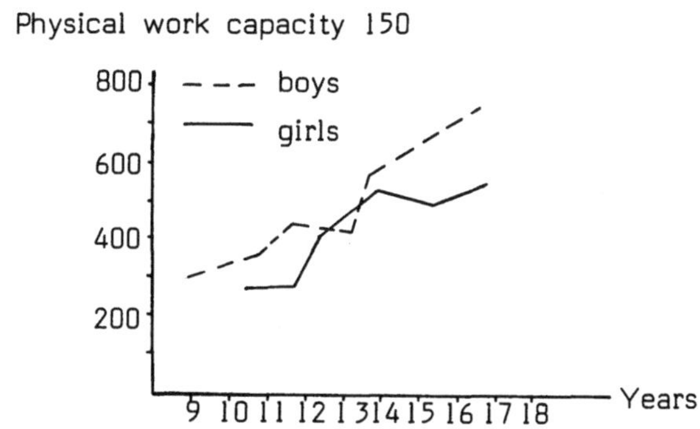

Fig. 1. The physical work capacity according to age and sex in normal weight boys and girls

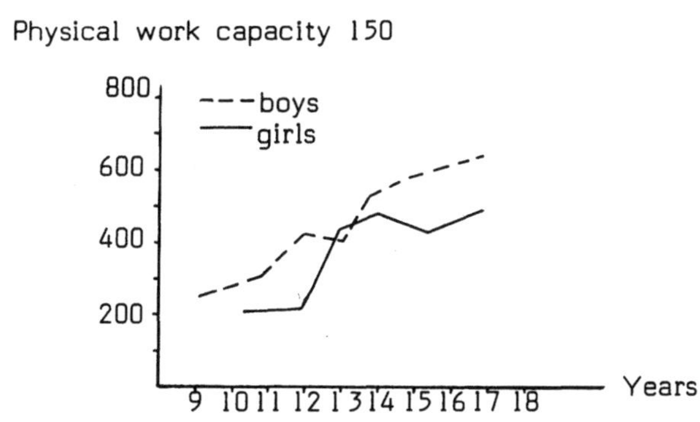

Fig. 2. The physical work capacity according to age and sex in obese boys and girls

Table 1. The mean values ±SD for physical working capacity (PWC) at a pulse rate of 150 and 170 in normal weight children and adolescents

Age group (years)		PWC	150	PWC	170
8.0–11.4	Boys (6)	324	±102		
	Girls (10)	276	±109		
11.5–14.4	Boys (6)	450	±108	649	±112
	Girls (10)	397	±126	660	±135
14.5–17.4	Boys (8)	687	±177	836	±136
	Girls (10)	459	±128	574	±166

Table 2. The mean values ± SD for physical working capacity (PWC) at a pulse rate of 150 and 170 in obese children and adolescents

Age groupe (years)		PWC	150	PWC	170
8.0–11.4	Boys (8)	309	± 83		
	Girls (15)	273	± 68		
11.5–14.4	Boys (10)	404	± 101	589	± 102
	Girls (15)	287	± 127	615	± 125
14.5–17.4	Boys (9)	654	± 164	798	± 124
	Girls (15)	441	± 120	547	± 145

Table 3. Coefficients of correlation between PVC 150 and SFT, according to sex and age group

Age group	Obese				Normal weight			
(years)	Boys	(*n*)	Girls	(*n*)	Boys	(*n*)	Girls	(*n*)
8.0–11.4	–0.73**	(8)	–0.44*	(15)	–0.43	(6)	–0.18	(10)
11.5–14.4	–0.49*	(10)	–0.23	(15)	–0.29	(6)	–0.17	(10)
14.5–17.4	–0.33	(9)	–0.59	(15)	–0.25	(8)	–ö0.39	(10)

* $P<0.01$; ** $P<0.001$

Table 4. The coefficients of correlation between PWC 150 and daily energy, protein, fat and carbohydrate intake in obese and normal weight boys and girls

Obese		Normal weight		Controlling for:
Boys (27)	Girls (45)	Boys (20)	Girls (30)	
0.54	0.53	0.11	0.15	Protein intake
–0.49	–0.49	–0.25	–0.13 (NS)	Energy intake
0.06	–0	0	0.07	Fat intake
0.02	0	0	0.05	Carbohydrate intake

* $P<0.01$; * $P<0.001$

The PWC 150 was negatively correlated with the SFT score (for obese boys $r - 0.73$, $r - 0.49$; for obese girls $r - 0.44$), indicating that the fat children were less fit than the normal weight children of the same age group ($P < 0.01$, $P < 0.001$) (Table 3).

The relationship between PWC 150 and nutritional intake is shown in Table 4. There was an overall inverse relationship between PWC 150 and the daily food energy intake (for obese boys and girls $r - 0.49$; $P < 0.01$ and $P < 0.001$). This suggested that the fitter children ate less than those who are less fit. The daily protein intake was positively associated with the PWC 150 ($r+0.54$, $r+0.53$; $P<0.01$ and $P<0.001$). There was no relationship between PWC and carbohydrate and fat intake.

Summary

The report aimed to investigate the usefulness of determining PWC as an indirect measurement of fitness. According to our experience with obese children, we may conclude the following: PWC was greater in normal weight boys and girls of the same age. Fat children were less fit than normal weight children. There was an overall inverse relationship between PWC and the daily food energy intake. The daily energy protein intake was positively associated with PWC. Carbohydrate and fat intake was negatively associated with PWC. This suggests that PWC could be used in controlling the actual level of physical activity in obese children, and as a measure in the course of dietary therapy.

References

1. Borgeson M (1962) Overweight children. Acta Pediatr Scand [Suppl] 132:59
2. Brodarec A (1979) Tables of composition of foods. Pliva, Zagreb
3. Brook CGD (1971) Determination of body composition from skinfold measurement. Arch Dis Child 46:182
4. Cullens KJ, Week PT (1978) Sporting activity and exercise habits of the 1975 Buselton population. Med J Aust 1:69
5. Cumming GR, Keynes R (1967) A fitness performance test for school children and its correlation with PWC and Max O_2. Can Med Assoc J 96:1262
6. Jelliffe BB (1969) Appreciation de l'etat nutritionel des populationes. OMS, Geneva
7. Nie NA, Hull CH, Jenkins JG (1975) Statistical package for the social sciences, 2nd edn. McGraw-Hill, New York
8. Mocellin R, Rutenfranz J (1971) Investigation of the physical working capacity of obese children. Acta Paediatr Scand [Suppl] 217:138
9. Montoue HJ, Frantz MF, Kozar AJ (1972) The values of age, height, and weight in establishing standards of fitness for children. J Sports Med Phys Fitness 12:174
10. Rose CL, Cohen ML (1977) Relative importance of physical activity for longevity. Ann NY Acad Sci 301:671
11. Simić BS (1977) Medical dietetics. Belgrad 78
12. Van Döblen W (1954) A simply bicycle ergometer. J Appl Physiol 1:222
13. Williams M (1979) Fitness testing for adolescents and young adults. Aust Fam Physician 8:279

Knowledge, Habits and Standpoints of Novi Sad Adolescents in Relation to Cardiovascular Diseases and Possibilities of Their Prevention as Part of a Comprehensive Community Cardiovascular Control Programme

B. Legetić, M. Planojević, V. Grujić, and J. Pisarev

Cardiovascular diseases (CVDs) form the major public health problem in the industrialised world. It is a fact that the incidence of these diseases is very high in Yugoslavia, and especially in the province of Vojvodina. In 1976 Novi Sad, the capital of Vojvodina, joined the Comprehensive Community Cardiovascular Control Programme under the auspices of the WHO, as a pilot area. Since that time effective methods have been developed to reduce the CVD risk among adults, and in the last year interest has been directed to the programme for adolescents. The main interest was how the risk factors developed in childhood and whether their development could be influenced. Early adolescence is the age when it might be possible to teach young people how to maintain their health and live free of major disease in the future. The aims of this programme are:

- To examine the knowledge, habits and standpoints of Novi Sad adolescents (14–15 years of age) towards CVDs
- To obtain epidemiological information about the cardiovascular risk factors
- To establish the health education programme in all elementary schools (42), working with children, parents and teachers
- To evaluate a comprehensive community intervention programme concerning the reduction and prevention of CVD risk factors

This paper concerns only the knowledge, habits and standpoints of Novi Sad adolescents (14–15 years of age) in relation to CVDs. The questionnaire (which was anonymous) consisted of 27 questions and was completed by 500 adolescents (about 20% of all those aged 14–15). The questions were divided into three groups. The first group was drawn up to show the adolescents' knowledge of the anatomy and physiology of the cardiovascular system and the main risk factors. The second group of questions considered the different opinions on the treatment of CVDs and possibilities of their prevention. The third group of questions was about habits (smoking, nutrition, physical activity, alcohol consumption etc.) and about personality structure.

Results

Of the 2424 adolescents aged 14–15 years in Novi Sad, 500 completed the questionnaire. Of these 500, 51% were boys and 49% girls.

Primary Health Care in the Making
Ed. by U. Laaser, R. Senault, H. Viefhues

First Group of Questions

About 90% of adolescents had some knowledge of the anatomy and physiology of the cardiovascular system. In addition:

- 56% of those tested knew what atherosclerosis is.
- 84.8% of those tested knew what blood pressure is.
- 97% of those tested knew what diabetes mellitus is.
- 77.4% of those tested knew what stress is.

On the other hand, 80.8% of the examined pupils could not mention any of the risk factors for CVDs.

Second Group of Questions

About 60% of adolescents thought that their health is good, but 21.6% considered themselves able to do a lot to improve it. It is interesting to note that about 75% of adolescents thought that most CVDs can be prevented.

It can be seen from Table 1 that about 20% of the adolescents smoked cigarettes either every day or occasionally. Table 2 shows the percentages of those investigated who were classified as very active, active or non-active. The very active were considered to be those who go in for sports at least four times a week, while active were those who ride a bicycle or play football or basketball during their free time. The non-active are those who watch TV, read and sleep during their free time. About one-third of adolescents are very active, one-third active and one-third non-active. This finding is not favourable, because at that age they should almost all be very active or active.

Table 3 shows that about 60% of families used vegetable oils, and the rest animal fats.

Alcohol consumption is shown in Table 4. It was noticed that the number of children who smoked was significantly higher among those who also consumed alcohol.

Observing the personality structure of the questioned adolescents, it is noticeable that more than 50% considered themselves responsible, about 10% very frequently got angry, and almost 27% tried to act as though nothing had happened. 8.6% claimed that they have no real friends, and 34% thought it is hard to say.

Table 1. Percentage of regular smokers, occasional smokers, ex-smokers, and non-smokers among Novi Sad adolescents

	%
Regular smokers	8.0
Occasional smokers	12.8
Ex-smokers	19.6
Non-smokers	59.6

Table 2. Percentages of very active, active, and non-active Novi Sad adolescents

	%
Very active	35.2
Active	36.4
Non-active	28.4

Table 3. Percentages of adolescents using visible fats and sweets in their food

Answers	Fats (%)	Sweets (%)
Yes	36.3	98.6
No	63.6	1.4

Table 4. Alcohol consumption

Answers	%
Yes	14.4
No	85.6

This investigation showed that the adolescents of Novi Sad would be a good base for a health education programme that is planned for the forthcomming period. After 2 years of intervention the same questionnaire and the same survey will be carried out. The same sample will be examined. We hope to present the results of the programme at one of the future meetings.

Review of the Results and Recommendations of the Cologne Study

U. Laaser and P. Allhoff

In 1975 6302 15- to 19-year-old adolescents of 8252 (76.4%) attending all high schools and 10% of vocational schools in Cologne were medically examined in order to determine their cardiovascular risk profile. About a year later in 1976 3004 of 3692 (81.4%) remaining students at those schools were examined again. In 1980 a second follow-up was carried out on 1342 of 2018 (66.5%) attainable former students.

Results

1. Adequate preventive examinations of adolescents in schools with a participation rate of 75% can be carried through without great difficulty.
2. A follow-up examination with sufficient participation can be organized, even after the students have left school and in part moved to other cities. The range of the follow-up essentially depends on the funds available.
3. A cardiovascular risk profile in adolescents can reliably be determined by simple methods taking into consideration eight parameters (systolic and diastolic blood pressure, heart rate, total cholesterol, serum urine acid, postprandial serum glucose, body mass index and smoking).
4. To determine the most important laboratory values, taking capillary blood is sufficient. Quality control of blood pressure measurements is possible similar to the procedures used for laboratory examinations.
5. Increased values of the examined risk parameters from a clinical point of view are also significantly frequent among adolescents.
6. The most important risk parameters (especially systolic and diastolic blood pressure, total cholesterol, cigarette smoking and the body mass index) prove to be relatively stable over a total examination period of 5 years; this is especially true for elevated values.
7. Applying multivariate statistical procedures, all three examinations show an unexpectedly high association among elevated risk parameters. The summary of the analyses carried through hitherto permits the characterization of potential risk groups, the composition of which remains relatively stable during the whole period of examinations. With regard to these risk groups, it should be noted that:

Primary Health Care in the Making
Ed. by U. Laaser, R. Senault, H. Viefhues

a) Students of vocational schools tend to consume more cigarettes and alcohol, and female students of vocational schools use oral contraceptives more frequently. These behavioural characteristics are traceable through several years after the students have left school.
A more heavily burdened life-style compared with that of high school students may be assumed on the basis of the increase of cholesterol values and the diminished chance of participating in preventive examinations after leaving school.
b) It is characteristic of girls using oral contraceptives that they are heavier smokers, drink more alcohol, and have increased values of total cholesterol and lower values of HDL-cholesterol (standardized for age). With regard to total cholesterol, the risks of young women taking very strong oral contraceptives are especially high.
c) In the case of a positive family history, blood pressure and total cholesterol should be examined at least once while children are growing up.
d) Health education, especially with regard to smoking and drinking behaviour as well as to the use of oral contraceptives, should be intensified in the transitional period between elementary and vocational school.

References

1. Laaser U (1978) Quality controls of blood pressure measurements in the Cologne Study. Acta Cardiol (Brux) 33:80
2. Laaser U (1980) Die Kölner Adoleszentenstudie: Rahmenkonzept und Durchführung. In: Borgers D, Tietze KW (eds) Anwendungsgebiete epidemiologischer Methodik. Berlin, Reimers-Verlag
3. Laaser U, Allhoff P (1982) Prävention im Wachstumsalter: Das kardiovaskuläre Risikoprofil bei Jugendlichen in Köln. Monatsschr Kinderheilkd 130:760
4. Laaser U, Allhoff P (1983) Zur Epidemiologie der Hypertonie bei Adoleszenten: Ergebnisse der Kölner Studie. Arbeitsmed., Sozialmed., Präv. med. 18:153
5. Laaser U, Schütt A (1978) The cardiovascular risk-profile in Cologne; a representative study including 6302 pupils. Z Kardiol 67:837
6. Laaser U, Schütt A (1980) Cardiovascular risk factors in the adolescent population in Cologne. In: Kesteloot H, Joossens JV (eds) Epidemiology of arterial blood pressure. Den Haag, M. Nijhoff-Verlag
7. Laaser U, Roegele F, Meurer KA, Kaufmann W (1977) Die Verbreitung des Nikotinabusus bei Schülern; ein Teilergebnis der Kölner Studie zum kardiovaskulären Risikoprofil bei Jugendlichen. Verh Dtsch Ges Inn Med 83:1727
8. Laaser U, Assmann G, Simantke O, Kaufmann W (1979) HDL-cholesterol and contraception in adolescent girls: The Cologne Study. Trans Eur Soc Cardiol 1:2, 20
9. Laaser U, Allhoff P, Denner A, Lemke P, Schütt A (1982) Kölner Studie zum kardiovaskulären Risikoprofil bei Jugendlichen 1975-76-80. Bonn, BMJFG
10. Schütt A, Laaser U (1980) Risikoaggregation bei Jugendlichen. Untersuchungen mit Hilfe der Konfigurationsfrequenzanalyse. In: Borgers D, Tietze KW (eds) Anwendungsgebiete epidemiologischer Methodik. Berlin, Reimers-Verlag

Analysis of Suicides in Adolescents and Young Adults: Implications for Prevention

S. G. Gerberich, M. Hays, J. S. Mandel, R. W. Gibson, and C. J. Van der Heide

Introduction

Between 1970 and 1978, the suicide rate among United States residents, 15–24 years of age, increased by 41%, from a rate of 8.8/100 000 population in 1970 to 12.4/100 000 in 1978, while the rate for the remainder of the population remained generally stable. In this age group, the increase is associated primarily with an increasing number and rate of suicides among males [1]. Similar increases in the suicide rates have been observed in the State of Minnesota (Fig. 1). Again, this increase is especially evident in the young male.

Throughout the United States, the method of suicide has changed dramatically from 1968 to 1979. While the rate for suicide by firearms increased by 30% during this time, the rate for suicide by all other means decreased by 2%. Moreover, the largest increase was in males, 15–24 years old, whose firearm suicide rate more than doubled [2].

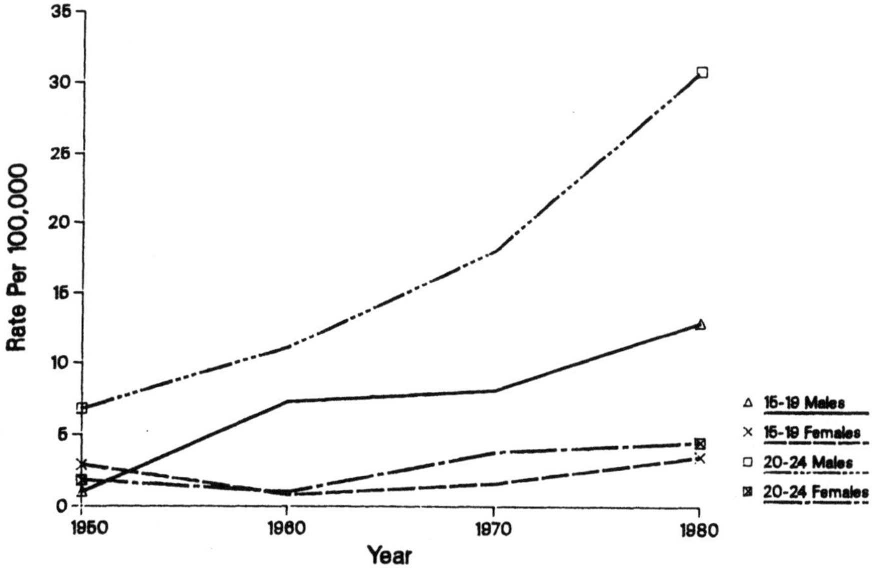

Fig. 1. Suicide death rates by selected age group and sex – Minnesota residents, 1950–1980 (Source: Center for Health Statistics, Minnesota Department of Health, Minneapolis, Minnesota – 1983)

Primary Health Care in the Making
Ed. by U. Laaser, R. Senault, H. Viefhues

In response to these changes, the United States Department of Health and Human Services has established, as a priority, the objective to reduce the rate of suicide among people 15–24 years of age from 12.4 to less than 11 cases per 100 000 population by 1990. To accomplish this, it was determined that further research was needed to explain the marked increase in suicides among young white males and to characterize their deaths more precisely [1].

The purpose of this epidemiological study was to determine the rate of suicides among adolescents and young adults in two large Minnesota counties and to analyze the variables associated with these suicides. In this manner, potential strategies for prevention could be identified more realistically.

Methodology

Following approval to conduct an archival study, by the Committee on Human Subjects in Research at the University of Minnesota, data relevant to all suicide cases that occurred during 1980 and 1981 were abstracted using a specially designed tool that incorporated all case-file data. These cases were identified through the Medical Examiners' offices in Hennepin and Ramsey Counties. Subsequently, these cases were checked against all cases identified by the State Health Department for completeness. Utilization of these two counties accounted for 34% of the total state population. In this portion of the study, 83 cases, ranging in age from 12 to 24 years, were included from a total of 366 cases. Univariate analyses were conducted through computer application, utilizing the Statistical Package for the Social Sciences (SPSS) [3]. To identify a typology of suicide cases, a cluster analysis [4] was conducted. In addition, a preliminary multivariate analysis was done, using a discriminant function technique.

In general, an epidemiological model that considers the interaction of the *host* (or individual), the *agent,* which is transmitted by a *vehicle* or *vector,* and the *environment,* provided a framework for this investigation and subsequent development of strategies.

Host variables include age, sex, genetic, cultural, mental, and physical characteristics. Only some of the host variables relevant to suicides are addressed in this paper.

Agents associated with suicides may include chemical, thermal, mechanical, or electrical energy. Mechanical energy, as an example, is the agent involved in firearm deaths. Transmittal of this energy is facilitated by the vehicle. As opposed to a vector, associated with illness, an example of a vehicle associated with suicides in firearm deaths is the bullet – generated by the gun. Consideration of the vector or vehicle is especially important, since preventive measures are often directed most successfully against the vehicles and vectors rather than against the physical or chemical agents they transmit [5–7].

Conditions within the environment play an important part in the total model. Interactions of the host and agent within the environment determine the final outcome – in this case, suicides.

Results

Of the 83 cases identified between the ages of 12 and 24, 79.5% were males; 86% of all cases were single. While no statistically significant difference in the mean age (19 years) was found in this subgroup between males and females, large differences between the sexes were observed for other variables.

Age and Sex

Through analysis of the data by age and sex for each year, it was noted that males, in particular between the ages of 15 and 19, experienced a significant increase in rate: from 11.0 to 25.2/100 000 population (Table 1).

Race

According to race, 94% were Caucasian; the remaining 6% included Blacks and American Indians. This percentage is not significantly different from the average Minnesota population.

Methods of Suicide

The most frequent methods of suicide were by gunshot, by hanging or strangulation, and by gas; differences in the utilization of these methods between the sexes are shown in Table 2. Through this breakdown, it is seen that gas is the most frequent method used by females, followed by equivalent use of gunshot and drug overdose. In addition, the mode of jumping also accounted for 12% of female cases.

Table 1. Suicide rates[a] by sex and age, 1980–1981

Year/ sex	Age 12–14	15–19	20–24
1980	($n=3$)	($n=10$)	($n=24$)
Male	3.9	11.0	27.9
Female	2.0	4.8	3.8
1981	($n=0$)	($n=21$)	($n=25$)
Male	0.0	25.2	26.6
Female	0.0	7.9	6.3

[a] Cases per 100 000 population

Table 2. Suicide methods by sex, ages 12–24, 1980–1981

Method	Male ($n=66$)	Female ($n=17$)
Gunshot	48.5	23.5
Hanging/strangulation	24.2	5.9
Gas	15.2	29.4
Jumping	4.5	11.8
Overdose	1.5	23.5
Drowning	3.0	0.0
Electrocution	1.5	5.9
Other	1.5	0.0
	99.9	100.0

Table 3. Use of firearms by suicide victims in Minnesota in 1980–1981 by age

Year	Age			Total
	10–14 ($n=3$)	15–19 ($n=31$)	20–24 ($n=49$)	
1980	0	3	9	12
1981	0	10	14	24

A further breakdown of the use of guns by sex and age reveals a much greater percentage of the youths aged 20–24 who used firearms. In addition, it was found that the increase in cases in 1981 was solely associated with the use of firearms (Table 3). Analysis by type of gun indicated that 64% were either rifles or shotguns; only 36% were handguns (Table 4).

Further attention to the most frequent methods of suicide revealed that, in those cases involving drug overdose, 63% involved the use of antidepressants. Furthermore, 50% of these had been prescribed for the individual.

Location of Suicide Action

The primary location of the suicide action was within the home (60%). Other buildings, including hospitals and prisons, accounted for 17%; bridges accounted for 16%. Of interest was the fact that two cases were associated with the Washington Avenue Bridge, which is located in the heart of the University of Minnesota campus. Furthermore, of the total cases involving all ages that were identified during 1980 and 1981, five were associated with this bridge, which has a long history of such cases.

Suicide Note/Previous Attempts and Threats

As shown in Table 5, while approximately 40% of both males and females between the ages of 15 and 19 left a suicide note, a greater percentage of 20- to 24-

Table 4. Type of firearms used in suicides, ages 12–24, 1980–1981

Type of gun ($n=36$)	Percent	
Shotgun	44.4	64.0
Rifle	19.4	
Handgun	36.0	
Total	99.8	

Table 5. Suicide note by sex and age, 1980–1981

Sex	Age		
	12–14	15–19 (Percent)	20–24
Female ($n=17$)	0	38	63
Male ($n=66$)	0	39	41

year-old females left a note. It was further observed that at least[1] 24% of the suicide events were preceded by previous attempts, or parasuicides; 53% of the females and 17% of the males were identified as having at least one previous attempt. In addition, at least 25% of the individuals involved had threatened suicide (females, 29%; males 24%).

Reasons for Suicide Action

Major reasons identified for the suicidal action included: family interaction problems (28%); social interaction problems (24%); break-up with a significant other (24%); isolation/loneliness (39%); and minor violations of the law (11%). These will be discussed subsequently in more detail, relevant to their inclusion in the cluster analysis.

Significant Underlying Conditions

Significant underlying conditions identified from the death certificates indicated that 28% of the suicide cases had underlying mental disorders. Alcohol and/ or other drug use and sexual problems, including homosexuality, were associated with 12% of the cases. Fifty-five percent of the cases were not associated, apparently, with a significant condition. However, these data need to be differentiated from other case-file data that indicated some type of history of drug or alcohol problems accounting for at least 35% and 25%, respectively, of the suicide cases. In addition, at least 40% had some history of mental disorder.

Cluster Analysis

Cluster analysis involved the identification of four significantly different groups of suicide cases ($P < 0.05$) that exhibited similarities in the reasons for suicide, methods used, and age. In Table 6, characteristics of cases in these groups and the original percentages of cases within those groups are identified. Analyses, incorporating variables of previous suicide attempts, the number of attempts, and the history of drug and alcohol problems, cannot be completed until a follow-up study is conducted to complete the information on all cases for these variables. However, the modeling that has been completed to this time reveals the ability to develop typologies of suicide cases that are useful in identifying the underlying variables associated with suicidal behavior. These underlying variables can then be evaluated as to how well they can predict the actual observed type of suicide.

---

[1] Data relevant to previous attempts and previous threats were missing in 64% of the cases

Table 6. Typology[a] of suicide cases

Characteristics		Number/ percent
I.	Mild legal/miscellaneous problems Violent and nonviolent method used, primarily drug overdose Ages 20–24	21 (*25.6*)
II.	Current family/social interaction problems; no history of mental illness or significant underlying condition Violent method used (e.g. firearm, hanging) Not age-dependent	25 (*30.5*)
III.	Current family/social interaction problems Nonviolent method used (e.g., drugs, gas) Not age dependent	19 (*23.2*)
IV.	Interaction problems; history of mental illness Violent method used Ages 20–24	17 (*20.7*)

[a] Derived through use of cluster analysis technique ($p < 0.05$)

Implications for Prevention

Based on both univariate and multivariate analyses, to this time, it is possible to identify *implications for prevention.* Although it is not realistic to believe all suicides can be prevented, it is appropriate to develop strategies that can facilitate reductions in the rates of suicide.

In the realm of injury control and, in this case, prevention of suicide, Haddon's strategies [5–7], developed in the early 1960s, serve as a means for developing realistic strategies for all types of hazard. These strategies are based on considerations of the epidemiological model, whereby the goal is to prevent the energy or other agent from interacting with the host at levels that exceed the injury threshold. Of further importance is consideration of the use of mixed strategies that will benefit the greatest number of people – with priority being given to those strategies that do not involve individual action. Applications of Haddon's strategies [5–7] in the prevention of suicide are presented in Table 7 and discussed in the following.

Applications of these strategies to suicide prevention include limiting the manufacture and/or distribution of firearms. Of particular relevance in this study was the finding that the majority of firearms used were not handguns – as identified in a previous study [8] – but rather shotguns and rifles, which very likely relates to a high utilization of guns in Minnesota for hunting. Therefore, the suggestion that the rise in suicide rate might be controlled by restricting the sale of handguns [9] requires re-evaluation.

In particular, it is essential to involve architects and engineers in designs that facilitate safety. By designing barriers that not only prevent impulsive suicidal acts but also prevent accidents/injuries in general, we can eliminate the

Table 7. Application of Haddon's strategies [5–7] in the prevention of suicide

Haddon's strategies	Examples of potential applications in the prevention of suicides
1. To prevent the creation of the hazard in the first place *or* 2. To reduce the amount of the hazard brought into being	Limit the manufacture and/or distribution of firearms
3. To prevent the release of the hazard that already exists	Ban the sale of guns in certain populations
4. To modify the rate or spatial distribution of release of the hazard from its source	Initiate the use of individual tablet packaging of drugs to prevent the rapid consumption of large quantities of drugs; use judicious prescribing techniques
5. To separate in time, or in space, the hazard and that which is to be protected	Separate the ammunition from the guns; separate the drugs – by use of a locked cupboard
6. To separate the hazard and that which is to be protected by interposition of a material barrier	Utilize fences/barriers on bridges and high buildings to prevent impulsive suicidal acts and inadvertent falls
7. To modify relevant basic qualities of the hazard	Alter pharmacologic agents to reduce side-effects of drug ingestion
8. To make what is to be protected more resistant to damage from hazard	Involve the school systems in educational programs, in the facilitation of strong support systems, in early detection and in the use of counseling programs. Initiate clinical psychotherapeutic programs. Incorporate the use of exercise in primary and secondary prevention programs; promote interests in other activities
9. To begin to counter damage already done *and* 10. To stabilize and repair the object	Parasuicidal cases: Administer emergency measures. Initiate those strategies identified in Strategy Number Eight that will raise the level of resistance by utilizing more intensive programs, including clinical psychotherapeutic programs

mortality and morbidity associated with such locations as the Washington Avenue Bridge in Minnesota.

At least 24% of the suicide events were preceded by parasuicides or previous attempts. In addition, at least 25% of the individuals had threatened suicide previously. Evidence of this behavior provides an opportunity for aggressive intervention strategies. Such strategies include the utilization of comprehensive counseling programs and psychotherapy. Most importantly, the involvement of school systems in early detection, in the provision of relevant educational programs, and in the promotion of strong support systems among students of all ages further provides the potential for a concomitant reduction in anomie and frequency of suicide events as the adolescent progresses toward adulthood. The identification of the mean age of 19 years for both males and females between 12 and 24 years of age who committed suicide indicates a need to strengthen coping mechanisms and an individual sense of self-worth while they are in a system that can facilitate these outcomes most realistically.

Of further importance is the finding by some researchers that the perception of death could facilitate suicidal behavior [10, 11] which also has implications for appropriate approaches. Furthermore, given the fact that many of the suicidal victims in this study had a history of some degree of mental illness, it would appear appropriate, based on the scientific literature, to incorporate the use of exercise in both the primary and secondary prevention programs. Although the mechanisms underlying such changes remain unclear, there seems to be little doubt that both acute and chronic exercise can affect emotional well-being in a positive direction, especially in individuals who are moderately depressed or anxious [12]. Participation in running which can be comfortably sustained for 1 hour, three to four times per week for 10 weeks, seems to be as effective for the treatment of moderate depression as traditional psychotherapy according to Griest [13]. Also, bouts of exhaustive maximal treadmill runs as well as exercise stress tests performed to 80% of an individuals predicted maximal capacity have been shown to result in reduced anxiety [14]. Similarly, it is essential to promote interest and involvement in other activities that provide opportunities for creative expression and physical activity.

Haddon's ninth and tenth strategies can be used to deal with the parasuicide case or the suicide attempter, once the individual has been stabilized in the acute phase. Strategies like those identified to raise the level of resistance in the individual (eighth strategy) can also be applied here, together with more intensive clinical psychotherapeutic programs.

Most important is the continued effort in research of variables associated with suicide. In particular, continued investigation in the development of typologies of suicide cases through modeling (as in the present study) will facilitate progress in the identification of other relevant strategies.

McIntire and Angle [10] reported that many of the adolescent suicide deaths are unintentional; the victim did not really intend to die. In a poison control center study [15], none of the deaths could be classified as intentional. Rather, the adolescents were victims of pharmacologic roulette. While the suicide decision itself is not usually impulsive, it may be done on impulse. Therefore, it is possible to initiate relevant strategies.

While the data presented are from a short period of time, they provide many implications for the development of prevention strategies. Further, they provide a basis for additional study.

Acknowledgments. The authors thank the following individuals for their significant contributions to this study:

John I. Coe, M.D., Chief Medical Examiner, and Joan Willet, Manager, Hennepin County Medical Examiner's Office, Minneapolis, Minnesota

James Essling, Chief Investigator, and Carol Koop, Medical Office Supervisor, Ramsey County Medical Examiner's Office, St. Paul, Minnesota

Paul Gunderson, Ph.D., Director, Carol Vargas, M.A., Research Analyst, and James Wiggington, M.P.H., Senior Research Specialist–Center for Health Statistics, Minnesota Department of Health, Minneapolis, Minnesota

Colleen Renier, B.S., Applications Programmer, and Barbara A. Elliott, Ph.D., Assistant Professor, Behavioral Sciences, University of Minnesota, Duluth, Minnesota

References

1. Centers for Disease Control (1983) Violent deaths among persons 15 – 24 years of age – United States 1970 – 1978. MMWR 32/35:453 – 457
2. Baker SP, O'Neill B, Karpf R (1984) The injury fact book. Heath, Lexington, MA
3. Hull C, Nie NH (eds) (1981) Statistical package for the social sciences. McGraw-Hill, New York
4. Loesch JH (1977) Cluster analysis package, version 1.0. University of Minnesota, Social Sciences Research Center, Minneapolis
5. Haddon W Jr (1963) A note concerning accident theory and research with special reference to motor vehicle accidents. Ann NY Acad Sci 107:635 – 646
6. Haddon W Jr (1967) The prevention of accidents. In: Clark DM, MacMahon B (eds) Preventive medicine. Little Brown, Boston, pp 591 – 621
7. Haddon W Jr (1980) Advances in the epidemiology of injuries as a basis for public policy. Public Health Rep 95/5:411 – 421
8. Browning CH (1974) Epidemiology of suicide: firearms. Compr Psychiatry 15:549 – 553
9. Boyd JH (1983) The increasing rate of suicide by firearms. J Engl J Med 308/15:872 – 874
10. McIntire MS, Angle CR (1980) Suicide attempts in children and youth. Harper and Row, New York
11. Orbach I, Glaubman H (1978) Suicidal, aggressive, and normal children's perception of personal and impersonal death. J Clin Psychol 34/4:850 – 856
12. Morgan WP (1982) Psychological effects of exercise. Behav Med Update 4:25 – 30
13. Griest JH, Klein MH, Eichens RR, Faris J, Gurman AS, Morgan WP (1979) Running as treatment for depression. Compr Psychiatry 20:41 – 54
14. Morgan WP (1979) Anxiety reduction following acute physical activity. Psychiatr Ann 9/3:36 – 45
15. McIntire MS, Angle CR (1971) Suicide as seen in poison control centers. Pediatrics 48:914 – 922

"Health Education" – A New Subject in the Secondary Schools of SR Slovenia, SFR Yugoslavia

D. Repovš

Introduction

In federatively organized Yugoslavia there are certain differences among socialist republics and autonomous regions in the organization and performance of health education. General directions are given by federal legal regulations and principles which are supplemented by the republics and regions according to the actual situation and concrete needs of the population. The social republic of Slovenia is one of the smaller republics, but is quite developed (ca. 1/12 of Yugoslav territory and population, ca. 1/7 of national income). The stage of development of the health services and national pathology is very close to the situation in Central Europe.

Therefore, the principal trends of health educational work are directed towards prevention, early detection and active co-operation of the population in treatment and rehabilitation. The emphasis is on stimulating conscious decisions to adopt a healthy life-style and on providing a healthier close and wide environment.

Health Educational Approaches

Health educational work takes a variety of forms:

- Permanent and especially organized health educational work in the framework of the health services
- Health education of children and youth in the school system,
- Health education of the general population, especially in local communities (i.e. the basic sociopolitical territorial formations)
- Health education of the working population at work
- Health education performed in social-political organizations and associations (e.g. Red Cross),
- Healt education through the mass media (TV, local and republic-wide broadcasting, daily papers, journals and especially the newspapers of working organizations).

Primary Health Care in the Making
Ed. by U. Laaser, R. Senault, H. Viefhues

Present Position of Health Education in the Slovene School System

Health education contents are included first in kindergartens, infant schools and primary schools (1st–8th school year). During this period, health education contents are integrated into different subjects, such as biology, physical culture and sociopolitical education.

In new, so-called oriented education (9th–12th school year, i.e. secondary school), health education is an independent subject in the first two years.

In some schools at higher levels there is also health education, mostly as an independent subject (schools for higher medical personnel, faculty of medicine, faculty of biology for future teachers of health education in primary and secondary schools). Selected health educational items are also included in postgraduate curricula for medical and paramedical workers.

A New Approach in Secondary Schools

In the school year 1981/82 health education became an independent part of the new compulsory programme. This solution was decided upon bearing in mind the importance of this school age for the forming of behavioural patterns and for a more responsible attitude towards the community health. It forms the basis for a new approach at the national level too. Through children we also reach their parents and so we can influence their thinking about health.

The second, no less important reason for the change, was the fact that we were not satisfied with the health condition of our school-children and youth. The majority of defects and illnesses can be prevented or quickly improved with appropriate education at this age.

We were also obliged to do something because of the poor condition of elementary knowledge about health and the lack of hygienic life-styles.

Themes and Concrete Programme

The programme comprises 52 teaching hours (i.e. 45 minutes each) and is divided into five thematic domains:

In the *first school year* there are 17 hours:

1. *Health and healthy life-style* (10 hours)
   - positive health
   - health protection of schoolchildren and youth
   - body hygiene – washing
   - hygiene of clothing and footwear
   - dental health
   - nutrition
   - environmental health
   - principles of healthy living

2. *First aid* (7 hours)
   - accidents and their prevention
   - four actions for life saving
   - reanimation
   - bleeding
   - wounds
   - bone and joint injuries
   - other important injuries or sudden illnesses

   In the *second school year* there are 35 hours:
3. *Health and diseases* (14 hours)
   - first symptoms of diseases
   - prevention and control of infectious diseases
   - sight protection
   - hearing protection
   - care of locomotion system
   - classical and modern social diseases
4. *Mental health* (14 hours)
   - development of a healthy personality
   - adjusted and unadjusted behaviour
   - humanisation of relationship between sexes
   - parenthood preparation
5. *Sociopathological phenomena* (7 hours)
   - unhealthy behavioural patterns in adolescents
   - addictions (tobacco, alcoholism, drugs)
   - uncommon sexual behaviour

The programme in the first year is adapted to the basic personal hygienic needs of pupils. In hours devoted to first aid they repeat their basic knowledge and above all become aware of the fact that it is possible to prevent accidents. In the second year they first receive instruction in the basic problems of health and disease, with special emphasis on active care for better health. They then deal with and search for solutions to their own problems in adolescence and also some unhealthy behavioural phenomena.

There are two textbooks for this programme, and two manuals for teachers were prepared.

Unsolved Problems

Irrespective of the fact that the programme of "oriented" secondary education started in the school year 1981/82, we have not completed the preparation of detailed methodology and didactic procedures.

The second problem is motivating the young to participate actively in this subject. In fact, however, even we have been pleasantly surprised: pupils and teachers have found the programme interesting and attractive. Until now, no difficulties have been reported. One important reason for this is that the teaching process is based on discussions and group work.

Owing to the brief period of operation of the programme, a detailed evaluation has not yet been undertaken. Basic data showed quite good success in the first two years of the new subject, though the project is long-term oriented.

We are extremely interested in an interchange of ideas, information and experiences in this domain. We are especially interested in recent achievements in the methodology of health educational courses at schools (at all levels – not only secondary!) and in written or audiovisual aids for this type of health education.

Yugoslav Perspectives

Similar programmes will soon be introduced in the secondary schools' of other Yugoslav republics and autonomous regions. Thus with time we can expect an increase in the health knowledge of the total population, more responsible lifestyles, better self-care and an improvement in community health.

Some Results of the "Schülerstudie Gesundheitserziehung Hamburg"

R. Fehr and E. O. Krasemann

The "Hamburg Study on Health Education of Pupils and Their Families" started in 1981 and will run for at least 3 years [1, 2]. Seven hundred and twenty pupils (of four different schools) as well as their parents are taking part in this study, which is jointly sponsored by the Ministry of Health of the FRG and the Hansestadt Hamburg. At two schools, health-directed intervention is carried out, which is founded in part on the "coping" concept and stresses social learning as well as the training of problem-solving capabilities. The other two schools are taking part for reasons of comparison.

The scientific investigations within this study serve two purposes:

a) Evaluation of the specific intervention after a sufficient period of time – this time has *not* passed yet
b) To gain knowledge on the health status and the personal risk factors of the population being studied, including the influence of some psychological and social factors on the distributions observed

Both aims are meant to contribute to the primary prevention of chronic diseases.

At the beginning of the study, the pupils were physically examined mainly in regard to nutritional state and arterial blood pressure, and they were requested to answer a questionnaire concerning smoking, eating and drinking habits, leisure activities, physical exercise, personal interests and other psychological factors. Their parents received a set of questionnaires concerning similar topics as well as questions on their working and living conditions. Physical examination of the pupils and administration of questionnaires to them is repeated at yearly intervals.

The response rates to the investigations carried out up to now has amounted to about 80% of the pupils and about 75% of the parents (i.e. at least one parent filling out the questionnaires).

When entering the study, 94% of the pupils were aged 10 or 11 years; only 6% were already 12 or 13 years of age. The boys predominated slightly, with 53% vs 47% of girls in this population.

For illustrating the use of data gathered up to now, I am going to give two examples. The first one implies a cross-sectional analysis of questionnaire data, while the second makes use of longitudinal data of the physical examinations to investigate the "tracking" phenomenon.

Primary Health Care in the Making
Ed. by U. Laaser, R. Senault, H. Viefhues

One basic assumption of the Hamburg Study on Health Education of Pupils implies that the paradigm of personal risk factors should be completed by taking into account some individual and social factors which may play a role in causing or favouring risky behaviour of the individual. Particular importance is being attached to the influence of self-assurance (*Selbstsicherheit, Selbstwertgefühl*) as part of a person's self-concept.

Let us consider smoking, which undoubtedly is one of the most important personal risk factors of adult life. Assuming that smoking at an early age is correlated with smoking habits later in life, it seems relevant to investigate the circumstances of smoking onset in early youth. The hypothesis to be tested is: Pupils with a higher degree of self-assurance tend to have their first smoking experiences at a later point in time than do pupils with lower degrees of self-assurance. Since a sex effect on smoking habits was known for both adult and growth age and since an effect of social class seemed plausible, we felt bound to control for both sex and social class. Because of the small variance in this population, age was excluded from the analysis.

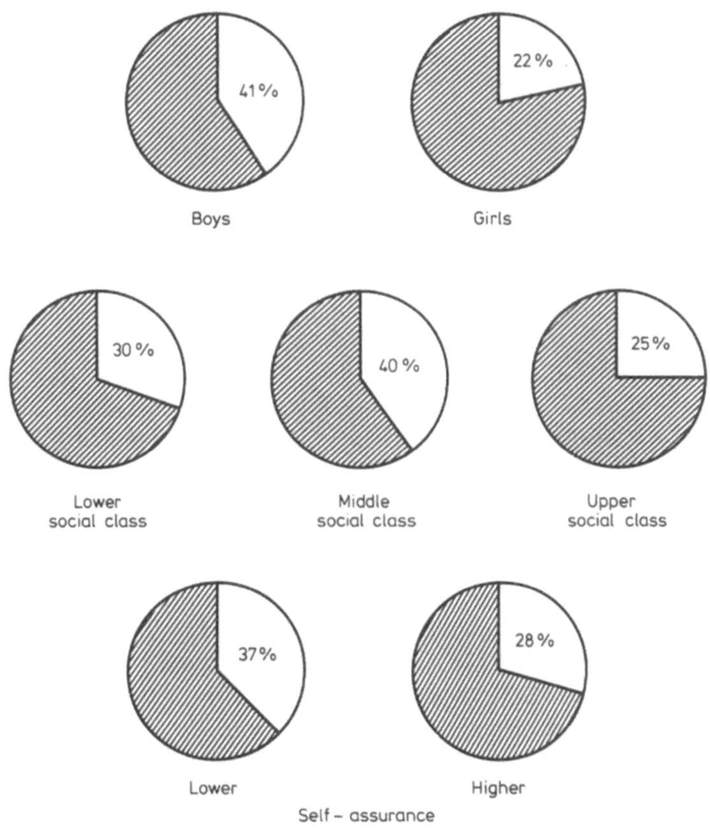

Fig. 1. Smoking experience in relation to sex, social class and self-assurance (considered separately). *Open area,* smoking experience (%); *shaded area,* never smoked (%)

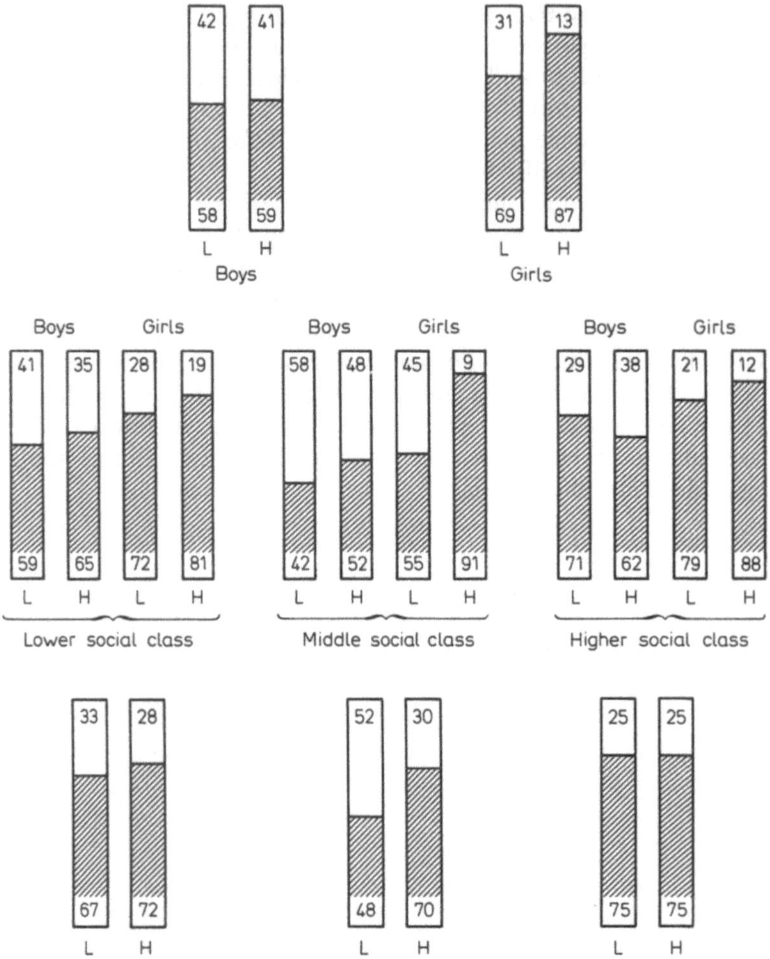

Fig. 2. Smoking experience in relation to sex, social class and self-assurance (considered together). *Open area,* smoking experience (%); *shaded area,* never smoked (%); *L,* lower self-assurance; *H,* higher self-assurance

Self-assurance was measured by a ten-item subscale of a standardized psychological test instrument [3]. The resulting test score was dichotomized to "lower" and "higher" degree of self-assurance. Social class was judged by a slightly modified standard scale of socioeconomic status [4], classifying the professional status of the pupils' fathers. The 18 degrees of this scale were trichotomized to (1) "workers", (2) "qualified employees" and (3) "managers", academic people etc.

Four hundred and six pupils had valid values for all four variables analysed. Of these, 68% claimed *no* smoking experience whatsoever. Figure 1 shows the influence of sex, social class, and self-assurance from a bivariate point of view, to begin with. Smoking experience is more widely spread with: boys, middle third of social ranking, lower self-assurance.

Even though the three variables sex, social class and self-assurance did not show any significant correlations in our population, we held that a multivariate analysis was necessary. Figure 2 (middle part) shows the data of the corresponding four-dimensional contingency table: each subpopulation, e.g. boys, lower social class and lower self-assurance, is represented by a column. The fraction of pupils without any smoking experience is shown by the shaded area (e.g. 59% of the first subpopulation).

Ignoring the factor "social class" leads to the structure shown at the top of Fig. 2, where for the boys there is hardly any effect of self-assurance left. Ignoring the factor "sex" leads to the structure shown at the bottom of Fig. 2.

Following the approach of Grizzle, Starmer and Koch (see in Küchler [5]), the multivariate dependency analysis of the complete four-dimensional table showed that

a) independent *main* effects can be assumed for sex, social class (but restricted to middle vs upper fraction) and self-assurance, and
b) there is a marked *interaction* between self-assurance and social class, which *enhances* the effect of self-assurance in the middle class, and *diminishes* it in the uppermost fraction.

"Nonmet"-model (Grizzle, Starmer, Koch)

	Effect	Probability
1) $\bar{X}$	0.69	–
2) Sex	–0.11	0.001
3) Middle vs. upper social class	–0.07	0.010
4) Self-assurance	–0.06	0.008
5) Interaction self-assurance vs middle social class	–0.07	0.010
Goodness of fit: $P=0.480$		

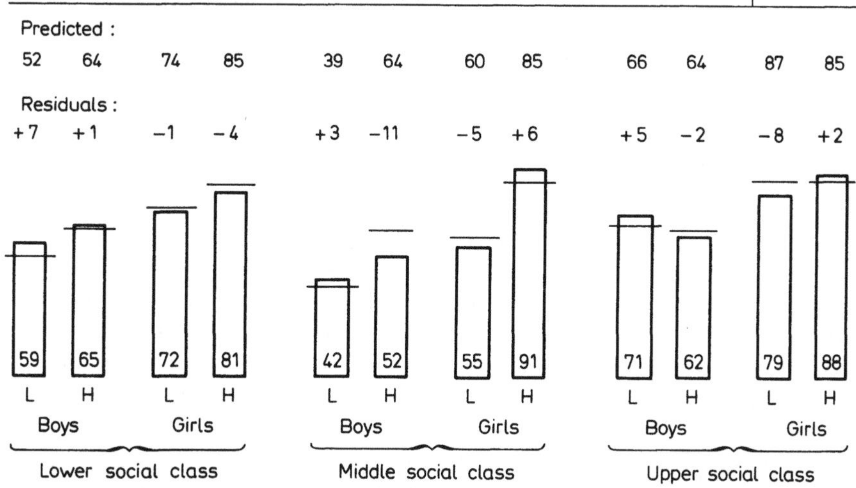

Fig. 3. Smoking experience in relation to sex, social class and self-assurance; results of the NONMET analysis. *Columns,* observed rate of "never smoked" (%); *bars,* predicted rate of "never smoked" (%)

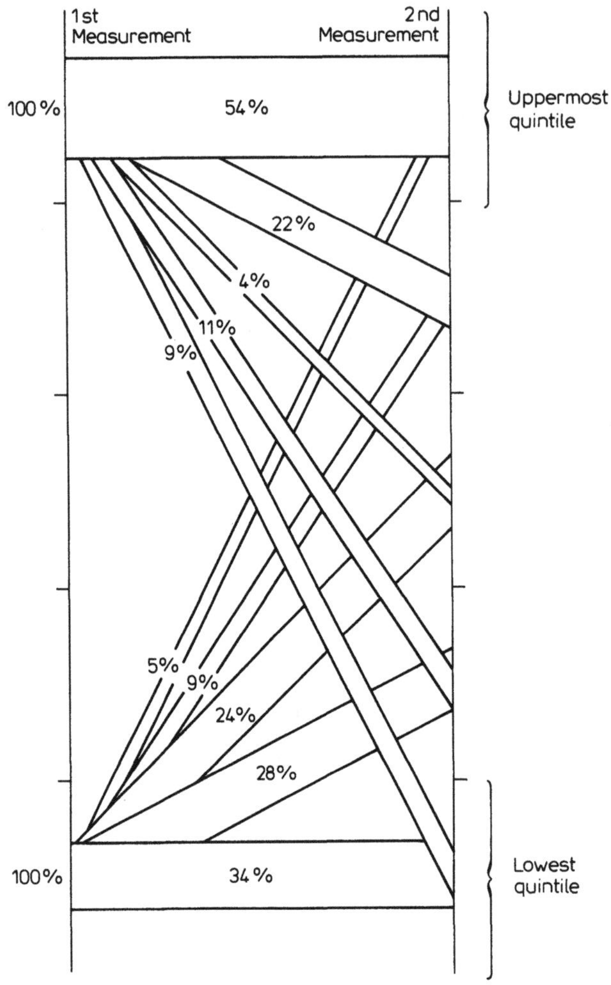

Fig. 4. Tracking of arterial blood pressure (entrance examination vs follow-up): transitions from extreme quintiles

Figure 3 shows this model, which has a satisfying goodness of fit.

It can be summarized that – controlling for age and social class – the pupils' self-assurance shows a significant effect on their very early smoking habits, at least as far as the lower and the middle social classes are concerned. We judge this result as a backing for the educational concept underlying health intervention in this study, which attaches much importance to the development of a positive self-concept as a protective factor against risky behaviour.

Finally, I shall make some comments on the "tracking" of systolic blood pressure in our population. Without a certain amount of tracking it would be rather pointless to use this item in the context of screening and primary prevention in childhood. Because of different dates of entry to the study, up to now only two of the four schools have got their first follow-up examination.

In this cohort of about 300 pupils, the results of the first and second examination (1 year later) were compared. The arterial blood pressure was

Table 1. Tracking of arterial blood pressure (entrance examination vs follow-up 12 months later)

	Correlation coefficient r_{12}	% remaining between 4th and 5th quintile	% remaining between the *same* quintiles
RR syst.	0.487	54.5%	34.7%
RR diast. IV	0.337	30.3%	30.3%
RR diast. V	0.360	32.1%	30.9%

measured by random-zero sphygmomanometry under defined conditions. The middle column of Table 1 shows the fraction of pupils who *continued* to belong to the uppermost 20% of the distribution. As far as systolic blood pressure is concerned, more than half of the pupils with an entrance value above the 4th quintile were found to have a similarly high value at the first follow-up. Figure 4 shows the transitions when comparing systolic blood pressure at the entrance examination with that at the first follow-up examination.

We conclude that in spite of numerous factors potentially disturbing the data quality of the systolic blood pressure measurement there is a remarkably high degree of tracking. Further investigations in the future will show to what degree this holds true for a longer period of time.

References

1. Krasemann EO, Lewerenz J (1982) Modellvorhaben zur Primär-Prävention von Krankheiten über die Veränderung von Einstellungs- und Verhaltensweisen – Bericht über die Vorstudie. Bundesgesundheitsblatt 25:173–180
2. Lewerenz J, Fehr R, Krasemann EO (1982) Beeinflussung gesundheitsrelevanter Einstellungen und Verhaltensweisen bei 10- bis 14jährigen Schülern – Ein Modellversuch zur Primärprävention. Prävention 5:51–55
3. Wagner JWL (1977) Fragebogen zum Selbstkonzept für 4.–6. Klassen (FSK 4–6). Beltz, Weinheim
4. Handl J, Mayer KU, Müller W (1977) Klassenlagen und Sozialstruktur. Campus, Frankfurt
5. Küchler M (1979) Multivariate Analyseverfahren. Teubner, Stuttgart

An Ecological Concept of Health Promotion in Child and Youth Work – Projekt Gesundheit/Bund Deutscher Pfadfinder

H. Hildebrandt

"Projekt Gesundheit"[1] – Origin and Context

Within the practical work of the "Bund Deutscher Pfadfinder"[2] during the past couple of years we have noticed a lot of problems connected with both physical and mental health (e.g. sickliness, drug addiction, self-destructive and aggressive impulses). On the other hand the voluntary workers, the so-called "teamers", developed an increasing interest in "health food", the use of herbs instead of allopathic medicine, and new approaches to the body and body awareness. Traditional organizations of health education do not offer adequate material or counselling, so some of us developed an action research project aimed at improving our understanding of and ability to deal with the problems mentioned above during our everyday work with children. In contrast to highly sponsored prevention programmes, the German Federal Government provided only a small fund for our semi-professional project, thus limiting both its duration and the intensity of work.

What Has Been Done

Within 2 years of commencing the project work (only 10 months of which was funded), our activities covered the following areas:

1. We collected a wide range of material on projects and concepts in the field of health, body and children and evaluated them. Intensive discussion of traditional and modern methods and theories made possible the development of our own concept.
2. We organized a self-awareness/self-help group for ourselves and some befriended mothers, exploring and discussing the "history" of our bodies and diseases and their biographical, social and environmental contexts, and looking also for patterns of reacting to the sickness of other people.
3. On a nearby adventure playground organized by a group of parents we worked together with them (children and adolescents both being present).

[1] Literally translated: "Project Health"

[2] Literally translated: "League of German Scouts". Since 1970 this body has been developing into a libertarian, ecologically oriented youth organization

Primary Health Care in the Making
Ed. by U. Laaser, R. Senault, H. Viefhues

We tried out and developed body-oriented games, role-plays on sickness and life, and "photo interviews" to explore personal body image, arranged theatre playing, applied massages to our own bodies and others', scouted the environment with children, and organized festivals and camps.

4. We interviewed German and immigrant parents and children on their opinions with regard to sickness, living conditions and health promotion.
5. In some workshops with other "BDP-teamers" we confronted our ideas and experiences with the practical conditions in ordinary work with children and tested the chances of transfer.
6. We evaluated and documented all these various experiences [1, 3] and introduced them into the discussion of the World Health Organization [2].

Some Results Relevant to the Discussion on Health Promotion and Life-Styles

Speaking About Health Implies Speaking About Society

Professional and lay opinions on health always imply underlying ideologies of society, which will usually not be voiced. In expert–client interaction conflicting ideologies will rarely result in direct confrontation but rather lead to various forms of indirect resistance on the side of the clients. This mechanism seems understandable. Sensing that somebody who declares himself an expert is trying to change one's life according to his own concept of a healthy life and how life in general has to be, one must produce resistance because one's way of life is not a pleasure; rather it is a result of long conflicts and arrangements with social conditions, individual and collective experiences and ideals. In simple terms, this is why health education so often fails.

If we want to speak about health we must publicly clarify our own concept of life and society; for example what health promotion is all about. If somebody wanted to reduce the working days lost by sick leave, it is only natural that workers consciously or subconsciously resist [compare Parsons 1958]. We noticed similar processes involving children and days off school.

Our concept is explicitly based on *not* wanting to impose our own values and definitions on the people we worked with, but to develop the neighbourhood, which we also are a part of, together with them. In other words: Our practical work is aimed at the development of a non-standardizing "culture of life" (*Lebenskultur*), which implies liveliness and something multivarious instead of monolithic and dull: the opposite of the "culture of death" produced by fanatics of economic and military growth. We intend to attain this culture of life via a process of appropriation (or acquirement) of body, spirit and environment in social community action, a process which is at the same time health promoting.

Health promotion in this context cannot mean eradicating illness altogether despite all our efforts. Illness, like birth and dying, is part of the socioecological cycle of human life, and consequently should be socially accepted.

Warning of Too Frequent Use of the Word "Healthy"

"Healthy lifestyles", "make the healthier choice the easier choice"; such expressions are willingly used by health educators, hiding artfully their own uncertainty about what really is healthier and using a word with positive connotations. Another ethical problem is that defining something as "healthy" automatically stigmatizes the opposite as "sick" and banishes it into the competence of doctors, psychologists and psychiatrists.

Everybody Knows or Has a Presentiment of What They Are Suffering

In many interviews with children and parents we could see that people connect their sickness with their contexts of life using suggestions, associations and ascribed meanings. But this presentiment of a wholistic, systemic view is obstructed by various social and medical mechanisms. A very important source for understanding aetiology and opening up new ways of dealing with or preventing illness thus remains unutilized, and health promotion can perform a great task in confirming and supporting these wholistic ideas.

Integration vs Separation

There is no need for increasing specialization of youth, drug, sexual and educational counselling services but rather a great need for everyday supportive networks which allow autonomy and individuality and provide security and certainty. Strengthening lay competence has to be the main task of health promotion.

Learning from the Alternative Movements

One of the basic tenets of the increasing wholistic health movement and also the self-help groups is that the individuals must be actively involved in the process of maintaining and recovering their own health. The importance given to the unity of body, mind and spirit by most alternative therapies opens up a socio-psychosomatic understanding of illness as a part of life. Health-promoting strategies can learn a great deal from the self-help and wholistic health movements but should avoid their tendencies towards individualistic orientations.

Tenets of an Ecological Concept of Health Promotion in Child and Youth Work

Within the limited scope of a youth organization like ours the realization of a wholistic, ecological concept seems utopian. Defining our aim as the development of a non-standardizing culture of life by appropriation of body, spirit and environment in social community action, we can propose some principles:

1. Sensitization and qualification of voluntary workers and staff to a more wholistic understanding of illness, realizing that diseases are the physical expression of a network of social experiences of conflict and suffering and the socio-psychosomatic abilities of coping, is necessary and possible by means of a self-help group.
2. We recommend augmented use of body-oriented games derived from new body therapies, the use of massage, yoga etc., but in a very careful manner. Emphasis is to be laid on self-determination of the children in response to the signals of their body; manipulation by these methods has to be avoided.
3. Integration instead of separation also has effects on ordinary work with children. The integration of male and female, German and immigrant children in our groups is self-evident nowadays; a new effort has to be made to integrate the children into the community life, e.g. by creating places for all, like adventure playgrounds that are open to adults too, neighbourhood centres etc.
4. In building up a sociopolitical initiative to change health-damaging living conditions, voluntary workers, children and parents are on the same side and have common interests in their own well-being. Co-operation with other community groups, social movements and traditional organizations may help in this process and strengthen the possibilities for children to develop their own inherent abilities.
5. In such a context practical work with children can strengthen and confirm their own subconscious or conscious wholistic understanding of their life, their problems and their diseases as being part of a network. They must not see sickness to be their individual fate; they can, together with others, actively move into a process of changing, acquiring self-confidence.

Further Plans

Together with parents, initiatives and friends we want to create a centre of neighbourhood help with a café and rooms for meetings and various activities. We are planning to start with intensive interviews and to employ methods from the field of body therapy, thus researching the network of causes underlying our diseases and developing strategies to fight against or alleviate them. Additionally we want:

1. To thoroughly evaluate the taped material from our self-awareness group in order to stimulate and deepen the work of self-help groups
2. To hold an exhibition about our project and to discuss results and experiences with a wider public audience
3. To build up a working group on health promotion in Frankfurt
4. To develop our idea of health workshops
5. To organize a 6 months' excursion to the USA to visit and work for some time in health projects, especially those which are concerned with community activities, neighbourhood, self-help or mutual aid groups, holistic health movements and health maintenance organizations.

References

1. Gubinsky G, Hildebrandt H, Schultz ML (1983) Projektdokumentation: Krank werden, um sich vom Leben zu erholen – Gesundheitsbildung in der außerschulischen Kinder- und Jugendarbeit. Unpublished, available from Bundeszentrale für gesundheitliche Aufklärung, Köln
2. Hildebrandt H (1983) Gesundheitsförderung integriert in Jugendverbandsarbeit; Jugendliche und Gesundheit. Überlegungen zu riskantem Verhalten und Gesundheitserziehungskonzepten. WHO-Euro-Workshop "Gesundheitsförderung für Jugendliche", 4. – 6. 7. 83, Heidelberg
3. Hildebrandt H, Schultz ML (1984) Wenn ich traurig bin, dann bin ich auch krank – Kinder, Körper, Gesundheit. Jugend und Politik, Reinheim
4. Meanwhile (Dec. 1984) the "Self help and Neighborhood Center" has been started. Selbsthilfe- und Nachbarschaftszentrum. Frankfurt
5. Parsons T (1958) Definitionen von Gesundheit und Krankheit im Lichte der amerikanischen Werte und der Sozialstruktur Amerikas. In: Parsons T (1964) Sozialstruktur und Persönlichkeit, Frankfurt

Growing Up into the 1980s: An Ecological Framework for Health Promotion for Youth

P. Franzkowiak

Youth in the 1980s: Life and Perspectives

Youth is a phase in any individual's life-cycle that is characterized by manifold problems and conflicts. For adolescents, growing up, incorporates at least four problematic issues: puberty and maturity; the detachment from parental influence; getting work and learning how to labour; long periods of status insecurity while trying to build up a proper identity.

Young people between 12 and 20 (and even 25, if we refer to the growing population of post-adolescents) experience a strong discrepancy between their own, self-attributed competence for daily life, work, relationships etc. and the adults' attribution of incompetence and restricted independence in personal and cultural matters. The increasing orientation of adolescents towards social contacts outside their families makes them organize in peer groups and subcultures. The *subcultures* as a whole constitute the "youth culture" of a modern society at a given time. Their function is to give young people the space to act out their generational problems collectively and to work out successful ways of completing their "passage of status" into the dominant adult subcultures [2].

What affects the adolescent and post-adolescent population as a whole in the Central and North European countries are social changes that make youth researchers speak either of a "*locked-out generation*" [7] or a "generation with a new deficiency". A recent United Nations Report in preparation for the International Youth Year 1985 predicts that a major part of the young population will have to face radical restrictions concerning their options for individual development and their chances for social and economic integration. The future holds a number of alarming prospects: underemployment or no employment at all, threats to national and global peace, and fears about how to secure a personal income and satisfying social status – to name but a few.

Recently, two German pedagogues have defined the "new deficiency" by pointing to an overall lack of cultural space that the youth can occupy to engrave their individual and collective traces onto [14]. This is due to a historically new form of cultural expropriation of individuals in the industrialized countries which has been developing with regard to a collective relative satiation with goods and social (welfare) services. Nearly all institutions and agents for "making sense" that are made available by the traditional post-war culture appear to be used up when approached by the younger generation. The

Primary Health Care in the Making
Ed. by U. Laaser, R. Senault, H. Viefhues

transfer of cultural patterns is disturbed nowadays. So, in the course of adolescence, the peer-group replaces the adults' institutions as *the* "identity workshop": it is now the dominant social and cultural framework for young people.

Adopting to a Life-style

Peer-groups and subcultures distinguish themselves by specific collective *life-styles* that any member can (and with regard to certain features: must) attain to. The term "life-style" here is not used in the traditional medical sense, as merely a synonym for behaviour or risky behaviour in general. In essence life-styles represent the way in which individuals and social groups come to terms with their immediate and wider environment [12].

In sociological terms life-styles are regarded as mediating structures; an expression of the way in which the broader values of society are transmitted down to the individuals. Individual behaviour choices can be limited or expanded by environmental factors and also by the extent to which the individual feels in charge of his or her own life. The crux of this approach is the reciprocal nature of the individual/environment relationship. The way in which an adolescent lives his or her own life may produce behaviour patterns which are either health promoting or detrimental to health. To affect a young person's life-style, however, comprehensive activities are required to change the individual, collective and environmental components of his or her life.

The Issue of Health in Adolescents' Life-styles

A fair number of sociological and epidemiological studies show that health is a positive social value for teenagers (as for the majority of adults, too). Yet this attitude apparently has no consequences for their everyday performance. Young people see *long-term health issues as irrelevant,* or at best marginal, to the important priorities of their lives. Health, for them, is one of several available options. And it is not the most attractive one, because it is often associated with personal restraint or even asceticism. To lead a healthy life is regularly associated with leading a dull, even intolerable life [3].

Health is not a pragmatic value or a behavioural determinant for young persons, at least up to the age of 20–25. Their motto is: "What I do with my body is my own affair." Treating their mental and physical resources in a risky manner is an integral part of their growing up, of their labouring for integration and identity. There seems to be a hardly bridgeable gap in any youth life-style between their definition of body consciousness and body experience compared with the medical or educational idea of health consciousness and individual prevention.

Up to their mid-twenties, young people do not develop a preventive, health-conscious life-style. For them other matters count more than possible but fairly distant health damage in the future. They strive to enjoy and consume their present, by definition youthful, life.

A Functional Perspective on Youth Risk Behaviour

Epidemiological risk behaviours, such as cigarette smoking and abundant alcohol consumption, are the major targets of contemporary prevention trials. All measures to encourage young people to break away from such patterns have, however, shown moderate short-term effects or no substantial effects at all.

Evidence from recent youth research in this area should explain why medical and/or epidemiological thinking cannot be easily translated into acceptable life-style alternatives for the adolescents themselves. For low and middle class youngsters from the age of 12, smoking, drinking and also visiting a pub are of the same superior importance as making friendships or gaining sexual experience. These matters may even become pivotal affairs in the adolescents' self-respect. They are elementary because of their *symbolic value* as "adult matters". When doing so, young people can quite easily obtain adult-like experience and competence. Not being able to exercise the adult role in reality, they go for its symbolic substitutes: smoking, drinking and access to public places [10].

This, in the long run health-damaging, risk behaviour has a lot of meaning for the people involved; they are functional for their subjective well-being. Risk behaviour (when we estimate it from this viewpoint), is a rational and sensible form of everyday behaviour – and it is performed by the majority of people in our industrialized societies, young and old. In its manifold forms it is used to act out conflicts in a compensatory way. The risk is generally defined in subjective terms, according to notions of its approximately calculable personal benefits. The aims of performing risk behaviour are twofold: to cope with actual personality or interaction conflicts but also to re-establish the person's mental and physical faculties [5].

The young actor's perspective on risk behaviour is fundamentally different from the health educator's view. Such behaviour patterns have to be estimated as *functional elements of the given life-styles,* hereby following a distinct, biographical logic: not a medical one. That is why to quit risk behaviour is so hard for those who are the "targets" of today's preventive programmes – they are challenged to change their whole lives, not just an isolated habit.

A New Paradigm for Health Education

There are strong signs of a paradigmatic shift in health education towards the concept of health promotion. *Health promotion* can be defined as a social and political strategy to provide a wide range of life-style options for individuals and social groups alike. The main targets of this strategy are the elements of the social support system which influence individuals in their personality development and thus in their personal decisions on how to become or stay healthy [11].

Available experience from recent Western and North European programmes confirms that health promotion for youth should employ different strategies according to the different "living spheres" of young people. In schools and work-places, the focus should be on the setting up of psychosocial support networks for young people by influencing the existing curricular and personal (teachers, trainers etc.) resources. In the less institutionalized social settings of the community, health promotion efforts must concentrate on the participation and self-organization of adolescents according to their felt needs and priorities. Generally, high priority must be given to the youths' self-study of their situation and their self-determination of positive values and modes of individual and collective change [4, 6].

As outlined above, long-term health issues (in the medical sense) have only a marginal impact on adolescents and young adults. Due to this, health promotion is obliged to meet their everyday life problems and expectations with non-paternalistic offers of advice and practical support. The priorities of young people in modern societies are undeniably different from those of a professional health educator. Health promotion will therefore have to leave the narrow path of risk factor warnings and corresponding behavioural change; rather it must develop comprehensive methods for supporting young people in dealing with the following *paramount social and cultural issues:*

- adolescents' problems in school and at work; threats of anticipated or actual unemployment;
- the issue of peace and perceived threats of military or nuclear catastrophes;
- problems in friendships and partnerships; developing positive body and sexual experiences; other problems of maturity;
- working out a personal identity; integration vs. independence in family, school, at work and in the peer group;
- dealing competently with leisure time offers, especially the wide range of electronic entertainment; and
- managing physical and mental well-being and its subjective disorders.

From a Social to an Ecological Framework of Health Promotion

In the current scientific and political discussion, the life-style concept is regarded as *the* conceptual framework for health promotion. Life-styles, however, can serve as indicators for analysing and influencing the social dimensions of health only. A comprehensive concept, on the other side, that reflects the interaction of physical and mental and social options for the health of individuals as well as groups is the *human ecology approach.* This holistic or systems approach (to put it in other words) takes account of the fact that all human situations involve a constant interplay between variables of many different kinds: physical, chemical, biotic, social, cultural and economic. It provides a rational means of studying and improving the understanding of these patterns of interplay. Human ecology represents the study of the dynamic patterns of interaction in human situations between these different kinds of variable [1, 13].

The approach offers a broad perspective on human beings, focussing particularly on the interdependencies of the physical, natural and social environment and the individual and its social groups. Human ecology is basically an interdisciplinary, not a specializing concept, which fits well into the scientific explanation and legitimation of health promotion.

The Practice of Ecological Health Promotion for Youth: The Body and Health Workshop Model

Health promotion on a human ecology background combines methods for body experience and mental growth with collective social action. Promoting health in this sense incorporates a complex of strategies which aim at the development and support of a comprehensive and unanimous "culture of living". The overall objective is the individual's self-determination over his or her own physical, mental and sociocultural resources for proper motives.

This philosophy has been realized with considerable success in a German Boy Scouts' project over the past 2 years [8]. Comprehensive "body and health workshops" were introduced to 8- to 14-year-olds in their local playgrounds and adjacent leisure-time activities. Relying on the example of "future workshops" [9] and supported by neighbourhood parents, a wide and imaginative range of human growth and sensitivity-raising methods were employed. Thus, the boys and girls were encouraged to *gain experience and familiarity with their own bodies:* their potentials and limitations but also susceptibilities for weakness or illness. These efforts were embedded into collective social action of the young people, such as playground construction, a problem-oriented community diagnosis, and also parents' participation or counselling.

This comprehensive model of body and health workshops, directed by the needs and priorities of the participating youth, works as a means of health promotion, too, when introduced to adolescents and young adults [4]. The workshops can be carried out in schools and other institutionalized social settings as well as in the more informal, peer group governed spaces and areas of the community.

The model itself is not a new one, not even to health education. Its employment in the ecological framework of an "appropriation of body and environment by social action" [8], however, promises to open new horizons for youth-oriented health promotion. Children and adolescents can be successfully motivated to work on those aspects of their life-styles that are relevant to health and the prevention of future damage – but: as perceived and rated as important by themselves. The basis of the young people's engagement must be *their self-perceived need* for a self-determined physical, mental and/or sociocultural change. The relevant issues of their engagement may differ with age, social setting, background culture and sex: it has to be accepted, though, that they are hardly those of the traditional, risk-oriented health education.

By adopting the human ecology approach as a conceptual framework and the body and health workshop model as its practical means, one of the main foundations of health promotion should be realized: its orientation towards non-authoritative support of people who are struggling to come to terms with their social, personal and also (not only) health-related problems – without reducing them to patients, pupils or even "targets".

References

1. Boyden S, Millar S (1978) Human ecology and the quality of life. Urban Ecol 3:263–287
2. Brake M (1980) The sociology of youth culture and youth subcultures. Routledge and Kegan Paul, London
3. Doubrawa R (1978) Gesundheitsverhalten und Einstellung zur Gesundheitsvorsorge bei jungen Menschen. Offentl Gesundheitswes 40:84–93
4. Franzkowiak P (1983) Perspectives of health promotion for youth in the European countries. Workshop "Youth lifestyles, risk behaviour and health" of the WHO Regional Office for Europe, Spitzingsee, Bavaria 26–28 October, 1983
5. Franzkowiak P, Wenzel E (1982) Risikoverhalten und Gesundheitsförderung. HYGIE 1/1:30–40
6. Green LN (1983) New policies in education for health. World Health. April/May:13–14
7. Hartmann J (1982) Youth in industrialized societies during the 80s, a locked-out generation? 10th World Conference of Sociology, Mexico-City, August 16–20, 1983 (Research Committee 34: Sociology of youth)
8. Hildebrandt H, Schultz ML (1984) „Wenn ich traurig bin, dann bin ich auch krank" – Kinder, Körper, Gesundheit. Jugend und Politik, Reinheim
9. Jungk R, Müllert NR (1983) Zukunftswerkstätten: Wege zur Wiederbelebung der Demokratie. Goldmann, Munich
10. Projektgruppe Jugendbüro und Hauptschülerarbeit (1977) Die Lebenswelt von Hauptschülern. Juventa, Munich
11. WHO-Euro (1982) Health promotion and lifestyles: perspectives of the WHO Regional Office for Europe. HYGIE 1/3, 4:57–60
12. WHO-Euro (1983) Intervention studies related to lifestyles conducive to health. Report on a workshop, Copenhagen, 9–11 March (ICP/HED 019 (3)/2)
13. Wustlich R (1980) Ökologische Psychologie. In: Asanger R, Wenninger G (eds) Handwörterbuch der Psychologie. Beltz, Weinheim Basel, pp 299–304
14. Ziehe T, Stubenrauch H (1982) Plädoyer for ungewöhnliches Lernen. Rowohlt, Reinbek

C. The Occupational Setting

Industrial Jobs and Coronary Heart Disease

W. Maschewsky

At the Science Center Berlin the relation between industrial jobs and CHD has been empirically studied since 1977. Among other things, a retrospective survey was performed on 964 male and female workers in West Berlin. The infarction patients were between 30 and 64 years of age and were all German nationals. They had had their first (and only) myocardial infarction between autumn 1977 and spring 1980. We collected them from hospitals, a rehabilitation clinic and the membership files of the state insurance agency (LVA) in Berlin. The contrast group was also drawn from the membership files of the LVA, using a representative selection scheme based on age and sex. Here I will only present results about male industrial workers:

1. It could be shown that working conditions are relevant for myocardial infarction (MI). Their impact is comparable to the impact of medical risk factors. Conditions outside the work sphere show an even higher impact (see Table 1).
2. Present working conditions show a smaller effect than past conditions. This results to some extent from an over-representation of future MI patients in "sheltered work-places": Even before the outbreak of MI a considerable number of future patients show severe health impairment and they therefore have to accept lateral transfer or demotion within the firm. Accordingly, these workers report little stress for the job where the MI happened. Because stress accumulation in the past is normally disregarded, it appears as if stress reduction correlates with increasing MI risk. *Conclusion:* Studies about MI have to take into account occupational mobility, biographical changes/reductions in work-load, and the time-lag between impairment of health and onset of illness ("sleeper effect").
3. Among those workers who have not yet lost their old job, status and competence, MI seems to be caused or facilitated by psychosocial stress (see Table 2). Responsibility without sufficient control, time pressure, high demands on emotional discipline and bad social relations seem to have a pathogenic impact: The individual experiences stress, but can neither control the situation nor avoid it.
4. Working conditions show less effect than leisure conditions. On the one hand, leisure activities seem to aggravate and not to reduce MI patients' work problems: MI patients experience little social support, but many conflicts; they have many duties outside work; and they take stimulants (like

Primary Health Care in the Making
Ed. by U. Laaser, R. Senault, H. Viefhues

Table 1. Discriminant analysis of the differences between MI-patients and a contrast group for male industrial workers (first 15 factors; IG, infarction group; CG, contrast group)

Dimension/variable	Rank order	Conformity to hypothesis	Kind of difference	Significance
Medical risk factors				
Consumption of alcohol	9	+	CG>IG	1%
Duration of smoking	11	+	IG >CG	10%
Other risk factors (without smoking)	12	+	IG >CG	10%
Work				
Nervous overload	3	+	IG >CG	10%
Frequency of disturbances	4	–	CG>IG	10%
Difference between achieved status and qualification	5	+	IG >CG	10%
Active coping	13	+	CG>IG	20%
Leisure				
Social support	1	+	CG>IG	1%
Activity in leisure time	2	+	IG >CG	10%
Sexual frustration	6	+	IG >CG	1%
Number of children	7	+	IG >CG	1%
Overload in leisure time	8	+	IG >CG	1%
Financial resources	14	–	IG >CG	10%
Net income	15	+	CG>IG	10%
Personality				
Avoiding conflicts	10	+	IG >CG	10%

Table 2. Selected work characteristics for male industrial workers (IG, infarction group; CG, contrast group)

Characteristics	CG ($n=62$)	IG ($n=86$)	Significance	Odds ratio
Responsibility for other workers' faults	5	20	1%	4.75
Change of job/employer/profession in the last 10 years (only unskilled/semi-skilled workers)	32	69	1%	4.73
Night-shift 10 years ago	4	11		2.97
Nervous stress 10 years ago	31	50	5%	2.23
Changing work-place	24	41	5%	2.20
Suppressing anger when stressed	47	65	5%	2.09
Fast reaction demanded	32	48	10%	1.96
Sitting position at work	37	52	10%	1.84

coffee, cigarettes and alcohol) in order to increase their efficiency, not to reduce tension; etc. On the other hand, problems in the work sphere seem to be "shifted" to the leisure sphere: Frustration with the job turns into frustration with the family: conflicts with the boss are relieved at home; exhaustion is attributed to family duties, not to work-load.

5. A very general condition for the onset of MI seems to be a growing discrepancy between external demands and internal resources. If the worker tries to keep up with the output standards, he has to produce the same output at a deteriorating cost-benefit ratio. This accelerates the exhaustion of his psycho-physical resources, and develops into a vicious circle. The growing discrepancy between external demands and internal resources is dependent on loss of qualification (rationalisation), increasing intensity of work and lack of a sufficient number of work-places that are suitable for the impaired health and work efficiency of older workers.
6. This gradual erosion of psycho-physical capability to cope with work stress is accelerated when external demands change. Both upward mobility and downward mobility increase suddenly the demand to adapt to a new environment. Even if stress reduction is intended, a change of environment produces a destruction of attitudes, habits, competence and gratification, which actually increases stress – at least for some time.

References

1. Maschewsky W (1982) The relation between stress and myocardial infarction: a general analysis. Soc Sci Med 16/4:455–462
2. Maschewsky W, Schneider U (1982) Soziale Ursachen des Herzinfarkts. Campus, Frankfurt

Coronary Prone Behaviour Related to Occupational Stress in a Sample of Male Workers

M. T. Tenconi, A. Taccola, C. Mercuri, G. B. Gotti, M. R. Spina, and G. Bellotti

Introduction

Type A coronary prone behaviour has been indicated to be an important risk factor for coronary heart disease (CHD) since 1959 [1]. Case control and cohort studies [2–4] have shown a significant association between behavioural pattern and CHD. Moreover, an enhanced reactivity of Type A subjects to behavioural stress has been demonstrated [5, 6]. At present there are no data about the assessment and the prevalence of coronary prone behaviour in Italian population samples.

Aims

This research was carried out in order to study:

1. The specific behavioural pattern of a group of male workers and its possible relationship with some coronary risk factors.
2. Occupational stress apparently related to behavioural features, and its effects on the cardiovascular system.

Materials and Methods

The sample consisted of 70 male urban policemen of Pavia (Italy) aged 20–59. Their occupation differed in that 28 were appointed to road traffic, 21 to city patrol, and 21, at higher career levels, to office duties. The behavioural type was assessed by means of an Italian form of the Rosenman and Friedman Structured Interview (SI) [7]. The interviewers were trained by a professor of psychology at the Medical Faculty of Pavia, and under his supervision, administration and evaluation criteria were systematically standardized. The following traits were analysed: competitive drive, hostility, speed, impatience and "stylistics", i.e. mannerisms during the interview. Each interview was recorded and separately evaluated by at least three interviewers (the total and the partial scores are the result of averaging the three evaluations). Theoretically the score

Primary Health Care in the Making
Ed. by U. Laaser, R. Senault, H. Viefhues

range of the SI is from 10 to 50, subjects who score in the lowest group being classified as type B, and those who score in the highest group as type A.

Data on smoking, alcohol and coffee habits were collected, together with the measurement of systolic blood pressure, diastolic blood pressure, and body mass index. Moreover, total cholesterol, HDL-cholesterol and triglycerides were determined, and a basal ECG and an ECG after exercise were recorded. In the road traffic and city patrol group (36 subjects), a 6-h dynamic ECG registration by Holter was performed while they were working at a specific crossroad. We used this device because the possible cardiovascular modifications induced by stress are generally transient and could arise when the subject, during daily activity, is heavily involved with work.

Results and Discussion

Table 1 shows the means of some coronary risk factors in the two age groups considered. They are similar to those found in larger epidemiological studies on the male Italian population of same age [8]. The difference between the means of each variable in the two age groups was not statistically significant.

In Table 2 we can see the mean of the partial and total scores at the evaluation by SI on the whole sample.

Table 1. Mean and SD of some haematological and functional variables in the study sample by age (CH-tot, total cholesterol; CH-HDL, high density lipoprotein; SBP, systolic blood pressure; DBP, diastolic blood pressure)

Age	CH Tot (mg/dl)	CH-HDL (mg/dl)	Triglycerides (mg/dl)	Basal heart rate (min)	SBP (mm Hg)	DBP (mm Hg)
20–39	216.5	46.06	133.46	62.20	130.16	85.13
(30)	±49.45	±8.49	±90.19	±8.81	±12.63	±10.34
40–59	238.3	44.85	144.97	62.82	135.67	87.57
(40)	±40.68	±7.81	±64.72	±9.27	±15.23	±10.37
Total	228.95	45.37	140.04	62.557	133.31	86.52
(70)	±45.62	±8.07	±76.28	±9.022	±14.34	±10.35

Table 2. Mean and SD of partial and total scores at the evaluation of the SI on the whole sample

No.	Stylistics	Competitive drive	Hostility	Speed	Impatience	Total
70	26.43	28.81	33.89	33.97	34.55	31.57
	±8.54	±7.14	±8.06	±6.57	±6.6	±4.63

In the analysis of mean scores in the three groups (Table 3) with different duties (road traffic, city patrols, office) we can notice, as already reported in the literature, that subjects at a higher career level scored higher than those assigned to road traffic for total SI score, stylistics and competitive drive.

The quintile distribution of total SI score (Table 4) placed 17.14% of the examined sample in the lowest quintile (type B) and 15.7% in the highest quintile (type A). The prevalence of type A in our sample is higher than that reported by Kittel et al. [9] in Belgian workers (5.4%) and by Koskenvuo et al. [10] in the adult Finnish population. However, on comparing the prevalence of behavioural types in different populations, we should consider that in our sample policemen are preselected for special aptitudes and a healthy constitution.

Signs of ischaemia by basal ECG recording were found in three subjects who scored in the 4th and 5th quintiles.

The analysis of linear correlation coefficients shows a significant positive relationship between age and stylistics and between basal heart rate and SI total score, hostility and impatience. No significant relationship was found between total or partial SI score and BMI, systolic or diastolic pressure, or total and HDL-cholesterol (Table 5). The number of cigarettes per day appears positively related to SI total score and significantly related to stylistics (Table 5).

Finally, in a subgroup of 36 road traffic and city patrol volunteers, the relationship between the cardiovascular effects of their occupational stress and be-

Table 3. Means and SD of partial and total SI score in three groups with different duties

Occupational sphere	Age	SI total score	Stylistics	Competitive drive	Hostility	Speed	Impatience
Road traffic ($n=28$)	35.14 ±6.31	30.55 ±3.84	24.81 ± 6.37	26.96 ±6.06	34.25 ±7.92	32.91 ±5.81	33.70 ±6.57
City patrols ($n=21$)	39.42 ±4.84	31.00 ±5.66	24.62 ±10.67	28.33 ±7.12	32.79 ±8.88	34.14 ±7.87	34.80 ±6.07
Office ($n=21$)	49.61 ±5.19	33.48** ±4.03	30.30*** ± 7.64	31.73** ±7.84	34.50 ±7.65	35.21 ±6.16	35.40 ±7.26
Total ($n=70$)	40.77 ±8.21	31.57 ±4.63	26.43* ± 8.54	28.81 ±7.14	33.89 ±8.06	33.97 ±6.57	34.55 ±6.6

* $P<0.05$: vs office; ** $P<0.02$: vs road traffic; *** $P<0.01$: vs road traffic

Table 4. Quintile distribution of total SI scores, numbers and percentages of subjects in each quintile

Quintiles	I	II	III	IV	V	
Total SI score (range)	21.6–26.92	26.93–30.75	30.76–32.89	32.9–35.52	36.23–43	
No.	12	16	16	15	11	70
%	(17.14)	(22.86)	(22.86)	(21.43)	(15.71)	100

Table 5. Linear correlation coefficients (r) between the considered parameters and total and partial SI scores (BMI, body mass index; SBP, systolic blood pressure; DBP, diastolic blood pressure; CH-tot, total cholesterol; CH-HDL, high density lipoprotein)

	Age (70)	BMI (70)	Basal heart rate (70)	SBP (70)	DBP (70)	CH-tot (70)	CH-HDL (70)	Smoking (70)
SI total score	0.191	–0.035	0.277*	0.128	0.022	–0.084	–0.0073	0.229
Hostility	–0.102	0.074	0.344***	0.158	0.181	0.158	–0.058	0.189
Speed	0.148	–0.124	–0.046	–0.027	–0.079	–0.020	0.0004	0.171
Impatience	0.048	–0.096	0.301**	0.070	0.0153	0.071	0.096	–0.013
Competitive drive	0.174	0.041	0.158	0.129	0.011	–0.049	–0.029	0.100
Stylistics	0.281**	–0.036	0.080	0.114	0.009	0.030	–0.008	0.303**

* $P<0.05$; ** $P<0.02$; *** $P<0.01$

Table 6. Linear correlation coefficients (r) between percent increases (Δ) in heart rate (HR) and total ECG scores, and total and partial SI scores

	Mean Δ % HR	Δ % Basal HR B. Holter HR	Δ % Basal HR Max. Holter HR	Δ % B. Holter HR Max Holter HR	Max. HR as % max. theoretical HR	Total ECG score
Total SI score	–0.079	–0.029	–0.116	0.012	0.118	0.269
Stylistics	0.008	0.061	–0.168	0.030	–0.049	0.0024
Competitive drive	0.023	–0.140	–0.108	0.076	–0.068	0.234
Hostility	0.092	–0.004	–0.126	–0.001	0.144	–0.195
Speed	0.298	0.015	0.153	0.254	0.077	0.277
Impatience	–0.026	–0.126	–0.128	0.107	0.330	0.449***

*** $P<0.01$

havioural features was examined by dynamic ECG registration (Holter) (Table 6). Although no significant relationships were found between behavioural scores and percent increase (Δ) of heart rate considering either basal heart rate or maximal heart rate at the Holter registration, we observed a positive relationship between SI total score, competitive drive, speed, impatience (highly significant) and total ECG score, formulated for each subject using basal ECG, ECG after exercise and dynamic ECG results. Increased heart rate, arrhythmias and/or aspecific or specific P wave, QRS, S-T and T wave changes were found during dynamic ECG registration in 35.7% of subjects classified as normals at basal ECG and ECG after exercise.

The above results seem indicative of the influence of situations involving occupational stress on the cardiovascular system; carriers of "coronary prone" behavioural features may be unable to modulate their anxiety, with the consequent arousal of psychosomatic reactions. A possible neuroendocrine and metabolic involvement might give rise to functional or even organic changes at the cardiovascular level.

References

1. Friedman M, Rosenman RH (1959) Association of specific overt behavior pattern with blood and cardiovascular findings. JAMA 169:1286–1296
2. Jenkins CD, Zyzanski SJ, Rosenman RH, Cleveland GL (1971) Association of coronary prone behavior scores with recurrence of coronary heart disease. J Chronic Dis 24:601–611
3. Rosenman RH, Brand RJ, Jenkins CD, Friedman M, Straus R, Wurm M (1975) Coronary heart disease in the Western Collaborative Group Study: final follow-up experience of 8.5 years. JAMA 233:872–877
4. Rosenman RH, Brand RJ, Sholtz RI, Friedman M (1976) Multivariate prediction of coronary heart disease during 8.5 year follow-up in the Western Collaborative Group Study. Am J Cardiol 37:902–910
5. Rosenman RH, Friedman M (1974) Neurogenic factors in pathogenesis of coronary heart disease. Med Clin North Am 58:269–279
6. Dembroski TM, MacDougal JM, Shields JL (1977) Physiologic reactions to social challenge in persons evidencing the type A coronary prone behavior pattern. J Human Stress 3:2–9
7. Rosenman RH (1978) The interview method of assessment of the coronary-prone behavior pattern. In: Dembrowski M (ed) Coronary prone behavior. Springer, Berlin Heidelberg New York
8. Gruppo di ricerca ATS-RF_2 del C.N.R. (1980) I fattori di rischio dell'arteriosclerosi in Italia. G Ital Cardiol [Suppl 3] 10
9. Kittel F, Kornitzer M, Zyzansky SI, Jenkins CD, Rustin RM, Degre C (1978) Two methods of assessing the type-A coronary prone behavior in Belgium. J Chronic Dis 31:147
10. Koskenvuo M, Kaprio J, Langinvainio H, Rano M, Sarna S (1981) Psychosocial and environmental correlates of coronary-prone behavior in Finland. J Chronic Dis 34:331

Work Stressors and Coronary Risk: Two Perspectives

I. Weber and J. Siegrist

Epidemiological results concerning job characteristics and risk of coronary heart disease (CHD) are still contradictory or at least ambiguous. Thus their predictive power in explaining new cases of CHD in combination with traditional coronary risk factors is limited. This dilemma is partly due to the fact that poorly differentiated status indicators are applied instead of meaningful characteristics of work and occupation. Too often, oversimplified indicators of workers at risk produce contradictory findings due to opposite effects of single characteristics.

In order to reduce this kind of difficulty, Karasek et al. (1982, Job characteristics, occupation and coronary heart disease, unpublished resp. [7]) have proposed a new job strain model in which two basic dimensions of work situations are combined: the extent of situational demands and the extent of situational control. Karasek supposes psychophysiological strain at work to be the result of the joint effects of these dimensions: strain arises if a person facing heavy job demands has low decision latitude. Decision latitude means the margin of control the worker has over the demands of the work-place. This is the core of Karasek's job strain model.

However, this approach has its limitations as well. It seems adequate in analysing work situations of the relatively higher qualified employees. In these groups experiences of overload combined with low control at work seem to be of importance for stress-related disease susceptibility. However, low decision latitude seems to be of relatively little importance in work situations with narrowly defined and largely pre-structured tasks. Blue-collar workers with tasks which can be described as simple, repetitive and highly routinized seldom experience situations which require high decision latitude to accomplish their tasks.

We can illustrate this with our own survey data [5]. In a case control study we put the question whether the fact of being controlled at work results in subjective strain. The proportion of unskilled workers with myocardial infarction reporting strain with respect to control is low if compared with demand characteristics (Table 1). The same holds true for higher socioeconomic groups: unskilled workers do not experience strain due to lack of control more often than do workers and employees in the middle management, although we can suppose real differences of margins of control between these groups (Table 1).

The findings shown in Table 1 are based upon self-report data of patients with myocardial infarction. But there is similar evidence if we take self-report

Primary Health Care in the Making
Ed. by U. Laaser, R. Senault, H. Viefhues

Table 1. Self-ratings of job characteristics by occupied men[a] with first myocardial infarction[b]

Strain due to	Unskilled workers ($n=115$)	Superiors/middle management ($n=68$)
Control in execution	17%	13%
Control of outcome	21%	16%
Problems with superiors	29%	44%
Time pressure	63%	75%
Noise	50%	43%
Heat/cold	60%	49%

[a] Men aged 30–55 years
[b] Interviewed within at least 6 months after MI

data of healthy industrial blue-collar workers from an ongoing prospective study on cardiovascular risk [cf. 4], as shown in Table 2. The distribution of frequencies in Table 2 shows that experiences of overload due to time urgency (high demand) play a dominant role in the workers' daily experience of work stress. Emotional reactions of anger and irritation are admitted to a considerable degree, although the corresponding question is related to highly routinized experiences. As compared with time urgency, being controlled at work is a problem of minor importance: it is mentioned as a potential source of subjective strain by a minority of blue-collar workers only, and a still smaller proportion reacts to these experiences with emotional upset and irritation.

Thus, empirical evidence from self-rating data in two different groups of workers (MI patients and healthy blue-collar workers) points to the role of high demand as an important source of work-related subjective strain. On the other hand, low decision latitude as a low margin of control does not seem to be related to a comparable degree to strain. Does this mean that the two-dimensional model introduced by Karasek is of limited use? Our answer to this question is as follows.

Table 2. Self-ratings of job characteristics by industrial blue-collar workers ($n=416$)

Characteristic	Frequent[a] occurrence	Strong[b] emotional response
Quantitative overload	54%	49%
Troubles in execution	45%	33%
Disagreement with co-workers	30%	40%
Incorrect treatment by superior	14%	61%
Strict control	12%	16%

[a] Frequent = scores 3, 4 or 5 on a 5-point scale
[b] Strong = scores 3, 4 or 5 on a 5-point scale

The work dimensions of demand and control, on which the model of Karasek sheds light, represent only one side of job experiences which are relevant for coronary risk. Such experiences are restricted to the *context of performance.* In this context, job strain is the result of excessive and repetitive job demands.

Another dimension related to occupational career is often neglected in the analysis of work stress and CHD. Individuals at work are not only involved in daily tasks; they also pursue selfish ends, looking for promotion, income, security and approval. This aspect of occupational work can be called the *context of gratification* [6]. It is our argument that a low degree of control in the context of gratification is a much more powerful stressor than a low degree of control in the context of performance. Threat to control over achieved social status in a long-term perspective, poor opportunities to gain promotion or even to maintain an achieved position, experiences of cutdown in personnel and forced downward mobility are thought to affect emotional well-being much more than low decision latitude during daily work performance, epsecially among members of lower socioeconomic groups or groups with low chances for occupational mobility. We propose to adapt the two-dimensional model of job strain to conditions of low long-term control: active coping without success, continuous struggle without reward, overwhelming demands upon one's adaptive capacities – these are patterns of experience that we call *"active distress"* and which might be critical for cardiovascular pathology [4].

Social epidemiology provides preliminary evidence with regard to this argument. Kornitzer et al. [2] found an incidence of new coronary events twice as high in employed men of a private bank as compared with men working in a semi-public bank. Traditional risk factors at the beginning of this prospective study were unable to explain excess morbidity and mortality. Additional exploration revealed significantly higher psychomental workload and a higher degree of occupational instability, including cutdown in personnel in the private company [3]. A similar finding was reported from the Kennedy Space Center [1]. An unusually high rate of sudden cardiac death was observed in a group of young, highly specialized aerospace professionals. Again, traditional risk factors were unable to explain excess mortality, and additional exploration revealed an extremely competitive work environment due to the fact that after each successful space launch a cutback in budget and personnel by 15% was executed.

Finally, we present data from our own retrospective case control study on patients with premature MI [5, 6]: The occupational careers of 380 men who had survived an acute myocardial infarction and of healthy occupied men have been analysed. In the case group there were significantly more individuals who had experienced events of involuntary occupational change, such as change of company after job loss or dequalification of tasks, than in the control group of comparable age: 21% vs 9% ($P < 0.01$). In addition, risky coronary prone coping patterns were more pronounced in individuals whose status was threatened by such events [6].

Preliminary results of the ongoing prospective study indicate that the incidence of new coronary events in the blue-collar study population is higher than expected for the age-standardized male population in West Germany. This higher incidence to some degree reflects marked experiences of status threat in the occupational setting. It is along these lines that further analysis will be carried out in our group.

References

1. Eliot R, Clayton F, Pieper G, Todd G (1977) Influence of environmental stress on pathogenesis of sudden cardiac death. Fed Proc 36:1719–1724
2. Kornitzer M, Thilly C, Vanroux A, Balthazar E (1975) Incidence of ischaemic heart disease in two cohorts of Belgian clerks. Br J Soc Med 29:91–97
3. Kornitzer M, Kittel F, Dramaix M, de Backer G (1982) Job stress and coronary heart disease. Adv Cardiol 29:56
4. Siegrist J (1984) Threat to social status and cardiovascular risk. Psychother Psychosom 42:90–96
5. Siegrist J, Dittmann K, Rittner K, Weber I (1980) Soziale Belastungen und Herzinfarkt. Enke, Stuttgart
6. Weber I (1984) Berufstätigkeit, Belastungserfahrung und koronares Risiko. Ph. D. dissertation, Minerva, München
7. Karasek RA, Baker D, Marxer F, Ahlbom A and Theorell T: Job decision latitude, job demands, and cardiovascular disease. Am J Pub Health 71:694–705

Some Aspects of the Return to Work After Myocardial Infarction

K. Undeutsch and C. Halhuber

Myocardial infarction rehabilitation today consists of medical treatment as well as of psychosocial care. Rehabilitation is intended to compensate irreparable consequences by still present functions of the organism. Rehabilitation comprises all somatic and psychosocial endeavours to preserve for the person, afflicted with a chronic heart disease, the same position within society that he occupied before his affliction. Problems of keeping his job, of being re-employed, of modification of the work-load and, finally, of being retired and how to cope with it, are of the greatest importance for those endeavours.

What is the present situation vis-à-vis returning to work after myocardial infarction? The return to work is not only of importance from the point of view of social medicine or of national economy or of health politics, but also in terms of the patient's quality of life.

Figures relating to the number of patinets returning to work after myocardial infarction vary from 40% to 90% in the national and international reports; the following factors may account for this discrepancy.

1. The *kind of work:* Studies in Germany [16] have shown a higher rate of return to work for white-collar workers (sedentary or moderate work) than for blue-collar workers (physical work). Often, white-collar workers seem to have more chance to arrange their work with more flexibility and to adapt their job to the new health situation. Weiß [20] showed that the percentage of patients performing heavy physical work who returned to work was smaller than among patients with moderate physical work. Studies from Israel [1] and the U.S. support this finding.
2. *Medical reasons* also influence the rate of return to work. In German, English and American papers there is consensus about a number of medical factors that influence reintegration into work: severe angina pectoris, ventricular dysrhythmias, extent of obstructive coronary artery disease, heart failure, aneurysms. Non-cardiac diseases, e.g. diabetes, also reduce the rate of return to work [6].
3. The *waiting time for further medical procedures* is another important factor influencing return to work after myocardial infarction; this is especially so when coronary surgery is involved. Walter et al. [18] found a reduction in return to work with increasing waiting time for coronary surgery. Hammermeister et al. [8] showed that the most important predictor of return to

Primary Health Care in the Making
Ed. by U. Laaser, R. Senault, H. Viefhues

work is whether the patient was employed 3 months before surgery or catheterization.

4. Individual *psychosocial factors* play an important role in the return to work after myocaridal infarction. According to Samek [14] the return to work after myocardial infarction increases with the level of school education. Shapiro et al. [15] and Kentala [9] found a negative effect of low social class on return to work. Another interesting paper was that by Kottke et al. [10]. Major activity status (return to work for those previously employed, and return to other major pre-infarction activity for those not employed) was significantly poorer for the lower class patients than for the upper class patients. Only 35% of the lower class patients returned to major activities, while almost 90% of the upper class patients did so. Employer attitudes or the lower class patients' lack of incentive to return to work may have influenced the work status. The definitive answer cannot be obtained from this study. Behar et al. [1] reported that family support increases the return to work after myocardial infarction. Kushnir et al. [12] reported that cardiac patients who attributed their disease to work stress were less likely to return to work than those who did not. Danchin et al. [4] reported in a study from Canada that annual income and social class influence the return to work. The first results of a study by Lehmann [13] showed an influence of job position; moreover the physician's advise concerning return to work after myocardial infarction was of not less importance. The patient's own opinion regarding the capability of performing the old job was also of importance. On the other hand, family problems did not influence return to work.
5. Present *sociopolitical and economic trends:* There is little doubt that rehabilitation and coronary surgery can alleviate symptoms and improve exercise performance. Therefore failure to return to work must often be caused by non-medical factors. Possible reasons include the patient's fear; economic incentives to remain retired because of pension, disability insurance and social security benefits; economic disadvantages to the employer because of the workman's compensation insurance; and competition for jobs from younger, healthier people. Donat et al. [5], Krasemann and Jungmann [11], Weidemann and Finberg [19] and Walter et al. [18] all reported reduced return to work after the age of 55.

The above-mentioned factors, which influence the return to work after myocardial infarction, also influence the length of time before returning to work after myocardial infarction.

On the other hand, measures have been demonstrated during the past 10 years which increase the return to work:

1. *Step-wise return to work* (increasing working hours from 4 to 6 to 8 hours). Studies by Brost et al. [3] have shown a higher rate of return to work after myocardial infarction when step-wise return was performed.
2. *Comprehensive medical and psychosocial care* according the "Hamburg Model" or the concepts of Prof. Halhuber. Krasemann and Jungmann [11] for the "Hamburg Model" and Halhuber and König [7] for the "Höhenried Rehabilitation Clinic" reported a higher rate of return to work among pa-

tients with intensive follow-up treatment in a rehabilitation clinic than among patients without organized rehabilitation. After the establishment of coronary groups in the vicinity of the patients' homes for the continuation of therapy, the percentage of patients able to return to work increased even more [11]. Several studies from the U.S. have also shown an increase in return to work after myocardial infarction when a rehabilitation centre was visited.

3. *Co-operation and dialogue with the general practitioner.* A study by Stein and Krasemann [17] showed the importance of good co-operation between the physician of the rehabilitation clinic and the general practitioner. If there is good co-operation, then the percentage of patients who return to work is greater and also the time before return to work is shorter. The same authors also showed that a precise patient/physician dialogue as to the patient's prospects and the exact date of return to work upon discharge from the rehabilitation clinic has positive effects on the percentage returning to work and on the time before return to work. Lehmann [13] also reported a positive effect of patient/physician dialogue on return to work. The recommendation of the physician of the rehabilitation clinic as well as that of the general practitioner is of much importance for the patient. Positive motivation increases the number of patients returning to work, while anxiety and uncertainty on the part of the physician decrease the return to work.

To improve the return to work in the future and for further follow-up, the occupational health services should play a bigger role, because their doctors know their patients suffering from myocardial infarction and also the patient's working conditions. The prognosis of coronary heart disease is not negatively influenced by an early return to work [1, 17]. In addition, it is necessary to establish general criteria to answer the question of whether coronary patients should return to work. Furthermore, it is important to carry out more research in the psychosocial field to learn more about its influence on return to work.

References

1. Behar S, Cohen E, David P, Wolyvovics M, Almog H, Friedman Y, Agmon Y, Nenfeld HN (1981) Return to work after acute myocardial infarction. J Isr Med Assoc 1
2. Boulay FM, David PP, Bourassa MG (1982) Strategies for improving the work status of patients after coronary artery bypass surgery. Circulation [Suppl 3] 66:43–49
3. Brost R, Krasemann EO, Stolley B (1982) Untersuchungen zur stufenweisen Arbeitsaufnahme nach langer Krankheit. Rehabilitation 21:45–50
4. Danchin N, David P, Robert P, Bourassa MG (1982) Employment following aortocoronary bypass surgery in young patients. Cardiology 69:52–59
5. Donat K, Weiß B, Ziegeler WJ (1983) Schicksal nach Herzinfarkt in der Großstadt. Herbsttagung der Deutschen Gesellschaft für Herz- und Kreislaufforschung, Ulm
6. Gutmann MC, Knapp DN, Pollock ML, Schmidt DH, Simon K, Walcott G (1982) Coronary artery bypass patients and work status. Circulation [Suppl 3] 66:33–42
7. Halhuber MJ, König K (1982) Institutionalized, residential rehabilitation of patient with ischemic heart disease? In: Mathes P, Halhuber MJ (eds) Controversies in cardiac rehabilitation. Springer, Berlin Heidelberg New York, pp 128–138

8. Hammermeister KE, De Rouen TA, English MT, Dodge HT (1979) Effect of surgical versus medical therapy on return to work in patients with coronary artery disease. Am J Cardiol 44:105–111
9. Kentala E (1972) Physical fitness and feasibility of physical rehabilitation after myocardial infarction in men of working age. Ann Clin Res [Suppl 9] 4
10. Kottke TE, Young DT, McCall MM (1980) Effect of social class on recovery from myocardial infarction. Minn Med 8:590–597
11. Krasemann EO, Jungmann H (1979) Return to work after myocardial infarction. Cardiology 64:190–196
12. Kushnir B, Fox KM, Tomlinson IW (1975) The influence of psychological factors and an early hospital follow-up on return to work after first myocardial infarction. Scand J Rehabil Med 7:158–165
13. Lehmann H (to be published) Erste Ergebnisse der Oldenburger Longitudinalstudie zur Rückkehr zur Arbeit.
14. Samek L (1983) Welche Faktoren beeinflussen die Wiederaufnahme der Arbeit nach Herzinfarkt? Herbsttagung der Deutschen Gesellschaft für Herz- und Kreislaufforschung, Ulm
15. Shapiro S, Weinblatt E, Frank EW (1972) Return to work after first myocardial infarction. Arch Environ Health 24:17–25
16. Stabl M, Stocksmeier U, Natus W (1980) Arbeitswiederaufnahme und Berentung sozialversicherter Herzinfarktpatienten. MMW 122:512–516
17. Stein G, Krasemann EO (1981) Prospektive Untersuchungen zur Dauer der Arbeitsunfähigkeit nach Herzinfarkt. Herz Kreisl 13:526–532
18. Walter P, Thies B, Gerhardt U (1983) Wieviele Patienten nehmen nach einer Koronaroperation ihre Arbeit auf? Med Klin 78:276–280
19. Weidemann H, Finberg J (1983) Mehrjährige Verlaufsbeobachtung der medizinischen und beruflichen Rehabilitation nach Herzinfarkt bei Frauen im Vergleich zu Männern. Herz Gefäße 3:83–93
20. Weiß B (1982) Wiederaufnahme der Arbeit nach erstem Herzinfarkt. Ergebnisse der Hamburger Infarkt-Nachsorge-Studie. Dtsch Med Wochenschr 108:1872–1876

Vocational Rehabilitation in Hypertension and Renal Diseases

W. Huber, E. Marquard, and W. K. Schreiber

Arterial hypertension is the most frequent single or contributory cause of early invalidity due to coronary and circulatory disorders. This fact turns the question of maintaining hypertensive persons in employment – in regard to their rehabilitation – from being a purely individual problem into an economic one, too.

In this connection, it is imperative to identify stress factors existing at the place of work and their effect on the person. These are:

1. Physical strain
2. Mental and emotional stress
3. Environment factors

On 1: In particular, work having a high proportion of static activity (for example, lifting and carrying heavy loads) causes the mean pressure to rise and should therefore be avoided [8].

On 2: When exposed to mental stress under time pressure or external distressing factors, the hypertensive person will react with an increase in blood pressure which persists longer than in normotonic persons [4]. Work involving continuous concentration under time pressure and/or pressure due to responsibility [4], monotonous work entailing a high proportion of repetitive activity [3], work dissatisfaction and noise [1, 6] lead to chronic stress; it can be assumed that this type of stress will lead to hypertension in predisposed persons.

On 3: Noise and heat as well as other unsuitable working [4, 7] surroundings can also be considered environmental factors which may promote hypertension.

The kind of work that is not suited to a person with hypertension and reduced physical capacity (hypertension, stage II WHO) is the kind where the symptoms of the disease or the side-effects of therapy (vertigo, impaired vision, tendency towards orthostasis, tiredness) may put the patient or other persons at risk. Thus, there are certain jobs or working conditions which must be considered unsuitable for the hypertensive person:

- heavy physical work,
- work involving driving, controlling and supervisory activities,
- work on scaffolding and ladders,

Primary Health Care in the Making
Ed. by U. Laaser, R. Senault, H. Viefhues

- work at moving machines and electrical installations,
- work at blast-furnaces, open fires or intense heat, and
- work with 24-h shifts.

The aim of rehabilitation therefore should be to remove these factors or at least to reduce them. In this case an attempt should first be made to transfer the person within the company or to adapt the work-place. It should also be taken into account that certain types of stress are not confined to working life, while other types cannot be basically eliminated. The aim, therefore, is to achieve occupational restrictions in the right proportion to the need, which, in most cases, is proportional to the severity of the disease. When undergoing retraining, due consideration should be given to the prospects the future profession will have on the open labour market, since the objective of our efforts cannot be to give the patient, after a successful rehabilitation, a profession which suits his disability when he is unable to obtain work.

In hypertensive persons, limitations in their physical capacity can be expected to occur as from stage II WHO as a result of other organs becoming affected. Hypertension is thus recorded in statistics relating to vocational rehabilitation under those diseases for which the hypertension was also responsible or which have hypertension as a sequelae.

Due to the complexity of the disability, renal insufficiency as a result or cause of hypertension represents a first-class example of the problem facing vocational rehabilitation. In the case of the sequelae which are nearly always present in chronic renal insufficiency, the disability is brought about by the concurrent involvement of several organ systems. This applies also in the case of a successful transplantation. The sequelae may be: renal anaemia, myopathy and peripheral neuropathies, osteopathy and a reduction in defence against infections (especially due to the immune suppression after transplantation).

Considerable limitations in physical capacity are partly the result of this, requiring the following conditions to be fulfilled by a job and by a work environment [2]:

- no physically demanding work,
- no unilateral static strain,
- no fine motor skills (may vary from case to case)
- no work involving exposure to heat, humidity and cold,
- no work involving a high risk of infection,
- no work at machinery with open moving parts,
- no work involving toxic substances (for example, cadmium, mercury),
- no working under time pressure, and
- sufficient pauses for rest.

If the patient has to undergo dialysis, then it is essential to co-ordinate working hours and dialysis times. It would also be helpful if the place of employment and place of dialysis were not too distant from each other.

Despite this multifaceted disability, the dialysis patient is well capable of taking up employment, provided the job fits his abilities. The reality, however, shows a considerable discrepancy between the number of persons potentially able to work and those actually in employment. According to statistics compiled by EDTA in 1979, in the Federal Republic of Germany only 46.5% of dialysis patients able to work actually exercise an occupation. Of these, 27.7% are in full-time and 18.7% in part-time employment. This in itself low percentage is 13% below the European average [10].

Two investigations by the Stiftung Rehabilitation in Heidelberg confirm this finding. We carried out a survey of 713 dialysis patients from 15 centres and enquired about their occupational background [9]. Of 483 respondents who supplied details about their employment, 38.9% were working full-time and 22.6% part-time. The study shows that in addition to physical and psychic factors, the social environment has a vital influence on the actual occupational status of dialysis patients. Working patients do not enjoy greater immunity from sequelae than do non-working patients. Thus, the somatic status does not appear to be the major factor determining whether a patient takes up employment or not. The only exception thereto are severe additional disabilities such as diabetes mellitus.

Of major importance are factors such as work satisfaction, work motivation, opportunities for promotion and restrictions imposed by dialysis treatment. In contrast to patients undergoing dialysis in a centre, a distinctly larger number who are in employment are those with home dialysis. To a certain extent, this patient group might be pre-selected in regard to intellectual, economic and educational conditions.

Patients who work full-time tend to do their dialysis in the evening or even at night. This underlines the necessity for increasing the opportunity for evening or night dialysis.

According to their physicians, most patients are capable of working part-time (43%); 18% are considered capable of full-time employment, while 39% are seen as unemployable. This leads to the demand for the creation of more part-time jobs.

In a second study we were able to show that especially craftsmen undergoing dialysis give up their jobs. The reason for this could partly be the physical strain of the activity which cannot be coped with any longer and partly also unfavourable circumstances. Craftsmen are often employed in small firms where there are no opportunities for transfer. Only 23.8% of craftsmen under dialysis maintain their employment, in contrast to 49.3% of white-collar workers and civil servants, and 33.3% of self-employed persons. One can generally state that a higher education and occupational status in a trained profession tend to favour continuation of employment during dialysis. There are no statistics to show that there is a relationship between sex, age, school education and employment of dialysis patients who were in employment before dialysis treatment commenced. Numerically, there is only a slight relationship between the medical assessment of work capacity and actual employment.

It has been postulated, on the basis of the EDTA statistics and a paper by Pach et al. [5], that there has been an improvement in the proportion of employed persons following successful kidney transplantation. Our survey shows, however, that vocational rehabilitation following kidney transplantation is disappointing. Of the 69% of patients who were employed before commencement of dialysis and who later underwent a transplantation, only 24% were still in employment after the transplantation. This means that the above rate is little better than that of patients undergoing dialysis at a centre, and less than half as good as that of home dialysis patients. Nearly all the patients who took up employment following successful transplantation (altogether, 95 patients with functioning kidney transplants were surveyed) had previously undergone training or had already been in employment. Nearly half of the successfully transplanted respondents claimed that, if necessary, they could take up employment.

Successfully transplanted patients felt they were in a better position to enter employment, though they apparently felt no need to do so. Rather they tend to satisfy their own interests, are more active in their free time and have greater social contacts. Thus, their regained productive power following transplantation is most likely to be employed in the pursuit of leisure.

Findings from the Heidelberg Vocational Retraining Centre go to prove that the vocational rehabilitation of chronically ill persons, in this case dialysis patients, can be successful. Out of 30 dialysis patients who were retrained there, 18 had not been in employment before retraining, 22 were in employment 24 months after retraining (of whom 17 were full-time and 5 part-time) and one was still studying. Eight patients were not employed, but six of them were willing to work. Of these 30 patients, 17, that is more than one-half, had applied for retraining themselves. This corresponds to statements made by handicapped persons in vocational rehabilitation generally. This gives rise to the suspicion that the road leading to vocational resettlement is not being smoothed out for the handicapped but, rather, made more difficult. It is obviously easier and more convenient to send a patient into retirement than to rehabilitate him or her vocationally. This criticism is directed not only at the pertinent institutions but also at physicians. In fact, a survey of physicians – dealing with the vocational situation of their patients – showed that the physicians knew all the details of their patients' medical condition but that they had relatively little information about questions concerning training, work performance and occupational status. The physician's information on and/or interest in the vocational rehabilitation of patients could be an important factor in determining the patient's attitude towards remaining in employment. It is, therefore, essential to make physicians aware of the fact that vocational rehabilitation – after a patient has been recognised as incurable – can *also* mean treatment in the curative sense.

References

1. Andren L, Hansson L, Björkmann M, Jonson A (1980) Noise as a contributory factor in the development of elevated arterial pressure. Acta Med Scand 207:493
2. Huber W, Marquard E (1983) Der chronisch Nierenkranke im Betrieb. Zentralbl Arbeitsmed 33/1:16
3. Johannson G, Aronson G, Lindström BO (1978) Social, psychological and neuroendocrine stress reactions in highly mechanised work. Ergonomics 21:583
4. Mustacchi P (1976) Arterial hypertension and the work environment. J Occ Med 18/8:561
5. Pach J, Waniek W, Dostal G, Merguet T (1977) Berufliche Rehabilitation unter Langzeitdialyse und nach Nierentransplantation. Inn Med 4:222

6. Parvizpoor D.: Noise exposure and prevalence of high blood pressure among weavers in Iran. JOM 18/11:730
7. Perry HM Jr, Perry EF, Erlanger MW (1980) Possible influence of heavy metals in cardiovascular disease: Introduction and overview. J Environ Pathol Toxicol 42/3:195
8. Rost R, Hollmann W, Liesen H (1976) Körperliches Training mit Hochdruckpatienten, Ziele und Probleme. Herz Kreisl 8/12:680
9. Tews HP, Schreiber WK, Huber W, Zelt J, Ritz E (1980) Vocational rehabilitation in dialyzed patients. A cross-sectional study. Nephron 26:130
10. Wing AJ, et al. (1980) Combined report on regular dialysis and transplantation in Europe XI. XVIIIth Proc. EDTA

Occupational Performance of Patients with Multiple Sclerosis

S. Poser, P. Denecke, H. Friedrich, and R. Schipper

Recent reports from the United States and Great Britain suggest that the majority of patients with multiple sclerosis (MS) are unemployed. According to Scheinberg et al. [7] and Elian and Dean [2], a great many of them have an untapped ability and willingness to work. With stronger vocational rehabilitation efforts many patients were considered capable of working, a statement which was also true for patients from Israel [6].

Earlier German and British studies gave a more favourable picture of occupational status, 30% still being employed after a mean duration of MS of more than 20 years [1] and 50% 15 years post-diagnosis [4].

Our present study analyses the occupational situation of an epidemiological sample in a time of economic recession. The neurological status of 92 patients with a clinically definite or probable diagnosis of MS [5] was assessed in a standardized way at least three times between 1972 and 1983. The course was characterized as relapsing/remitting, remitting/progressive or progressive from onset and the speed of deterioration was evaluated each time. A progression index was devised by dividing the grade of disability according to Kurtzke [3] by the duration of the disease. For example, a patient with a present stable disability of grade 3 after a duration of 6 years has a progression index of 0.5. The smaller the quotient, the better the prognosis. Patients who deteriorated by not more than one grade within 5 years (progression index equal to or less than 0.2) were considered to have a benign course, while those who deteriorated by at least five grades within 5 years (progression index equal to or greater than 1.0) were called malignant cases; the ones in between were regarded as intermediate. The psychosocial situation was assessed by a detailed interview in 1978 and followed up until 1983.

In 1978 20 of the 92 patients, or 22%, were still employed after a mean duration of the disease of 18 years. Twenty-five (27%) were not working for reasons such as marriage, childbirth or old age. Of these 25, 23 were women taking care of their families. We called this group "housewives", disregarding the two men with old-age pensions. Of the 92, 42 (46%) were receiving a pension on medical grounds; five young patients were temporarily unemployed.

The sex ratio for the whole sample was 55 : 37 (women to men). The mean present age was 48 years, the mean duration of the disease 18 years and the mean progression index 0.3. Forty-eight patients (52%) had a benign, 38 (41%) an intermediate and 6 (7%) a malignant course. The employed patients were

Primary Health Care in the Making
Ed. by U. Laaser, R. Senault, H. Viefhues

more often male; they were younger, had a shorter duration of the disease and a smaller progression index compared with the other groups (Table 1). There was no correlation between employment and the educational level or type of training. The "housewife" group consisted of women who had no claim to a pension irrespective of disability or too mild a disability to warrant a benefit. This heterogeneity makes proper evaluation of employment status impossible. The following comparisons take only the employed and pensioner groups into consideration.

Table 1. Comparison of groups of MS patients with different vocational status

	Employed (n=20)	Not employed for diverse reasons (n=25)	Pension due to MS (n=42)
Relation women: men	9:11	23:2	21:21
Mean present age	44.5 years	48.9 years	52.1 years
Mean duration of disease	13.9 years	19.4 years	21.1 years
Mean progression index	0.126	0.265	0.392

In the employed group 17 out of 20 (85%) belonged to the benign, 3 to the intermediate and none to the malignant category, whereas the distribution of the pensioners was 14 : 23 : 5. The course of the disease was more often relapsing/remitting in the employed group, whereas chronic progression predominated in the retired group; here 12 (29%) had a chronic progressive course from onset, which is known for its unfavourable prognosis and only one of the employed group had this type of course.

In the employed group 18 out of 20 (90%) were only slightly disabled (grade 0–3 according to Kurtzke [3]), but 9 out of 42 (21%) of the pensioners belonged to this category also.

Eight patients were only slightly disabled at the time of retirement but have reached a moderate or severe disability in the meantime. Together with the 9 slightly disabled pensioners they are considered as a group of patients with a working potential for several more years.

Three main reasons were found to explain the early pension in this group:

1. Doctors or other members of health services, in some cases the employer, suggested the application for a pension, sometimes even against the patient's will.
2. The patient made the claim on the National Insurance Scheme because of dissatisfaction with his job.
3. Non-restricted housewives tried to improve the financial budget of the family by applying for a pension because of MS. We know of only two cases who did not succed with their application. In some instances the National Insurance officers seem to base their decision on such a claim only on the diagnosis MS and irrespective of the disability and course of the disease.

The possibility that women get a pension after a considerable time of housewife status is a remarkable feature of the German Social Security System. It is about to be abrogated in the present situation of economic recession.

That an early pension does not necessarily please patients is obvious considering the social network and coping behaviour: The 17 patients with early pension were more often isolated, and had more family problems and more difficulties in coping with the disease than any other group. It cannot be determined whether these patients had a pre-existing difficult personality structure which contributed to early retirement and the negative consequences or whether life as an early pensioner was the main source of dissatisfaction.

On the other hand, we found two patients still working in spite of considerable disability (grades 6 and 7). They are highly motivated and doing extremely well.

During the follow-up period of 5 years six more patients became pensioners: 2 in the employed group, 3 in the temporarily unemployed group and 1 in the housewife group. One employed woman had not paid insurance contributions and changed to the housewife group. One man receiving unemployment benefits in 1978 had found a job in the meantime. Three of the new pensioners were only slightly disabled. Eleven patients had died in the meantime (seven of the pensioners group, 4 of the housewives), 2 from suicide.

Altogether 18 out of 92 (20%) of the patients were still employed in 1983 after a mean duration of 23 years. This figure is similar to the recent American and British reports mentioned above [2, 7] and less favourable than previous German findings [1], studies from Israel [6] and Great Britain [4]. The varying prognoses of working ability in these studies arise from the different selection of patients, different treatment of housewives, different social security systems and a rapidly changing job marked. There is remarkable agreement between the studies, however, as to the ratio of patients who are unemployed but still have a working potential: 30% – 40% of the unemployed group were considered able to work provided that individual measures had been taken. Among these, vocational rehabilitation efforts and transportation services are most important, but psychosocial help to improve motivation and coping behaviour is necessary also. Essential prerequisites for these measures to be successful are:

1. Modification of the popular misconception that all patients with MS will end up in a wheelchair; 52% of our patients had a benign course.
2. Better information for patients and health personnel about the services and benefits available and the ways to attain them.
3. Easier access to rehabilitation programs for patients with a benign course, stable disability and high motivation. At present it is hard to convince vocational rehabilitation personnel that it is worthwhile to retrain any patient with MS.

In a time of recession these measures will not improve the present occupational status but they must be taken for the sake of a future generation of MS patients.

References

1. Bauer HJ, Firnhaber W, Winkler W (1965) Prognostic criteria in multiple sclerosis. Ann NY Acad Sci 122:542–551
2. Elian M, Dean G (1983) Need for and use of social and health services by multiple sclerosis patients living at home in England. Lancet 1:1091–1093
3. Kurtzke JF (1961) On the evaluation of disability in multiple sclerosis. Neurology (Minneap) 11:686–694
4. Mitchell JN (1981) Multiple sclerosis and the prospects of employment. J Soc Occup Med 31:134–138
5. Poser S (1978) Multiple sclerosis. Springer, Berlin Heidelberg New York
6. Rozin R, Schiff Y, Cooper G, Kahana K (1982) Vocational rehabilitation of multiple sclerosis (MS) patients. Int Rehabil Med 4:75–79
7. Scheinberg L, Holland N, Larocca N, Laitin P, Bennett A, Hall H (1981) Vocational disability and rehabilitation in multiple sclerosis. Int J Rehabil Res 4:61–64

Mortality and Accidents in the Electrical Industry

S. Koifman, V. L. G. Blank, and J. A. M. Souza

Many physical changes have been reported after exposure to electricity fields. In the main they have been related to the central nervous system, cardiovascular system and the gastrointestinal tract. Soviet researchers have reported a decreased red cell count, high blood pressure, arrythmia, sexual disturbances, nervousness, nausea and other symptoms after exposure to 5 kV [3]. In Germany, Hauf [2] studied acute manifestations of these disturbances and found that they disappeared after exposure had ceased. In Mexico, Ajenjo et al. (1979, Work process and health standards of workers exposed to electrical risk, unpublished) confirmed these findings and demonstrated that survivorship after retirement of workers not exposed to electricity was 10 years longer than that of exposed workers (93.4% and 61.6%). Raynor et al. [5] pointed out a possible association between blood pressure and renal carcinoma among electrical workers in the U.S.A.

An investigation based on information collected in 700 industries in Brazil has shown that 90% of the occupational accidents resulting in incapacity were produced by electricity. This, together with the lack of safety measures in general, has stimulated the electrical labour union to fight for better working conditions. However, it is important to appreciate that Brazil is a country in which the majority of the population, including even the skilled workers, is primarily concerned with aspects of its daily maintenance. Unemployment is widespread and as a result only a few unions have solid ground on which to fight for improved labour conditions. Further, there is a consensus that individual error plays a large role in occupational accidents. This approach to the problem tends to conceal the important underlying social framework: poor living standards, low wages, the continual threat of unemployment and, as a consequence, the need to work overtime. In this context, the struggle initiated by the electrical labour union in Rio de Janeiro can be seen to gain a special dimension.

This study can be seen as a small step in this process and it is hoped that it will help the electrical workers to discuss their health and working conditions, and to take action to bring about changes. The objectives of the research have been to measure the mortality risk and accident risk among electrical workers in Rio. The data were collected from the reports of accidents and deaths of union members, who represent 60% of this group of workers. In general, the information on accidents has been analysed by a commission made up of workers and industrial representatives, and the reports are available at the union.

Primary Health Care in the Making
Ed. by U. Laaser, R. Senault, H. Viefhues

Mortality data were analysed using the standardized mortality ratio, and the age-specific mortality rates for the male population of Rio de Janeiro were used as a standard. An increased mortality risk of 47% among electrical workers in relation to the general population was observed. Nevertheless, when the observed and expected deaths among workers under 50 years of age are compared, a higher number of expected deaths is observed (30 observed to 44 expected). This may be due to a higher socioeconomic level and consequently better health conditions of these workers, as compared with those of the population in general. Further, this group is generally subject to a physical examination prior to admission and this factor may exert an important selective influence. Only after the age of 50 does the trend change and the observed deaths (72) are seen to be three times higher than expected (Table 1).

Probably, with stratification of the over 50 age group (which was not done because the data on the older workers were not available) it would be possible to decrease the SMR. However, even in this case it is difficult to imagine that the SMR would decrease to a value of 100%, in other words to a value which indicates identical risk of mortality among the electrical workers and the population in general. The existence of an increased number of deaths among those over 50 years of age may suggest a cumulative process after exposure, which begins to present manifestations later in life. This hypothesis is reinforced by the analysis of death certificates. The electrical workers in 1980 presented a proportional mortality ratio of 50% for cardiovascular diseases and 28% for cancer; for both groups, the Brazilian national data are 25% and 10% respectively. The cases of cancer among electrical workers included the following localizations: lung (two cases), and colon, vessel, prostate, stomach, leukemia and melanoma (one case each). The majority of cases were probably related to occupational exposure despite the fact that control for smoking was not carried out. Future studies are being planned to investigate the possible exposure to chemical solvents during the routine activities of these workers.

In relation to accidents, a marked geographical distribution was observed, with high rates in the central area of Rio (Table 2), which is characterized by a large quantity of obsolete equipment in underground installations. The more obvious difficulties of working in confined underground areas are further in-

Table 1. Observed and expected deaths for electrical workers, Rio de Janeiro, 1979

Age (years)	Male electrical workers (*n*)	Mortality[a]	Expected deaths	Observed deaths
20–29	4 179	3.1	13	3
30–39	3 334	4.3	15	16
40–49	1 844	8.8	16	11
50 or more	700	35.4	25	72
Total	10 057	12.3	69	102

[a] Death rates per 1000 inhabitants, Rio de Janeiro, male population. SMR = 102/69 · 100 = 147.8% (147.5–148.1)

Table 2. Time and space distribution of casualty frequency rates[a] in electrical areas, Rio de Janeiro, June 1979 to May 1980 (Source: Casualty Statistics, Light and Power Company)

Area		Month												Median
		Jun.	Jul.	Aug.	Sept.	Oct.	Nov.	Dec.	Jan.	Feb.	Mar.	Apr.	May	
I	Central	53.3	18.4	56.5	28.6	42.0	17.8	32.2	25.1	25.9	45.7	25.0	20.6	27.2
II	Cachambi	12.7	10.2	18.8	15.6	25.6	40.2	19.5	15.9	15.9	35.1	24.3	9.1	17.4
III	Campo Grande	15.2	8.0	–	–	7.6	–	–	–	7.8	31.8	–	–	–
IV	Nova Iguaçu	11.1	29.4	23.3	16.6	10.9	15.7	27.4	22.2	11.1	11.3	5.3	32.1	16.1
V	Barra do Piraí	22.6	18.5	5.7	11.2	22.4	27.1	11.3	23.8	5.9	11.6	5.6	22.5	15.0

[a] Per 1 000 000 hours worked

Table 3. Fatality rates in electrical production areas, Rio de Janeiro, June 1979 to May 1980 (Source: Casualties Statistics, Light and Power Company)

Area		Accidents	Deaths	Fatality rate (%)
I	Central	292	5	1.7
II	Cachambi	121	1	0.8
III	Campo Grande	11	–	–
IV	Nova Iguaçu	88	1	1.1
V	Barra do Piraí	51	1	1.9
Total		563	8	1.4

Table 4. Severity of accidents in electrical production areas, Rio de Janeiro, June 1979 to May 1980 (Source: Casualties Statistics, Light and Power Company)

Area		Severe accidents		Non-severe accidents		Total	
		No.	%	No.	%	No.	%
I	Central	180	62.7	107	37.3	287	100.0
II	Cachambi	75	62.5	45	37.5	120	100.0
III	Campo Grande	9	81.8	2	18.2	11	100.0
IV	Nova Iguaçu	38	43.7	49	56.3	87	100.0
V	Barra do Piraí	32	64.0	18	36.0	50	100.0
	Total	334	60.2	221	39.8	555	100.0

Table 5. Casualties in Brazil, 1969–1978 (Source: Escosteguy [7])

Year	Employees	Accidents		Workers involved
	(*n*)	No.	Increase (%)	(%)
1969	7 268 449	1 050 296	–	14.6
1970	7 284 022	1 220 111	+15.2	16.7
1971	7 764 486	1 330 523	+ 9.0	17.1
1972	8 148 987	1 504 723	+13.1	18.5
1973	10 956 956	1 632 696	+ 8.5	14.9
1974	11 537 024	1 796 761	+10.0	15.6
1975	12 996 796	1 916 167	+ 6.6	14.7
1976	14 945 489	1 743 825	− 9.8	11.7
1977	16 589 505	1 614 750	− 7.4	9.7
1978	18 500 000	1 564 380	− 3.1	8.5

creased by risks resulting from the collection of water due to rainfall or sewage disposal. The geographical distribution of accidents overlaps with the fatality rates: 1.7% in the central area and 1.4% in Rio de Janeiro generally – both higher than the fatality rate for accidents in Brazil, i.e. 0.3% (Table 3).

Finally, it is important to comment on the degree of severity of the accidents reported in the electrical industry. Most electrical production plants in Rio report only the severe accidents or those which prevent the worker from carrying out his labour activities (Table 4). This phenomenon is not confined to the electrical industry but is also present in other branches of Brazilian industry. The uncontrolled exploitation of the labour force through overtime and low wages has resulted in an increased number of labour accidents. By 1975, this number had reached nearly 2 million (Table 5). In 1976, two changes in the laws relating to the prevention of accidents were introduced:

1. The National Security Service payments were restricted to cover the care of workers only for the period commencing 15 days after the date of the accident. The costs resulting from care before that date became the responsibility of the industry. Consequently, industries are now only interested in reporting severe accidents.
2. The small payment made to workers who suffered minor accidents (those in which labour activity was not affected) was cancelled.

These two measures have resulted in an artificial decrease in the notification of accidents, including those in the electrical production areas.

References

1. Gotlieb SLD (1981) Differential mortality by causes, São Paulo, Brazil. Rev Saude Publica 15:401–417
2. Hauf R (1976) L'influence des champs alternatifs électriques et magnétiques à 50 H2 sur les hommes. Rev Gen Electr:31–50
3. Knave B, Gamberale F, Bergstrom S, Iregren A, Kolmodin-Hedman B, Wenberg A (1979) Long-term exposure to electric fields. Scand J Work Environ Health 5:115–125
4. Lilienfeld AM (1976) Mortality statistic. In: Lilienfeld AM (ed) Foundations of Epidemiology. Oxford University Press, New York
5. Raynor WJ, Shekelle RB, Rosso FHA, Maliza C, Apul O (1981) High blood pressure and 17 years cancer mortality, in the Western Electric Health Study. Am J Epidemiol 13:371–377
6. Young LB, Young HA (1974) Pollution by electrical transmission. Bull At Sci 34–38
7. Escosteguy apud Possas, C. Health and Work. The Social Security Crisis. Rio de Janeiro, Edicões Graal, 1981, pg 133

Nutritional Habits and Their Relation to Health in the Occupational Environment *

J. S. Vobecky, J. Vobecky, and D. Shapcott

Introduction

Recent years have witnessed increasing attention to occupational health, in great measure due to the close association between the well-being of workers and their productivity. In industrialized countries, both inadequate and excessive nutritional intakes contribute significantly to morbidity and mortality. Because only limited data are available on the nutritional status of industrial workers in relation to occupational exposure to environmental hazards, we investigated this relationship in a cohort of 252 industrial workers.

Methods

Nutritional status was evaluated three times at 6-month intervals:

- by a 7-day dietary record and by assessment of food habits;
- by biochemical determinations of 18 components in fasting venous blood, urine and hair, performed at the beginning and at the end of the study; and,
- by anthropometric measurements (consisting of weight, height, tricipital and subscapular skinfold thickness).

The assessment of life-style was also done at 6-month intervals.

Occupational exposure to noise, dust, chemical agents and high temperatures was continuously recorded for each worker, by an industrial hygienist, directly at the working site.

The assessment of the nutritional status will focus on:

- the mean daily nutrient intake per kg of body weight;
- alcohol consumption;
- the mean nutrient intake and dietary habits with regard to occupational exposure and working hours; and, finally,
- on selected biochemical parameters.

---

* Supported by grant No. 780-400, Conseil de la Recherche en Santé du Québec

Primary Health Care in the Making
Ed. by U. Laaser, R. Senault, H. Viefhues

The studied group consisted of workers mostly of French Canadian origin selected in four different plants, manufacturing asbestos textile, paper pulp, heavy machinery and textile. Their mean age was 39.7 years, ranging from 20 to 53 years; the length of employment varied from 1 to 20 years.

Results

The mean intake of almost all 29 studied nutrients exceeded the RNI level; however, some values were below RNI, varying in a large range from 2.8% for phosphorus to 100% for fibre. Some workers had an intake below the recommended levels even for protein (3.7%), vitamin C (6.8%), iron (7.9%) and others. Using as a limit < 75% of RNI as an indicator of possible deficiency, their proportion decreased, but for some nutrients such as fibres, vitamin E and folates the proportions still remained higher than 50% (Table 1).

Alcohol consumption was of particular importance. The mean daily intake was 14 g of ethyl alcohol, ranging from 0 to > than 50 g/day; consequently, up to 17% of calories were supplied by alcohol; those consuming > 50 g of alcohol daily had a lower intake of vitamin C, folates and calcium but a significantly higher intake of riboflavin and niacin (Table 2).

The relationships between nutrient intake and alcohol consumption also showed dose-related patterns (Fig. 1). Vitamin C decreased below the level of

Table 1. Proportion of workers with nutrient intake below RDA

Nutrient	Unit	RDA	< RDA (%)	< 75% RDA (%)
Calorie	kcal	2300	32.8	6.8
		2700	58.2	17.9
Protein	g	56	3.7	0.6
Fibre	mg	8	99.4	93.1
		14	100.0	99.8
Ca	mg	800	58.4	31.7
Mg	mg	300	53.2	16.2
P	mg	800	2.8	0.5
Fe	mg	10	7.9	0.9
Zn	mg	10	12.4	1.9
Vit. A	IU	3000	13.8	5.8
D	IU	100	33.8	24.6
E	mg	8	79.3	54.0
C	mg	30	6.8	2.7
B_1	mg	1.4	54.6	20.4
B_2	mg	1.7	46.5	14.6
B_6	mg	2.0	68.6	26.2
B_{12}	mcg	3.0	9.6	3.1
Niacin	mg	18	18.2	3.3
Folate	mcg	200	96.9[a]	90.6[a]

[a] Given as free folate

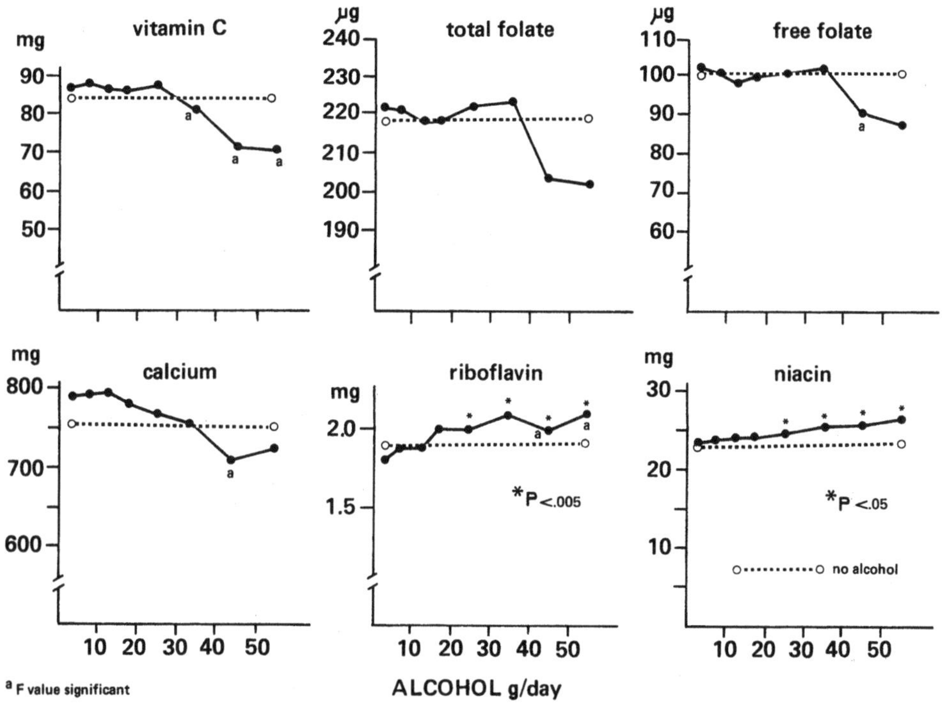

Fig. 1. Food intake of selected nutrients according to alcohol consumption

Table 2. Food intake of selected nutrients according to alcohol consumption

Nutrient	Alcohol consumption			
	≦50 g		>50 g	
	x̄	s	x̄	s
Vitamin C (mg)	87.0	66.4	70.4	40.0
Folate (µg)	221.0	85.0	201.0	80.0
Free folate (µg)	103.0	47.0	88.0	42.0
Calcium (mg)	784.0	340.0	728.0	229.0
Riboflavin (µg)	1.8*	0.6	2.1*	0.5
Niacin (mg)	23.1**	6.0	26.7**	7.0

* $P<0.01$; ** $P<0.001$

those not consuming alcohol when alcohol consumption exceeded 30 g/day. For folates and calcium, the decrease became evident when alcohol reached 40 g/day. Once again, the significant increases of riboflavin and niacin were noted very early, i.e. as soon as the alcohol intake rose above 20 g/day. (To test the differences Student's *t*-test and ANOVA were used.)

To identify the changes in nutrient intake with regard to occupational exposure, the workers were divided into two groups: those exposed to one or more of the mentioned hazards, and those without any exposure (Table 3).

There were no differences in the relative weight, nor in alcohol consumption but the significantly higher mean intake of calories, protein, carbohydrates and fat was always in the exposed group. According to the number of risks to which the workers were exposed, all examined items, i.e. calories, proteins, carbohydrates and fat (Table 4), showed a statistically significant gradient from zero risk to three risks. But for those exposed to four risks, a slight decrease was observed.

The relationships of food habits to occupational exposure corroborated with the previous observations (Table 5).

The higher proportions of non-exposed workers were found below 75% of Dietary Guide Recommendations. In other words, it seems that those exposed to selected occupational hazards consumed principal food items in sufficient quantities, i.e. above 75% of the recommendations. For milk and cereals, most differences were statistically significant.

Considering the consumption < 75% level as an indicator of an inadequately balanced diet, the risk of nutritional inadequacy increased according to the number of food groups consumed below this level. In relation to occupational hazards (Table 6), the percentage of exposed workers without any deficient food groups was always higher. Also those deficient for four groups were al-

Table 3. Mean energy, nutrient and alcohol intake according to the occupational exposure to the selected risks[a]

	Exposure to risks			
	One or more[b] (n=203)		None present (n=23)	
	$\bar{x}$	s	$\bar{x}$	s
Relative weight	1.06	0.14	1.08	0.16
Calorie (g/kg)	36.3*	10.1	33.1*	7.8
Protein (g/kg)	1.34**	0.38	1.28**	0.24
Carbohydrates (g/kg)	3.96***	1.31	3.43***	1.03
Fat (g/kg)	1.47***	0.47	1.37***	0.39
Alcohol (g/day)	0.28	0.29	0.27	0.24

[a] 26 workers exposed to other risk were excluded

[b] One or more of selected risks present: noise, chemical agents, dust, temperature

To test the difference between two means, Student's t-test was used: * $P<0.05$, ** $P<0.01$, *** $P<0.001$

Table 4. Mean daily energy and nutrient intake according to the number of risks[a]

Number of risks	Calories (cal/kg)		Proteins (g/kg)		CHO (g/kg)		FAT (g/kg)	
	$\bar{x}$	s	$\bar{x}$	s	$\bar{x}$	s	$\bar{x}$	s
0	32.6	9.2	1.28	0.25	3.43	1.27	1.33	0.40
1	32.0	10.0	1.13	0.36	3.55	1.29	1.21	0.51
2	33.7	9.7	1.30	0.34	3.47	1.08	1.41	0.44
3	36.5	11.1	1.38	0.40	3.98	1.39	1.50	0.50
4	35.5	7.5	1.26	0.28	3.91	0.95	1.48	0.42
Total	35.0	9.8	1.31	0.35	3.76	1.22	1.44	0.46
ANOVA: F	3.34		4.76		5.17		3.70	
P	0.01		0.001		0.001		0.006	

[a] Any combination of exposure to dust, noise, temperature and chemical agents; mean values are based on three dietary records collected at 6-months intervals ($n=553$)

Table 5. Proportion of workers consuming $\leqq$ 75% of recommended daily allowance according to occupational hazards (test of proportion was used)

Exposure		Milk	Fruits	Vegetables	Potatoes	Meat	Cereals, bread
Noise	Yes	21.7[a]	56.3	42.8	22.9	28.7	76.5[b]
	No	34.2[a]	56.0	39.9	24.7	29.4	86.5[b]
Dust	Yes	22.4	55.9	42.7	22.0	28.5	75.9[c]
	No	28.7	57.7	41.4	28.0	30.2	86.6[c]
Chemical hazards	Yes	15.9[d]	51.8	30.3[e]	14.8[f]	25.9	77.8
	No	26.4[d]	57.9	46.8[e]	26.2[f]	29.9	78.2
Temperature	Yes	19.3[g]	56.0	39.1	23.2	28.9	75.2[h]
	No	28.6[g]	56.5	46.7	23.2	28.6	81.4[h]

[a, b] $P<0.01$ [e] $P<0.001$ [g] $P<0.002$
[c, d] $P<0.009$ [f] $P<0.005$ [h] $P<0.05$

Table 6. Proportions of workers consuming one or more food groups at $\leqq$75% level of daily allowance according to occupational hazards (test of proportion was used)

Exposure		Number of deficient groups				
		None	One	Two	Three	Four
Noise	Yes	9.4	33.6	33.8*	17.2	5.7**
	No	6.6	38.0	24.7*	16.1	14.2**
Dust	Yes	9.5	34.8	32.5	17.1	5.8*
	No	6.6	32.5	31.8	17.0	11.8*
Chemical hazards	Yes	12.1*	36.4	35.3	12.1*	3.8*
	No	7.8*	33.6	31.3	18.9*	8.2*
Temperature	Yes	10.6	35.6	33.4	14.2*	6.0
	No	7.0	32.9	31.3	20.4*	8.3

* $P<0.05$; ** $P<0.005$

ways less frequent among the exposed workers, with significant differences for exposure to noise, dust and chemical hazards; but for those deficient in three food groups, less consistent patterns were observed.

According to working hours (Table 7), those working in daytime only had a mean intake of calories, carbohydrates and alcohol significantly higher than those in rotating or night shifts.

Furthermore, the metabolic response to the nutrient intake measured by biochemical parameters presented some variations in relation to the specific occupational risks (Table 8). In most cases, there were no significant differences between the exposed and non-exposed workers. But when focusing on selected vitamins (A, C, E and folate) which reflect more rapidly the food intake, their serum levels tended to be higher in the non-exposed workers with the exception of those exposed to chemical agents for vitamin E and folate and in those exposed to high temperature for vitamin C.

To determine whether exposure to specific occupational environment could increase the metabolic needs, the frequency of deficient values of selected vitamins (Table 9) was examined. Deficient serum levels of vitamin C, E and folate were more frequent in the exposed workers excepting for vitamin E and folates in those exposed to chemical agents, but vitamin A was always more frequently deficient in the non-exposed.

The deficient values for one or more vitamins were more frequent (Table 10) in those exposed to any one of the risks studied. On the other hand, the highest proportion of workers without any deficienct values was almost always in those not exposed. No one worker was deficient for all four vitamins.

Finally, the workers deficient in selected vitamins were compared according to the number of risks (Table 11) from zero to four: 43.5% of workers without any deficient value were found in the group "0 risk" and this decreased to 31.8% in the group "three and four risks"; but workers deficient for two or more vitamins increased from 13% in the "0 risk" group to 25.6% in the "three and four risk" group.

Table 7. Daily energy, nutrient and alcohol intake according to working hours

	Working hours				P^a
	Day-time (n=149)		Other (n=76)		
	$\bar{x}$	s	$\bar{x}$	s	
Calories (cal/kg)	35.1	±7.3	31.9	±7.6	<0.001
Protein (g/kg)	1.36	±0.34	1.29	±0.37	NS
CHO (g/kg)	3.81	±0.98	3.33	±0.99	<0.001
Fat (g/kg)	1.49	±0.46	1.41	±0.43	NS
Alcohol (g/kg)	0.28^b	±0.28	0.19^c	±0.20	<0.005

[a] Student's t-test was used
[b] n=103
[c] n=55

Table 8. Mean level of biochemical parameters according to occupational hazards

Exposure		Vitamin A (μg/dl)		Vitamin C (mg/dl)		Vitamin E (mg/dl)		Folic Acid (ng/ml)		Iron (μg/dl)	
		x̄	s	x̄	s	x̄	s	x̄	s	x̄	s
Noise	Yes	59.8	16.4	0.59	0.28	0.53	0.19	5.0	3.2	138.9	35.7
	No	60.1	15.9	0.62	0.28	0.57	0.24	5.7	3.6	130.3	32.6
Dust	Yes	58.8	15.8	0.59	0.28	0.53	0.19	4.8	2.7	171.6	52.1
	No.	65.1	18.4	0.63	0.29	0.56	0.22	6.2	4.1	138.9	35.7
Chemical hazards	Yes	57.2	15.3	0.57	0.26	0.58	0.26	5.5	2.4	132.2	28.4
	No	60.8	17.0	0.60	0.28	0.52	0.18	4.9	3.5	134.2	40.9
Temperature	Yes	58.1*	14.9	0.60	0.29	0.54	0.21	4.8**	2.7	137.0	26.2
	No	62.0*	18.5	0.59	0.26	0.53	0.19	5.4**	3.8	129.6	48.3

* $t=2.52$, $P<0.02$; ** $t=2.31$, $P<0.05$

Table 9. Mean level of selected biochemical parameters in blood, hair and urine according to the number of risks

Number of risks	*n*	Vit. A (μg/dl)		Vit. C (mg/dl)		Vit. E (mg/dl)		Folic Acid (mg/ml)		Iron (μg/dl)	
		x̄	s	x̄	s	x̄	s	x̄	s	x̄	s
0	24	59.6	16.9	0.61	0.23	0.54	0.21	5.5	2.5	131.3	33.1
1	17	70.7	21.4	0.75	0.34	0.59	0.24	7.3	5.9	127.6	35.5
2	73	61.4	17.7	0.53	0.25	0.54	0.19	5.1	3.9	134.2	60.6
3	82	58.9	14.2	0.65	0.29	0.48	0.14	4.0	1.9	134.2	24.2
4	52	55.9	15.9	0.55	0.25	0.60	0.26	5.7	2.5	134.4	28.7

Table 10. Proportions of workers with deficient serum level of selected vitamins according to occupational exposure

Exposure		Vitamin A[a] <30 μg/dl	Vitamin C[a] <0.4 mg/dl	Vitamin E[a] <0.5 mg/dl	Folic acid <2.5 ng/ml
Noise	Yes	0.5	31.6	48.4	14.2
	No	2.9	18.2	44.1	3.0
Dust	Yes	0.5	30.7	48.5	14.6*
	No	2.1	26.1	44.7	4.3
Chemical hazards	Yes	0	31.7	41.5	4.8*
	No	1.1	29.1	50.0	15.3
Temperature	Yes	0	31.9	47.9	17.6*
	No	1.8	27.3	47.7	6.4

[a] According to Nutrition Canada

* $P<0.05$

Table 11. Proportion of workers with deficient level for none, one or more selected vitamins according to occupational exposure

Exposure (number of risks)	Number of deficient vitamins		
	None	One	Two or more
0 (23)	43.5 (10)	43.5 (10)	13.0 (3)
1–2 (90)	37.8 (34)	41.1 (37)	21.1 (19)
3–4 (129)	31.8 (41)	42.6 (55)	25.6 (33)
Total (242)	35.1 (85)	42.1 (102)	22.8 (55)

Conclusion

The presented results indicated:

1. That the nutritional status of workers varied according to the type of industry
2. That the daily mean intake was higher than RNI for most of the studied nutrients; but an important proportion were below the RNI levels, including such nutrients as vitamin C, iron and protein, while other nutrients were even below the 75% level of RNI
3. That alcohol consumption evidently influenced the intake of some nutrients; in particular it was associated with a decreased intake of vitamin C and folates, and an increased intake of riboflavin and niacin
4. That the mean nutrient intake was almost always higher in workers exposed to selected occupational hazards, namely to the chemical hazards
5. That the rotating shifts influenced significantly the intake of calories, carbohydrates and alcohol

Based on these data, we concluded that nutrient intake as well as biochemical parameters were modified as a metabolic response to the specific needs in workers exposed to the studied occupational hazards, and that these hazards strongly influenced energy and vitamin needs.

Finally, we would like to emphasize that the relationship between nutritional status and working conditions underlined the importance of assessment of nutritional status for prevention and health promotion in an industrial setting, and the need for more detailed studies.

Alcohol in the Working Environment *

U. Canaris and J. Töppich

Introduction

Within the framework of a representative repetitive study on health norms and health behaviour of the population in the Federal Republic of Germany, we also investigated in 1980, for the first time, the connection between work-induced stress and health-abusive behaviour. The results of the study show that, particularly with regard to the consumption of alcohol, there exists a significant relationship between stress at the work-place and regular health hazardous alcohol consumption. Eleven per cent of all employees, i.e. about 3 million, drink alcohol daily at work. Where employees feel content at work, this rate decreases to 4%, whereas under stressful working conditions the figure increases to 23%. Similar results were obtained by interview concerning the quantity of alcohol consumed. Whereas only 8% of low stressed employees admit to drinking more than 280 g of alcohol per week, this figure increases to 17% for high stressed employees, and probably even more, since interviews tend towards understatement. These findings have been corroborated and qualitatively extended by a study carried out simultaneously by the Swiss Agency for Alcohol Problems.

After we published our results, we received an overwhelming demand for information and co-operation from industry, research and related fields of activity. This made it possible for a long-intended pilot intervention project concerning alcohol prevention in the working environment to be planned in a more detail way. Talks with industrial representatives enabled us to develop, test and evaluate a preventive intervention concept directly at the place of work. The objective was to make the daily consumption of alcohol an everyday topic and so influence it to prevent alcohol-induced diseases.

Our preventive intervention concept is based on a hypothetical systematization of a firm's structure regarding the consumption of alcohol. We identified three levels:

1. The working process
2. The availability of alcohol on the firm's premises
3. The communication within a firm concerning alcohol

---

* A health education intervention project of the Federal Centre for Health Education (FCHE), Federal Republic of Germany

Primary Health Care in the Making
Ed. by U. Laaser, R. Senault, H. Viefhues

The Intervention Concept in Detail

The Working Process

Within the working process, the consumption of alcohol has a functional meaning both for the individual employee and for the social system within the firm, as described below:

- Firstly, alcohol is used as just one psychoactive means of regulating psychic and/or physical tensions. Thus, activities which are characterized by a low level of achievement and activities which offer few possibilities to avoid working stress are both connected with a statistically significant high habitual consumption of alcohol. Likewise, activities with long periods of relatively low stress alternating with short periods of high stress give similar results.
- Secondly, alcohol is also of importance within the informal working organization, for example as a means of mobilizing energy reserves, a reward for achievement and to establish and maintain social contacts. Also, alcohol plays an important part, especially on a higher hierarchical level, in creating a climate beneficial to negotiations. Alcohol, in this context, serves as a "social lubricant".
- Finally, alcohol has a symbolic and ritual meaning. Being "hard drinking" is considered a sign of strength, maturity and masculinity. In introductory rites for "newcomers" alcohol plays an important role. For office parties, alcohol is considered a means of demonstrating solidarity irrespective of status. Many professions have traditional drinking patterns.

As a working hypothesis for the planned intervention on this level, we have formulated the following: Preventive interventions must offer acceptable and realistic alternatives which replace the functional meaning of alcohol consumption and reduce the underlying tensions by changing the activities and/or by reinforcing the capacity to cope with tensions and to relax.

Availability of Alcohol in the Firm's Canteens, Shops, Drink Machines etc.

The availability of alcoholic beverages is, in our view, a decisively important factor in determining the pattern of alcohol consumption in the firm. Alcohol, permanently available and accessible without any effort or high cost, creates a permanent reason for drinking and is also a continual temptation for persons having problems of alcohol control. The easy availability supports in addition the previously described functional use of alcohol.

The starting points for intervention therefore take account of the following determining factors in a firm: the quantities available; the variety and form of the products; the container size; the number of sale points, the cost and the non-alcoholic alternatives.

There are indications that changes in alcohol availability may reduce the overall consumed quantities and that they are important with respect to the credibility of other individual-oriented intervention measures. The often practised isolated prohibition strategy has not proved to be effective. According to reports based on practical studies, the upgrading and cheapening of non-alcoholic beverages seems to be more efficient.

Communication Within a Firm Concerning Alcohol

In the working world, as everywhere else, people talk about alcohol only in a quite specific, legitimizing way which tends to minimize its health-endangering effects. The causes and effects of its functional consumption are still largely taboo, being only a subject of discussion in the context of alcoholism. These communication patterns thus support the problematic approach to alcohol. Our intervention concept aims at breaking down these communication patterns by the following means:

- Firstly, by assuming a thematic approach to the causes and effects of the everyday consumption without moralizing or blaming the individual, as a prerequisite for the individual to self-examine his or her pattern of consumption.
- Secondly, by offering health knowledge. This should comprise practical rather than theoretical suggestions which take account of the personal and social situation of the persons concerned and their drinking patterns.
- Thirdly, by making guidance available to colleagues and superiors as to how they should deal with heavy permanent drinkers. The combining of a firm's welfare programmes for alcoholics with preventive, communicative measures is regarded as particularly effective, since it then links therapy and prevention in an overall programme.

It is the objective of all communicative measures to create conditions for the self-consciousness of one's own consumption of alcohol and behaviour vis-à-vis other persons. However, such individual-oriented interventions must be completed within the framework of a firm's overall prevention programme by structural measures. For such a firm's prevention programme to be effective, it must relate to all three levels of the firm's structure as described above.

The Role of the Federal Centre for Health Education as Regards Alcohol Prevention in Industry

In two pilot firms having different structures the FCHE is carrying out company-related intervention projects, the results of which will be generalised and made available in the form of prevention programmes to other interested firms. The FCHE therefore sees its principal role as an advisor to firms which have already shown an interest in such prevention programmes.

Within the framework of a firm's prevention programme, the FCHE is, above all, active in:

- counselling with respect to the development of health education measures, i.e. primarily communicative measures;
- producing various material for a firm's internal preventive campaign;
- making available research results, health education advisors, etc.; and
- carrying out the evaluation, associated with the pilot programme and its financial aspects.

In this connection, the following conditions must be fulfilled:
- The firms should be prepared to develop, test and carry through programmes with respect to the three aspects of the conditions for health-endangering alcohol consumption.
- Such alternatives cannot be determined on a remote theoretical basis, i.e. detailed intervention measures must be established in close association with the firm's requirements. Changes must be harmonized, credible and understandable. This requires a communicative programme development that involves all relevant participants in the firm.
- For a programme to be successful and firmly established, it should involve the firm's employees as much as possible and with a minimum of outside intervention.

In order to meet these conditions, the following measures have been taken in the currently running pilot projects:
- Development of joint objectives
- Creation of working groups in the firm with the participation of the management and the employees' association
- Initial analysis in the firm in respect of: work procedure, internal sale points, communication patterns and investigations into potential alternatives/interventions.

By early 1984 these steps are intended to lead to an overall strategy. Afterwards will follow a 2–3 year implementation phase so that detailed results can be expected by approximately 1986.

References

1. Bundeszentrale für gesundheitliche Aufklärung (1981) Effizienzkontrolle 1980 der Bundeszentrale für gesundheitliche Aufklärung, Cologne
2. Weiss (1980) Beruf, Arbeitssituation und exzessiver Konsum von Alkohol. Arbeitsbericht der Forschungsabteilung der Schweizerischen Fachstelle für Alkoholprobleme, no 6, Geneva

D. Environmental Risks

Air Pollution and Health Indicators: Regional Findings for the Netherlands

J. van Reek

Introduction

The relationship between prolonged exposure to air pollution and health indicators has been investigated for adults in several Dutch studies [1]. In four studies highly polluted areas were compared with slightly polluted control areas [2–6]: Vlaardingen and Vlagtwedde in 1965 until the present, Amsterdam and Den Helder in 1971 and Amsterdam, Vlaardingen and Hoorn in 1976. The respondents in the polluted areas had more respiratory complaints and decreased lung function values. The same method has been used in several other countries.

Another method has been used by Lambert for Great Britain [7]. He correlated regional air pollution data with nationwide survey data. A similar approach will be used in this paper. First it will be investigated whether the use of regional air pollution data and a Dutch nationwide survey will yield a similar result to those found in the mentioned Dutch studies. Then the air pollution data and the health indicators will be correlated at the aggregated level. Finally, calculations will be repeated at the individual level.

Material and Methods

The data concerning subjective complaints and visits to the general practitioner were derived from the survey *Health of Partners* by Hans Philipsen. Actually, this was a secondary usage of data, which might even be beneficial, because the respondents were not influenced by questions on pollution.

In June 1973, 781 couples who were representative of Dutch couples within the age of 21–65 years were interviewed for this survey. Subjective complaints were measured with the Inventory of Subjective Health [8]. The total number of complaints, not including the respiratory complaints, was a summation of 34 items (yes = 1/34; no = 0). The Inventory of Subjective Health included the following five questions regarding respiratory complaints:

- Are you regularly bothered by coughing? yes/no
- Do you get short of breath easily? yes/no
- Do you often have to clear your throat? yes/no

Primary Health Care in the Making
Ed. by U. Laaser, R. Senault, H. Viefhues

- Do you often have sneezing fits? yes/no
- Is your nose often blocked? yes/no

The score for respiratory complaints was calculated after coding yes = 1/5 and no = 0.

Information about the last visit to the general practitioner during the previous 5 years was obtained by using the following two questions:

- When did you pay your last visit to your family doctor for reasons other than influenza, a common cold or routine pregnancy control?
- What was the reason for that visit?

The answers to the last question were coded for the 17 main groups of the International Classification of Diseases. The codes of some other variables were:

- Smoking yes = 1
  no = 0
- Prosperity high = 1
  low = 2
- Age 21–30 years = 1
  31–50 years = 2
  51–65 years = 3
- Sex male = 1
  female = 2.

Nationwide measurements of some air pollutants have been made in the Netherlands. The 98th percentile of SO_2 for the Netherlands was measured during the period 1 October 1975–1 October 1976 [9]. Though these measurements were rather crude, ten provincial estimates in μg/m³ could be derived (see part of Table 2). The resulting scores were plausible, considering the sources of SO_2 pollution. For the calculations the categories were changed in the following way:

- < 100 μg/m³ = 1
- 100–124 μg/m³ = 2
- 125–149 μg/m³ = 3
- ≥ 150 μg/m³ = 4.

Unfortunately there were no nationwide measurements of SO_2 for 1973. In a comparison of three areas in Zuid-Holland, the differences in SO_2 values between the periods 1973/1974 and 1975/1976 appeared to be similar [9, note 9, p. 11].

The 98th percentile of SO_2 is often used as an indicator of air pollution because it is caused by many sources of air pollution (industrial emissions, car traffic and heating of residences and glass-houses) and its measurement is relatively cheap. It is highly related to the 50th percentile SO_2 and other air pollution indicators. Aggregated data were calculated for two different regional distributions of the Netherlands. Firstly, the above-mentioned distribution into ten regions was used. To enable the calculation of correlations over a larger number of areas, the ten regions were then divided into agrarian rural, industrialized rural and urban areas (excluding the three largest cities). As a result of this distribution and separate inclusion of Amsterdam, Rotterdam and The Hague, there were 33 areas. Unfortunately, the data available in *Health of Partners* were based on less than 20 respondents for seven areas. After omission of these areas, 26 areas remained.

The 98th percentile of SO_2 could be estimated for the 26 areas with the following information. According to maps concerning Zuid-Holland, the 98th percentile of SO_2 is a category (25 μg/m^3) higher in urban areas [9, note 9, pp. 65, 67]. It is assumed that this difference also applies to the other provinces. In Noord-Holland the SO_2 air pollution is a category lower in the agrarian rural area [9].

Results

Firstly, a result similar to the well known comparison of Vlagtwedde and Vlaardingen [2] was achieved. The respiratory complaints of couples in the agrarian rural area of Groningen and Friesland were compared with those of couples in the urban areas of Zuid-Holland. The respiratory complaints were significantly higher in the more highly polluted area (Table 1).

There was also a significant correlation between the 98th percentile of SO_2 and the respiratory complaints when the data based on ten areas were used (Table 2). The respiratory complaints were low in the agrarian northern provinces and high in the industrial western provinces. The southern provinces were polluted by local and foreign industry. Though the high air pollution in the southern provinces was not well known, the number of respiratory complaints was high.

The correlations between air pollution, subjective complaints and the last visit to the general practitioner were then calculated for 10 and 26 areas. The values of the zero order correlation coefficients differed little for the two calculations (Table 3). In the 26-area calculation the 98th percentile of SO_2 also correlated significantly with the total number of complaints, not including respiratory complaints and the last visit to the general practitioner because of respiratory diseases, due to the larger number of data points.

The third order correlation coefficients also differed little. They were calculated by holding smoking, prosperity and age constant. Unfortunately occupational exposure at air pollution could not be included.

Table 1. A comparison between a slightly and a heavily polluted area

	Respiratory complaints
Agrarian rural areas in Groningen and Friesland ($n=52$)	0.13 ± 0.17
Urban areas in Zuid-Holland ($n=382$)	0.18 ± 0.22
t-test difference	$t = -1.88$*

* $P \leqq 0.05$ (one-sided test)

Table 2. Provincial data on air pollution and respiratory complaints

	98th percentile of SO_2 (in μg/m³)[a]	Respiratory complaints
Groningen and Friesland	< 100 (1)	0.12
Drente	100–124 (2)	0.18
Overijssel	125–149 (3)	0.15
Gelderland	125–149 (3)	0.15
Utrecht	100–124 (2)	0.16
Noord-Holland	100–124 (2)	0.17
Zuid-Holland	125–149 (3)	0.17
Zeeland	100–124 (2)	0.14
Noord-Brabant	≧ 150 (4)	0.17
Limburg	125–149 (3)	0.19
	$r=0.56$ ($P<0.05$)	

[a] In parentheses: values after recoding

Table 3. Correlations between air pollution, subjective complaints and visits to the general practitioner (during partial correlations, smoking, prosperity and age remain constant)

	Respiratory complaints	Total number of complaints, not including respiratory complaints	Visits to the G.P. because of respiratory diseases	Visits to the G.P. because of diseases, not including respiratory diseases
Mean value	0.16±0.22	0.19±0.14	6%±24	54%±28
Zero order correlation coefficient (based on 10 areas)	0.56*	0.32	0.40	–0.10
Zero order correlation coefficient (based on 26 areas)	0.58**	0.45**	0.33**	–0.17
Third order correlation coefficient (based on 26 areas)	0.58**	0.46**	0.35**	–0.14

* $P \leqq 0.05$
** $P \leqq 0.01$

Discussion

Though a clear correlation between the 98th percentile of SO_2 and respiratory complaints was found, an important methodological problem remained. Hammond showed two sources of error in ecological correlations. The ecological correlation will often be higher than the individual correlation, but if the individuals are grouped homogeneously on the independent variable, the regression equations will be equal. Aggregation bias should also be considered [10]. Both sources of error were studied by means of regression analysis.

The equation of the relationship between respiratory complaints (y) and air pollution (x) based on data of 26 aggregates was:

$$y = 0.02x + 0.09 \quad (\beta = 0.58; P < 0.01)$$

After the air pollution data for these aggregates were added to the survey data through the place of residence, it was possible to calculate the equation on the individual level:

$$y = 0.02x + 0.11 \quad (\beta = 0.08; P < 0.001; n = 1562)$$

The two equations differed little and it could be concluded that the first-mentioned ecological error was absent.

The second ecological error was studied by analysing the influence of cigarette smoking, age, prosperity and sex on the correlation. For this purpose multiple regression was run for the 26 aggregates and the 1562 respondents (Table 4). No second ecological error was found for the correlation between air pollution and respiratory complaints. However, the high correlation between cigarette consumption and respiratory complaints on the individual level had disappeared on the aggregated level. This finding shows that analysis on the ag-

Table 4. Multiple regression analysis of respiratory complaints and explanatory variables based on individual and aggregated data

	Beta	*F*
Individual data ($n = 1562$)		
Cigarette consumption per day	0.22	71.56***
98th percentile SO_2	0.07	8.45**
Age	–0.04	2.32
Prosperity	–0.01	0.12
Sex	–0.01	0.04
Aggregated data ($n = 26$)		
98th percentile SO_2	0.56	10.34**
Prosperity	–0.25	2.06
Age	–0.04	0.06
Cigarette consumption per day	0.04	0.05

** $P \leq 0.01$
*** $P \leq 0.001$

gregated and the individual level might lead to different results. The aggregated method of analysis has to be used with great prudence.

References

1. Knipschild P (1980) CARA en luchtverontreiniging in Nederland. University of Limburg, Maastricht pp 14–32
2. Van der Lende R (1969) Epidemiology of chronic nonspecific lung disease (chronic bronchitis). Diss. Groningen. Van Gorcum, Assen
3. Van der Lende R, Visser BF, Wever-Hess J, Tammeling GJ, De Vries K, Orie NGM (1973) Epidemiological investigations in the Netherlands into the influence of smoking and atmospheric pollution on respiratory symptoms and lung disturbances. Pneumologie 149:119–126
4. Van der Lende R, Kok TJ, Peset Reig R, et al. (1981) Decreases in VC and FEV_1 with time: indicators for effects of smoking and air pollution. Bull Eur Physiopathol Respir 17:775–792
5. Van der Maas PJ, Van Leeuwen P, Biersteker K, Noordam AL (1973) De invloed van luchtverontreiniging in Amsterdam-Noord op de luchtwegen van 10- en 11-jarige schoolkinderen. GGD Amsterdam
6. Van der Maas PJ (1973) Cara bij kinderen. Diss. Amsterdam, pp 91–93
7. Lambert PM (1973) Smoking air pollution and bronchitis in Britain. Lancet 1:853–857
8. Van Reek J, Diederiks J, et al. (1982) Subjective complaints and blood pressures.. J Psychosom 26:155–165
9. Raad inzake de luchtverontreiniging (1978) Overzicht van de luchtverontreiniging in Nederland over 1975 en 1976. Ministerie van Volkgezondheiden Milieuhygiëne, Leidschendam, p 63
10. Hammond JC (1973) Two sources of error in ecological correlations. Am Sociol Rev 38:764–777

Possibilities and Limits of Data Drawn from the "Gesundenuntersuchung" for an Epidemiological Study of the Connection Between Air Quality and Chronic Bronchitis

P. Lercher and W. W. Kofler

Introduction

Thirty years of epidemiological research into the contribution of social and environmental factors to morbidity and mortality from chronic respiratory disease have shown the difficulty of establishing consistent relationships. Cassel and co-workers [1] name as a reason for this difficulty the tendency of health effects research to investigate the network environment by isolating the effects of their components. This approach neglects the fact that the relationships of the components to each other vary and that the effect of the whole is greater than the effect of the sum of the known parts.

Verführt and Smidt [8] found that there was a considerable longitudinal variability of anamnestic, clinical and lung function data. They pointed out that these variations present a serious obstacle if one wants to search for the effect of a certain factor on chronic bronchitis. Therefore a successful identification should be taken all the more seriously. In Austria very little information is available on the effects of air pollutants on the morbidity of the population.

Our objective was to test the suitability of data drawn from the "Gesundenuntersuchung" for epidemiological research as well as for health planning purposes with special regard to air pollution.

Population and Methods

It was for this purpose that 86 116 participants of the "Gesundenuntersuchung" living in the Tyrol, Salzburg and Carinthia were allocated to four zones of increasing air pollution.

Their anamnestic prevalence of chronic bronchitis was taken from standardized questionnaires. SO_2 was used as an indicator for defining the different zones. The method, which is adapted to the special needs of the Alpine region, was described by KOFLER in 1977 [2]. Its basis were data gained from over 1600 lead dioxide candles as well as 28 continuous monitoring stations.

The type of load by point sources of emission, which differs from the type of load by area sources of emission, was taken into consideration to a larger extent because of the higher peak concentration which occurs in the former

Primary Health Care in the Making
Ed. by U. Laaser, R. Senault, H. Viefhues

Table 1. Stress categories by sources; total sulfation; wintertime (after Kofler [2])

Category	SO_3 level by area sources	SO_3 level by point sources	Short description
I	Less than 5.0 mg SO_3 per 28 d/dm^2	Less than 5.0 mg SO_3 per 28 d/dm^2	SO_3 level is negligible from a hygienic viewpoint
II	5.0–14.9 mg SO_3 per 28 d/dm^2	5.0–11.9 mg SO_3 per 28 d/dm^2	An impact on health is not likely
III	15.0–34.9 mg SO_3 per 28 d/dm^2	12.0–24.9 mg SO_3 per 28 d/dm^2	The possibility of adverse health effects cannot be excluded
IV	More than 35.0 mg SO_3 per 28 d/dm^2	More than 25.0 mg SO_3 per 28 d/dm^2	Adverse health effects must be taken into account in unfavourable weather conditions

(Table 1). The allocation of the participants was carried out by means of the postal code of their home address and was based on the worst lead dioxide candle measurement of the winter months (November–April).

A more detailed allocation was not possible because of data protection, just as we could not carry out multivariate analysis. We only obtained computed contingency tables whose significance was tested by the χ^2 test.

Results and Discussion

We focussed our attention on those 58 482 participants who are current non-smokers. But first we shall take a look at the overall prevalence among smokers and non-smokers with regard to air pollution.

Table 2: The predominant effect of smoking is evident and confirms earlier research. The prevalence of chronic bronchitis (CB) in smokers is two and a half times higher than in non-smokers without taking into account different smoking status. Therefore it is not surprising that – contrary to non-smokers – no association with air pollution can be observed.

Table 3: Sex is a significant factor in the occurrence of CB. Men get CB more frequently than women. However, the relationship between the rates of CB and air pollution is only apparent for women, especially if one looks at the age-adjusted rates. The confounding influence of occupational hazards may be one factor, another could be that women usually stay longer in their place of residence than men, who often work out of town. The difference in the prevalence of CB between men and women becomes less significant in the zones III and IV.

Table 4: If sex as well as age are taken into account, the apparent relationship between the prevalence of CB in women and air pollution is still evident. Such a trend could not be observed in men. It is noteworthy that in the age group

Table 2. Prevalence (%) of chronic bronchitis by current smoking category and by air pollution

		Zone I	Zone II	Zone III	Zone IV	Relation zone I:IV	χ^2
Smokers	no.	1 095	3 755	4 830	3 259		
	%c	17.08	14.78	12.69	15.99	1:0.9	NS
Non-smokers	no.	5 142	15 734	17 402	10 552		
	%c	4.96	5.16	6.07	7.07	1:1.4	***
	%a	5.02	5.43	6.09	6.48	1:1.3	
Smokers and non-smokers	no.	6 237	19 489	22 232	13 811		
	%c	7.09	7.01	7.51	9.17	1:1.3	***
Relation non-smokers: smokers		1:3.4	1:2.9	1:2.1	1:2.3		

%c, crude prevalence rates
%a, age-standardized rates
NS, no significance
*** significant at the 0.001 level

Table 3. Prevalence (%) of chronic bronchitis among non-smokers by sex and by air pollution

		Zone I	Zone II	Zone III	Zone IV	Relation zone I:IV	χ^2
Women	no.	3 564	10 693	11 580	6 907		
	%c	4.04	4.06	5.15	6.41	1:1.6	***
	%a	4.10	4.26	5.17	5.86	1:1.4	
Men	no.	1 578	5 041	5 822	3 645		
	%c	7.03	7.50	7.90	8.31	1:1.2	NS
	%a	6.93	7.85	7.90	7.76	1:1.1	
Relation women:men		1:1.7	1:1.8	1:1.5	1:1.3		

%c, crude prevalence rates
%a, age-standardized rates
NS, no significance
*** significant at the 0.001 level

40–59 the highest difference in the rates of CB between men and women can be observed. This difference lessens again for men and women over 60. In zone IV it vanishes altogether. The biasing effect of occupational burden should also be taken into consideration in explaining these inconsistencies.

Figure 1: Gives a graphic representation of the above results.

Table 5: The educational level is a significant factor for the prevalence of CB. In the highest level the lowest prevalence of CB occurs. There is a close relationship between the prevalence of CB and air pollution in level I. This relationship lessens in level II and cannot be observed in the highest educational level.

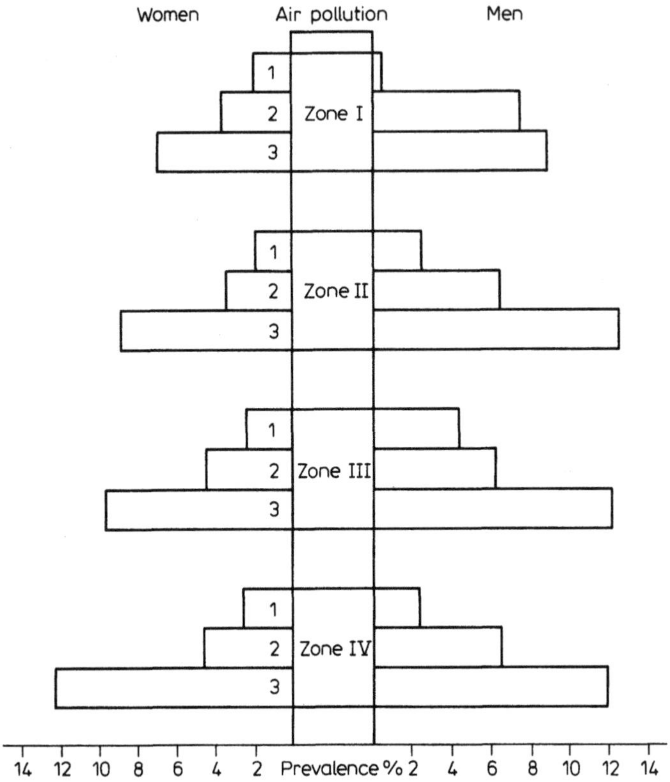

Fig. 1. Chronic bronchitis among participants in the "Gesundenuntersuchung" in the Tyrol, Salzburg and Carinthia. Prevalence (%) by age (1, 19 – 39; 2, 40 – 59; 3, 60 –), sex and air pollution

Table 6: Very little changes if one considers both education and sex. However, it is remarkable that in this case, there is a similarly close relationship between educational level I and air pollution for men as well as for women. This would be a further indirect hint on the importance of occupational exposure. But there is a remaining difference between the sexes which cannot be explained by age and educational level. This requires further investigations.

Figure 2: The above results are graphically presented.

Table 7: A connection between the number of children living in the household and the frequency of CB with regard to air pollution can only be regarded as a preliminary result, since an extensive evaluation has not yet been made. However, our attention must be attracted by the fact that CB is more prevalent in people with no children. Psychosocial factors may play a role.

Table 8: The same applies to the indicator marital status. The unduly high rates of CB in widowed and divorced persons deserves further analysis, although the small size of the subsample will be a limiting factor. As long as the influence of smoking and age (especially in the case of widowed persons) has not been clarified, every statement remains speculative.

Table 4. Prevalence (%) of chronic bronchitis among non-smokers by age, by sex and by air pollution

			Zone I	Zone II	Zone III	Zone IV	Relation zone I:IV	χ^2
19–39	Female	no.	806	2617	2921	1470		
		%	2.11	2.03	2.46	2.72	1:1.3	NS
	Male	no.	196	787	936	491		
		%	0.51	2.54	4.27	2.44		*
40–59	Female	no.	2093	6183	6209	3516		
		%	3.82	3.41	4.62	4.72	1:1.2	**
	Male	no.	943	2843	2933	1613		
		%	7.53	6.37	6.21	6.57	1:0.9	NS
60–	Female	no.	665	1893	2450	1921		
		%	7.07	8.98	9.67	12.34	1:1.7	***
	Male	no.	439	1411	1953	1541		
		%	8.88	12.54	12.19	12.01	1:1.4	NS
Relation	Female		1:3.4	1:4.4	1:3.9	1:4.4		
19–39:60–	Male			1:4.9	1:2.9	1:4.9		

NS, no significance
* significant at the 0.05 level
** significant at the 0.01 level
*** significant at the 0.001 level

Table 5. Prevalence (%) of chronic bronchitis among non-smokers by educational level and by air pollution

		Zone I	Zone II	Zone III	Zone IV	Relation zone I:IV	χ^2
Educational level I	no.	3552	9412	7388	3780		
	%c	4.90	5.25	6.24	7.94	1:1.6	***
	%a	5.00	5.49	6.20	7.03	1:1.4	
Educational level II	no.	1299	5185	8027	5218		
	%c	5.00	4.96	6.03	6.84	1:1.4	***
	%a	5.51	5.51	6.00	6.20	1:1.1	
Educational level III	no.	139	729	1687	1371		
	%c	5.76	5.21	5.57	5.62	1:1.0	NS
	%a	6.09	5.53	5.58	5.35	1:0.9	
Relation level I:III		1:1.2	1:1.0	1:0.9	%c 1:0.7 %a 1:0.8		

Level I, those who left school at the age of 15
Level II, those with additional schooling
Level III, those with A-levels and university graduates

%c, crude prevalence rates
%a, age-standardized rates
NS, no significance
*** significant at the 0.001 level

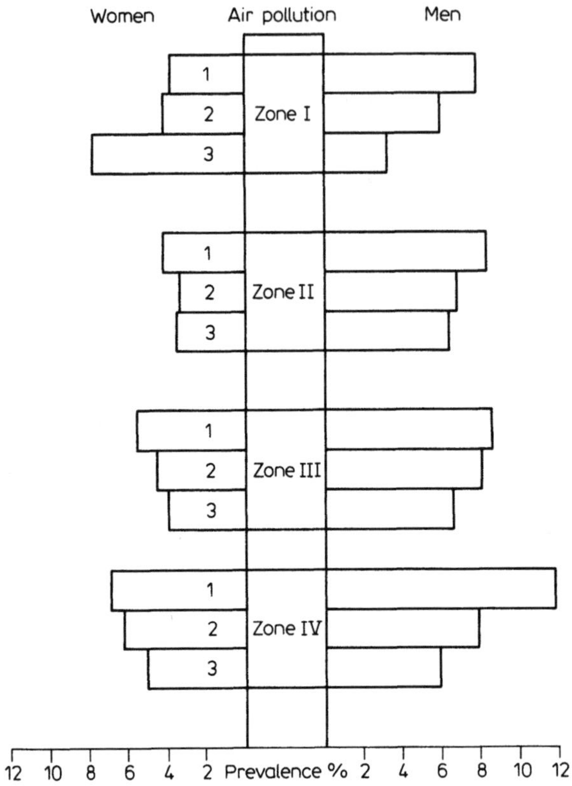

Fig. 2. Chronic bronchitis among participants in the "Gesundenuntersuchung" in the Tyrol, Salzburg and Carinthia. Prevalence (%) by schooling, sex and air pollution. *1*, those who left school at the age of 15; *2*, those with additional schooling; *3*, those with A-levels and university graduates

Table 6. Prevalence (%) of chronic bronchitis among non-smokers by educational level, by sex and by air pollution

			Zone I	Zone II	Zone III	Zone IV	Relation zone I:IV	χ^2
Level I	Female	no.	2665	7138	5850	3002		
		%	3.94	4.27	5.62	6.93	1:1.8	***
	Male	no.	887	2274	1538	778		
		%	7.78	8.31	8.58	11.83	1:1.5	*
Level II	Female	no.	725	2961	4813	3218		
		%	4.28	3.51	4.65	6.18	1:1.4	***
	Male	no.	574	2224	3214	2000		
		%	5.92	6.88	8.09	7.90	1:1.3	NS
Level III	Female	No.	76	305	684	570		
		%	7.89	3.61	3.95	5.09		NS
	Male	no.	63	424	1003	801		
		%	3.17	6.37	6.68	5.99		NS
Relation level I:III	Female			1:0.8	1:0.7	1:0.7		
	Male			1:0.8	1:0.8	1:0.5		

NS, no significance
* significant at the 0.05 level
*** significant at the 0.001 level

Table 7. Prevalence (%) of chronic bronchitis among non-smokers by number of children and by air pollution

		Zone I	Zone II	Zone III	Zone IV	Relation zone I:IV	χ^2
No child	no.	769	2824	5194	3297		
	%	7.28	7.19	8.32	9.19	1:1.3	*
One child	no.	843	3040	3692	2405		
	%	5.58	5.23	5.85	5.49	1:1.0	NS
Two children	no.	1138	3710	3941	2155		
	%	3.51	3.64	3.86	4.36	1:1.2	NS
More than two children	No.	1901	4590	2709	1191		
	%	4.31	3.83	4.02	5.04	1:1.2	NS
Relation two children: no child		1:2.1	1:2.0	1:2.2	1:2.1		

Defn.: Children refers only to those currently living with their own parents
NS, no significance
* significant at the 0.05 level

Table 8. Prevalence of chronic bronchitis by marital status and by air pollution; smokers and non-smokers

		Zone I	Zone II	Zone III	Zone IV	Relation zone I:IV	χ^2
Never married	no.	542	1 615	2 360	1 486		
	%	5.72	6.44	6.27	8.41	1:1.5	*
Married	no.	6 741	20 870	21 472	12 830		
	%	7.05	6.92	7.20	8.37	1:1.2	***
Widowed	no.	575	1 729	1 968	1 490		
	%	6.96	7.00	10.82	14.36	1:2.1	***
Divorced	no.	97	480	1 119	996		
	%	10.31	10.00	9.12	11.24	1:1.1	NS
Relation married: widowed		1:1.0	1:1.0	1:1.5	1:1.7		

NS, no significance
* significant at the 0.05 level
*** significant at the 0.001 level

Limitations

It is not possible to transfer the results directly to the general population since the "Gesundenuntersuchung" is undertaken on a voluntary basis. Unknown factors of the thus gained data are the memory of the participants and the non-standardized setting of diagnosis (many investigators).

It is not possible to estimate the proportion of obstructive disease in the participants since spirometric analysis was not available. The influence of possible confounding factors like indoor air quality, infection of the lower respiratory tract in early childhood or selective migration cannot be controlled, nor was the length of time individuals had lived in their place of residence known. The influence of cohort effects cannot be excluded due to the cross-sectional design of the study.

The limitations in defining the levels of personal exposure and the restriction in data analysis by the legal protection of data suggest that these findings should partly be looked upon as preliminary.

Conclusions

The problem in the epidemiological research of health hazards caused by air pollution is that due to the confounding factors, large samples and many demographic, social and socioeconomic data are required. Some of these problems could be solved; others could not. However, the methods described above seem to offer a chance to monitor the long-term effects of air pollution on chronic respiratory morbidity of the population in a certain region by means of time-series analyses. Thus it also becomes possible to evaluate the effectiveness of pollution abatement with regard to health effects.

An important prerequisite for this task is easy access to all the data of the "Gesundenuntersuchung" for the epidemiologist and the release of data collections by the local councils. Furthermore the "Gesundenuntersuchung" should include valid respiratory indicators to identify those who are at high risk of developing serious disease later. Some of this is partly realized in the US by different "health-related mapping projects" [6, 7] and in North-Rhine-Westphalia (Federal Republic of Germany) by air pollution control plans [3, 4, 5].

References

1. Cassel EJ, Lebowitz M, McCarroll JR (1972) The relationship between air pollution, weather, and symptoms in an urban population. Am Rev Respir Dis 106:677–683
2. Kofler W (1977) Die Abgrenzung von Erholungsgebieten und Belastungszentren auf Grund ihrer Luftverunreinigung. 1. und 2. Mitteilung. Zentralbl Bakteriol Hyg [B] 164:159–192
3. MAGS (1976) Luftreinhalteplan Rheinschiene Süd (Köln), 1977–1981
4. MAGS (1977) Luftreinhalteplan Ruhrgebiet West (Duisburg-Oberhausen-Mülheim), 1978–1982
5. MAGS (1982) Luftreinhalteplan Rheinschiene Mitte, 1982–1986
6. NCHS (1979) Proceedings of the 1976 workshop on automated cartography and epidemiology. DHEW Publication, no (PHS) 79-1254, Washington, DC
7. Stebbings JH, Voelz GL (1981) Morbidity and mortality in Los Alamos County, New Mexico. Environ Res 25:86–105
8. Verführt J, Smidt U (1980) Längsschnittvariabilität der anamestischen, klinischen und lungenfunktionsanalytischen Daten eines Erhebungsbogens für die chronische Bronchitis und das Lungenemphysem. Prax Pneumol 34:414–434

Biological Effect of the Air Quality Measured at the Population Level

W. Jedrychowski, M. Krzyzanowski, and B. Wojtyniak

The role of atmospheric air pollution in the aetiology of chronic respiratory diseases has been studied in many epidemiological surveys, but until now their results have been rather controversial. It seems that further investigations in this field should take into consideration factors that possibly confound the effect of air pollution. The definition of "chronic" respiratory symptoms employed may have some impact on the results obtained. In several studies, spontaneous remission of symptoms believed to be "chronic" was observed. As the diagnosis of chronic chest diseases may be biased by the temporary occurrence of cough or phlegm and by a short-term variability in lung function, it was decided to define as chronic the persistence of chest symptoms over a 5-year period.

Two examinations of the probability sample of Krakow inhabitants performed at an interval of 5 years included interviews using a standardized questionnaire based upon one developed by the Medical Research Council in Great Britain. Interviews were followed by invitations to participate in spirometric evaluation of lung function.

Chronic bronchitis was diagnosed in those persons who reported symptoms of both chronic cough and phlegm production. Persistent chronic bronchitis was diagnosed when symptoms of chronic bronchitis were present in both surveys over the 5-year period. The obstructive syndrome was diagnosed in persons among whom the value of FEV_1/FVC was equal to or less than 70%. Persistent obstructive syndrome was diagnosed when lung obstruction was confirmed in both surveys. Taking into account the low rates of chest symptoms among women, the analysis was limited to men only. In addition, men changing their smoking habits, i.e. ex-smokers or those who started smoking during the study period, were excluded from the analysis.

The data on air pollution were collected daily over the 5-year period using a network of 20 sampling stations situated in the study area. The concentration of the suspended particles of a diameter of less than 10 μm was measured reflectometrically and concentrations of sulphur dioxide were measured using an electrocolorimeter. On the basis of the air pollution measurements it was possible to single out two areas in the city – one with a lower air pollution and another with a higher pollution level. Average daily air pollution concentrations were about twice as high in the centre of the city as in the remaining areas (Table 1). After the classification of the city into areas with different air pollu-

Primary Health Care in the Making
Ed. by U. Laaser, R. Senault, H. Viefhues

Table 1. Average daily air pollution concentrations in Krakow (based on 5-year survey data)

	Highly polluted area	Less polluted area
Respirable dust	180 μg/m³	109 μg/m³
Sulphur dioxide	114 μg/m³	53 μg/m³

Table 2. Logistic regression coefficients for chest symptoms in relation to age, smoking and air pollution (1240 males)

Independent variables	Dependent variables		
	Persistent chronic bronchitis	Exacerbations of chest symptoms	Obstructive syndrome
Age (yrs)	0.0579***	0.0816***	0.1064***
Smoking	2.6593***	1.4266 NS	1.5901***
Air pollution	0.4750*	0.9218*	0.0513 NS

NS, non-significant
* significant at 0.10 level
** significant at 0.05 level
*** significant at 0.01 level

tion levels, it was possible to follow the population experience with regard to persistent chronic chest symptoms.

To assess the separate and joint effects of chosen environmental factors on the respiratory symptoms, multiple logistic regression analysis was carried out. Table 2 presents the results of the logistic analysis in the whole group. It can be seen that besides age, persistent chronic bronchitis was related significantly to both smoking and air pollution, exacerbations of chronic chest symptoms to air pollution, and obstructive syndrome (by contrast) to smoking. The effect of air pollution when age and smoking were controlled was stronger for exacerbations than for other chest symptoms. The risk of acute exacerbations in persons with chronic chest symptoms who were residents in the highly polluted area was 2.5 times greater than in the residents of the other part of the town. Cigarette smoking had the strongest impact on the persistence of chronic bronchitis.

When we included occupational variables in the logistic model, it appeared that for people exposed to occupational hazards it was of importance whether they lived in the more or the less polluted area. Comparing the odds ratios for chronic bronchitis, the effect of occupational exposure to chemicals was about four times greater among people living in the more polluted area than in all others exposed (Fig. 1).

The prevalence of persistent obstructive syndrome among residents of the highly polluted area was similar to that among residents in the less dusty area. However, there was significant interaction between air pollution and occu-

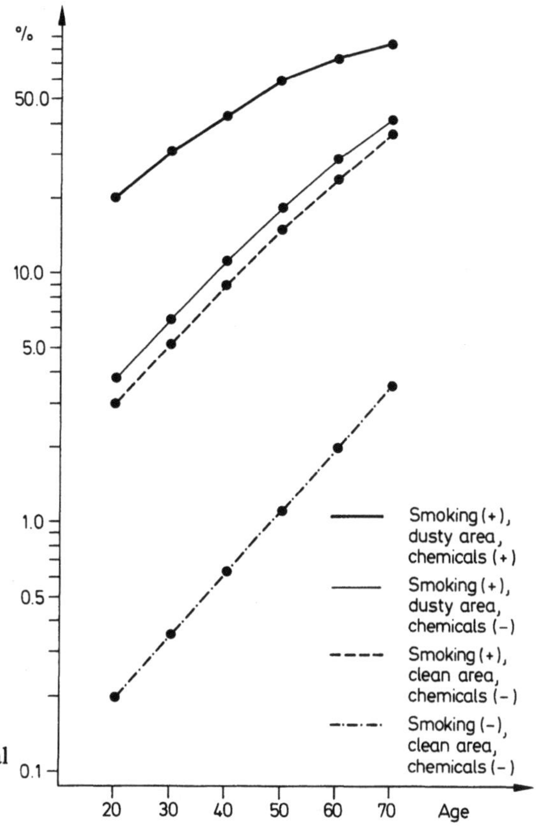

Fig. 1. Probability of persistent chronic bronchitic symptoms in relation to age, smoking, atmospheric air pollution and exposure to chemicals in the occupational environment (based on logistic multiple regression)

pational exposure to high or variable temperature. In residents of the highly polluted area this factor was associated with a sharp increase in the prevalence of obstructive syndrome, whereas its effect on the residents of remaining areas appeared negligible (Fig. 2).

The most intriguing result of our study regards the strong combined affect of atmospheric air pollution and thermal stress at work on the development of chronic obstructive lung disease. This might suggest that under constant thermal stimuli the bronchioles tend to narrow, and as the surface area for deposition of particles becomes much smaller so the concentration of potentially adverse air pollutants becomes much higher. This in turn may lead to further inflammatory airway obstruction and thus to weakening of bronchiolar wall and disruption of alveoli and emphysema.

In considering the biological significance of the results, we have to bear in mind that the measurement of smoking and other factors was carried out at the individual level whereas air pollution is at the population level. The other difficulties in the interpretation of data arise from the fact that it was not possible to use very precise exposure indicators of air pollution (duration of residence in the particular area). In addition, we should not forget that the smoking effect was measured practically against "zero" level (non-smoking), but the effect of air pollution was not assessed in comparable terms because in all parts of the

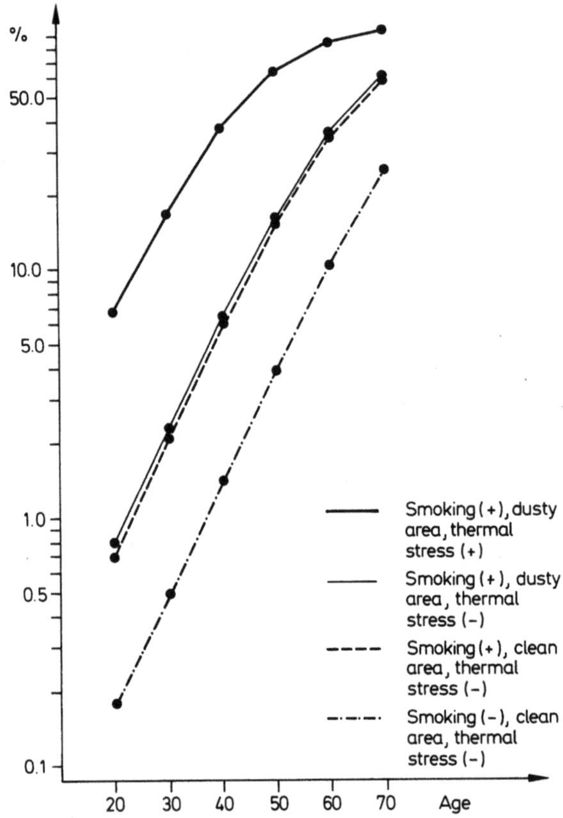

Fig. 2. Probability of persistent chronic lung obstruction in relation to age, smoking, atmospheric air pollution and exposure to thermal stress in the occupational environment (based on logistic multiple regression)

city we observed a somewhat elevated level of pollution. One should expect that the effect of air pollution was actually underestimated in this study. Perhaps in reality the difference between the effect of air pollution and that of smoking is much smaller.

Acknowledgements. This research was carried out under the patronage of the Scientific Program Council for Studies on Chronic Respiratory Disease in Kraków (Chairman: Prof. Jan Kostrzewski). The study was performed in part under the agreement between the National Institute of Hygiene, Poland, and National Centre for Health Statistics, USA (the field study was partly supported by the grant under the contract NCHS PL 1, and analysis was done within the agreement on joint scientific and research co-operation).

E. The Chronically Ill

Family Rehabilitation in Chronic Illness

U. Gerhardt

The sociological literature on chronic illness focusses on the issue that a "re-designing of life-styles" is essential for successful rehabilitation. My main proposition is that rehabilitation is a family process which leads to changes in a family's role composition and way of life. The hypothesis is raised that differences in family rehabilitation are conducive to differences in the quality of life with chronic illness and, moreover, that the prospect of survival depends on the quality of the newly found equilibrium, or disequilibrium, in the family's role structure.

The hypothesis is discussed here on the basis of data procured from the total group of male married patients with end-stage renal failure in the south-east of England who were between the ages of 20 and 50 years at the onset of their dialysis treatment and who had not been patients for more than three years at 1 January 1978. Of the total study population of 76 cases, 68 were interviewed once, and 56 twice, after a 1-year interval, yielding a total of 234 interviews from husbands and wives, amounting to over 600 hours of tape-recorded material. As may be seen from Table 1, the original distribution of treatment types in our study population was similar to that of the general United Kingdom treatment population 1 year previous to the study. Over time, the distribution of treatment types among the surviving cases reversed the proportion of transplant and dialysis cases. The figures under III are based on the data of a 5-year follow-up completed in 1983.

Through an elaborate procedure of data processing using a technique of qualitative interpretation adapted from Max Weber's idea of an "ideal type", four idealized typified versions of the division of labour between the spouses were found to characterize the occupational side of the patient careers:

1. *traditional* family rehabilitation where the husband remains the sole or main breadwinner despite his severe disability
2. A similar situation with male dominance but with the husband's being unemployed
3. A *dual-career* marriage where both spouses secure the family's income
4. An arrangement where the wife alone secures the livelihood, often in "rational" anticipation of the family's need to survive after the husband's eventual death.

In our sample, the tendency is remarkably stable to stay with one of two composite types, namely, either a male-centred type of family structure with

Primary Health Care in the Making
Ed. by U. Laaser, R. Senault, H. Viefhues

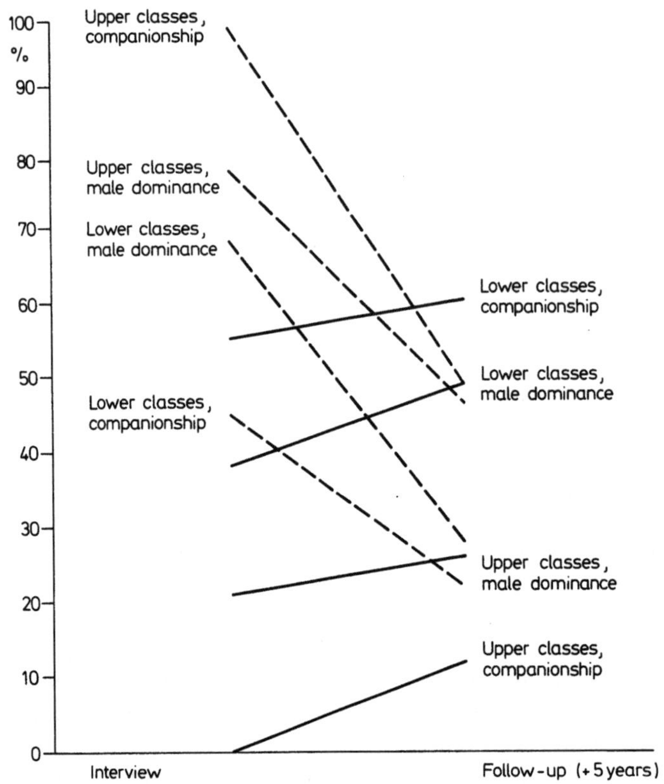

Fig. 1. Proportion of surviving patients by treatment group, social class and long-term type of family rehabilitation, at interview I and 5 years later, in percentages ($n = 68$, $n = 52$). * Percentages calculated after omission of social class V and cases that were unclassified in British social class terms

sexual role differentiation (1 and 2), or a companionship type of family structure with role blurring between the sexes (3 and 4). Among the 77% of our study population who survived, only 5% changed from one of the two composite types to the other, and the proportion of male-centred cases rose slightly from 42% to 45% while that of companionship-type families dropped from 35% to 32%.

The picture of stability does not prevail in the figures relating to survival and treatment over time (see Table 1). However, the marked decline in the proportion alivc on home dialysis and the increase in the proportion alive with a transplant are not only due to differences in mortality rates but also to frequent transplantion of dialysis patients, often after years of treatment on the machine. It emerges that, over time, social class and type of family rehabilitation acquire a prominent role as relevant factors connected with type of treatment among the surviving patients (Fig. 1).

Returning to the initial statement that chronic illness requires a "re-designing of life-styles", a concluding remark may be in order. It ought to be mentioned that our data give answers regarding *survival;* not, however, death rates

Table 1. Distribution of treatment types at interviews I and II ($n=68$, $n=62$) and today ($n=52$), as compared with the total treatment population of the United Kingdom at 31 December 1976. (Percentages)

	UK	I	II	III
Hospital dialyses	22	17	9	10
Home dialyses	40	50	46	32
Total dialyses	62	67	55	48
Cadaver donor transplants	33	23	32	38
Live donor transplants	5	10	13	14
Total transplants	38	33	45	52

since the study population itself was selected on the basis of the criteria of survival until up to 3 years after the inception of treatment.

Therefore, our data give information on the processes and factors connected with survival. Among them, social class and family rehabilitation are of prime importance. The rate of survival in the upper classes is lower than that in the lower classes (class V excluded). This may be due to the treatment since more dialysis cases, in a long-term perspective, are among the upper classes because more lower-class cases acquire transplants. But it may also be due to family rehabilitation since the survival chances with dual-career family rehabilitation are nearly twice as good as with a traditional family role structure; however, the former is seven times and the latter is four times better than that of cases in which the patient is unemployed, regardless of the type of marriage. Although the companionship type of family rehabilitation increases the family's protection against financial losses, its protective effect, when the husband-patient is not working, is no better than both spouses' unemployment. Thus, our study shows that the chances of survival which presumably are connected with the family's successful "redesigning of life-styles" are better for patients who manage to stay at work. While the traditional and dual-career families show a survival ratio of 5.7, the unemployment and "rational" type of family rehabilitation only achieves a survival rate of 1.3.

Acknowledgements. I wish to express my gratitude to Dr. Anthony Wing, M.D., F.R. C.P., Consultant, St. Thomas' Hospital, London S.E.1, for his encouragement and support throughout this study. The Social Science Research Council, London, provided funds under project Nr. 5013, 1977–1982, and the German Research Council (Deutsche Forschungsgemeinschaft) supported the data analysis and methodological work in a follow-up project, 1981–1982. I also wish to thank the many collaborators and researchers who participated in the work in England or Germany. The final project report, entitled "Patientenkarrieren. Eine medizinsoziologische Studie", is as yet unpublished, Giessen 1983, 752 pp.

Family Psychology and "Family Confrontation"

B. Luban-Plozza

The persons around the psychosomatic patient usually regard him either as seriously ill with some organic disease, or as a trivial case, a hypochondriac or malingerer. The patient's symptoms are often aggravated as a direct *consequence;* he feels deserted and alone.

Even today, 'protection against affronts' is primarily extended to the patient with organic disease, less so to the functionally disturbed and least of all to the psychiatric patient and hence, of course, also the psychosomatic sufferer. Indeed, the latter faces an increased tendency to 'discriminate' against him. Socially and in health the weakest member of his group, he must submit to the role of patient offered him by society. The manifestly ill patient then plays a role in relation to the family that resembles the neurotic situation in relation to the individual concerned. The individual psychosomatic symptoms often represent the tip of the iceberg in the sense of the family's delegate pathology (Stierlin).

Michael Balint applied psychoanalytic principles in his group work with general practitioners. They succeeded in giving an accurate illustration of the doctor–patient relationship by clinical methods. Detailed observations are made. Much thought is given to understanding their significance and to the possibilities they offer for treatment. What sort of findings are involved? First they listen to what the patient has to say. His thoughts, feelings and opinions are taken seriously and not dismissed as the incorrect ideas of a layman. Indeed, the patient's message often has first to be deciphered, decoded and translated.

The physical behaviour is observed. Basic conflicts may be manifested in this aspect of behaviour. The comparison of pre-verbal and verbal observations provides an initial opportunity for verification.

The doctor also observes his own emotional reactions to the patient. Following this an attempt is made at the integration of both interactional and somatic complaints into one single picture, namely the *overall diagnosis*, to quote Balint. This overall diagnosis may be related to the patient's life history. The general practitioner, who usually has known the patient for a long time, does not have to ask for the case history first. However, the general practitioner is usually unaware of how much he already knows and is unable to mobilize his preconscious knowledge. The above were some preliminary remarks to the psychosocial dynamics of the family.

Primary Health Care in the Making
Ed. by U. Laaser, R. Senault, H. Viefhues

The following circumstances lead to artificial, "trumped-up" family ties:

1. Mutual mental infection – weekend neurosis. No defense against an eventual infectious psychotic nucleus
2. Greater opportunity to get divorced, which weakens mutual responsibilities
3. Nearly no identification with the family group and peer group
4. The battle of one generation against the other
5. Increase of sibling rivalry
6. Early distortion and fortification of Oedipal ties because of precocious sex information
7. Many mothers are not the centre of the home anymore
8. Insecurity of parents regarding how to discipline their children because of an excess of psychological advice
9. Increase of the tyranny of complaining (injustices collecting) and the ease of looking for scapegoats
10. Crowded housing, which spoils modesty and intimacy
11. Growing lack of mutual understanding and emotional communication
12. Mutual alienation in the family
13. Children do not want to take care of their aged parents
14. Intrusion of the philosophy "I don't care" – mutual detachment
15. Contagion with anger and violence from the outside
16. Too early sexual experience, which takes away individuality; the children are precociously tied to deep, grasping emotions

We have tried to use the dynamics in a therapeutic way by introducing the *concept of family confrontation* (Luban-Plozza 1971). This concept was taken over by E. Petzold and his colleagues (Heidelberg). We make use of this concept within a psychosomatic *hospital setting*, but here we should like to concentrate on the *practitioner's surgery*.

This concept includes:

Firstly: A clear understanding of the patient's needs.

Secondly: Therapy should have produced (substantial) improvement before the patient is confronted with members of the family. This can well wait until he is somewhat better.

Thirdly: The members of the family are cautiously acquainted with the patient's symptoms and, ideally, also with the core of the conflict situation if the circumstances permit.

Fourthly: the doctor abstains from passing moral judgements and giving advice

Together with the patient the doctor works at an attempt to let him sense the palpable connection between his somatic symptoms and the mental obstacles. Allies capable of insight are of great help to the doctor (even a child may be such a confidant and assume useful key functions). Help of this kind could take the form of a joint suggestion to have constructive discussions aimed at restructuring the family constellation. This makes it easier for the family member previously singled out and branded as sick to make his way back into the group. Having learned to revise its thinking, the family will understand the patient better and may be able to review old family patterns. It would be difficult to overemphasize the fact that, far from being a waste of time, family confrontation is most valuable for all concerned. Moreover, responsibility is shared and more clearly defined – also vis-à-vis the doctor – if the family as a whole empathizes with the patient's predicament and therapy is able to relieve him of part of the stress of suffering.

Not all the familial interactions perceived by the doctor need be brought out into the open. Quite often it is enough for him to form an idea of the family interrelationships on his own, with the aid of the material assembled. In so doing he may at times catch really grotesque glimpses of the pathogenic situation; for instance, during a separate interview the husband called his wife a dragon. Later the dragon wife enters the consulting room and turns out to be a frail little woman. Observations of the ecological network and interrelationships in the family concerned are also of interest. The same person may adopt totally different attitudes: for instance, one of great concern on the telephone and a tone of callous, even sadistic reproachfulness in face-to– face conversation with the doctor. The therapist may have to deal with a constructive and friendly or a destructive and hostile attitude on the part of the rest of the family. The former makes things easier for him; confrontation with the family gives him ample opportunities to penetrate to deeper levels of insight. If, however, the 'healthy' members of the family relate negatively to the patient, the doctor needs to handle them more circumspectly so as to protect the sick member against further injury from his relatives. This, of course, brings up the question of confidentiality. How much latitude, if any, is there for the doctor? Regarding destructive stances of other family members: hostility to treatment on the part of the seemingly healthy partner is more often found in men than in women.

Lack of communicative rapport is sometimes known as 'emotional illiteracy' or 'emotional anaesthesia'. Below an example is given of a "family psychosomatic disturbance":

The Syndrome of the Silent, Impassive Husband

The husband is often absent and too busy – and when he is there, does not talk. When asked to give, say, the date of his wedding anniversary or his wife's birthday, he is most likely not to know or, in striking contrast with his normal presence of mind, will need a pause to cover his embarrassment (ostensibly to reach for a cigarette, for instance!).

The wife feels deprived of sympathy and suffers psychosomatically. She communicates – unconsciously – by body language, her symptoms of weakness, frigidity and lumbago. The marriage partners mete out reciprocal 'punishment'.

The husband makes a great show of doing things for his wife: he goes along when she has her laboratory tests, clinical examinations and X-rays. However, *she* alone sees the neurologist. After all, it is not *he* that is ill (nor does he feel ill). 'No time for the family' is one of the most often heard complaints these days, and many a reader's ears may be burning as if his own wife had once again observed the fact with a sigh of resignation. Modern society at this moment appears to include more and more 'Don Juans of achievement and success'! A frank exchange comes as a release to all concerned. The patient is afforded the important realization that the therapist sees the particular family member (say, the autocratic father or the impassive husband) in his true light and does not hesitate to say as much.

The doctor's independence and willingness to make admissions should be manifest to the patient from the start. This will help him to acquire a sense of assurance that is indispensable to the maintenance of his confidence. This includes learning how to stand up for himself and even being permitted to criticise and attack his partner in the session with the doctor – for the sake of emotional relief. The doctor, too, must be able to express himself equally freely, since it is important that he should be in a position to articulate and interpret negative feelings – with all their weaknesses. In all of this there is only one precaution to be strictly observed: the doctor should not contribute to guilt feelings.

It is inadmissible that a diagnosis of psychosomatic disturbance should entitle a doctor to make condemnatory remarks any more than does a diagnosis of cardiac or pulmonary disease (or, for that matter, of venereal infection). It is part of the therapist's task to make the other family members refrain from condemning the sick member as "only" psychosomatically ill. He must grasp this and treat the patient accordingly.

Yet 'family confrontation' is not identical with 'family therapy'; rather it may pave the way for the latter. In both cases the family – the 'true patient' – is approached as a unit. The psychosomatic disorders of one member may be a sufficient indicator that the whole 'family organism' is sick in spite of a facade of make believe. It is far from possible for the general practitioner to seize all the details of a familial conflict situation (indeed, as the family doctor he is often already fully aware of them as they have evolved through the generations). In most cases it is, however, possible for him to relax the tension of a tangled conflict and to get a hold on an individual family member.

The family members could learn that differences in character are differences and not faults and that although they are perhaps not reversible, they may be adapted to if all members agree. Little, annoying habits can be very irritating to others and can be dealt with without a change of personality. H. Stierlin described this process as a "positive spiralling mutuality" which eventually affects all parts of the family system, balancing relational individuation dynamics and motivating each family member to change while reforming the family structure to allow change. Essential sources of motivation which the therapist needs to tap, he said, are curiosity, the striving for competence and the wish to belong to a desirable group or team. These intrinsic motivations are the therapist's most powerful allies in altering the family game in a positive direction.

Neurotic role distribution in the family has a detrimental effect not only on the first generation of offspring but also on their eventual partners and families as well. The kind of conventional behaviour and emotional reaction a woman acquires in childhood are bound to influence the way in which she behaves towards her husband and brings up her children. With due alteration of details, the same holds for the male spouse, who is even more manifestly a product of the imprinting influence exerted by the parent of the opposite sex.

It is estimated that one in three children who present for treatment exhibit symptoms that include psychosomatic features. Clearly, facilities for treatment are not available in sufficient numbers for that reason alone; thus the preventive role of family therapy assumes special importance. It requires teamwork, however, and this is where the general practitioner comes in first and foremost. His opportunities to study family problems in detail (or his chances of being drawn into them) are more numerous than those of the specialist or a member of other professions. Hence he is under a special duty, indeed a moral obligation, to act in conflict situations and thereby to prevent behavioural disorders from evolving into a set of psychosomatic symptoms. He is, in fact, presented with an extraordinary opportunity to give preventive aid to jeopardized children by bringing his influence to bear on the family group as a whole.

Far-reaching changes have meanwhile come about in methods of treating psychosomatic disorders in response to social and psychological problems. It may seem as if customs peculiar to totally different cultures are being borrowed when we are told that in Vikersund, Norway, the family always visits the psychiatric clinic together with the patient concerned. The unit consists of bungalows where the families can stay and live as at home; the doctor, however, has access at any time of day or night. The financial side of the arrangement is entirely taken care of by the social security system. Those in charge of the clinic are convinced that they are moving in the right direction since change and readjustment are, in fact, rarely required of the patient exclusively, but usually of the 'healthy' family members as well and at the same time.

References

1. Balint M (1965) Primary Love and Psycho-analytic Technique. Tavistock, London
2. Biermann G (1969) Psychotherapeutische Probleme bei psychosomatischen Erkrankungen im Kinder- und Jugendalter. Praxis 10, pp 451 – 458
3. Fromm E. Personal Communication
4. Luban-Plozza B (1970) Aspects psychosomatiques de la médecine de famille. Med Hyg 28, pp 154 – 157
5. Luban-Plozza B (1972) Preventive medical and psychosocial aspects of the family practice. Psychiat Med 3, pp 327 – 332
6. Luban-Plozza B, Comazzi A (1973) The family as a factor in psychosomatic disturbances. Psychother Psychosom 22, pp 372 – 377
7. Luban-Plozza B, Pöldinger W (1980) Der psychosomatisch Kranke in der Praxis. Springer-Verlag, Berlin, Heidelberg, New York, Tokyo (1985) 4. Auflage, English (Roche Edition)
8. Luban-Plozza B, Spiess W (1982) Die Familie: Risiken und Chancen. Antonius-Verlag, Solothurn
9. Pinter E (1970) Ueber Familienpsychotherapie. Praxis 59, Hallwag-Verlag, Bern, pp 1066 – 1069
10. Richter HE (1970) Patient Familie. Rowolth-Verlag, Reinbek
11. Stierlin H (1975) Von der Psychoanalyse zur Familientherapie. Klett-Verlag, Stuttgart

Who Treats the Chronically Ill: The General Practitioner or the Internist?

G. Mall

An increasing number of internists are engaged in the primary care provided by the West German Health Service. More and more patients go with their ailments – without an appropriate referral certificate – to the specialised physician who, in their opinion, is the one best equipped to deal with their ailment. Chronic diseases are in most cases diseases of the inner organs and, thus, fall within the competence of the internist. However, general practitioners treat on average more patients than internists do. For this reason, it is of interest to know which of the two groups of physicians has to deal particularly frequently with certain types of chronic disease.

For this purpose, health insurance certificates represent a useful source of information. 2626 health insurance certificates of general practitioners and internists – presented for settlement to the AOK (Local Sick Fund) in the first quarter of 1980 – were thus selected according to random criteria. It was found that general practitioners had on average 362 AOK patients, and internists 275. The diagnoses on the health insurance certificates were coded in accordance with the ICD. Out of 912 different diseases, 81 of the most important chronic diseases were picked out. It was possible to allocate to these 81 diseases 32% of all diagnoses entered on health insurance certificates.

The general diseases of the ICS are compared in Table 1 with the total number of diagnoses made by each group of physicians, and the corresponding organ diseases with the number of patients. The reason for proceeding in this manner is that during the course of a general disease several diagnoses can be attributed to one patient; in the case of a corresponding disease of the organs this is less likely to be the case. In addition, the percentage of each disease in relation to the overall morbidity and mortality is shown.

The object is to find the answer to three questions:

1. What is the proportion of a disease in relation to the average diagnostic spectrum of general practitioners and internists?
2. With which chronic diseases do patients visit more frequently the general practitioner or the internist?
3. To what extent does the spectrum of disease of both groups of physicians correspond to the overall morbidity and mortality statistics?

Primary Health Care in the Making
Ed. by U. Laaser, R. Senault, H. Viefhues

Table 1. Who treats the chronically ill: the general practitioner or the internist? Absolute and relative frequency of diagnoses entered on health insurance certificates relating to chronic diseases diagnosed by 46 general practitioners and 35 internists, settled by the AOK Stuttgart during the first quarter of 1980. The ratio of general practitioner to internist in the random sample corresponds to the ratio of the basic total number. The percentage share of the overall morbidity and overall mortality was computed for 1980 on the basis of the *Statistical Yearbook 1982*

Pos. no. of ICD	General disease/ organic diseases	General pract. ($n=45$)		Internists ($n=36$)		% share of all patients	% share of all diagnoses	% share of overall morbidity	% share of overall mortality
		% share of all patients ($n=1665$)	% share of all diagn. ($n=5480$)	% share of all patients ($n=961$)	% share of all diagn. ($n=2892$)	($n=2626$)	($n=8372$)		
390–459	*Circulatory diseases*	–	411 7.5%	–	350 12.1%	–	9.1%	26.1%	28.4%
400–405	Hypertension	262 15.7%	–	222 23.1%	–	18.4%	–	3.4%	2.0%
410–414	Ischaemic heart diseases	58 3.5%	–	75 7.8%	–	5.1%	–	3.6%	11.8%
430–438	Diseases of cerebral vessels	91 5.5%	–	53 5.5%	–	5.5%	–	–	14.3%
140–208	*Malignant tumors*	–	26 0.5%	–	27 0.9%	–	0.6%	– –	21.9%
150–159	Digestive organs	9 0.5%	–	9 0.9%	–	0.7%	–	–	6.7%
174, 175	Mammary gland	12 0.7%	–	6 0.6%	– –	0.7%	–	–	1.7%
161, 162	Respiratory organs	1 0.1%	–	5 0.5%	–	0.2%	–	–	3.5%
179–189	Sexual organs	4 0.2%	–	7 0.7%	–	0.4%	–	–	1.8%
490–493	*Diseases of respiratory organs*	–	228 4.2%	–	160 5.5%	–	4.6%	4.7%	3.1%

490, 491	Bronchitis	188 11.3%	–	121 12.6%	–	11.8%	–	–	1.9%
492, 493	Asthma due to emphsema	40 2.4%	–	39 4.1%	–	3.0%	–	–	1.2%
250	*Diabetes mellitus*	152 9.1%	2.8%	121 12.6%	– 4.2%	10.4%	3.3%	6.4%	1.9%
571–578	*Diseases of the digestive organs*	–	187 3.4%	–	164 5.7%	–	4.2%	2.4%	2.3%
571–573	Chronic liver disease	108 6.5%	–	103 10.7%	–	8.0%	–	1.2%	–
574–576	Biliary tract	61 3.7%	–	55 5.7%	–	4.4%	–	1.2%	–
577, 578	Pancreas	18 1.1%	–	6 0.6%	–	0.9%	–	–	–
710–739	*Rheumatic diseases and diseases of the bones and joints*	–	686 12.5%	–	216 7.5%	–	10.8%	15.7%	×
710–719	Arthropathies	188 11.2%	–	92 9.6%	–	10.7%	–	–	×
720–724	Dorsopathies	245 20.7%	–	157 16.3%	–	19.1%	–	–	×
725–729	Rheumatism	93 5.6%	–	31 3.2%	–	4.7%	–	–	×
730–739	Osteopathies	60 3.4%	–	17 1.8%	–	2.9%	–	–	×
	Total	–	30.9%	–	35.9%	–	–	–	–

The results are shown in detail in Table 1: Diseases of the circulatory system are the most important for the internist, and rank second amongst general practitioners. Nevertheless, overall general practitioners treat more patients suffering from this disease. Only in the case of ischaemic heart diseases do more patients go to the internist. The proportion of hypertension in relation to the overall morbidity is unusually low compared with the corresponding proportion of diagnoses found in health insurance certificates. There is one possible explanation: this statistic is based on data furnished by a microcensus which surveyed only the most severe diseases.

It is striking that malignant tumours have hardly any relevance compared with their proportion as regards the overall mortality (for the overall morbidity this question was not put). Since – after these types of diseases have been detected – the further diagnosis and therapy thereof fall within the responsibility of hospitals, these patients 'disappear' from out-patient care. Other specialist physicians, too, are, to some extent, competent to deal with diseases falling under this group. However, it is still worthwhile considering whether it would not be desirable to provide for these patients a greater intensive care through the family physician.

Chronic diseases of the respiratory organs make up a high proportion of an internist's average diagnosis spectrum; overall, however, more patients go to the general practitioner.

Physicians generally diagnosed diabetes mellitus in roughly every tenth patient; internists relatively more frequently than general practitioners. Nevertheless, a greater number of diabetics are treated by general practitioners. Unfortunately it is not possible to distinguish between juvenile diabetes and diabetes in adults, since such a distinction is not made by health insurance certificates or the ICD. From a sociomedical and health economics point of view, however, such a distinction would be of considerable relevance.

For the general practitioner the most important group of diseases are rheumatic diseases, and bone and joint disorders; for internists this group of diseases ranks second. Patients suffering from these diseases consider the general practitioner to be the competent person; the general practitioner also has the greater relative proportion of all diagnoses.

The above data show that the individual internist deals with chronic diseases more frequently than the general practitioner. Only rheumatic diseases and diseases of the bones and joints fall within the domain of the general practitioner. However, a different picture emerges if one asks which of the two groups of physicians the majority of patients with chronic diseases go to. Since more general practitioners than internists are involved in out-patient care and the individual practitioner treats on average more patients than the internist, the proportion of general practitioners treating various chronic diseases is always greater than that of internists. Only the ischaemic heart diseases remain the domain of the internist.

This gives rise to the following consequences: if questions relating to diagnosis, therapy and health policy of chronic diseases are to be discussed with individual physicians, then the internists are the more important partners with whom to deal; general practitioners are relatively more frequently the competent physicians for acute diseases. However, if, in an analogous case, the aim is to address a whole group of physicians, then the general practitioners have a much greater say in the matter. Their share in the out-patient care of chronic diseases is overall that much greater than that of internists; the former deal relatively less but, viewed in absolute numbers, still more frequently with this type of disease.

Compliance – A "Risk Factor" for Chronic Diseases?

A. Füller

From a medical point of view, treatment and prevention of some chronic diseases seems possible, as we know something about the causative factors, the disease processes and effective therapeutic and preventive strategies. Nevertheless, the anticipated great success of the measures taken is frequently not forthcoming; again and again the *inadequate compliance* of treated patients is named as the essential cause of failure; this means that patients do not submit sufficiently to the advice, recommendations and prescriptions of the medical professionals. Research shows that such behaviour has grown over the last few years [1].

On the basis of some considerations and studies about the conditions and causes of insufficient compliance, the promotion of compliance is proposed by means of facilitating and supporting measures like:

- Changes in the dosage of drugs
- Improvement of information with regard to medication and its effects
- Formation of groups of patients
- Negative sanctions against insubordination vis-à-vis medical prescriptions

It is expected that an improvement of compliance by physicians in the long run will lead to higher success rates of treatment and the prevention of chronic diseases. On the other hand it can be realistically presumed that not all medical personnel will be able to influence the compliance of patients, as health behaviour is conditioned by a complex network of psychic and social causes.

Many reasons for insufficient compliance are quoted:

- The insignificant regard paid by physicians to the feelings and personal experiences of patients [2]
- Inter-role conflicts of patients [3]
- Conflicts between physicians and patients [5], or, more exactly, between the different expectations towards behaviour
- The submission of personal emotions to the technical authority of physicians
- The growing critical attitude towards the claim to authority made by physicians and towards their manner of prescribing drugs [1].

Moreover, *insufficient compliance* may be seen as *intelligent and rational behaviour* (Weintraub 1976). Some reasons for this thesis are [15]:

Primary Health Care in the Making
Ed. by U. Laaser, R. Senault, H. Viefhues

1. In public discussions the dangers and side-effects of medical prescriptions are pointed out (e.g. dependence and the side-effects of sedatives, such as thalidomide, and hormonal drugs).
2. Patients sometimes experience the effects of medication upon their health more clearly than does the prescribing physician.

Therefore, one may ask whether an improvement in the compliance of patients with chronic diseases is always *desirable*. In fact, the compliant role (i.e. the conforming behaviour of a person, prescribed by a doctor for a limited time) seems more suited to acute than to *chronic diseases;* from the latter patients one expects [13, 14]:

1. Self-observation, self-control and self-responsibility
2. Technical and dietetic readiness
3. Knowledge and competence
4. Activity and co-operation with treatment

Mere reactive submission to a traditional doctor–patient relationship seems inadequate and ineffective for people with chronic diseases – and also for healthy people whose behaviour is to be influenced to prevent such diseases. This means that the traditional *model of compliance* in the medical field as an aspect of the traditional doctor–patient relationship is contrary to some prerequisites of coping with chronic diseases. On the other hand, competent, self-confident and in some cases non-compliant behaviour by chronically ill people suits the demands of physicians for self-responsibility of people for their own health.

The traditional, and in the treatment of acute diseases usual, relationship of doctor to patient seems to be a special case of a *relation of authority* between competent and mighty experts and incompetent laymen [12]; this relation is similar to the relations of authority in industrial life. Such a relation of authority becomes evident in the language and sometimes in the behaviour of physicians towards their lower-class patients. This is described by the Italian physician and author *Carlo Levi*, when reporting how the doctor in the southern Italian village in which Levi lived in exile considered medical treatment to be a *feudal right* over the life and death of the so-called *cafoni*, the despised poor farmers [8].

Such a relation of authority is based upon confidence in the judgements and decisions of experts – these experts expect such an attitude; therefore, they often overestimate the compliance rates of patients [3]. Hence deviance from such a relation is characterized as "querulous" or "know-all" [10]. In fact, non-compliance is a danger for the expansive but always precarious authority structures in health care.

One can suggest with some legitimacy that a relation of authority includes some dangers for the treatment and prevention of chronic diseases, *not only in individual but also in social and political terms.* The main danger may be called *"medicalization"* [4, 16]. *Medicalization* has some effects on society and health:

1. Expansion of social control by using the definition of illness in many instances of deviance and the accumulation of authority by physicians.

2. "Production" of new diseases by creating new definitions of diseases (e.g. psychic diseases, hypotension, very mild hypertension etc.). This is supported by the pharmacological industry, which can be characterized as "ingenious in inventing illnesses and cures for questionable complaints" [7] – in relation, for example, to tranquillizers and antihypothensives.
3. Individualization of social and political problems (by using medical thinking more and more), the consequence being to blame the victim instead of changing conditions.
4. Preferring technocratic solutions to health problems (by medication). In this case medical interests are often allied with the economic interests of some industries [11].
5. Through the expansion of medical services the dependency of people grows and personal activities concerning health decline. As a consequence, adequate health behaviour by the population may be impaired.

Concerning these considerations about the effects and dangers of compliance in the case of chronic diseases, substitution of the traditional, compliant behaviour in the doctor–patient relationship by another, more competent and self-confident type of behaviour seems to meet the conditions for coping with such diseases. Such a new relationship based upon open information and participation may include:

- Reduction of authority without legitimation
- The right to insubordination
- Reciprocity of the relationship: physicians can learn from their patients and vice versa
- Provision of information to patients by physicians with regard to their intentions and decisions
- Including the social environment in the co-operation
- Considerating the patient a part of the therapeutic team [2, 6, 9].

Though non-compliance seems to be a danger for treatment and prevention of diseases, for the relation of authority between doctors and patients and for economic interests, developments in morbidity (growth of chronic disease), partly caused by better health care, demand at least the partial substitution of compliance by more adequate attitudes and behaviour.

References

1. Anderson R (1980) Prescribed medicines. Who takes what? J Epidemiol Community Health 34:299–304
2. Beckmann D (1979) Wesentliche Voraussetzungen für ein langfristiges Arbeitsbündnis zwischen Arzt und Patient. In: Bock KD (ed) Arzt und Hypertoniker. Braunschweig
3. Hermann U (1979) Forschungsfragen zur „Compliance" – Datenauswahl und Datenanalyse anhand eines rollentheoretischen Modells. In: Mackensen R (ed) Soziologische Analysen, TU Berlin. Berlin, pp 288–292
4. Illich I (1978) Die Nemesis der Medizin. Rowohlt, Reinbek
5. Kasl SV (1975) Issues in patient adherence to health care regimens. J Human Stress 1:5–17

6. Kickbusch I (1979) Laiensystem and Krankheit. Med Mensch Ges 4:2–8
7. Lennard HL, Epstein LJ (1971) Mystification and drug misuse. Jossey-Bass, New York
8. Levi C (1982) Christus kam nur bis Eboli. dtv, Munich
9. Martin JF (1978) The active patient, a necessary development. WHO Chron 32:51–57
10. Pfeiffer W (1981) Plädoyer für ein effektiveres Arzten. refero-med Bayer 35:2–9
11. Pflanz M, Basler HD, Schwoon D (1977) Use of tranquillizing drugs by a middle-aged population in a West German city. J Health Soc Behav 18:194–205
12. Popitz H (1968) Prozesse der Machtbildung. Mohr-Siebeck, Tübingen
13. Redler E (1979) Selbsthilfegruppen. Med Mensch Ges 4:8–13
14. Szasz TH (1972) Geisteskrankheiten – ein moderner Mythos. Walter, Freiburg
15. Weintraub M (1976) Intelligent Noncompliance and capricious compliance. In: Lasagna L, (ed) Patient compliance. Futura, Mount Kisco, N.Y.
16. Zola IK (1979) Gesundheitsmanie und entmündigende Medialisierung. In: Illich I, et al. (eds) Entmündigung durch Experten. Rowohlt, Reinbek

Non-fatal Myocardial Infarction in Women Under 50 Years of Age, with Reference to Oral Contraceptive Use in Belgrade*

J. Ananijević-Pandey and H. Vlajinac

Although it seems well established that women have an increased risk of myocardial infarction while taking oral contraceptives (OCs), and that the effect on the risk persists after discontinuation of long-term use [6], authors often conclude that these data should be replicated in other settings, because the background risk of that disorder and the distribution of factors predisposing to it vary appreciably in different parts of the world [7]. That is why we decided to do a small case control study of risk factors for myocardial infarction in our setting, with special reference to OC use. Our setting differs from western countries in that OC use is not so common: in Yugoslavia it rose from 2.5% in 1969 to 5.0% in 1978 in women of reproductive age (15–44). OC use in Belgrade falls into the same range.

Patients and Methods

Our case series consisted of women under 50 years of age who were hospitalised for myocardial infarction (code 410 according to the eighth revision of the ICD) between 1976 and 1980, in any of three hospitals in Belgrade. Altogether 65 patients were identified from hospital records. Complete information was available for 45 patients. Control series consisted of women hospitalised for different surgical conditions (benign tumours, appendicitis, hernia, different trauma, cholecystitis). Four patients were taken as controls for each patient with infarction. Controls were matched individually for age (plus/minus 1 year), year of admission and place of residence (only Belgrade). 180 controls were identified but complete information was available for only 142 of them.

The mean age of cases and controls was the same (46.3 years). Only one-third of both groups were younger than 44. Information from both groups was obtained through home visits and the completion of questionnaires by 17 female medical students. Questionnaires were designed to obtain information on the following variables: marital status, ethnic group, education, occupation, weight and height, history of hypertension, hypercholesterolaemia, diabetes,

* Funded by the Scientific Community of the Republic of Serbia through the contract No 4.11/3-579, 1981–1983

Primary Health Care in the Making
Ed. by U. Laaser, R. Senault, H. Viefhues

family history of myocardial infarction, gravidity, parity, history of pre-eclamptic toxaemia, menopausal state, past use of OCs, cigarette smoking and physical activity. Information was sought from each patient about all the items included but the response was not always complete. Blood pressure, blood glucose, level of cholesterol, and height and weight were not measured individually and our figures are likely to underestimate the prevalence of hypertension, diabetes, hypercholesterolaemia and obesity in both groups.

Individual matching was not taken into account in the statistical evaluation. For the analysis we used the Mantel-Haenszel [3] method to calculate the approximate risk ratio (RR) for each variable separately. Confidence limits (95%) were computed with Miettinen's simple interval estimation of RR [5]. Standardisation on possible confounding factors was computed [4].

Results

A similar proportion of cases and controls were married and both groups were mostly of Serbian nationality (Table 1). Cases had a higher educational level (defined as having completed 12 years of school or more) than controls, but the significant difference disappeared after standardisation on cigarette smoking as a confounding factor. Differences according to occupation (employed vs unemployed, including housewives) disappeared after standardisation on three pos-

Table 1. Socio-demographic, medical, obstetric and life-style variables of myocardial infarction and control patients at time of admission, Belgrade, 1976–1980

	No. and percentage of patients		Crude RR	*P*
	Myocardial infarction	Controls		
1. Married	36 (80.0)	118 (83.1)	–	–
2. Serbian	38 (84.4)	124 (87.3)	–	–
3. Higher education	27 (60.0)	35 (24.6)	4.6	0.01
4. Employed	31 (68.9)	59 (41.5)	3.1	0.01
5. Hypertension	24 (53.3)	29 (20.4)	3.0	0.01
6. Diabetes	8 (17.8)	3 (2.1)	10.0	0.01
7. Hypercholesterolaemia	10 (22.2)	8 (5.6)	4.8	0.01
8. Family history of MI	21 (46.7)	31 (21.8)	3.1	0.01
9. Obesity	22 (48.9)	58 (40.8)	1.1	0.1
10. Nulligravidity	9 (20.0)	13 (9.1)	2.5	0.05
11. Nulliparity	13 (28.9)	19 (13.4)	2.6	0.05
12. Postmenopausal	16 (35.6)	44 (31.4)	1.2	0.1
13. Pre-eclamptic toxaemia	5 (15.6)	13 (10.6)	1.6	0.1
14. Past OC use	2 (4.4)	13 (9.1)	0.5	0.1
15. Cigarette smoking	24 (53.3)	16 (11.2)	12.1	0.001
16. Physical inactivity	25 (55.5)	97 (68.3)	–	–

sible confounding variables simultaneously (smoking, hypertension and hypercholesterolaemia).

Blood pressure readings were not available for individual patients and hypertension was defined as being present if the women herself reported elevated blood pressure (diastolic pressure 90 mmHg/12 kPa or more). For 26.7% of cases and 71.0% of controls the value of blood pressure was not known. In the analysis we supposed that the non-reporting of blood pressure value is equal to the absence of hypertension in the patient's history. Elevated blood pressure was present in 53.3% of cases and 20.4% of controls, giving the value of crude RR 3.0 to 1 (CI 2.2 – 8.6). Standardisation on other possible individual risk factors did not affect the value of the RR, though simultaneous standardisation on all three (smoking, diabetes, hypercholesterolaemia) reduced it.

A history of diabetes was reported by 17.8% of cases and 2.1% of controls, giving the value of crude RR of 10.0 to 1 (CI 5.1 – 19.3). After standardisation on possible confounding factors individually (smoking, hypertension, hypercholesterolaemia) the RR diminished, and its significance disappeared after standardisation on these three factors simultaneously.

For 44.5% of cases and 84.5% of controls blood cholesterol value was not known. Here also we supposed that non-reporting meant non-existence of elevated cholesterol, and both categories, "unknown" and "normal values", were combined into one in the analysis. According to these rough data, elevated cholesterol (270 mg/100 ml or 7.0 mmol/litre or more) was reported by 22.2% of cases and by 5.6% of controls, giving the crude RR value of 4.8 (CI 3.1 – 7.4). After individual and simultaneous standardisation on possible confounding factors (smoking, hypertension, diabetes), significant difference disappeared.

A family history positive for myocardial infarction (measured as MI experienced by patient's mother, father, brother or sister) was reported by 46.7% of patients and by 21.8% of controls, giving the value of crude RR of 3.1 (CI 1.5 – 4.7). After simultaneous standardisation on possible confounding factors (smoking, diabetes, hypercholesterolaemia), significant difference disappeared.

Obesity, measured by the Quetelet index (weight in grams/height in cm^2), was reported by 48.9% of cases and by 40.8% of controls to be of value 2.57 or more; the difference was not statistically significant.

Nulligravidity was reported by 20.0% of cases and 9.1% of controls. Nulliparity was reported by 28.9% of cases and 13.4% of controls. Significant differences (*P* less than 0.05) disappeared after standardisation on possible confounding factors (smoking, hypertension, hypercholesterolaemia) simultaneously and individually.

A similar proportion of cases and controls were postmenopausal (35.6% and 31.4%) and reported history of pre-eclamptic toxaemia (15.6% of cases and 10.6% of controls).

No one women in either group was a current user of OCs. Past use was reported by 4.4% of cases and 9.1% of controls, giving an RR below 1. Among controls, only four women had used OCs for more than 12 months, and none had done so for more than 5 years. All other patients (including cases of MI) had used OCs for less than 12 months.

Cigarette smoking appeared as the only risk factor which remained significantly more present in cases than controls after standardisation on possible confounding factors (hypertension, diabetes, hypercholesterolaemia) individually and simultaneously. Smoking 15 cigarettes a day or more was reported by 53.3% of cases and 11.2% of controls, giving the RR value of 12.1 to 1 (CI 5.9–24.5).

Physical inactivity (measured by absence of any recreational or sporting activity in the patient's history) was reported by 55.5% of cases and 68.3% of controls, the difference not being significant. In comparison with patients without any risk factors, the RR increased from 5.0 to 1 in women with one factor (hypertension, hypercholesterolaemia, diabetes or smoking) to 30.0 to 1 in women with two or more factors at the same time.

Discussion

Although the overall use of OCs in our setting was as low as 2.5–5.0%, according to the hypothesis we expected that the proportion of current users or long-term past users of OCs would be higher in the case group. However, this was not so. Our study has some shortcomings, such as the small number of patients in both groups (compared with the last study from US) [6] and the fact that some medical indices were not measured in individual patients (with the consequent underestimation of their prevalence). But we consider information bias concerning OC use unlikely, since the prevalence of past use of OCs among cases and controls does not differ grossly from that reported by the general population of women of reproductive age in our setting. Also, there was no selection in the choice of cases, other than the fact that these patients had, of necessity, survived. The method of selecting the controls ensured that the patients in both groups were comparable for age, year of admission and place of residence. They were found to be comparable in marital status and ethnic group. We consider, then, that the main result of our study – that past use of OCs of short duration (less than 5 years) does not present a risk factor for myocardial infarction in women under 50 years of age – is in accordance with the papers of Mann et al. [2] and Slone et al. [6].

Considering the distribution of other known risk factors in our study, we found, as expected, the following variables to be more common in the cases: smoking more than 15 cigarettes per day, history of hypertension, hypercholesterolaemia and diabetes. The synergistic effect of more than two factors simultaneously was also confirmed in our study. Concerning the independence of risk factors for MI, we found only heavy cigarette smoking to act as an independent risk factor. The explanation of the failure of hypercholesterolaemia to act independently in our study might lay in under-reporting, as blood cholesterol was not measured individually. The supposition that patients not known to have the condition do not, indeed, have it was based on the results of Krueger et al. [1]. They showed that for obtaining the data for risk factors such as diabetes, hypertension and high cholesterol, questionnaires are as good as hospital abstracts. The same considerations apply to the explanation of the failure of hypertension and diabetes to act independently.

References

1. Krueger DE, Ellenberg SS, Bloom S, et al. (1981) Risk factors for fatal heart attack in young women. Am J Epidemiol 113/4:357–370
2. Mann JI, Vessey MP, Thorogood M, et al. (1975) Myocardial infarction in young women with special reference to oral contraceptive practice. Br Med J 2:241–245
3. Mantel N, Haenszel W (1959) Statistical aspects of the analysis of data from retrospective studies of disease. J Natl Cancer Inst 22:719–748
4. Miettinen OS (1973) Standardization of risk ratios. Am J Epidemiol 96/6:383–388
5. Miettinen OS (1974) Simple interval estimation of risk ratio. Am J Epidemiol 100:515–516
6. Slone D, Shapiro S, Kaufman DW, et al. (1981) Risk of myocardial infarction in relation to current and discontinued use of oral contraceptives. N Engl J Med 305/8:420–424
7. Vessey MP (1982) Oral contraceptives and cardiovascular disease: some questions and answers. Br Med J 284:615–616

Rehabilitation After Surgery for Chronic Vascular Disease: Goal and Reality

M. Arndt, D. Rühland, R. Keferstein, and W. Pircher

The increasing number of people suffering from arterial vascular disease in recent years has led to an explosion of costs in the branches of surgery dealing with these patients. Due in particular to the development of smoking habits, the number of younger patients affected by vascular disease is steadily increasing.

In the context of discussions about either diminishing social security benefits or raising the age of retirement, the actual effectiveness of surgical treatment is gaining more and more importance, especially in view of the patient's rehabilitation. As the majority of operations are performed because of claudication and rest pain and/or transient ischaemic attacks, *rehabilitation* from the surgeon's point of view means above all to return the patient to full employment, and, if possible, to enable him to resume his normal social life. This goal is to be achieved by medical measures in combination with technical and social initiatives.

The objective of medical, i.e. surgical, measures is to restore the interrupted blood flow. This can be achieved by:

- Intraluminal angioplasty
- Desobliteration in combination with a patch plasty
- Transplantation or implantation of autologous vein or artificial material like vascular grafts

In order to secure functioning or patency, especially in the case of grafting, follow-up treatment with several drugs is necessary for most patients. In most of our cases this is supervised by the general practitioner. Especially vitamin K antagonists, indispensable in peripheral bypasses with artificial material, are apt to limit occupational rehabilitation in many cases, because their specific risks forbid the employment of these patients in jobs with a high risk of injuries.

A must for any patient after surgery is to give up smoking altogether. This is really the only factor that might help to slow down disease progression and to improve the patency of grafts.

In some cases, especially when larger operations have been performed to restore blood flow, a special rehabilitation programme is indicated; this will normally be carried out in specially selected centres. Such measures, however, appear indicated only in patients who were in employment before the operation and who may expect to be re-employed after treatment.

Primary Health Care in the Making
Ed. by U. Laaser, R. Senault, H. Viefhues

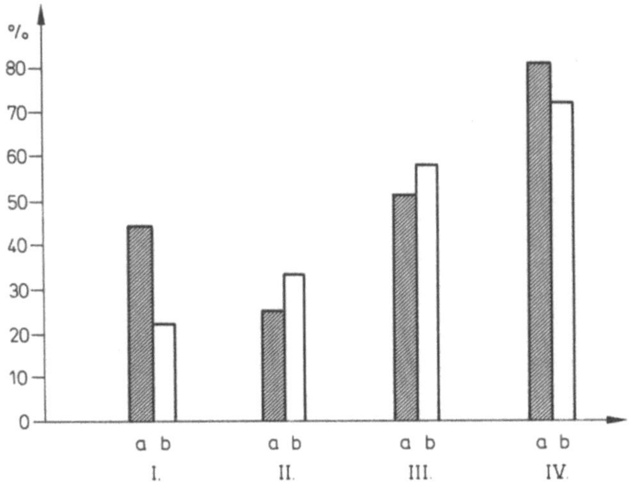

Fig. 1. A comparison between the ability to work before (*a*) and after (*b*) operation. I, professionals; II, civil servants; III, employees; IV, labourers

Due to the different types of operation performed, the period of physical recovery which, from the surgical point of view, involves inability to work, varies from 2 weeks to 3 months. For the surgeon the question of whether rehabilitation can be achieved must influence his assessment of the indication for surgery in many cases. To put it plainly, this means that a person still able to walk 300 m without pain, and generally willing to retire, should not necessarily go through an operation with an overall lethality of 4% or more.

Considering their differing pre-operative conditions, patients with peripheral bypasses are rather hard to evaluate in terms of their ability to return to work. The same problem is seen in patients with occlusive disease of the supra-aortic branches, of whom many are above or near the age of retirement.

Among the patients with aortofemoral bypass there will be – judging by our own experience – a large number with comparable pre-operative conditions and surgical outcome who had been working before the operation. In addition, the surgical outcome can be ascertained by sphygmopalpation in most of these cases. We were therefore interested to find out whether the hope of returning to work, professed by the majority of vascular patients, was actually fulfilled.

We investigated 120 patients with aortofemoral bypass with a minimum follow-up of 1 year after surgery. The mean age of patients in this group was 54 years. Only patients in employment before operation, and in whom surgical procedures had been successful, were included in the study.

It was disappointing to see that 40.8% were still smoking although they had been warned about the risk. 85% of the patients stated that they had been handicapped before operation with regard to their social life. 83.8% of the patients were completely content with the outcome of the operation and were prepared to go through with it once more under the same circumstances. It has to be noted that a large number of these patients suffered from impotence due to lesion of the sacral nerves during the operation.

The most disappointing fact revealed in our investigation was that, in contrast to the good surgical results 73.9% of patients had not returned to work. Looking for the reason for this critical social result of our efforts, we feel that it lies in the occupational distribution of our patients. The fact that those who retired after the operation were recruited from the group with the highest social security benefits, i.e. the civil servants, whereas independent professional men and labourers tended to return to work (Fig. 1), shows that it cannot be the surgical outcome nor any other condition that decisively influences rehabilitation.

The main incentive to retire seems to come from personal social security provisions. A high standard of social benefits enables and even encourages the patient not to return to work. It is obvious that these observations, disappointing for the surgeon as they are, will have some future influence on the indication for surgery.

As a conclusion we feel that closer contact between the surgeon, the general practitioner and the official institutions for rehabilitation is required for improving the effectiveness of work and money invested in vascular surgery.

Multiple Sclerosis and Geophysical Factors

J. Resch

Multiple sclerosis has a prevalence in middle and northern Europe of about 40 to 80 cases per 100 000 persons. One sees that it is not a rare disease. The disease has a significant social importance, as the majority of those affected are still relatively young. Thus the average age at manifestation is about 30 years, and among women under 35 years old, multiple sclerosis is the second most prevalent diagnosis leading to premature pensions in the Federal Republic of Germany (the first being schizophrenia).

Nothing definite is known about the cause of multiple sclerosis. Risk factors which could make prevention possible are not known. However, the results of epidemiological science surely tell us something about the aetiology of the disease. Two things seem to be very important, and these represent the basis of our examination.

First there is the geographical distribution throughout the world, which is confirmed by hundreds of epidemiological studies. They indicate a clear decrease from North to South in Europe and North America and a decrease from South to North in Australia. Figure 1 shows 80 prevalences against geographic latitude. These values have been denoted as methodologically comparable by Kurtzke [2]. Most values are from Europe. As can be seen, the values from North America and Australia are shifted about 10 ° to the equator in relation to those of Europe. In contrast the values ascertained from East Asia are shifted about 10 ° away from the equator. So there is a difference at low prevalences of about 20 °, i.e. more than 2000 km at the surface of the earth, between North America and East Asia. The differences between the continents disappear if the prevalences are drawn against the geomagnetic instead of the geographic latitude. This is shown in Fig. 2. The better correlation of the prevalence of multiple sclerosis with geomagnetic latitude is of major significance. This still does not mean that the geomagnetic latitude is aetiologically relevant. Nevertheless, as a result of this correlation Barlow [1] put forward the hypothesis of an aetiological meaning of cosmic rays. The cosmic rays are closely correlated with geomagnetic latitude.

There is a second important result of epidemiology: People, who immigrated for instance to South Africa, Israel or Hawaii, have the same prevalence of multiple sclerosis as the population in their mother countries, although the disease often does not become manifest until decades following immigration. However, this is only the case if the immigrants have been adults at the time of

Primary Health Care in the Making
Ed. by U. Laaser, R. Senault, H. Viefhues

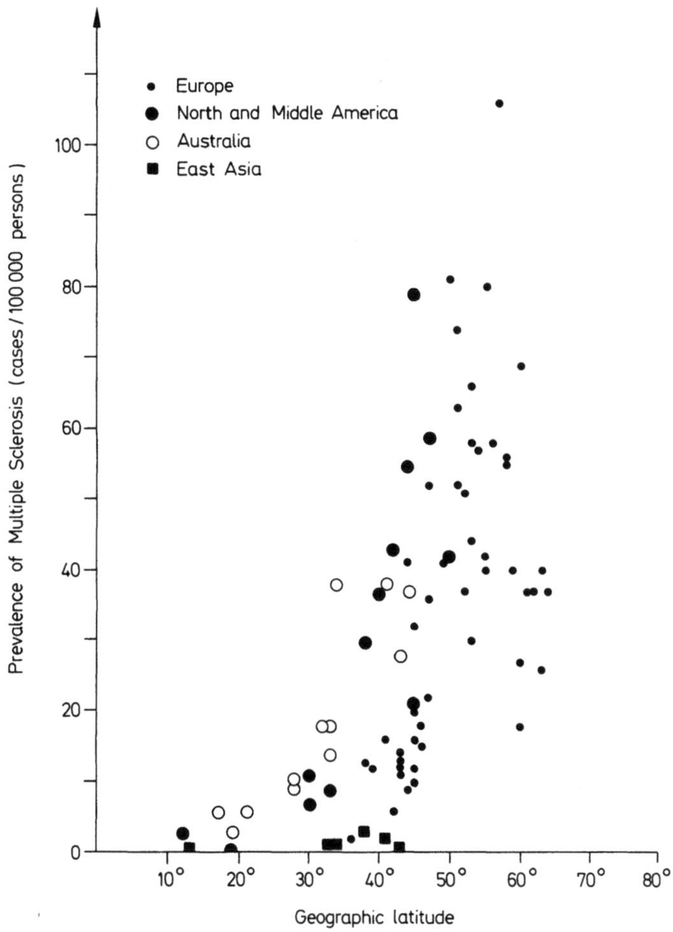

Fig. 1. Prevalences of multiple sclerosis in relation to geographic latitude

immigration. If they have been children, then the prevalence of multiple sclerosis among the immigrants will be the same as the prevalence among the original inhabitants. The reason for this seems to be that a causal factor (or factors) of the disease is working in the age between childhood and adulthood, although the disease manifests itself on average at about the age of 30 years. The critical time seems to be between age 10 and age 15.

Starting from the hypotheses of a causal meaning of cosmic rays or magnetic activity, which both correlate with geomagnetic latitude, these influences seem to be operative between ages 10 and 15. It is known that the magnitude of these geophysical factors changes in dependence on the solar cycle. Figure 3 shows the 11-year period of the solar cycle. If the cosmic rays or the geomagnetic activity is a causal factor for multiple sclerosis, then it would follow that the risk of multiple sclerosis at successive age classes of youth changes in an 11-year rhythm.

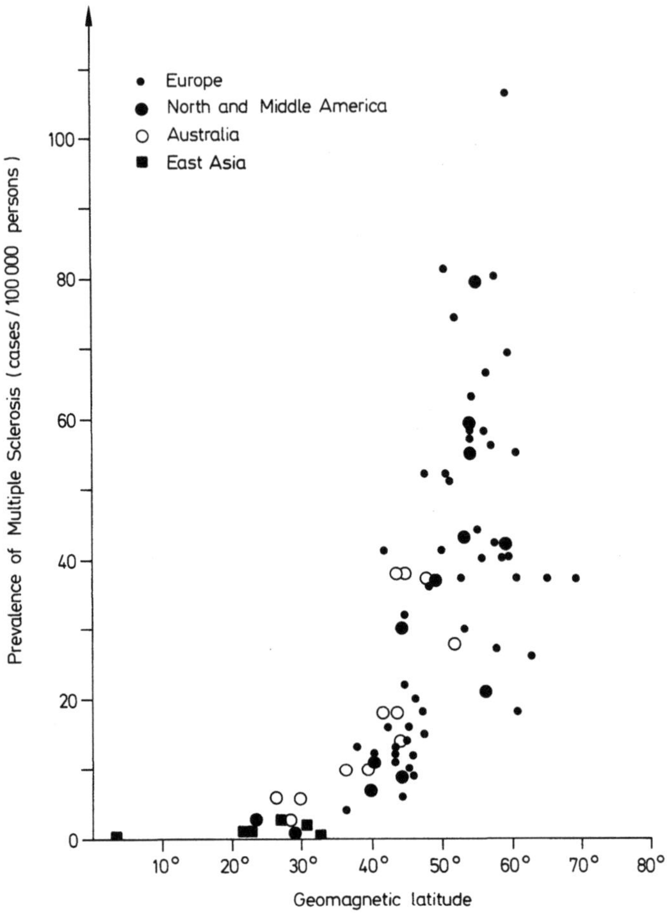

Fig. 2. Prevalences of multiple sclerosis in relation to geomagnetic latitude

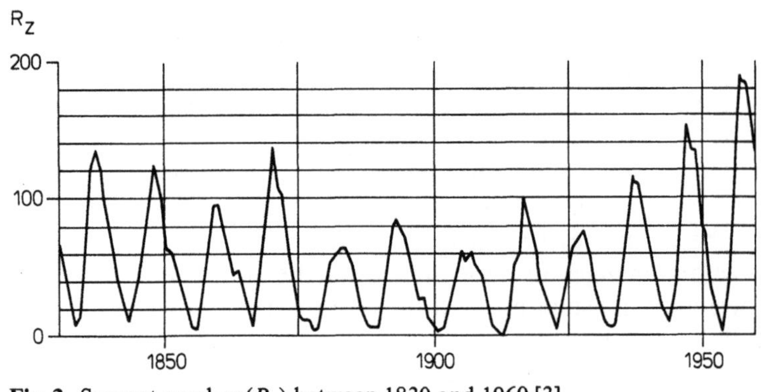

Fig. 3. Sunspot number (R_z) between 1830 and 1960 [3]

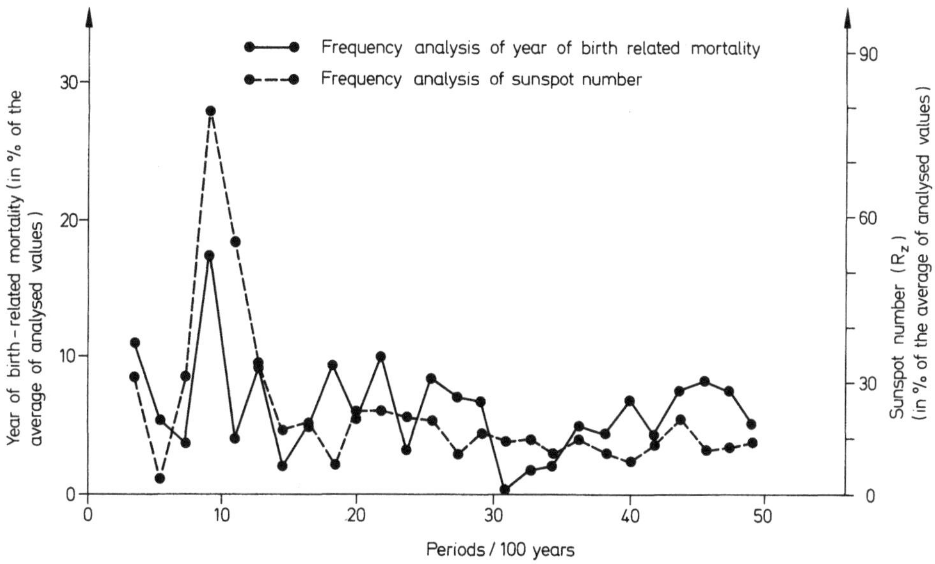

Fig. 4. Fourier analysis of birth-related multiple sclerosis death rates (1889–1943) among women in Baden-Württemberg and Rheinland-Pfalz and number of sun spots (1902–1956)

In order to evaluate whether scientific data supporting our hypothesis exist, we have examined the multiple sclerosis death rates of women in the years 1968–1975 in the German Bundesländer Baden-Württemberg and Rheinland-Pfalz. 1215 cases were included. We calculated the average death rate of the years 1968–1975 for every year of birth between 1889 and 1944. A Fourier analysis has been done with this sequence of death rates. Figure 4 shows the result (straight line). There is a clear maximum at a frequency of nine periods per 100 years, i.e. a period comprises 11 years. The dotted line shows the frequencies of the sunspot number itself. A high correspondence of both curves related to the period of 11 years is clearly demonstrated. At other frequencies no correspondence is visible.

Not only is there a geographical relationship of multiple sclerosis to geomagnetic latitude but also a temporal relationship to the solar cycle. It follows that the hypothesis of a causal relevance of geophysical factors for multiple sclerosis is increasingly likely to be correct.

References

1. Barlow IS (1960) Correlation of the distribution of multiple sclerosis with cosmic-ray intensities. Acta Psychiatr Scand [Suppl 147] 35:108
2. Kurtzke JF (1975) A reassessment of the distribution of multiple sclerosis. Acta Neurol Scand 51:110
3. Waldmeier M (1961) The sunspot activity in the years 1610–1960. Schulthess, Zürich

Chronic Mental Illness: Social Factors and Rehabilitation Outcomes

J. Kunow

Re-integration into work and gainful employment is a central aim of rehabilitation. This goal is also supported by German legislation. If the client is not able to attain this goal, employment in a protected working situation is desirable: The working situation provides structure for the course of the day, and the opportunity for the client to communicate with other persons and find support for his self-confidence, thereby positively influencing the course of illness. Therefore, re-integration into gainful employment is, aside from independent living, social contact, active organisation of leisure time and general satisfaction with one's life, an essential aspect of the rehabilitation outcome.

In the last 4 years at the Weinsberg PLK we have conducted three studies in which the level of employment after hospitalisation was one topic of investigation. These three studies were:

1. A longitudinal study examining 60 schizophrenic patients living in the "Therapeutikum Heilbronn". Data were collected in the spring of 1978 and in the spring of 1980. (25% of these patients had been in a mental hospital for longer than 5 years)
2. A retrospective study in 1982 examining 171 ex-patients of a rehabilitation ward in the PLK Weinsberg who had been discharged in 1979. (Diagnosis: 90% schizophrenia and 10% affective psychosis)
3. A survey study in 1982 examining 128 clients of a social advisory agency in Cologne. (Diagnosis: 60% schizophrenia and 40% affective psychosis)

In these three studies the rehabilitation outcome was measured in terms of actual working conditions, i.e.:

- Without work
- Protected working situation or unemployed but looking for employment
- Working under normal conditions of the labour market, at least 20 hours/ week.

The outcomes of the aforementioned studies, as measured by our criterion of integration into work and employment, were extremely varied (due to the differences in the analysed populations). Within the group of the severely handicapped clients of the Therapeutikum Heilbronn, only 10% of all cases were considered a clear success (i.e. working under normal conditions of the labour market) (Table 1). In 14% of all cases there was a deterioration in their condition; the clients had become patients of a mental hospital again or were

Primary Health Care in the Making
Ed. by U. Laaser, R. Senault, H. Viefhues

Table 1. Working situation of the Therapeutikum Heilbronn clients after 1 year of training ($n=60$)

Without work	8	14%
Protected working situation or unemployed but looking for employment	46	76%
Working under normal conditions of the labour market at least 20 hours/week	6	10%
Total	60	100%

Table 2. Working situation of the PLK Weinsberg patients 3 years after discharge

Without work	27	16%
Protected working situation or unemployed but looking for employment	64	37%
Working under normal conditions of the labour market at least 20 hours/week	30	18%
Missing cases	50	29%
Total	171	100%

living in a nursing home. Of the clients under investigation, 16% were still in the protected working situation of the Therapeutikum (as Ciompi has pointed out, such a stabilisation is a success in itself).

From the 171 patients who were dismissed in 1979 from a rehabilitation ward of the PLK Weinsberg and examined in 1982 we obtained the following data (Traine 1983):

- 18% working under normal conditions of the labour market,
- 16% without work,

i.e. most of the clients were working in a protected working situation (Table 2).

The clients of the social advisory agency in Cologne were chronically mentally ill who through their handicap were covered by the law for the severely handicapped (SchwBG). The working situation of these clients in February 1982 was as follows: 38% were working under normal conditions of the labour market, while about the same number (44%) were working in a protected situation or were unemployed, but looking for employment. Sixteen per cent were without work (Table 3).

In all three studies variables which may explain why some patients are able to work again while others are not were measured. In other words: What factors influenced the patients' chances of rehabilitation? This question cannot yet be answered conclusively. "Rehabilitation is presently lacking a comprehensive theoretical framework which permits the integration of already existing knowledge" [5, p. 104]. The purpose of this paper is to contribute to the development of such a theoretical framework.

Table 3. Working situation of patients of a social advisory agency in Cologne

B:0:Without work	21	16%
Protected working situation or unemployed but looking for employment	57	44%
Working under normal conditions of the labour market at least 20 hours/week	48	38%
Missing cases	2	2%
Total	128	100%

We take here the social support approach [1] which was developed in the 1970s out of life event research. The life event approach assumes that a number of life-changing events which must be simultaneously dealt with can exert a strong influence upon the individual's health. With its "stress model" this approach also offers a plausible explanation for the biological effect of social events.

Altogether the explanatory power of this approach has proven disappointing: The correlation between life events and mental and/or physical impairment has at best reached $r = 0.3$. This correlation, however, varies greatly from study to study. One cause of the modest level of explanatory power lies in the failure to consider the varying initial conditions of the individual. Thus Brown was able to show that the extent and the quality of the social-psychological and material support which the individual received from his environment through social relations offered an important protective factor against the effects of life-changing events.

Recognising that the causes of life events are not always immediately obvious, psychological research has increasingly stressed a further protective factor. On the basis of learning theory Rotter developed the position that in such situations some individuals tend to seek causes in their environment while others seek them in themselves. He considered, the variable *i*nternal versus *e*xternal locus of *c*ontrol (IEC) – a relatively stable personality characteristic which, nevertheless, can be changed by learning experiences. He suggested that internal attribution provides effective protection against the negative effects of life-changing events.

Our approach must be expanded beyond the life event model, however. Recent socio-psychological theories, particularly behaviouristic approaches, interpret stress as a consequence of conflicting demands upon the individual. Apart from life-changing events, those conflicting demands include chronic overdemands of work (especially contradictory demands and time pressure), marital problems and the effects of other social contacts which are maintained despite negative evaluation. Contradictory expectations from various realms of life (role conflict) have to be considered in this context as well.

The simple linear hypothesis of life event research has been further developed in a model which consists of the following groups of variables [1, p. 9]:

- Social stressors: life-changing events (e.g. death of a spouse or loss of employment); chronic environmental demand such as work stress and marital problems.
- Psychosocial resources: the psychological ability and social competence necessary to cope with problems.
- Social resources: help and social support which the individual obtains from his social network.
- Stress reactions: short-term physiological and psychological stress, mental and physical impairment and illness, and eventually the shortening of life expectancy.

In this verbal form the model may be plausible, but nevertheless it is untestable. The interrelationships between the variables are not sufficiently elaborated. In order to draft a precise and testable model we suggest the following line of thought.

A high level of life-changing events leads to mental and physical illness. According to social-psychological theories, demanding social relations and persistent role conflict have a similar effect. We postulate a direct linear and nonrecursive relationship between illness as a reaction, and stress arising from environmental demands or life-changing events (see Fig. 1). On the other hand, the effects of the individual's psychosocial resources (personality-specific coping strategies) become evident only with the occurrence of demanding events: Coping strategies moderate the negative influence of demanding social relations and persistent role conflict, as well as that of life-changing events upon the individual's health. In order to develop a testable model we therefore postulate an interactive relationship. A necessary additional condition is the measurement of coping strategies on a scale ranging from well-articulated strategies (0.1) with a strong moderating effect to poorly articulated strategies

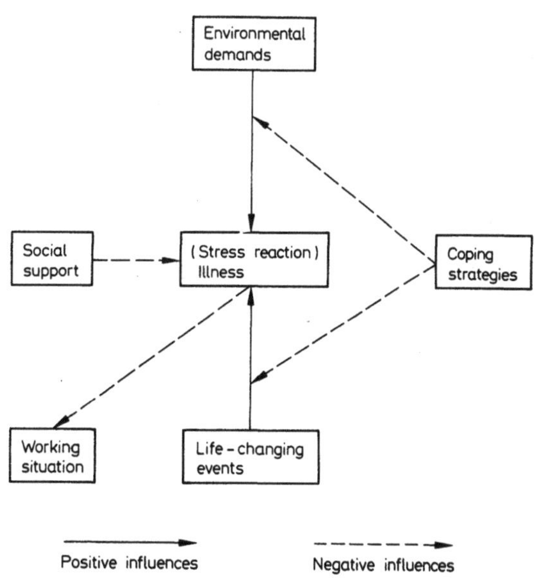

Fig. 1. The "social support model"

(1.0) with little effect. The theoretical importance of the factor "social support" must still be considered; does social support also weaken the effects of demanding life events and other stressors, or does it have its own specific effect upon (mental) health?

Here we take the view of Badura [1, p. 22]: "Social relations constitute a necessary condition for mental health, or put differently: these exert a direct effect." In this model the client's present working situation is taken as a dependent variable of mental health. We can express these specifications in the causal model given in Fig. 1. This model proves consistent with the results of all three studies. The variance explained thereby is at best 20%. The social support model as elaborated here can be considered as a meaningful complement to the medical model of illness.

In reference to the working situation of the clients, we must expand our model: On the basis of present data, working situation is also influenced by the following variables:

- The number of existing social contacts
- The individual's evaluation of his own ability to work
- A long period of time since the last hospitalisation

It is important to note here that the estimation of the coefficients is not consistent from model to model (regression approach). This can be a result of either of two causes: Either the model is incomplete, or, what we consider more probable, the operationalisation of the individual variables must still be improved. We are presently working on this improvement. Furthermore one must point out that the method of testing which has been used here (causal analysis) can only test whether a given model is consistent with the data or not. In order to obtain a satisfying degree of confidence in our findings, further studies on other samples are necessary.

References

1. Badura B (ed) (1981) Soziale Unterstützung und chronische Krankheit. Suhrkamp, Frankfurt
2. Brown G, Harris T (1978) Social origins of depression: A study of psychiatric disorder in women. Cambridge University Press, London
3. Reimer F (ed) (1977) Chronisch psychisch krank – Artefakt oder Krankheit? Thieme, Stuttgart
4. Rotter JB (1966) Generalized expectancies for internal versus external control of reinforcement. Psychol Monogr 80:1–28
5. Waltz EM (1981) Soziale Faktoren bei der Entstehung und Bewältigung von Krankheit – Ein Überblick über die empirische Literatur. In: Badura B (ed) Soziale Unterstützung und chronische Krankheit. Suhrkamp, Frankfurt, pp 40–119

Longitudinal Pattern of Aftercare in a Cohort of Recent Onset Schizophrenics

G. Krüger, H. Biehl, B. Krumm, and C. Schubart

Introduction

The question of "need and supply" in the field of psychiatric care has increasingly stimulated epidemiological research in the past decade [e.g. 4], while at the same time the main focus of attention in treatment has gradually shifted from hospital-orientated ("institutionalism") towards community-orientated care ("rehabilitation").

For several reasons, e.g. the different roles of general practitioners and psychiatrists in private practice compared with other countries, psychiatric aftercare in West Germany could not simply replicate the experiences in Scandinavia or Anglo-American countries.

Previously, two empirical studies in West Germany have reported comprehensively on the aftercare pattern of schizophrenic patients: Bosch and Pietzcker [3] recorded treatment over a catamnestic period of 1 year in two patient groups in a metropolitan and a rural region. Of the discharged patients, 45% did not have any psychiatric aftercare contacts, and only 32% in the urban region and 11% in the rural region had regular psychiatric contacts, i.e. at least once a month. Adding the contacts by general practitioners, these figures rose to 37% (city) and 46% (country).

A more recent study in Mannheim, which was performed prospectively with an epidemiologically defined schizophrenic patient cohort [9], showed that after about 5–6 months a pattern of utilization developed, with about 60% being out-patients, 25% in-patients and 15% not in any form of aftercare. These percentages remained relatively stable over an observation period of 18 months [5].

This paper will now describe the "natural course" pattern of aftercare of an epidemiologically defined cohort of schizophrenic patients over 2 years, starting with their first psychotic episode. It is one aspect of an ongoing WHO multicentre study on impairments and disabilities associated with schizophrenic disorders, whose main scope and objectives have been described elsewhere [2, 8, 11].

Patients and Methods

In the three psychiatric institutions in our region (State Hospital Wiesloch, Psychiatric University Clinic, Heidelberg, and Central Institute for Mental Health,

Primary Health Care in the Making
Ed. by U. Laaser, R. Senault, H. Viefhues

Mannheim), all patients with first onset of schizophrenia were continually included in the study if suffering from hallucinations, delusions (not based on affective disorders) and/or thought and speech disorder (different from retardation as in depression and acceleration as in mania). Patients were excluded:

- If they were below 15 or above 44 years old
- If they resided outside Mannheim, Heidelberg or the Rhine-Neckar district
- If there was evidence of organic brain disease, mental retardation, severe sensory defect or alcohol or drug dependence
- If onset of the above symptoms had been manifested more than 1 year previously

Seventy patients were followed-up for 2 years. Levels of aftercare were defined according to a hierarchical structure of intensity of management measures and recorded in monthly steps at the follow-up contacts (every 6 months) by the research team, using information from the patient, his/her "key person" (mostly mother or spouse), medical records and other sources (treating doctors, social workers and agencies).

Results

Figure 1 shows the longitudinal pattern of psychiatric care of all 70 patients over 2 years, divided into monthly steps. Following a method suggested by Häfner and an der Heiden [5], we defined the following categories or "levels of care" according to a presumed hierarchy of intensity:

1. In-patient status in a psychiatric hospital
2. Institutional rehabilitation with accommodation
3. Psychiatric specialist treatment *with* medication
4. General practitioner or "family doctor" treatment *with* medication
5. Out-patient treatment *without* medication (incl. psychotherapy, social workers)

Furthermore, the group without utilization of aftercare facilities was divided into those *without* evidence of psychotic symptoms (category *6* on the figure) and those *with* unequivocal evidence of delusions, hallucinations or thought disorder (category *7;* possibly "non-compliers").

Finally, the two patients who committed suicide during the 2-year period (category *8*) (their individual aftercare pattern will be anecdotically illustrated below) and one patient who did not contact any professional service after receiving a permanent pension (category *0*) should be mentioned to complete the picture.

Looking more closely at the longitudinal changes among the different levels of care, one can identify a sharp decrease in the rate of hospitalized patients in the early phase, leading to an approximate "levelling-off" or "plateau effect" after 6–8 months of observation. This applies not only to the hospital "level of care", where there is a brief intermediate peak around the 12th to 14th month, but also to the distribution among other levels of care.

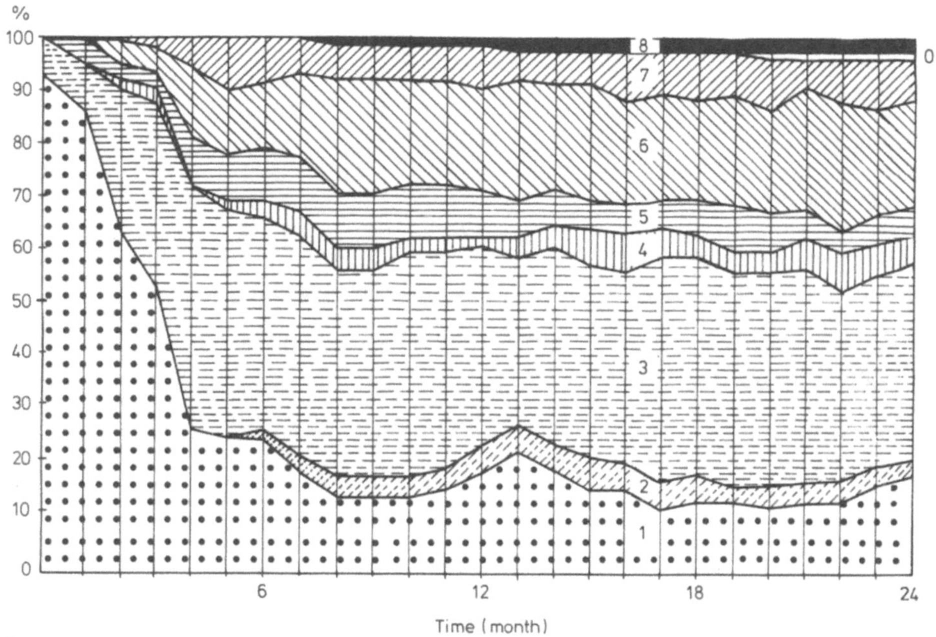

Fig. 1.

1: Psychiatric inpatient.
2: Institutional rehabilitation.
3: Outpatient, psychiatric specialist, *with* medication.
4: Outpatient, general practitioner, *with* medication.
5: Outpatient, *no* medication.
6: No treatment, *no* psychotic symptoms.
7: No treatment, productive psychotic symptoms.
8: Dead.
0: Permanent pension, no treatment.

Table 1 gives the numerical distribution at five different timepoints at half-yearly intervals (these coincide with the main study's follow-up assessments):

- Only 25% of the patients are hospitalized at the 6 months time point, a figure that decreases further during the course.
- At all timepoints about 43% use aftercare by psychiatrists, general practitioners or the clinic's out-patient department and take medication.
- Another smaller group (category 5; between 5% and 8%) has aftercare contacts *without* medication.
- Roughly 8%–10% of the patients live in the community and do not use psychiatric aftercare despite evidence of positive psychotic symptoms.
- After 1 year and later, another 18% do not have any treatment and do not show psychotic symptoms at the psychiatric follow-up interviews.

If we now calculate the average distribution of the levels of care after reaching some stability in the pattern (i.e. 8th to 24th month of observation) and base it on the incidence rate found in our study (93 new patients in 900 000 in-

Table 1. Status of 70 patients at follow-up contacts every 6 months (in percentages) follow-up after month

Status	0	6	12	18	24
1 Inpatient	94.29	25.71	18.57	12.86	17.14
2 Rehabilitation facilities with accommodation	–	1.43	5.71	5.71	2.86
3 Psychiatrists' outpatient facilities with drugs	5.71	40.0	37.14	40.0	37.14
4 General practitioners' outpatient facilities with drugs	–	2.86	1.43	4.29	5.71
5 Outpatient facilities (psychotherapy, social worker), but no drugs	–	8.57	8.57	7.14	5.71
6 No treatment no psychotic symptoms	–	11.43	18.57	17.14	18.57
7 No treatment in spite of overtly psychotic symptoms	–	8.57	8.57	10.0	8.57
8 Suicide	–	–	1.43	2.86	2.86

Table 2. Estimated need for treatment by schizophrenic patients (based on a 1-year-incidence cohort)

Level of care	Treatment places
Psychiatric inpatients	1.57/100 000
Institutional rehabilitation (with accommodation)	0.50/100 000
Outpatients *with* medication treated by psychiatrists	3.92/100 000
general practitioners	0.50/100 000
Outpatients *without* continued medication	0.76/100 000

habitants in 1 year), we can estimate the treatment demand for one year's cohort of schizophrenic patients, as shown in Table 2. These figures illustrate that in addition to the hospital sector (with a continuous demand for beds in the course of schizophrenic patient's careers), a high proportion of treatment places are required at rehabilitation institutions and with psychiatrists and general practitioners. In addition, one should mention the treatment rate of 0.83/100 000 which would be needed if active follow-up treatment, possibly with home visits, were to be given to those psychotic patients at present in the community *without* aftercare.

Rates of rehospitalization in patients depending on their aftercare pattern (e.g. compliance with long-term medication vs non-compliance) cannot be demonstrated due to lack of time, but to round off the illustration of the aftercare pattern in a "natural course" group of recent onset schizophrenics, the individual aftercare patterns of those patients in our study who committed suicide are shown in Fig. 2: The levels of care categories are numbered in the same way as mentioned above.

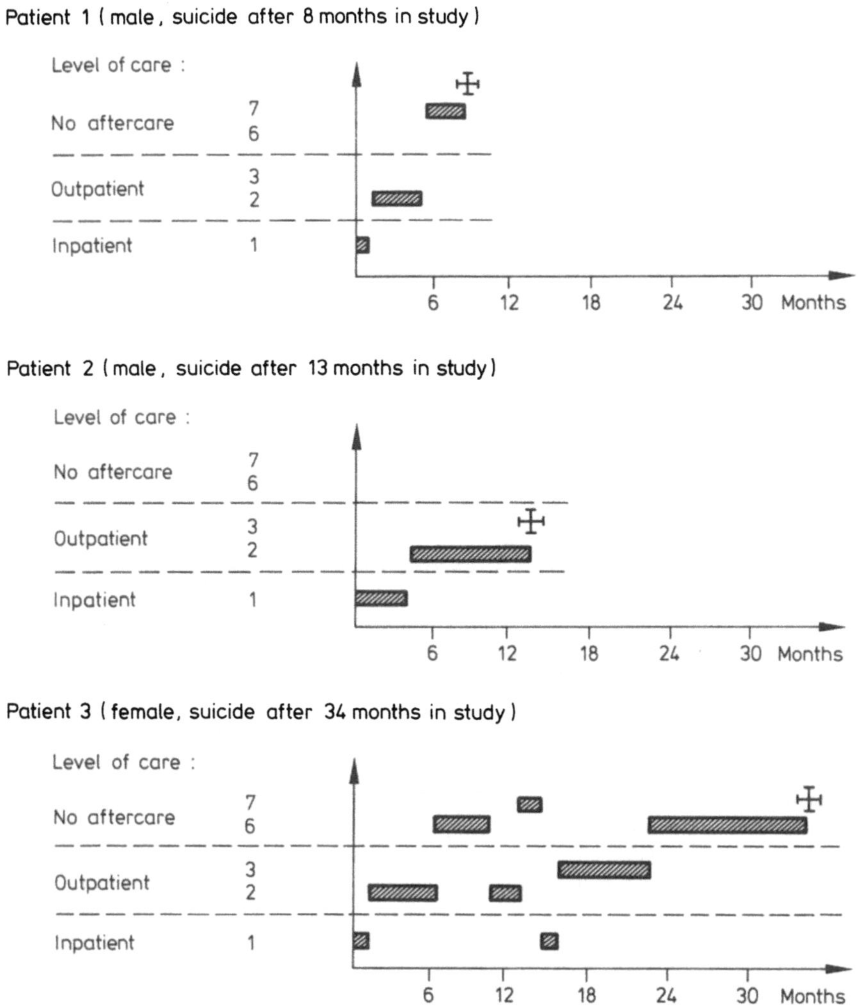

Fig. 2

Discussion

Any comparison of the demonstrated aftercare pattern and the estimated demand on different "levels of care" with the findings of other studies should be made only with the following reservations:

- Most former studies on schizophrenics report higher rates of hospitalized patients, whereas now, after the implementation of a more comprehensive community mental health service in this region, the average length of hospitalization and the number of long-stay patients (> 1 year) have decreased, as shown by Häfner and Klug [6].
- Another source of bias in many studies is the inclusion of patients with former hospital admissions, which inflates the reported in-patient rates [7].
- Still other influential variables are the distance to the next mental hospital, the number of psychiatrists in a region and the number of places in shel-

tered homes and workshops. A recent study in a rural Bavarian area [1] (Günzburg) reported that 34% of discharged first hospitalization schizophrenics were treated by their general practitioners, but there were only two practising psychiatrists in the catchment area of that mental hospital.

Outlook

Further analysis of the aftercare pattern will be possible after completion of the ongoing 5-year follow-up of the prospective disability study and will hopefully reveal the importance of aftercare and adaptive behaviour of patients in order to "survive in the community" [10].

References

1. Bell V, Aschoff-Pluta R, Blumenthal S, Lungershausen E, Vogel R (1983) Das Nachsorgeverhalten ersteingewiesener psychiatrischer Patienten im Jahr nach ihrer Entlassung. Psychiat Prax 10:24–27
2. Biehl H, Schubart C (1984) Werden die Weichen früh gestellt? – Zur Entwicklung von Behinderung bei neuerkrankten schizophrenen Patienten – Definition, Meßmethode und Verlauf über 2 Jahre. Spektrum 4:172–180
3. Bosch G, Pietzcker A (1975) Nachbehandlung krankenhausentlassener schizophrener Patienten – Ergebnisse einer empirischen Untersuchung. Anhang zum Bericht über die Lage der Psychiatrie in der BRD. Bundestagsdrucksache 7/4201, Bonn, pp 344–360
4. Häfner H (ed) (1979) Estimating needs for mental health care. Berlin
5. Häfner H, an der Heiden W (1983) The impact of a changing system of care on patterns of utilization by schizophrenics. Soc Psychiatry 18:153–160
6. Häfner H, Klug J (1982) The impact of an expanding community mental health service on pattern of bed usage: Evaluation of a four year period of implementation. Psychol Med 12:177–190
7. Heiden W an der, Klug J (1980) An integrated record system for the observation of the demand for medical and social aftercare as a basis for organizing extramural services. Acta Psychiatr Scand [Suppl 285] 62:54–59
8. Jablensky A, Schwarz R, Tomov T (1980) WHO collaborative study on impairments and disabilities associated with schizophrenic disorders: Objectives and methods. Acta Psychiatr Scand [Suppl 285] 62:152–163
9. Klug J, an der Heiden W, Scheel R, Kistner KH (1982) Inanspruchnahme psychosozialer Einrichtungen durch schizophrene Patienten im Langzeitverlauf. In: Beckmann H (ed) Fortschritte psychiatrischer Forschung. Stuttgart
10. Lamb HR (1976) Community survival for long-term patients. San Francisco
11. Schwarz R, Biehl H, Krumm B, Schubart C (1980) Case-finding and characteristics of schizophrenic patients of recent onset in Mannheim. Acta Psychiatr Scand [Suppl 285] 62:212–219

Efforts at Compensation with Regard to Basic Disorders Among Schizophrenics

H. D. Brenner, W. Böker, K. Andres, and W. G. Stramke

Introduction

A few years ago Zubin and Spring [10], in their well known synopsis of the models of illness derived from 80 years of research into schizophrenia, showed that these models, in their totality, correspond to a changed point of view.

In their "vulnerability model" they differentiated between "vulnerability to schizophrenia" as a relatively stable, time-independent "trait" and "episodes of schizophrenic disorder", which are unstable, changeable "states". It is towards the biological aspects of episodes of schizophrenic illness, but possibly also towards those of vulnerability itself, that pharmacotherapy – which predominates today – is aimed. This is especially so in the case of prophylactic treatment with depot neuroleptics. However, we know only too well that this pharmacotherapy – in spite of its undeniable merits – works purely symptomatically, and, in addition, is fraught with considerable risks.

Over many years we have attained the conviction from a large number of single observations, that social and psychological factors are also heavily involved in the interactional process implied by the vulnerability model referred to above. To be more precise, from these observations we have gained the clinical impression that numerous schizophrenic patients regularly demonstrate more or less clearly a temporary disorganisation of behaviour when they feel themselves in threatening situations of stress. They experience, so to speak, "psychotic mini-episodes". Surprisingly, many patients succeed in most such cases in averting a serious breakdown by means of conscious efforts aimed at self-stabilisation. Why and how they succeed and what is the precise nature of the individual efforts seem to us to be crucial questions for future research aiming at the development of corresponding preventive therapeutic measures [see 2].

Research Strategy

The mutual transactions between stressors, vulnerability, situational and personal variables and efforts at restabilisation which underly such a model are undoubtedly highly complicated and in the nature of a process. A simple struc-

Primary Health Care in the Making
Ed. by U. Laaser, R. Senault, H. Viefhues

tural model could, in our opinion, never cope with them. It therefore seems to us that extended research into this process is required, in preparation for which the individual components of the transaction process must be researched in purely descriptive terms.

In this sense we occupied ourselves first with compensatory efforts in regard to such psychic deficits, which can be assumed to be indicators, if not manifestations, of an increased vulnerability at the experimental-psychological research level [see 6, 7]. Involved specifically are disorders of attention, perception and thinking [see 4]. Since according to research by Süllwold [8, 9] these so-called basic disorders manifest themselves also at the level of subjective experience, it must be assumed that persons suffering from them will attempt, in the course of learning processes, to compensate for them. The degree of effectiveness of such attempts at compensation should have definite effects on the complex transaction process outlined above.

Methodology

In a first empirical descriptive study on 40 schizophrenic patients in remission after an acute schizophrenic episode we explored the question of whether there exists a connection between such autoprotective efforts and the basic disorders, and if so, what form it takes [3]. For this study we developed the methodology shown in Table 1. First the subject's accomplishment on various tests used as indicators of vulnerability to schizophrenia and the level of subjectively experienced basic disorders were measured. Then, during a semi-standardised interview of approximately 1½ hours' duration, an inquiry was made into consciously undertaken efforts at compensation with regard to the basic disorders. Four disorder factors have been separated analytically in addition to four phenomenologically defined disorder areas [8]. The interview data were classified by several raters into two specific categories of attempted compensation: "problem-solving oriented" and "non-problem-solving oriented". With regard to these two categories the category system showed adequate reliability. The results of this study showed that all patients were able to report that they made conscious efforts to compensate basic disorders. On average, compensation attempts were mentioned in regard to nearly 75% of the reported disorders. Surprisingly, definitely more problem-solving oriented compensatory efforts were reported than non-problem-solving compensatory efforts. Group comparisons revealed highly significant relations between the level of subjectively experienced basic disorders and both the total number of reported compensatory efforts and the number of problem-solving oriented compensatory efforts [see 3].

On the basis of these results we pursued in a second empirical descriptive study reported here the question of whether it might be possible to find differences in the attempts to compensate for basic disorders between patients whose course of illness was favourable and those whose was not. This research was carried out on 14 medium chronic schizophrenic patients who had all taken part in a previous evaluative study including a 2-year post-treatment period of

Table 1. Variables studied and measures used

Variables	Indicators of vulnerability	Subjectively experienced basic disorders	Compensatory efforts in regard to basic disorders
Measures used	Reaction time: – "cross-over paradigm" – "cross-modality shift paradigm" Span of Apprehension Test [1]	Frankfurter Complaint Questionnaire [8]	Semi-standardised interview: – disorders of normally automatic skills – perceptual disorders – depression, anhedonia – stimulus overload

observation [5]. These patients had a mean age of 34.92 years (SD = 17.47), a mean IQ (WIP) of 98.5 (SD = 11.88) and a mean duration of illness of 5.7 years (SD = 1.34). Eight of these 14 patients had shown a favourable course of the illness, six an unfavourable course.

The methodological approach was the same as that in our first study (see Table 1). Additionally, each patient supplied six weekly protocols. In these semi-standardised protocols, patients reported about situations which they subjectively experienced as most stressful or threatening and about their attempts to deal with these situations.

Results and Discussion

An overview of the most important findings of this study is presented in Tables 2–5. They can be summarized as follows. The findings of Table 2 support the relations, which were already significant in our first study, between subjectively experienced basic disorders and compensatory efforts. From this it would follow that the basic disorders accord to the meaning we have assigned to them in that they often apparently incite processes of self-stabilisation. Table 3 shows the findings of a comparison of the patients with a favourable and an unfavourable course of illness. The findings support our expectations to the extent that patients with a more favourable course have shorter reaction times, lower FCQ values and fewer basic disorders as determined by interview. Consequently they also report fewer compensatory efforts. The ratio between compensatory efforts and basic disorders in their case is, however, greater than among patients with an unfavourable course of their illness, and this is also so with the ratio between problem-solving oriented and non-problem-solving oriented compensatory efforts. Statistically significant, however, is only the number of basic disorders in the case of patients whose illness has an unfavourable course. Given the uniform tendency of the results in the direction of our theoretical expectations and the small sample size, type two errors are perhaps not unlikely. Such a cautious interpretation of the results in accord with the existing tendency is further supported by the results shown in Table 4. Again, these results reveal a clear tendency towards a greater problem-solving orientation among patients whose illness has a favourable course.

Table 2. Relations between basic disorders of the experimental psychological type (reaction time measures = RTM) or subjectively experienced basic disorders (Frankfurter Complaint Questionnaire = FCQ) and the other variables, by means of Spearman rank order correlations ($n = 14$)

	RTM	*t* value	FCQ	*t* value
FCQ	0.58 $P<0.05$	2.47	–	–
Total compensatory efforts	0.54 $P<0.05$	2.22	0.79 $P<0.05$	4.57
Problem-solving oriented compensatory efforts	0.46 $P<0.05$	1.79	0.80 $P<0.05$	4.62
Non-problem-solving oriented compensatory efforts	0.21 NS	0.75	0.28 NS	0.97
Reported disorders	0.61 $P<0.05$	2.67	0.70 $P<0.01$	3.43
$\frac{\text{Compensatory efforts}}{\text{Reported disorders}}$	0.30 NS	1.09	0.75 $P<0.05$	3.93
IQ (WIP)	0.24 NS	0.86	0.16 NS	0.56
Age	0.02 NS	0.07	0.15 NS	0.53
BPRS[a] (Brief Psychiatric Rating Scale)	0.18 NS	0.63	0.37 NS	1.38
D2-test[a]	0.03 NS	0.10	0.36 NS	1.34

[a] Measured at the time of discharge from the clinic, at the beginning of a 2 year post-treatment period of observation

Table 3. Comparison of schizophrenics with a favourable and unfavourable course of the illness by means of the Mann-Whitney *U*-test ($n = 14$)

	Patients manifesting a favourable course of the disease ($n=8$) Group means	Patients manifesting an unfavourable course of the disease ($n=6$) Group means	Difference by means of Mann-Whitney *U*-test
RTM	5.8	11.5	NS
FCQ	35.6	42.8	NS
Reported disorders	9.4	12.8	$P<0.05$
Total compensatory efforts	7.8	9.0	NS
Problem-solving oriented compensatory efforts	5.8	6.0	NS
Non-problem-solving oriented compensatory efforts	2.0	3.0	NS
IQ (WIP)	95.5	97.3	NS
Age	34.8	35.2	NS
BPRS[a]	33.3	29.8	NS
D2[a]	86.3	90.5	NS

[a] Measured at the time of discharge from the clinic, at the beginning of a 2-year post-treatment period of observation

Table 4. Relations between total efforts at compensation and total reported disorders, as well as between problem-solving oriented and non-problem-solving oriented compensatory efforts among patients of study 1 [3] ($n = 40$) and study 2 ($n = 14$)

	Relation between reported efforts at compensation and total reported disorders	Relation between problem-solving oriented and non-problem-solving oriented compensatory efforts
Patients of study 1	0.73:1	2.5:1
Patients of study 2	0.76:1	2.4:1
With good course of disease ($n = 8$)	0.83:1	2.9:1
With poor course of disease ($n = 6$)	0.70:1	2.0:1

It must be said that while the data presented do not definitely support the notion that an unfavourable course of the illness corresponds with unresolved basic disorders, the data are nonetheless compatible with such an idea. Little plausibility, by contrast, can be attached to the possibility that differences in the course of the illness could be due to differences in intelligence and age or to the global level of the illness and psychological achievement at the beginning of the 2-year post-treatment period of observation. These variables do not differentiate the two patient groups.

Finally, Table 5 shows that also from a content-oriented point of view, clear differences emerge between patients with favourable and patients with unfavourable courses in regard to the kind of compensatory efforts engaged in. The data show that patients with a favourable course primarily manifest compensatory efforts which can be characterised as "balancing", "reinterpretation" and "restructuring", whereas patients with an unfavourable course engage primarily in compensatory efforts that could be described as "behaviour displacement", "reality testing" and "stereotyping". The essence of the reported compensatory efforts contains an intentional and a strategic aspect as well. In regard to the intentional aspect it must be noted that the compensatory efforts are primarily focussed on reducing emotional tension provoked by the subjectively experienced basic disorders by means of appropriate cognitive or overt behaviour. In regard to the strategic aspect we have found thus far that similarities in the plan of action can be detected which cut across the qualitatively different categories of compensatory efforts (e.g. changes in the subjective evaluation of the disorders, changes in the structure of the present situation, a search for the familiar, collection of additional sensory information).

Critically, it must be said that whether our findings are specific to schizophrenic patients remains open till current studies with comparison groups of non-schizophrenics are concluded. Moreover, our samples so far have not been representative inasmuch as they were not randomly selected. We believe, how-

Table 5. Assignment to tentative, describing categories of problem-solving oriented compensatory efforts, as noted in six weekly protocols, by patients with a good and a poor course of illness ($n = 14$)

Descriptive categories / Group of patients	"Balancing"	"Reinterpretation"	"Restructuring"	"Structuring"	"Behaviour displacement"	"Reality testing"	"Stereotyping"	Problem-solving oriented compensatory efforts/total compensatory efforts
Patients with a favourable course of illness ($n = 8$)	11	7	5	6	4	4	2	39:48
Patients with an unfavourable course of illness ($n = 6$)	3	2	2	5	4	7	3	26:36

ever, that in spite of these limitations the findings support our research approach.

It it is possible to elucidate further the role of autoprotective efforts in the transaction process concerned with maintaining homeostasis and avoiding psychotic breakdown, then it should also be possible to increase the autoprotective potential of a highly vulnerable person so as to reduce the likelihood of future episodes of illness.

References

1. Asarnow RF, McCrimmon DJ (1978) Residual performance deficit in clinically remitted schizophrenics: a marker of schizophrenia? J Abnorm Psychol 87/6:597–608
2. Böker W, Brenner HD (1983) Selbstheilungsversuche Schizophrener: psychopathologische Befunde und Folgerungen für Forschung und Therapie. Nervenarzt 54:578–589
3. Böker W, Brenner HD, Gerstner G, Keller F, Müller J, Spichtig L (1984) Self-healing strategies among schizophrenics: attempts at compensation for basic disorders. Acta Psychiat Scand 69:373–378
4. Brenner HD (1983) Die Bedeutung experimentalpsychologischer Forschung für Theorie und Therapie der Schizophrenie. In: Brenner HD, Rey ER, Stramke W (eds) Empirische Schizophrenieforschung: Experimentalpsychologische Ergebnisse und Beispiele ihrer Anwendung in Behandlung und Rehabilitation. Huber, Bern Stuttgart Vienna
5. Brenner HD, Stramke W, Hodel-Oprecht B, Rui C (in press) A treatment program for impaired cognitive functions aimed at preventing chronic disability among schizophrenic patients: results of a two years field study. In: Sluss TK, Kramer M, Gruenberg EM, Cooper B (eds) The chronically mentally ill – an international perspective. Johns Hopkins University Press, Baltimore
6. Cromwell RL, De Amicis L, Hayes T, Briggs D (1979) Reaction time crossover, a vulnerability index: mean reaction time, a symptom severity index. Psychopharmacol Bull 15:24–25
7. Johnston MH, Holzmann PS (1979) Assessing schizophrenic thinking. A clinical and research instrument for measuring thought disorder. Jossey-Bass, San Francisco
8. Süllwold L (1977) Symptome schizophrener Erkrankungen. Uncharakteristische Basisstörungen. Springer, Berlin Heidelberg New York (Monographien aus dem Gesamtgebiet der Psychiatrie, vol 13)
9. Süllwold L (1981) Basisstörungen: Ergebnisse und offene Fragen. In: Huber G (ed) Schizophrenie: Stand und Entwicklungstendenzen der Forschung. 4. Weissmauer Schizophrenie-Symposium 1980. Schattauer, New York
10. Zubin J, Spring B (1977) Vulnerability. A new view of schizophrenia. J Abnorm Psychol 86:103–126

Identification of Specific Patterns of Work Incapacity Related to Chronic Illness: Analysis of Data Gathered by the Health Insurance Funds in Western Germany

L. von Ferber, H. J. Jesdinsky, A. Schröer, and H. J. Trampisch

Introduction

Up until now, our knowledge of what really happens in the field of primary health care has been rather limited. In particular, data on long-term follow-up is lacking. The aim of this paper is to identify and describe typical patterns of chronic disease based on data accumulated by the health insurance companies (health insurance is compulsory for 90% of the population in West Germany).

Some of the data in this area is "objective", such as absence from work, whereas others, such as medical diagnoses, are often questioned [6]. However, studies of the consistency of diagnoses in patients diagnosed by more than one physician, and computer analyses of the semantics of the diagnostic vocabulary used, both indicate that we are entitled to attach some validity to the diagnostic information obtained from health insurance files [4, 5].

The aim of the present study is to evaluate the validity of medical diagnoses by a formal statistical approach. We began by subdividing the available cases into three main groups of chronic disease. We then sought to identify pattern configurations typical for these groups exclusively using variables which are unrelated to the diagnostic vocabulary.

Methods

Selection of Cases

Data from nearly 5000 members of a health insurance scheme of a steel plant in Western Germany were screened. Use was made of computer files which record certified sicknesses and categorize them in a three digit ICD code. Data covering a period of 3 years were available when this study started. We selected those employees having at least two incidences of sick leave due to illness falling into one of the following groups:

- cardiovascular disease (CV)
- gastric or intestinal disease (GI)
- back problems (BP), including ischialgia and shoulder-arm syndrome

Foreigners and persons who entered the plant after 31 December 1978 and those who left the plant before 31 December 1980 were excluded.

We then traced back the non-computerized sick leave certificates in order to make the final selection of cases. We selected those who, in the 6-year period

Primary Health Care in the Making
Ed. by U. Laaser, R. Senault, H. Viefhues

Table 1. Selection of cases

	CV	GI	BP
Preselection	1388	948	1259
Final selection	111	113	143

between 1975 and 1980, had

- at least five diagnoses[1] falling into the group of back pain (BP), or
- at least three diagnoses[1] falling into the group of gastric or intestinal disease (GI), or
- at least three diagnoses[1] falling into the group of cardiovascular disease (CV) (as an exception, only one diagnosis of heart infarction or apoplexia was considered to be a chronic disease).

Cases falling into more than one group were excluded.

The unexpectedly large reduction in cases in the final selection (Table 1) was due to the high turnover in personnel and to the exclusion of foreigners and cases falling into more than one diagnostic group.

Definition of Variables

Table 2 displays the record of a patient included in the study.

Table 2. Record of patient no. 59. Born: 24 August 1933. First day of work: 20 April 1959

No. of periods of incapacity	Beginning	End	Duration (days)	Diagnosis
1	15 Feb. 1960	17 Feb. 1960	3	Influenza
2	1 Jan. 1963	29 Jan. 1963	21	Influenzal infection
3	14 Jan. 1969	19 Jan. 1969	6	Cold
4	2 Apr. 1970	8 Apr. 1973	7	Cold
5	2 Feb. 1973	9 Feb. 1973	3	Hypertension (CV)
6	27 Mar. 1978	4 Apr. 1976	9	Angina pectoris (CV)
7	30 Apr. 1979	22 Aug. 1979	115	Myocardial infarction (CV)

[1] ICD 8 categories constituting the group of back problems: 352*, 353, 713*, 717, 722*, 725, 727*, 728, 729*, 733*, 735*, 787; the group of gastro-intestinal disease: 009, 473, 531–533, 535–537, 560–564, 784, 785; the group of cardiovascular disease 305+, 400–404, 410–413, 427–429, 431, 433, 437, 440, 441, 443, 458, 782, 790+. With respect to the numbers marked *, the ICD does not distinguish between miscellaneous musculosceletal disorders and back morbidity. Especially, back problems are difficult to define by the ICD code. We therefore had to revise each record and to decide from the text whether there was a back problem or not. We had similar problems to solve with respect to the numbers marked + in the cardiovascular group

Data in the following list were obtained from Table 2:

List of variables No.	Name	Values derived from record		
(1)	Age in 1980	47 years		
(2)	Years working in the plant	22 years		
(3)	Latent period between entrance to the plant and first incapacity	10 months		
	Work incapacities are counted in periods of:	5	10	15 years
(4)	Frequency of work incapacity since entrance to the plant	2	4	5 cases
(5)	Total duration of incapacity since entrance to the plant	24	37	40 days
(6)	Frequency of incapacity since first incapacity	1		case
(7)	Total duration of incapacity since first incapacity	21		days

Statistical Procedure

A discriminant analysis of these variables was performed in order to estimate the fraction of correctly classified cases for several combinations of variables. We used the simplest discriminant rule – the multinomial rule. This rule requires all variables to be treated as qualitative. First, cut-off points were defined for all variables in order to reduce the number of possible outcomes. In this way most of the variables were dichotomized by their medians in the whole sample. For example, age was defined as low or high with respect to the cut-off point 47 years, which is the median of all 367 cases. Only for the variable "years in the plant" (2) were two cut-off points used. The allocation rule is then based on the estimated conditional multinomial distrubutions, i.e. the contingency table for the groups. A case falling into a certain cell of that contingency table is allocated to the group having the highest[2] percentage of all groups in those cells that have to be compared. In the case of unequal a priori probabilities, the highest product of the cell percentage and the a priori probability is used instead. By this simple application of the allocation rule it is abvious that it

- leads to easily interpretable results and
- makes no assumption regarding the distribution of the variables (e.g. normality).

The performance of the discriminant rule – and hence, the "separability" of the groups – is assessed by an unbiased estimation of the probabilities of correct classification, the "leaving one out" method. By this method, the discrimant rule is based on $n - 1$ cases instead of all n cases given, thus leaving one case out of the sample. This latter case is then allocated according to the rule resulting from all other cases, which is independent of the case being tested. The percentage of correctly classified cases was obtained by repeating this procedure with the remaining cases. The practical application of the method used in this paper has been described previously [8].

[2] With equal percentages a randomization procedure is used for allocation

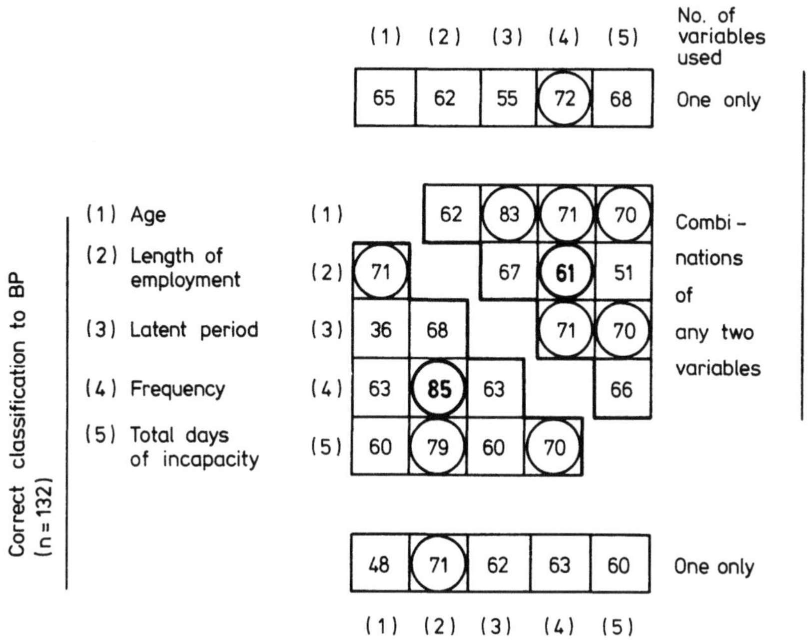

Fig. 1. Percentages of correct classifications (the "leaving one out" method) using a 5-year period after the first incapacity for work. *BP*, back problems; *CV*, cardiovascular diseases

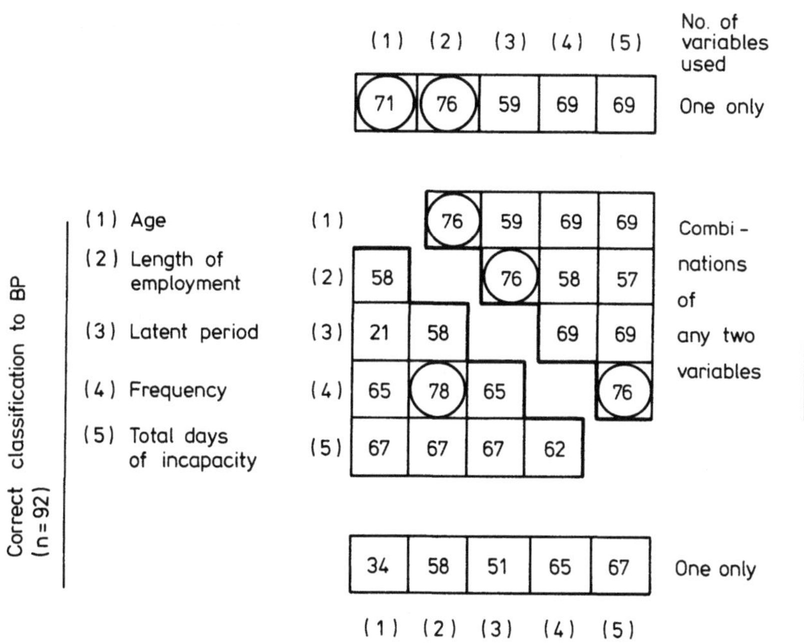

Fig. 2. Percentages of correct classifications (the "leaving one out" method) using a 15-year period commencing from entrance to the plant. *BP*, back problems; *CV*, cardiovascular diseases

Results

Figures 1 and 2 show the percentage of correctly classified cases when distinguishing between cardiovascular and back problem persons assuming equal a priori probabilities. The discrimination possible by one variable only is given in the upper row (percentage of correct classification to cardiovascular disease) and in the lower row (correct classification of back pain patients). The percentages obtained by any combination of two variables may be taken from the upper (cardiovascular disease) and the lower (back problems) triangle matrix.

Percentages above 70 are marked by light circles. When the average of the two corresponding correct classification percentages are above 70, the corresponding percentages are marked by heavy circles.

The highest percentage of persons correctly classified can be found when allocating back problem patients according to their frequency of incapacities and their length of employment at the plant – 85% are classified correctly. The corresponding percentage of cardiovascular cases which are correctly classified by the combination of these variables is only 61%. The overall percentage of correctly classified cases, i.e. the average of the two percentages cited above, is 73% (assuming equal a priori probabilities). This is the highest average percentage to be obtained from the data in Fig. 1. All the other average percentages are between 64 and 68. As a single variable, frequency of incapacities (variable 4) has the highest classification power (72% for the cardiovascular cases and 63% for back pain cases).

In terms of these percentages for correct classification, the results are similar when choosing other periods.

For example, Fig. 2, which gives the percentages for a period of up to 15 years of employment, is similar to Fig. 1 in its overall results. Again we find the

Table 3. Distribution of chronic patients according to length of employment and cases of incapacity for work in 5 years after the first incapacity (CV, cardiovascular diseases; BP, back problems)

Length of employment at the plant	Cases of incapacity in 5 years	CV		BP	
		n	(%)	*n*	(%)
Up to 12 years	Up to 7	10	(9)	2	(1)
	More than 7	5	(5)	29	(22)
	Total	15	(14)	31	(23)
From 13 to 23 years	Up to 7	11	(11)	29	(22)
	More than 7	14	(13)	33	(25)
	Total	25	(24)	62	(47)
More than 23 years	Up to 7	54	(51)	18	(14)
	More than 7	11	(11)	21	(16)
	Total	65	(62)	39	(30)
All people in the final selection	Total	105	(100)	132	(100)

highest percentage of correctly classified back pain cases when taking both years of employment at the plant and the frequency of sick leave into consideration.

A better understanding of the interaction between variables was obtained by examining the distribution of cases in 'multi-way' tables based on the variables screened by the above classification procedure.

Since the combination of length of employment at the plant and frequency of incapacity 5 years after the first incapacity (Fig. 1) has the highest resolving power, we chose this combination for a correlation in a 'multi-way' table. Table 3 shows the low frequency of certified sickness in the cardiovascular group. The cardiovascular group differs most from the back pain group when considering those who only worked in the plant for up to 12 years. An examination of the data for the length of employment at the plant reveals an obvious correlation with this variable. There are twice as many cardiovascular patients who were employed at the plant for 24 years or longer. The comparison of back pain and cardiovascular patients is especially favourable, as they show nearly the same age distribution. Thus we need not consider age as a disturbing factor.

Discussion

There are other combinations of two variables which led to a percentage of correctly classified cases nearly as high as the one described. However, for the purpose of this paper it was thought sufficient to obtain some variables which separate the groups of chronic illnesses and thereby lead to interpretable results, irrespective of which variables were actually included.

It is true that, by dichotomizing most of the variables – only the variable "years of employment at the plant" was split up into three periods, thereby permitting selection by length of employment – some loss of information is inevitably encountered. On the other hand, the use of the multinomial distribution exploits all the information in the resulting contingency tables, whereas any statistical procedure that utilizes the full range of the original variables imposes a "model" upon the data with the risk that the "model" inadequately reflects the real situation.

Another point which deserves comment is the use of the discriminant procedure with respect to the very problem in question. After having answered the question as to whether the possibility exists of finding different patterns for the various groups of chronic disease, there remains the problem as to which variables such a "difference" may best be ascribed. So, for our purposes, the use of discriminant analysis to develop a rule for the identification of subjects turns to the search for distinguishing variables.

At first glance, taking the "separating power" of only two variables may seem to be too restrictive. However, with the sample size available, the contribution of additional variables would not result in a higher percentage of correct classification using the "leaving one out" method.

Discriminant analyses were also done for CV versus GI and for BP versus GI. Here, age is a variable which accounts for some difference between the groups. Thus, the results are not so interesting from the sociological point of view and are not presented for discussion.

With these data and their presentation we open up a new scientific field, as to date no attempt has been made to systematically investigate health insurance data for typical pattern configurations.

As for cardiovascular diseases, we can show that people with these diseases have few certified sicknesses at different time periods, a long latent period without any certified sickness, and a long length of employment at the plant (61% more than 23 years). These results are consistent with clinical observations. Cases are published by Silomon [7], Bräutigam and Christian [2] and Adler [1]. The authors stress the high motivation to vocational work and the slight attention paid to bodily complaints by their heart patients. Dotzauer [3] stated that people who die of acute myocardial infarction have seldom been ill prior to the infarction, as far as their relatives and friends could recall. Accordingly, poor attention to bodily complaints and to frequent illnesses prior to myocardial infarction are reflected in our data as certified sickness.

Conclusion

With this method we were able to show that there is a close relationship between chronic illness and patterns in the data recorded by the health insurance companies. Moreover, it is possible to interpret the observed correlations from the point of view of the clinician as well as from that of the medical sociologist. These purely administrative data involving the frequency and duration of the work incapacity, the length of employment at the plant as well as the age of the person are not signs or symptoms of an illness in the traditional view of medicine. From the psychosocial point of view these data seem to characterize the pattern of illness behaviour: Whether or not a person applies for sick leave in response to his bodily complaints indicates how he views his illness.

Acknowledgements. We thank M. Knapp, Dipl. Math., for performing the statistical evaluations. This project was partly supported by BMFT in Förderungsprogramm: Forschung und Entwicklung im Dienste der Gesundheit, im Forschungsverbund: Laienpotential, Patientenaktivierung und Gesundheitsselbsthilfe.

References

1. Adler R, Rassek M, Schmidt TH (1979) Psychosomatische Aspekte internistischer Krankheiten. In: von Uexküll T (ed) Lehrbuch der Psychosomatischen Medizin. München
2. Bräutigam W, Christian P (1973) Psychosomatische Medizin. Stuttgart
3. Dotzauer G, Naeve W (1956) Statistische Erhebungen über Panoramawandel des akuten Herztodes. Dtsch Z Ges Gerichtl Med 45:30
4. von Ferber L, Slesina W (1981) Integriertes Verfahren zur Analyse arbeitsbedingter Krankheiten. Z Arbeitswissenschaft 35 (7NF):112–123
5. Heydthausen M, Koch F (1983) Diagnostic language in primary health care – a structural and semantical analysis of diagnosis on health service medical cards. 10th International congress of preventive and social medicine, 27. Sept. – 1 Oct. 1983, Heidelberg
6. Schwefel D, Brenner G, Schwartz FW (eds) (1979) Analyse der Wirtschaftlichkeit ambulanter Versorgung. Köln
7. Silomon H (ed) (1980) Herzinfarktrehabilitation. Stuttgart
8. Trampisch HJ, Jesdinsky HJ, Faber P (1982) Warum liefert die Diskriminanzanalyse so viele gute Ergebnisse? Dtsch Med Wschr 107:1730–1736

F. Migrants in Germany

Migration and Health

A. Geiger and F. Hamburger

In the Federal Republic of Germany, the topic of "foreigners and health" currently refers primarily to former "guest workers" and their families, bringing to mind the central role of medicine in the context of migratory labour policy from 1956 to 1973. Medical personnel in the Federal Employment Service's recruitment commissions in Italy, Spain, Portugal, Greece, Yugoslavia and Turkey carried out the central selection process: only healthy men and women, able to work and to submit themselves to stress, were of interest to German industry. This particular use of medicine for specific interests was never seriously examined, but instead accepted under the ideological cover of "preservation of national health". In contrast, this paper supports an understanding of medicine in which the norm of "health for every individual" is clearly the principle of orientation. This is the only way in which the currently perceptible tendencies in the Federal Republic to encourage medical contributions to a policy of "evicting foreigners" can be combatted.

The following main points can be listed concerning the involvement of medicine in the origin of the social problem of "foreigners" from the standpoint of a theory of social problems investigating the transformation of various situations (e.g. poverty) into generally recognizable social problems:

1. In the recruitment of workers the contribution of medicine to the process of selection seems harmless enough; however, from the standpoint of the home countries it becomes clear that this contribution guarantees the loss of substantial reproductive costs (nutrition of children, schooling, training etc.). The activity of the medical personnel serves as a means of sealing once and for all the relationship of exploitation between the heart of Central Europe and the peripheral countries of the Mediterranean.
2. In a later phase, when the once attractive "guest worker" becomes the social problem of the "foreigner", medical practice and research take on a "progressive" role: they uncover the fact that health risks accumulate in the position of foreigners' lives in general and that the former are excluded for systematic reasons – i.e. for reasons of the structure of the public health system – from adequate care. In sociopolitically favourable situations the revelation of disadvantages leads to sociopolitical pressure, culminating in organized help and medical assistance programmes. In fact, these can mean real assistance to their targets, the foreigners. It can be said without a doubt that the medical sub-systems which carry out such programmes are of use.

Primary Health Care in the Making
Ed. by U. Laaser, R. Senault, H. Viefhues

3. In the currently developing phase of a policy of evicting foreigners, the revelation of social and medical need is being used – often against the intention of those responsible for uncovering this need – against the disadvantaged themselves. Insight into the conditions leading to poor health in the migrants' situation is misused as a legitimation for forced repatriation. When the state programme of integration and tolerance towards minorities is reversed in a policy of isolation and competition, this obviously has an influence on the relationship of foreigners to medicine. Diagnoses of psychosomatic syndromes are openly reformulated in accusations ("lazy bones") and support that part of the German population which feels threatened by foreigners, including narrow-minded scholars ("Heidelberg Manifesto"). For the migrants in question, every illness becomes disproportionately threatening: in addition to the resulting physical and psychological stress, it also becomes a potential threat to life itself, leading as it can to unemployment, dependence on social welfare and, in legally correct compliance with § 10 of the Foreigners' Law, to eviction.

The objective dilemma between a humane social medicine and the possibility of its misuse in a policy directed against foreigners was the framework for the contributions and discussions of the Mannheim workshop. This was introduced in a general presentation of the current status of social medical research (Korporal). Here, the cumulative disadvantages in the social situation of foreigners (place of work, housing etc.) as well as medical care were made clear once again. The central question in the current discussion, namely just how necessary are measures directed primarily at foreigners (in the sense of ethnocentric orientation to problems), was discussed. Whereas the psychiatric standpoint (Blanco-Cruz) demanded that specific cultural traditions be considered, and the sociological standpoint (Zimmermann) demanded that ethnic customs be considered in hospital, a broadly based psychiatric-epidemiological study among children (Poustka) did not lead to demands for new consultation and treatment models.

The so-called "second generation" appears to have grown up in such a way that a medical orientation towards "foreigner" status has become obsolete; the sociopolitical problems would, however, appear to have become all the clearer. Considering the development of illness, there was consensus from the very beginning that a model for medical explanation is doomed to failure, particularly among foreigners. Two contributions (Theilen and Schöning-Kalender) traced the manner in which the family system comes under destructive pressures from the situation prior to migration and its consequences, especially the restrictions created in the country of migration (e.g. work restrictions, unemployment, employment and double burdening of women, housing etc.).

The practical projects and models presented have achieved a high sociopedagogic and sociomedical standard:

1. Health work has been integrated in other concepts for problem solving, particularly concepts involving social workers.
2. Contacts in the health care network are connected with primarily preventive measures and counselling in all areas (nutrition, preventive medicine, sexuality etc.)

3. Most contacts are directed at foreign women as the persons of primary contact for men and children.
4. Provision of the various services and contact with an otherwise socially isolated group of addressees are only possible through client-oriented women's work.
5. All of the functioning models work on the basis of experience and orientation to need and attempt to support or to revive traditional knowledge of popular medicine and to strengthen the addressees' competence to act and cope.
6. Counselling centres and health centres (especially those for Turkish women and mothers) co-operate with various agencies and individuals in the social and health sector and have revealed the latter's lack of unity, based on conflict of interests.

Particularly this disunity illustrates a central analytical point made by the workshop: a system of medical care which is structured to serve partial interests cannot serve to create health in an individual who is understood as a unity; the latter must put together the partial services of specialists, general and special clinics, general and particular insurance agencies, conflicting counselling, and experiences with lay personnel or professionals; that is to say, an individual should actually be healthy and fit in order to be able to take advantage of medical care properly!

The work with "foreigners" leads to a clearly ethnological view of one's own society, to a revelation of deep contradictions and to recognition of the possibilities for changing medical-social work with migrants. Potentially, this also implies a chance for German society to discover anew the traditions of self-help.

Sickness in the Process of Migration

C. Schöning-Kalender

The Background: Migration

"In the process of migration the migrant family develops specific orientations, which not only depend on the socio-cultural differences between country of origin and country of residence, but also on strategies and factual ways of coping with the experience of migration." This is one of the main theses of a research project entitled "Orientation Patterns of Turkish and Italian Families in the Process of Migration"[1]. The thesis is based on the fact that foreign workers' families have been living in Germany for up to 20 years now, so that migration has become a determinant factor in their everyday attitudes and decisions. Actually the "process of migration" has become a process of immigration without the families themselves being aware of it.

An example from immigration research in the USA shows the same phenomenon quite clearly: "We all thought we'd return in a few years. But obviously we never did." [1, p. 106]. These words of a Greek immigrant living in the USA in the 1940s could just as well be the words of a Turkish worker in Germany in 1983. The only difference, but an important one, is that Germany has never been recognized as a country of immigration, so that the fact of immigration is being neglected by officials in their political and administrative decisions.

Sickness: An Important Factor in Migrants' Everyday Life

This background has to be considered when sickness in the process of migration is dealt with in social research. During field work (intensive lifespan interviews and participant observation), sickness turned out to be one of the most important factors in families' everyday lives. I want to illustrate the important role of sickness for migrant families by referring to three major points:

---

[1] The research project referred to is sponsored by the Volkswagenwerk foundation and carried out at the Ludwig-Uhland-Institut für Empirische Kulturwissenschaft in Tübingen under the direction of Prof. Hermann Bausinger

Primary Health Care in the Making
Ed. by U. Laaser, R. Senault, H. Viefhues

The Insecurity of Migrants' Existence in Germany

Longer lasting disease of the supporter of the family in general leads to loss of employment. Although foreign workers are included in the general social system, in the present situation of restriction of social rights, caused mainly by the economic crisis, their asking for social help endangers the existence of the family in Germany. This is especially true for those whose home countries do not belong to the EC. A demand for social help by this group of people will usually be reported to the registration office, which leads to restrictions of their permit of residence.

While the traditional social network in their home countries (family, kinship) tightens up at the crucial point of fundamental need, in Germany this fundamental need and the demand for social help might have a price much too high: the loss of permit of residence. In this case family and kinship network can be helpful in different ways: they may help out with money, but also be helpful in finding jobs for other members of the family and be supporters in dealing with the officials. Especially in respect to the last mentioned ways of kinship and family help, personal intervention is more widespread and also more successful than Germans may even think of.

This, in consequence, leads to the thesis that the more families have succeeded to establish a family/kinship-network the less their existence will be endangered by long lasting disease and its consequences.

The Lack of Biographical Perspective

Foreign workers have been examined thoroughly by doctors before they came to Germany. When the traces of hard work become obvious without any goals having been reached, the feeling of having been abused takes over, demoralizing the whole family. In general these people are unable to consider their diseases as a result of the life cycle, i.e. of having grown older: indeed, they do work under miserable conditions, which lead to all kinds of disease, but they may also use the disease as an explanation or an excuse for not having achieved the original goal of going back to their native country as an economically revitalized family.

Another effect of this lack of biographical perspective is that causes of disease that are to be found way back in childhood and adolescence are not taken into account. This is especially true for women, whose working conditions in the village during the period of early girlhood must be considered in regard to a wide range of diseases that occur later. Two examples may illustrate this:

Case 1. A woman now almost 40 years old had to carry water from the age of 10 years. One day when she was doing her work she had a rectal prolapse. She never told anybody of this because she was ashamed and also because there was no money for a doctor anyway. Even her husband did not know about it for a long time after they were married. Hard working conditions in a factory in Germany caused renewed outbreak of the disorder, and she has now undergone at least five operations – without ever having told any doctor anything about the first occurrence and the length of time it has been going on.

Case 2. Another woman, whose husband left the village for Germany shortly after the marriage, was left on her own while pregnant. During the winter she had to clean the flat roof of the village house from huge amounts of snow so that it would not cave in. The child was born dead after 7 months. After that she lost a lot of blood with every birth or abortion. She told her German doctor that she was afraid of losing blood, but without telling him the "biographical" reason for this, so he interpreted it just as a general fear that southern European women are supposed to show to a greater extent than German women.

Discontinuity and Disorientation

A wide range of diseases seem to be the result of the special sociocultural situation of migrant families, which is determined by discontinuity in family life, changing of future perspectives, no possibility of long-term life planning etc. These special hardships can be summarized under two major topics:

Not Knowing Where Home Is. The facts that family, community and society in their native country have changed during their absence, that children are at least partially socialized in German (migrant) society, that there exist migrant colonies and networks, that work will be hard to find and that the decision to return will not be reversible (at least not for some nationalities), all lead to the feeling of not knowing where home is, of living between two worlds.

Having Failed in One's Goal. Originally, one member of the family left to work abroad to provide economic resources so that the family could then live together under acceptable economic conditions. The price that had to be paid was the temporary separation of the family. This "temporary" state has in many cases been going on for almost 20 years now, so that even if the economic goal is reached, the ideological aim of the family living together can hardly be achieved. The result is, for example, a lot of newly built appartment houses in Istanbul with nobody living in them – the families are spread over Turkey, Europe and even other continents.

Conclusion

The social factors and conditions of sickness in the process of migration, as pointed out above, are the first findings of fieldwork with Turkish migrant families. Although they need to be verified by wider and more systematic investigation, they suggest that sickness is in this case a specific reaction to – or even a part of – living conditions encountered in the process of migration which demand an orientation in permanent transition.

Some suggestions for practical measures can be made at this stage of investigation:

1. For medical treatment, analysis and therapy must be based on an insight into the migration process, which includes actual living conditions as well as cultural background.
2. It is necessary to realize that family-, kinship- or nation-orientated networks are necessary and valuable for migrant families, at least at this juncture. These networks should be employed to provide information about health, contraception etc.
3. Measures regarding the social health of migrants can only be successful when their status of residence is made clear by the government, and when they are able to live in Germany together with their families without the fear of being expelled at any moment!

Reference

1. Warner WL, Srole L (1945) The social system of American ethnic groups. New Haven (Yankee City Series, vol 3)

Illness and Health of Turkish "Citizens" in West Germany as Seen Against the Background of Their Personal Life Narratives *

I. Theilen

In this contribution I shall discuss several case studies from our field study[1] about Turkish men and women, their living conditions and their illnesses. Since I had better access to Turkish women, they are disproportionately represented in this study. The main points of this analysis concern the transformation of roles and relationships, particularly the aspect of loss and disintegration of familial life patterns. In some cases, the statement or indication of the disease is clearer; in other cases it is less so.

Disintegration of the family is a typical feature of Turkish nuclear families in the Federal Republic of Germany. Various forms of separation and phases of separation undergone by husbands and wives, by parents and children or by siblings can be found in almost all Turkish families. This has far-reaching consequences for the structure of communication and interaction within the family.

Case 1

The situation of 19-year-old Mustafa is as follows: His father has lived in the FRG for 14 years (1st loss); he himself stayed in Turkey with his mother, brothers and sisters. Three years later his mother died (2nd loss). The children lived with relatives in Turkey. Seven years ago, his father married again. His wife, Yasgülü A., who also stayed in Turkey, took care of the children from her husband's first marriage.

Mustafa spent a total of 10 years without his father. After these 10 years Ali A. brought his family to Germany. Mustafa, who was 15 at the time, came along against his will. Today there are frequent and massive conflicts between father and sons which are carried out openly.

Reproaches of the son directed against the father: "We don't have to listen to him. He is not really our father. For 10 years we were alone and he did not

* Translated by Rosemary and Brian Tracy

1 Working Group for Intercultural Health Research at the Institute for Tropical Hygiene of the University of Heidelberg; Study of the behavior of Turkish employees in health-related matters. Im Neuenheimer Feld 324, 6900 Heidelberg, West Germany. The study was financed by Stiftung Volkswagenwerk

Primary Health Care in the Making
Ed. by U. Laaser, R. Senault, H. Viefhues

care about us. Now he wants to determine our lives and play father. We cannot allow that . . . what did you do to us? We would have preferred staying in Turkey."

Comments of the father about his sons: "They are no longer Turkish: half Turkish, half German." He refers to the light color of his son's skin, but really means his rebellious behaviour.

The father cannot cope with these cultural and generational conflicts in the wake of the mutual estrangement. He has lost his role as a father. Before, his biography told of loneliness rather than of the stress which now exists within the family, the threat represented by his maturing sons who do not respect him. Half a year after the families moved to Germany Ali A. suffered a heart attack.

But Mustafa is also unhappy and depressed. Through his involuntary move to Germany, he lost his home, all his social contacts, his friends and relatives. At work, in the streets, in bars he is susceptible to and suffers from the hostility against Turkish people which is widespread in Germany. Through Turkish programmes on the radio, he learns that the figures for illnesses are higher for foreigners in Germany than for Germans, something which he comments upon as follows:

"We have more reason to be sick because of stress and difficult work and living conditions and everything . . . but heavy work alone does not make you sick . . . Look out of the window; there is the construction site of the firm where my father works. Four foreigners and one German work there; the German commands, the others work. Often when my father comes home in the evening he says that there is a lot of hostility and fighting going on. The hostility of the Germans makes us sick. Work alone does not make you sick."

Mustafa finds himself in a position where he can neither identify with his father nor with German society. With his strong Turkish identity on the one side and his relatively differentiated and distanced attitude to Germany, he fights in both directions to find his own way. For the past 6 weeks he has been treated for stomach problems.

In addition to the biographies of Turkish men and young adults, there seems to be an almost typical case history of the suffering of Turkish women. Throughout their lives runs a familiar pattern of role change, loss and separation. We shall consider the cases of two women.

Case 2

Yasgülü A., Mustafa's (step)mother is 30 years old and has been in Germany for 4 years. She was raised in a Turkish village and was married at the age of 16. Her husband owned a store in Istanbul and lived mainly there while she and the children who were later born stayed in the village. She only saw her husband for several days a year. Because of this separation she was alone a lot, but not lonely because she was tied into the net of village relationships with its resulting responsibility and protection.

She suffered her second, more drastic separation when her husband died. As a widow she remained with her children in the village, living with relatives.

Three years later she married Ali A., who shortly after his wedding went back to Germany. They lived apart for 3 years (3rd separation). She took care of his three children, but she had to give her own children from her previous marriage to relatives in Istanbul, because Ali A. would not tolerate them within the new family (4th separation). Since her wedding 7 years ago, she has neither seen her children nor heard about them.

Four years ago she and Ali A.'s children came to Germany. She had two more children of her own and now takes care of a family of seven. She hardly speaks any German. She is lonely and unhappy in Germany. She is homesick for the people in her village. She does not have any contact with German women, and with Turkish people only within the family framework, which means that the men dominate while the women passively listen.

Although I was a stranger to her in the beginning, she cried often, especially when topics like Turkey or children were mentioned. She said it was very difficult for her to live without her children and not to know how they were.

Recently she started a cleaning job several hours a day. She is very happy about this because it means a legitimate way of establishing and maintaining outside contacts.

The multiple separations and losses experienced by this woman, connected with mourning that she has not yet been able to emotionally come to grips with, can hardly be compensated. So far these experiences do not carry a message of illness. But according to available insights it is very probable that such massive events as the loss of a partner, of children – and therefore of the mother role – and loss of national, cultural, linguistic and family/social embedding will lead to depressions and other syndromes. The less human and personal satisfaction such women can find here within the German environment, the more likely this becomes. The situation of being thrown back onto the structure of the nuclear family with its encapsulation against the outside world enhances, in my opinion, the rise of illnesses.

Case 3

Fifty-year-old Nurhan C. has lived in the FRG for 8 years. Her husband and her three eldest sons had come to Germany 6 years before. The eldest daughter remained in Turkey, the youngest came with the mother. One of the sons died of cancer at the age of 22. Frau C. had a total of about 15 pregnancies. Several children died after birth or in early infancy. Today only four children live, three in Turkey, one here. Despite all these pregnancies she finds herself as mother of only one child. But even this has to be relativized, as we shall see shortly. Her role as woman and mother is empty.

She did not seem to suffer greatly from the loss of her newborns and infants. But she suffers from her times of separation from her sons and grandchildren, from her husband and her daughter. This suffering culminated with the death of her son Ehet. Still today, 4 years later, she grives this loss and suffers from depressions.

The family has no human, i.e. positive, relationships with Germans. Nurhan hardly speaks any German. She has friendly contact with only one other Turkish family. She feels isolated, lonely, unhappy. Since she finishes her housework relatively quickly, she spends a lot of time sitting on the sofa, thinking, crying. She is homesick, has no task important to her and little occupation.

Her relationship with her daughter H. is friendly, but ambivalent. This only child who has remained with her has developed beyond her. She is independent, capable of negotiating with bureaucratic institutions, she can translate when the mother goes to see a doctor. H. actively takes responsibilities upon herself which are normally taken care of by adults. She therefore turns out in many areas to be more powerful, more competent than the mother. On the one hand she places too many demands on her; on the other hand she has become her mother's rival. All the mother can do is take care of H.'s food and clothing. She cannot help her with her schoolwork, and she cannot take part in PTA meetings at school since, in a double sense, she does not understand what is going on.

Because of this loss of educational competence as a consequence of the described disempowerment of the mother, a disequilibrium develops: the traditional patterns of education are maintained, which results in tensions, fights, withdrawal and illness.

Tasks which Nurhan can perform do not exist in the immigrant situation – work in the fields, work in the home with other women, washing and sewing etc. – nor does she have the automatically resulting human, linguistic and emotional exchange which is crucial for overcoming grief. Nurhan is in a double sense without role, powerless, without skills and, what is worse, without positive life perspectives.

She suffers a lot from headaches, from pains in her back, sadness, itching all over her body, diffuse pains in her left lower stomach, gas and constipation, stomach aches, infections of the bladder and kidneys. She is constantly ill. The symptoms change all the time. Thus, she is constantly occupied. She goes to several doctors, from one check-up to another, spends hours in waiting rooms, takes medication all the time and constantly waits for some results.

Often the corresponding emotional environments of these states of illness are not clearly tangible for me as a German. I have become convinced that these illnesses have become part of Nurhan's life and that they fulfil substitute functions. This hypothesis concerning the psychosomatic nature of her illnesses is supported by the lack of any concrete outcomes of medical examinations. Already back in Turkey she had stomach problems, but we do not know within which contexts of relationships these manifested themselves. Her relationship with her husband is full of conflicts, as shown in her strategy of not telling him about her going out several hours a week to houseclean, an activity which allows her to break out of her isolation. This woman goes from one doctor to the next. These physicians cannot help her: on the one hand, they do not know anything about her background and they do not ask about it; on the other hand, the physician cannot be responsible for the solution of what is bascially a social problem.

Conclusion

The migration of these Turkish people to West Germany is a problem which is of considerable sociopolitical relevance. These case studies reveal that most of these men and women, besides other massive burdens, suffer from grave experiences of loss on the human level for which they could hardly develop strategies of compensation. These deficits are connected with the non-existent human exchange between the Turkish and the German population, with infamily and extrafamilial offences (i.e. increasing hostility against Turkish people). German laws and regulations concerning foreigners and their sociopolitical rights seem to pre-programme this suffering.

Almost each biography shows the recurring pattern of an experience of separation, loss, grief, social and personal animosity. In this paper, I have tried to point to the co-existence of certain aspects of illness and selected aspects of people's migration history. I support the hypothesis that there is a relationship between the two which may, however, only be captured individually on the basis of each person's biography, rather than collectively.

In addition to its sociological and sociopolitical relevance, this topic has therapeutic and preventive importance. The often deficient interaction between physician and patient and the low level of effectiveness in the treatment of Turkish patients are linked, in my opinion, to the following factors:

- The inability to overcome the language barrier
- Insufficient insight into further existing communication problems
- The inappropriateness of our Western therapeutic concepts which are based on different ideas of man
- The impossibility of treating human or social suffering through medication
- The inability of many phyicians to desist from revolving-door type treatments
- The widespread loss, on the part of the physician, of a large part of his traditional role as comforter and companion, and as one who offers emotional interaction
- The inadequate definition and categorization of these illnesses as "psychological" without further explication. Suffering is labelled as "psychological" or "masked depression", in which case nothing is done and no progress can be made
- The insufficient integration of other disciplines into medical practice

This problem of falling ill, behaviour while ill, the background biographical information and the additional hardship imposed through migration, is fairly well known.

Moreover, the people concerned are themselves competent enough to give important insights about themselves and their suffering. To conclude, I let two Turkish women express themselves on the topic "illness" (translated from "guest worker German"). This method of drawing on self-reflections as a source of important insights which I have put into practice shows that the often-cited problem of language barriers can clearly be overcome in everyday interactions as well as in physician–patient interactions if only one is prepared to listen with sensitivity and patience.

Ayse says:
Turkish women much much problems, always lots to think about . . . two children money send Turkey . . . two, three, four children Germany, always looking after them . . . Turkey kids no father and mother . . . always lots to think about, lots problems, lots of money give Turkey . . . much money need Germany . . . think kid Turkey maybe sick . . . maybe alone . . . always lots to think about, always worries, always problems . . . lots heavy heart . . . always alone . . . what do go Turkey . . . pay lots money ticket . . . again Germany go work . . . go here . . . go there . . . always, always, always . . . know nothing here, know nothing there; everything cost much money. Have lots, lots problems . . . all Turkish women much thinking . . . much ill.

Emine says:
"We aren't really at home anywhere. Not quite here, not quite in Turkey. Everywhere like foreigners. Half of my disease is homesickness. It is so heavy and so bad. Sometimes I think I am dead. I think now my legs and my spine. I think my nervous system left over. I think so heavy, so pain, my nervous illness destroy everything.

Body tired – much work. Soul kaputt – foreigners lots heavy. Our two lives. Oh strange land. Oh no desire. Think here – think there. So two. No desire. Problem with kids. If have kids, no more problems. Sons Turkey, mother Germany. Lots of thinking, lots of problems. Always two lives. Two thoughts . . ."

Studies on Social Hygienic Problems Appertaining to Foreign Children and Their Families in the Federal Republic of Germany

H. Mergerian and W. Bommer

Among the foreign children and foreign families living as guest-workers or refugees in the Federal Republic of Germany, the Turkish people evince the most medical, social and hygienic problems. On the one hand they are the most representative group (the number has increased in the last few years by 1.5 million) and on the other hand a very deep rift exists between the host country, which has highly developed medical, social and hygienic standards, and their state of health, their national and traditional way of living, their customs and their religion. Sometimes, these newcomers come across the same unhygienic and social conditions in the host country as those they have left behind. Naturally, other major difficulties are the language barrier, the climatic change and cultural distinctions. The children of these newcomers seem to be the ones mostly affected by these problems, i.e. when at school and in contact with persons of the same age. Only a small number of Turkish families and those of other guest-workers – those whose children were born in Germany and those who have lived there for several years – have been able to adapt to German everyday life, so that their social and medical problems have become similar to those of the indigenous population.

During the last 12 years we have carried out medical investigations especially on parasitic infections in Turkish people and their children of school age, and also in Vietnamese refugees. We were able to show that more than 45% of the newcomer Turks have a parasitic infection of the intestine. After 2 years the infection rate decreased to 30% and lower. For a time up to 45% of the Vietnamese refugees had parasitic infections, including strongyloidosis and severe giardiasis.

After considering our observations, surveys and experiences over several years, we have summarized the medical and social-hygienic aspects of the aforementioned groups into three main topics:

1. People coming from warm countries have the following medical problems: (a) infectious diseases with parasites such as intestinal helminths, echinococcosis and amoebiasis, and occasionally malaria, (b) bacterial diseases such as salmonellosis – also typhoid fever – or tuberculosis (old people!), or (c) viral diseases such as poliomyelitis or hepatitis A. Many children have no or insufficient protection by vaccination. Non-infectious diseases are blood disorders, deafness and visual disturbance. The medical problems of the newcomers have to be diagnosed immediately and cured. Attention

Primary Health Care in the Making
Ed. by U. Laaser, R. Senault, H. Viefhues

must be given to foreigners holidaying in their homeland, who risk infection or re-infection with echinococcosis, worms, malaria, hepatitis A, salmonellosis and occasionally cholera. Stool examinations of foreigners who have holidayed in a warm land and work in food supply are required.
2. Health education programmes for foreigners in their own language (e.g. in schools) on general hygiene, health nutrition, sexual hygiene, protection against sickness and ectoparasites, dental care etc. This is the precondition for finding out the specific problems of the foreigners in the host country and for carrying out controlled health education programmes with due respect for their national and religious pride, and their cultural and traditional customs.
3. Sanitation in their social environment. Better housing conditions, and playgrounds and fields for children are important and necessary. There is a need to restore and modernize, in accordance with currently accepted hygienic standards, the residential quarters of foreign families, who so often live in old, small, dark, humid, overcrowded apartments without bathroom and shower. Sometimes the WC is outside the dwelling and is used by many residents. Here we see the possibility for transmission of or re-infection by a parasitic or bacterial disease. To solve these problems one needs not only the co-operation and good will of the foreigners, but also the co-operation of the German population and, needless to say, administrative and financial support. Schools (school medical officers, teachers), firms (company physicians, work councillors), the church and other groups could organize events conducive to the solution of the above-mentioned medical, social and hygienic problems.

In the last few years one has seen more and more foreign employees – especially Turkish women – working as cleaning personnel in areas with high infection risks, for example in the operating theatres or on the intensive care units of hospitals. These persons need excellent training and instructions for their routine work, if possible in their native language. Because of daily handling of infectious materials, they have to be informed about the hazards, e.g. hepatitis B.

The number of foreign patients in hospitals has increased over recent years, particularly in districts with a high proportion of foreigners. The traditional customs of a hospitalized foreigner, e.g. body hygiene, religious duties, nutrition rules and contact with his family members or relatives, have to be respected by the nursing staff. According to German law, the patient has to be informed in detail about the diagnostic techniques, the specific treatment (surgical treatment with anaesthesia) and also the hazards and complications of that medical operation. He signs an agreement form in advance. Most foreign patients have language difficulties. Therefore they need a qualified interpreter with medical knowledge, e.g. a physician, a nurse or a medical student who is able to speak the same language can explain to the patient about the course of the disease, the prognosis etc. This person can also convey the patient's complaints or his individual social problems to the attending physician.

Foreign patients in maternity and gynaecological hospitals also present some medical and social problems. The gynaecologist again needs the assistance of a reliable interpreter when he explains to the patient and her husband the risks and hazards of a desired interruption of pregnancy, or the necessity of interruption and sterilisation although the family wishes a child.

Many pregnant foreign women do not know about the prenatal care services in the host country, or they do not want to attend the routine control examinations of prenatal supervision. This can lead to complications in the course of the pregnancy or to a complicated delivery, and later to negative social consequences for the family if the child thereby has a congenital defect.

Foreign parents often insist on the bedside care of their hospitalized child by a family member – mostly by the mother. Our experiences with sick children of Vietnamese refugees and Turkish families who have been accompanied by their mothers in the Children's Hospital in Goettingen have shown satisfactory results in the recovery of the infants over a short period.

Children from tropical and subtropical countries who have been adopted by German parents are often infected at the same time with different parasites or are suffering from acute or chronic infections due to bacteria or fungi. A rapid diagnosis and specific treatment is necessary, otherwise transmission to the other family members is possible.

The treatment of some chronic illnesses, e.g. coeliac disease, necessitates a specific gluten-free diet, which means prohibition of most cereals (exceptions are rice and maize) and restrictions on other food. The parents of the patient receive exact instructions on this diet from the paediatrician. Gluten-free food is more expensive and can be bought only in special stores. The diet differs very much from the traditional and national way of cooking at home. This is an additional handicap for the foreign housewife, especially in large families. Such diets cannot be followed exactly on vacations in the homeland.

The social and hygienic aspects of dialysis patients among the foreign population is another major problem. The number of foreign patients with kidney failure has increased in the last few years. Employees but also non-employed family members have to be taken into chronic dialysis programmes, which means permanent treatment by haemodialysis or peritoneal dialysis in hospitals, in dialysis centres (limited care) and at home (home haemodialysis, CAPD – continuous ambulatory peritoneal dialysis). The patient becomes dependent on an artificial kidney and has to change his way of life. He must take care of his personal hygiene, of nutrition and of his environment. Social and familial problems arise when the housewife who is a chronic dialysis patient cannot perform her "traditional" duties. Beside the medical care and rehabilitation of a foreign dialysis patient, the social supervision and welfare work are very important and necessary. Finally, the specific social, hygienic and medical problems of the kidney transplanted foreign patient have to be pointed out. The patient must also be informed in the host country about the possibilities of receiving specific medical care and treatment.

The Living Conditions and Education of Turkish Infants in the Federal Republic of Germany: Report on a Model Project in Nürnberg

M. Akkent, G. Franger, and N. Gültepe

Who is responsible for feeding Turkish infants, and how are they fed? Do they grow up mainly in their families. Do their mothers adapt knowledge about baby care and infant education which they have acquired in their native countries to their new situation? Do they change their educational behaviour?

These were the questions which we put to ourselves when, in the autumm of 1979, we started the project "Education of Foreign Infants in Early Childhood". It was financed for 3 years by the Federal Ministry for Youth, Family and Health and was carried out in Frankfurt and Nürnberg. The institution responsible is the Institut für Sozialarbeit und Sozialpädagogik in Frankfurt. The model project pursues the following tasks:

a) Analysis of socialization processes of Turkish children from 0–3 years of age in order to document the effects of different forms of infant care on socialization and to make pedagogically founded proposals for the development of aids for socialization and the qualification of counselling institutions.
b) The development and evaluation of concepts of counselling and further education.
c) The development of concepts of counselling and further education in order to improve the socialization conditions of foreign infants in the Federal Republic.

The support of infant education both inside and outside the family by way of advice to parents and foster parents is attempted through the installation of a centre for information and counselling of parents and German day-care "mothers" in a quarter in which a high percentage of the population is foreign. The centre has a mediating function between German and foreign socialization institutions and has the following aims: Testing new ways of addressing problems and information, eradication of the isolation of foreign families, giving medical advice to foreign families, offering facilities for further education which take their bearings from the everyday problems of the families, giving advice and further training to German day-care families, recruitment of foreign day-care mothers and mobilization of the latent potential of self-help. Further goals are the qualification of day-care institutions, the development of a co-operative model in order to bring together available subsidies and the creation of institutions for foreign families to further co-operation and co-ordinate

Primary Health Care in the Making
Ed. by U. Laaser, R. Senault, H. Viefhues

measures. In the project "Education of Foreign Children in Early Childhood", for the first time an attempt is being made to offer advice to pregnant Turkish women and mothers of small children confined to a certain quarter.

An example of our experiences in the "Mother-Child Counselling Centre" is given below.

Difficulties of Turkish Mothers in Participating in Cures

After 3 years of counselling activities with Turkish women in our mother–child counselling centre, we got to know a lot about the physical and psychological complaints of the women and wanted to organise a cure (i.e. stay in a health resort) for mothers and children with the Bavarian Foundation for Mother Recreation (Bayerischer Mütterdienst). The Bayerische Mütterdienst was in doubt whether such a cure could be organised, because they thought the husbands would not allow their wives to participate. After a short time it turned out, however, that the reason why the mothers would not participate was not their husbands, but much more the legal conditions, such as financing the cure.

When a female worker signs up for a cure, the pension scheme covers the full costs; however, the women, by so doing, lose the possibility of having their contributions to the pension scheme refunded if they want to return to Turkey. Women employed in firms were well informed about this regulation. Many of the women do not want to work in Germany until they are 60 years old. When the plans of the family have been realized, they want to return to Turkey and have their contributions to the pension scheme refunded, because they want to pay this sum into the Turkish pension scheme so that they can get their pension in Turkey. Or they want to use the money as capital for a new family existence. The different age limit for receiving pensions in Germany and Turkey plays a major role. In Turkey the age limit for women is 50.

When a woman employed in a firm does not want to make use of the pension scheme, she can apply for a recreational stay to be subsidized by the sick fund (Krankenkasse) if she can present a letter containing her doctor's opinion. She has to take a paid holiday or an unpaid holiday if she wants to participate in a 4-week cure. Many women, however, want to go to Turkey with their family for their holiday, which is very important for their psychological and physical well-being. Moreover, a large number of firms shut down their factories at a particular time of the year, so that all workers employed have to take their holiday at this particular time. The women do not like to take an unpaid holiday, firstly because of the pay they would have received during that time, but also because they are afraid of losing their jobs.

Housewives are usually insured in a sick found through their husbands and have the same claim to a cure in accordance with § 184a (RVO). This means that the sick fund will cover the entire cost. Because we planned a cure for mothers and children up to 6 years of age, the children over 6 years old could not be taken along. This presented a difficulty for mothers who did not work in firms. It was impossible to engage a German housekeeper, who could have been called in through a social care organization (Verband der freien Wohlfahrtspflege), since Turkish women hate seeing their household run by a German housekeeper. An example is that the German housekeeper could not cook the meals the way the family is used to or she would not comply with certain religious rules when washing clothes. On the other hand the mothers did not want to leave their children alone at home while nobody else in the family was there to look after them.

When a housewife applies for a cure purely for recreational purposes, part of the cost will be met by the sick fund; for the rest of the cost she can apply to the local benefit scheme. The families are very reluctant to apply for this benefit, however, which presents a problem for our initiative. They try as far as possible to avoid applying for social benefits, since they are afraid of negative side-effects. This is quite possible if they hand in several applications, but it is impossible if they apply just once.

On the other hand it is very difficult for the women to hand in applications and take the other necessary steps. In our case it took a member of the counselling centre 2 months to take all the necessary steps for only four women, starting with giving information to the women, accompanying the women to the doctors and carrying out all the formalities at the social benefit centre. How could the women have managed to do all these tasks alone?

For all these reasons, the cures which are necessary for the health of women cannot be made use of by Turkish women in the numbers that would be desirable. It is also possible that the situation will be misjudged further, the husbands being given as the reason why Turkish women do not make use of cures for mothers. In reality it is not the husbands who stop the women from participating in these cures. The reasons are far more complicated and are to be sought especially in German legal conditions.

Are New Counselling and Psychotherapeutic Patterns Necessary for Children of Foreign Employees (Guest-workers)? Results of an Epidemiological Study

F. Poustka

Introduction and Aims of the Study

Foreign children are clearly under-represented as in- or out-patients in child and adolescent psychiatric clinics compared with the German incidence figures. This has been demonstrated in hospital-based data in industrialized regions and towns that have a high proportion of foreigners, e.g. Frankfurt (analysing a 13-year period [6]), Berlin [8] and Mannheim [5].

This finding could be interpreted in different ways: Firstly, there could be a true low prevalence rate, reflecting healthy and efficient coping abilities related to a positive social selection of migrants who are willing to escape economic pressure in their homelands [4].

Secondly, one could suggest that there are high barriers to coming to the clinics, so that the true high prevalence rates of psychiatric disorders escape official attention. Reasons for this could be that immigrant families do not recognize their problems as such or feel that a special need would require a special treatment which cannot be achieved. Whereas this second possibility, in contrast to the first, is widely accepted, especially for adult disorders, the evidence supporting these conjectures is weak because it is mainly based on anecdotal material and/or treated cases only.

Generalization arising from this background could suffer from serious bias and will not be more reliable when entangled with theories of correctional social utopias.

According to a review of the literature of the early 1970s [1], it cannot be granted that migrant workers suffer more often from psychiatric disturbances than do control groups in the country of origin and country of residence, but they do more frequently display typical manifestations such as paranoid reactions, hypochondriac–depressive syndromes, psychosomatic conditions and sexual neurosis. Differences between the migrants' culture and the "immigration context", such as language, mystical beliefs and illness behaviour, influence other manifestations of psychiatric syndromes.

There is virtually no evidence that this is true for the second generation of immigrants according to results of epidemiological studies on immigrant children (see discussion in [5]).

So, especially for the situation in Germany, where there are nearly a million foreign school children, two main questions should be answered when inquiring

Primary Health Care in the Making
Ed. by U. Laaser, R. Senault, H. Viefhues

as to the needs of and adequate help for foreign children suffering from psychiatric disorders: What can be said about (a) prevalence rates and (b) the kind of disturbances and some main associations. Both aspects could seriously cause overloading of already established counselling and treatment facilities.

Method

All 13- and 14-year-olds with Turkish or Italian nationality, living for at least 5 years in Germany and registered in Mannheim, were investigated in the study, together with a German control group. This methodology should enable one to study a population not confronted with stressful life events shortly after migration but living under similar conditions (and nearly at the end of compulsory school age).

Interviews were taken at home at the same time with the parents in their native language and with the child, usually in German (also testing intellectual functioning and German language competence). Interviews with the parents and interviews with and testing of the children lasted approximately 2½–4 hours. The interviews contained questions about the individual (psychiatric symptoms, functioning in school), sociodemographic (living and working conditions) and familial characteristics (concerning migration, parental and parent–child interaction, and morbidity).

Results

Among the foreigners approximately 15% were refusers. The overall rate of psychiatric disorders among Turkish and Italian children in the age group studied (Table 1) is in line with rates in industrialized regions [7]. This is a rate which should cause neither alarm nor neglect. There are slight tendencies towards

Table 1. Psychiatric syndrome, nationality and sex ($n=212$)

ICD Nr.[a]	Turkish		Italian		German	
	m ($n=47$)	f ($n=45$)	m ($n=40$)	f ($n=41$)	m ($n=21$)	f ($n=18$)
313/300	3	4	0	4	1	1
312.0/314	2	0	6	3	3	2
312.3	4	1	1	4	2	1
307.6	3					
	17 (18%)		18 (22%)		10 (26%)	

[a] 313/300, emotional/neurotic disorder; 312.0/314, expansive disorder; 312.3, conduct and emotional disorder; 307.6, enuresis only

nationality-dependent patterns, such as a higher proportion of expansive (unsocialized, aggressive) disorders among Italian girls, and more emotional/neurotic disorders and a high rate of enuresis (in relation to age) among Turkish children. Further results showed that, compared with Italian children, Turkish children had emigrated later, experienced longer parental separation, had had more schooling at home but showed only the same level of school achievement (about half of them had to face serious negative results on school records), felt higher aspiration towards German assimilation and showed more handicaps in adaptation, e.g. towards German peers.

Other significant differences according to sociodemographic features showed that Turkish parents had, again in comparison with Italians, gone to school longer, had more experience in skilled work and earned higher wages. No differences were seen in relation to urban versus rural origin, work-load and living standards. On familial characteristics, Turkish families reported greater discrimination, a stronger relationship between the parents, less somatic complaints among the mothers and lees quarrelling with their children.

Despite these differences in background, patterns concerning psychiatric disorders among the foreign children (based on chi-square test statistics) showed no association with individual or sociodemographic characteristics, though they did show some associations with the familial items.

In Turkish families these associations were moderately but distinctly related to psychiatric disorders among other family members and to high symptom scores of somatic complaints in the mothers; in Italian families they were related to the parental relationship (quarrelling/isolation of the parents) the parent–child relationship (quarrelling/parents being worried about the child's difficulties at school/no parental support) and the wish to return to Italy within the next 5 years. (The associations were also confirmed in regression statistics.)

Conclusions

Among the Turkish and Italian children, compared with the Germans, neither so-called exotic patterns nor an alarmingly high rate of psychiatric disorders could be seen. Secondly, no migration- or assimilation-specific patterns of association could be demonstrated. There were no associations between the high rate of school failure and psychiatric disorders.

We can conclude, therefore, that special preventive and therapeutic strategies should not be established for foreign families. Of course, this plea involves serious limitations for the integrated treatment of second-generation foreigners by established child psychiatric-psychotherapeutic facilities. These facilities can only deal with the parents' needs through an active mediator who could manage to create confidence through explanation of the possibilities they have. This is in line with the situation regarding other provisions, such as sending their children to kindergarten [3] or to paediatric hospitals [2]. One method of overcoming barriers could be to train more young guest-workers with a good school education as social workers linked with schools and child guidance or psychiatric clinics.

References

1. Binder J, Simoes M (1978) Sozialpsychiatrie der Gastarbeiter. Fortschr Neurol Psychiatr 46:342
2. Collatz J, Natzschka J, Schwoon D (1977) Krankheiten, Einweisungshäufigkeit und Krankheitsverläufe bei ausländischen Kindern im Krankenhaus. Öff Gesundh-Wes 39:746
3. Liprecht W (1979) Ausländer zum Kindergartenbesuch ihrer Kinder. Mannheim, Büro für Städteentwicklung
4. Murphy HBM (1977) Migration, culture and mental health. Psychol Med 7:677
5. Poustka F (1984) Psychiatrische Störungen bei Kindern ausländischer Arbeitnehmer. Eine epidemiologische Untersuchung. Enke, Stuttgart
6. Schmidt MH, Ehrhardt K (1975) Psychiatrische Erkrankungen bei Gastarbeiterkindern. II. Ätiologie und Pathogenese. In: Poustka F, Spiel W (eds) Therapien in der Kinder- und Jugendpsychiatrie. Egermann, Vienna, p 1256
7. Schwartz Gould M, Wunsch-Hitzig R, Dohrenwend B (1981) Estimating the prevalence of childhood psychopathology. J Am Acad Child Psychiatry 3:463
8. Steinhausen H-C (1982) Psychische Störungen bei Gastarbeiterkindern im Rahmen einer Kinder- und Jugendpsychiatrischen Poliklinik. Z Kinder- Jugendpsychiatr 10:32

Migration and Health
– Thoughts on Past and Current Research

J. Korporal, J. A. Marmor, and A. Zink

It is not possible to discuss definitively the development of research into the consequences for health of labour migration to Germany within a brief paper such as this. Although a large number of research reports and papers that address general or particular aspects of the topic are now available, the treatment of migrant labour issues in the scientific and mass media makes it difficult to assess the true dimensions of the problem.

Scientific societies have waited until the past few years before devoting serious attention to this field. Journals or other fora of discussion are of recent vintage, and publishers can point to few authoritative publications.

Health-related topics were late and rare additions to the spectrum of research into the consequences of labour migration, primarily because, being selected on the basis of age and medical criteria, recruited migrants were not expected to present health problems. Scientific interest in health issues developed with the realization of a de facto immigration situation: the extended duration of residence in the host country.

The Volkswagen Foundation's provision of funds earmarked for research into the sociocultural consequences of migration has also helped to stimulate interest in this area [1]. Unfortunately, this financial aid may remain an exception: at the present time there seem to be no new funding sources developed explicitly to support migrant health research. Topical questions, however, are sometimes included in research projects whose major foci lie elsewhere.

Historical Development

Three phases can be identified in the development of migrant health research. First to appear were case reports by physicians concerning migrants appearing in their practices and in hospitals. Typical were the reports of gastro-intestinal ailments, primarily ulcers, which were seen with more than expected frequency in foreign-born men. Infectious diseases of every kind were also reported and discussed extensively.

A second phase was characterized by exploration of the relationship between the German doctor and the foreign patient. This approach broadened to include consideration of possible differential disease patterns, and analyses of inadequate structures or utilization of existing health care institutions.

Primary Health Care in the Making
Ed. by U. Laaser, R. Senault, H. Viefhues

The third and current phase can be said to focus on social and cultural factors that influence the causes, duration and recovery from illness.

The purpose of this paper is to define the central issues of migrant health research more precisely, and to present several important new results. The selection of material is guided more by the "availability" of results, or, in other words, by the interests of the researchers and their sponsors, than by consideration of the areas in which the most critical health problems might be expected.

The starting point of migrant health research was determined both by the unfamiliarity of the questions and by the distance between the researcher and the researched subject. Consequently, old sociomedical and sociohygienic questions, primarily concerned with infectious and parasitic diseases, which, with respect to the German population, had long been solved and rendered obsolete, were rediscovered and re-answered [2–4].

Another indication of the wide gap between the researcher/clinician and his subjects/patients is the, at times massive, at times thinly disguised, prejudice brought to the formulation of research problems.

The importance given to communication problems in the interpretation of research results is another characteristic of the earlier phases. That is, all communication problems between patient and physician were blamed exclusively on the "language barrier". Even today, informational deficits are blamed – without adequate evidence – for differences in care seeking and utilization behaviour, with the result that the influence of variations in culture and life-style is neglected.

Health care institutions have apparently learned to adapt to the problems presented by labour migration. Thorough, technically advanced diagnostics, broad but unspecific treatments, and a generous hand with drug prescriptions characterize this adaptation. Hospitals and private practices have adjusted to the special needs and concerns of their foreign patients; for other health care providers this seems to be less the case.

A certain lack of offical interest in migrant health issues can also be inferred from state and national statistical reports. Analyses grouped by nationality are the exception rather than the rule, which marks a retreat from the early 1970s, when differentiated social and health statistics were rather more routine [5, 6].

Current Migration Situation

As a result of the lack of analysis described above, many of the changes in the labour migrant situation in the 10 years since the end of the labour recruitment programme remain hidden or are difficult to recognize. Changes in age and social structures and the addition of family members and growing children have altered social reality to the point where it no longer conforms to official conceptions. These changes are partially reflected in social statistics in the changes in birth rates and reproductive behaviour, as well as in the increase of marriages between partners of differing nationality.

From 1975 to 1981 the birth frequency of German women in the ages between 15 and 50 remained approximately the same, while Turkish birth frequencies dropped to about 80% of the original figure [7]. At the same time, the age of child-bearing shifted from young and old to the middle range [8, 9].

The economic situation is also relevant to health issues. Non-German workers have been more affected by growing unemployment than their German colleagues. Foreign-born teenagers are especially hard-hit. Classic studies have documented the negative physical and psychological sequelae of unemployment [10]. However, with the exception of studies linking criminal behaviour and teenage unemployment, research into the consequences of unemployment among guest-workers for their health is a much neglected area [11].

As the average length of stay approaches 11 years for nearly 50% of the foreigners resident in Germany [12], chronic and degenerative diseases are becoming increasingly prominent. The typical labour migrant works in production, where high mechanical, physical and mental pressures are common. The same jobs are over-represented statistically as being responsible for involuntary medical retirements among German workers. Foreigners are exposed to these risks more often, and frequently without adequate safety precautions. A partial explanation for this might be that migrant workers were originally expected to leave after several years, and that, therefore, any exposure would be short term. Investigation into the consequences of decade-long exposure under hazardous working conditions came much too late.

Hazardous working conditions can also be responsible for industrial accidents and occupational diseases. Foreign workers have an accident rate that is double or triple that of their German colleagues [5]. (Information on the prevalence of occupational disease is not available.) Available figures date back to the early 1970s. It is, however, improbable that these ratios have changed significantly. This assumption finds support in the fact that overproportional numbers of rehabilitative measures for foreigners are paid for by the national accident insurance fund [13].

Only 3%–4% of all medical rehabilitative measures paid for by the national pension insurance fund between 1980 and 1982 were prescribed for foreigners, in contrast to 15%–18% of prescribed tuberculosis therapy. In the same time span, foreign workers accounted for only 2.4%–4.3% of career advancement programmes, with a smaller number of individual measures in comparison with Germans. Although the tendency has been in the opposite direction, occupational rehabilitation participation by foreigners increased in 1982 [14]. In comparison to the proportion of the work-force and the population who are foreigners, these figures remain below average and undoubtedly insufficient. It is difficult to assess the extent to which this is due to the fact that once a rehabilitative therapy has been carried out, the guest-worker can no longer receive the pension fund reimbursement he is otherwise entitled to on his return to his homeland.

The return to full employment by foreign workers following a rehabilitation programme has been less successful than with Germans. Approximately 15% of "rehabilitated" guest workers remain unemployable for personal or medical reasons [13, 15]. This is a significantly higher figure than for German workers.

Mortality

Mortality data for foreigners in the Federal Republic of Germany are difficult to obtain. While the total number of migrant workers increased, the death rate in Berlin (West) sank from 10 (1960) to 1.7/1000 resident aliens in 1981. However, the percentage of fatalities from Turkey, Yugoslavia and Greece rose from 5% (1960) to nearly 54% (1981) of all foreign deaths [16].

Resident aliens seem to be over-represented in traffic accident fatality statistics in comparison to the proportion of foreigners who drive. 1982 federal statistics, the first available with citizenship information, show that 5% of the traffic fatalities (and 6.4% of the seriously injured and 7% of the slightly injured) were foreigners living in Germany [17]. Berlin (West) figures for 1979 to 1981 showed an increasing rate of traffic accident involvement among foreigners: 7% to 11% of fatalities, 10% to 12% of serious injuries, and 10% to 11% of slight injuries [18].

Infant death rates for foreign children, including statistics for the early 1970s, have been published regularly since 1975/76. The infant death rates of foreign children have been higher than those of German children, especially in the latter half of the 1970s.

In Berlin (West) the average stillborn rate for Turkish births was twice as high as the German rate (1970–1980). In comparison with German stillbirths, Turkish stillbirths following a first pregnancy were over-represented. There seems to be a stronger relationship between increasing age and risk of stillbirth for foreign women than for German women [8, 9].

Low birth weight is a significant risk factor in infant mortality. Despite the fact that foreign infants are born underweight less frequently, they have a higher death rate in the first week of life. Causes of infant death merit a closing remark. Congenital malformations and complications of pregnancy and birth were over-represented, as were metabolic disturbances and disorders of the digestive tract [8, 9].

The differences in infant death rates are all the more significant because they would seem to indicate that prenatal care programmes have not been effective enough in reaching the foreign mother.

Morbidity

Information about the morbidity among foreigners resident in the Federal Republic is limited, for the most part, to the situation of children. High rates of infectious diseases – especially tuberculosis [19–22] – congenital and acquired handicaps [23, 24], scalds and burns [25–27], and poisonings [28, 29] are reported repeatedly.

An investigation in Lübeck reported that, in that region, 11 German an 14 foreign accident cases per 1000 children per year requiring treatment should be expected [30].

Higher rates of non-specialty medical care despite shorter geographic distances to specialty facilities, longer time spans before medical attention is sought, higher admission frequencies, and longer hospital stays following serious injuries and symptoms are the parameters that characterize the care situation of foreign children with accidental injuries.

It is well known that parents of foreign children are less likely to participate in the paediatric preventive care programme [31, 32]. As the number of privately practising paediatricians has increased, the proportion of general practitioners involved in the programme has decreased.

Less well known are the encouraging results obtained by the paediatric visiting nurse service in Berlin (West), which was able to treat serious diseases (severe scalds or chronic metabolic dysfunctions, for example) of both German and foreign children at home, with few communication problems between the German nurse and the foreign mother. One surprising result was that, despite adverse spatial and hygienic conditions, the rate of complications during treatment was the same for both groups [33].

Paediatric psychological and emotional problems will be discussed elsewhere in this volume. Women's health will be discussed only briefly, concentrating on prenatal care and delivery. Issues concerning migration/separation and health, and the effects of chronic exhaustion through the double load of household and job, will be discussed in other articles.

Blame for prenatal care problems, such as delayed programme entry or fewer visits to the doctor, is often laid at the feet of the foreign women. The role played by the structure of the German health care system – the fact that fewer diagnostic and consultative measures are recorded per prenatal visit for foreign women – is considered less often [34]. A study in Berlin (West) showed that, for identical diagnoses, foreign women were prescribed fewer, yet more problematic, medications than German women [34]. The study also showed significant differences in the prenatal care provided by general practitioners and gynaecologists/obstetricians. General practitioners tend to provide more consultative and fewer diagnostic and laboratory services. These differences do not, however, account for the differences between foreign and German women [34, 35].

Illnesses diagnosed during pregnancy show fundamental differences. German women tend to have more pregnancy complications or general illnesses, while foreign women had more complaints, psychosomatic illnesses and infections [34].

It is well known that foreign women have higher rates of surgical intervention and medication during delivery [36–39]. Both could be the result of less intensive prenatal care and/or an expression of the greater problems in cooperation between patient, midwife and physician during the delivery itself.

Foreign women are less influenced by "trends" in obstetrics (currently popular hospitals, alternative deliveries or programmed births). They are less likely to deliver their babies at home, and seem more likely to deliver at weekends than German women [9, 34].

We have refrained from discussing the critically important topics of health and illness behaviour, their social and cultural components, on the grounds that they will be taken up in other contributions. It will be seen that the emphasis of migrant health research has shifted – at least in part – from sociomedical/epidemiological to anthropological and medical sociological questions.

References

1. Korte H, Schmidt A (1983) Migration und ihre sozialen Folgen. Förderung der Gastarbeiterforschung durch die Stiftung Volkswagenwerk 1974–1981. Vandenhoek & Ruprecht, Göttingen, pp 92–95
2. Hein J (1966) Gefahren der Einschleppung von Tuberkulose durch Gastarbeiter und deren Angehörige. Internist 7:594–601
3. Germer WD (1966) Mit welchen in Deutschland wenig bekannten Infektionen muß man bei Gastarbeitern aus dem Mittelmeerraum rechnen? Internist 7:591–593
4. Aspöck H, Picher O, Flamm H (1975) Häufigkeit und Bedeutung des Parasitenbefalls von Gastarbeitern. Wien med Wochenschr 125:540–543
5. Leichsenring C (1972) Die Unfälle der ausländischen Arbeitskräfte in der Bundesrepublik Deutschland. Schriftenreihe des Hauptverbandes der gewerblichen Berufsgenossenschaften e.V., Bonn
6. Bundesanstalt für Arbeit (ed) (1973) Repräsentativuntersuchung '72 über die Beschäftigung ausländischer Arbeitnehmer im Bundesgebiet und ihre Familien- und Wohnverhältnisse. Nürnberg
7. Proebsting H (1983) Eheschließungen, Ehescheidungen, Geburten und Sterbefälle von Ausländern 1981. Wirtschaft Statist 2:79–85
8. Kolleck B, Korporal J, Zink A (1979) Totgeburtlichkeit und Säuglingssterblichkeit ausländischer Kinder in West-Berlin. Gynäkologe 12:181–190
9. Burmeister I, et al. (1984) Regionalanalyse von Totgeburtlichkeit und Säuglingssterblichkeit in Berlin (West) 1970–1980. Schriftenreihe des BMJFG, vol 138. Kohlhammer, Stuttgart
10. Jahoda M, Lazarsfeld PF, Zeisel H (1960) Die Arbeitslosen von Marienthal. Verlag für Demographie, Allensbach
11. Autorengruppe Ausländerforschung (1981) Zwischen Getto und Knast. Jugendliche Ausländer in der Bundesrepublik. Rowohlt, Reinbek
12. Arbeitsgruppe Bevölkerungsfragen (1983) Bericht über die Bevölkerungsentwicklung in der Bundesrepublik Deutschland. 2. Teil: Auswirkungen auf die verschiedenen Bereiche von Staat und Gesellschaft. Bonn
13. Statistisches Bundesamt: Rehabilitationsmaßnahmen. Fachserie 13, Reihe 5.2, 1975–1981
14. Verband Deutscher Rentenversicherungsträger: Statistik der deutschen Gesetzlichen Rentenversicherung. Die Leistungen zur Rehabilitation und die zusätzlichen Leistungen der Gesetzlichen Rentenversicherung im Jahre 1978 bis 1982. Frankfurt, 1979–1983
15. Bundesarbeitsgemeinschaft für Rehabilitation: Gesamtstatistik der Rehabilitation 1971 bis 1973. Frankfurt, 1971, 1973
16. Statistisches Landesamt Berlin (1983) Ausländer in Berlin (West) 1960 bis 1981. Berliner Statistik 342
17. Statistisches Bundesamt (1983) Straßenverkehrsunfälle 1982. Fachserie 8, Reihe 3.3
18. Statistisches Landesamt Berlin: Straßenverkehrsunfälle in Berlin (West) 1976 bis 1981. Berliner Statistik 265, 276, 290, 295, 313, 317. Berlin, 1977–1982
19. Stickl H, Wohlgemut M (1980) Infektionskrankheiten und Impfschutz bei Kindern ausländischer Arbeitnehmer. In: Hellbrügge T (ed) Die Kinder ausländischer Arbeitnehmer. Urban & Schwarzenberg, Munich, pp 197–212
20. Otto H-S (1973) Tuberkulose bei Gastarbeiterkindern. Bundesgesundheitsbl. 5:322–328
21. Collatz J, Natzschka J, Schwoon D (1980) Krankheiten, Einweisungshäufigkeit und Krankheitsverläufe bei ausländischen Kindern in der Hannoverschen Kinderheilanstalt. In: Hellbrügge T (ed) Die Kinder ausländischer Arbeitnehmer. Urban & Schwarzenberg, Munich, pp 29–47
22. Oeter K, Collatz J (1983) Gesundheitsprobleme der Kinder und Frauen ausländischer Arbeiter in der Bundesrepublik Deutschland. Öffentl. Gesundhwesen 45:534–539
23. Majewski E (1978) Behinderte ausländische Kinder. Darstellung der Problematik ihrer Versorgung am Beispiel der Abt. Jugendgesundheitspflege des Gesundheitsamtes Hannover. Dissertation, Hannover Medical School
24. Scholz D: Ergebnisse der Einschulungsuntersuchungen 1978/1981 in Berlin (West). Berlin, 1980, 1982

25. Zink C, et al. (1980) Epidemiologische und sozialpsychologische Aspekte von Unfällen im Kindesalter. Monatsschr Kinderheilkd 128:496–501
26. Zink C (1979) Zur Epidemiologie von Unfällen im Kindesalter: Psychosoziale Bedingungen ihrer Entstehung. Dissertation, Luebeck Medical School
27. Christen H-J, Zink C, Korporal J, Zink A (1984) Epidemiologie von Unfällen im Kindesalter. Monatsschr Kinderheilkd 331–339
28. Christen H-J, Korporal J, Zink A, Zink C (1981) Zur Epidemiologie von Vergiftungsunfällen im Kindesalter. Sozialpädiatrie 3:190–195
29. Christen H-J (1984) Zur Epidemiologie von Vergiftungen im Kindesalter. Eine empirische Studie. Dissertation, Luebeck Medical School
30. Zink C (1984) Stationär behandelte Unfälle von Kindern in der Region Lübeck. Auswertung von 1470 Behandlungsfällen der Jahre 1976 und 1977. (To be published)
31. Collatz J, et al. (1980) Psychosoziale Momente der Nutzung der gesetzlichen Früherkennungsuntersuchungen für Säuglinge und Kleinkinder durch ausländische Eltern. In: Hellbrügge T (ed): Die Kinder ausländischer Arbeitnehmer. Urban & Schwarzenberg, Munich, pp 225–247
32. Schmidt E, Collatz J, Betzner G, Hecker H (1978) Ursachen der hohen Nachsterblichkeit der Säuglinge in der Bundesrepublik Deutschland. In: Beck L, et al. (ed) Mütter- und Säuglingssterblichkeit. Schriftenreihe des Bundesministers für Jugend, Familie und Gesundheit, vol 67. Kohlhammer, Stuttgart
33. Burmeister I, Korporal J, Zink A (1984) Ergebnisse der sozialmedizinischen Begleitung des Modellversuchs: Externer Pflegedienst. Modell einer Hauskrankenpflege für Kinder. Abschlußbericht für die Robert-Bosch-Stiftung. Chap 6
34. Zink A, et al. (1984) Ausländische Schwangere – Vorsorge, Diagnosen und Therapie am Beispiel der Versicherten einer Ortskrankenkasse. De Gruyter, Berlin
35. Collatz J, et al. (1983) Perinatalstudie Niedersachsen und Bremen. Urban & Schwarzenberg, Munich, pp 214–240
36. Saurwein A (1969) Entbindung bei Ausländerinnen, zugleich ein Beitrag zur Frequenz und Indikationsstellung der abdominalen Schnittentbindung. Geburtsh Frauenheilkd 29:728–734
37. Schliemann F, Schliemann G (1975) Über den Geburtsverlauf bei Ausländerinnen. Therap Umschau 32:564–570
38. Wittlinger H, Hohlweg-Majert P, Sievers S (1977) Schwangerschaft und Geburt bei Gastarbeiterinnen. Med Klin 72:33–38
39. Schneider K-D (1977) Analgetikaverbrauch unter der Geburt. Vergleich zwischen Ausländerinnen und Deutschen. Dissertation, Freie Universität Berlin

Part III

Health Education in Primary Health Care

A. Education for Health through Participation

Health for All by the Year 2000: A Challenge for the Education of Health Personnel

T. Fülöp

The accumulated experience in international collaboration in general and in the health field especially, the conquest of smallpox, the great decision of the United Nations to set into motion a programme of action for the establishment of a new international economic order, and the increasing realisation of the great and growing inequities in the health field were some of the main factors which conditioned a historic resolution of the 30th World Health Assembly in May 1977. This resolution, after saying that "faced with the magnitude of health problems and the inadequate and intolerably inequitable distribution of health resources throughout the world today" and "considering that health is a basic human right and a world-wide social goal, and that it is essential to the satisfaction of basic human needs and the quality of life" and "reaffirming that the ultimate constitutional objective of WHO is the attainment by all people of the highest possible level of health", declared that "the main social target of governments and WHO in the coming decades should be the attainment by all citizens of the world by the year 2000 of a level of health that will permit them to lead a socially and economically productive life" [1].

The historic decision was made unanimously by all 152 States which were members of WHO at that time and which thus accepted the greatest challenge in the health field in the history of humanity: to remove the inequalities which the resolution so rightly calls "intolerable" and ensure "health for all by the year 2000". It is easy to understand the enthusiasm with which countries, governments and, first and foremost, people of the world greeted the prospect of "health for all by the year 2000". It is more and more clearly understood that health for all is *not* a single, finite target: it is rather a process leading to progressive improvement in the health of people.

The concept of health for all in this process will be interpreted and adapted differently by each country in the light of its social, economic and even political characteristics, the health status and morbidity patterns of its population, and the state of development of its health system. It is a moving target: as a certain health status is reached, people will set a target to reach a higher level, and so on. However, it is now a common understanding that "there is a base-line below which no individuals in any country should find themselves" and "by the year 2000, *all* people in *all* countries should have a level of health that will permit them to lead a socially and economically productive life" [2, p. 31]. What does this imply? "The level of health of all people should be at least such that

Primary Health Care in the Making
Ed. by U. Laaser, R. Senault, H. Viefhues

they are capable of working productively and of participating actively in the social life of the community in which they live" [2, p. 31].

Health for all is certainly not an unrealistic concept. It "does not mean that in the year 2000 doctors and nurses will provide medical care for everybody in the world for all their existing ailments; nor does it mean that in the year 2000 nobody will be sick or disabled. It does mean that health begins at home, in schools and in factories. It is there, where people live and work, that health is made or broken. It does mean that people will use better approaches than they do now for preventing disease and alleviating unavoidable disease and disability, and have better ways of growing up, growing old and dying gracefully. It does mean that there will be an even distribution of whatever resources for health are available. It does mean that essential health care will be accessible to *all* individuals and families in an acceptable and affordable way, and with their full involvement. And it does mean that people will realise that they themselves have the power to shape their lives and the lives of their families, free from the avoidable burden of disease, and aware that ill-health is not inevitable" [2, pp. 31, 32]. In essence this means freedom from avoidable suffering, pain, disability and death for all people by the year 2000.

This is clearly not only a most highly desirable but also a realistic and realisable concept, and therefore it could and should fire the imagination of people throughout the world. They certainly did not delay action. In September 1978, an International Conference on Primary Health Care was held in Alma Ata, USSR, where governments of WHO Member States were represented at a high level. The Conference declared solemnly that "health for all by the year 2000" is a main social target and "primary health care is the key to attaining this target as a part of development in the spirit of social justice" [3].

In 1979 the Health Assembly endorsed the Alma Ata Report and Declaration and invited Member States to act individually in formulating national strategies and collectively in formulating regional and global strategies. In response to that invitation, Member States of WHO formulated their national strategies for "health for all by the year 2000" as broad lines of action required in all sectors to give effect to the new health policy. Based on these national strategies, and in support of them, regional and finally global strategies were worked out. The Global Strategy for Health for All by the Year 2000 was discussed and adopted by the 34th World Health Assembly in May 1981. It reflects the national and regional strategies as seen from a global perspective. It is not a separate "WHO strategy", but an expression of individual and collective national responsibility, and of ways and means, and a plan of action, to support it by WHO.

The "health for all" concept and the Global Strategy are global in a number of different senses of this term. One obvious dimension of globality is that it equally refers to and is valid for both develop*ed* and develop*ing* countries. However, the Global Strategy is global not only in the geographical sense, concerning *all* WHO Member States, but also in the sense of inviting the globality of the people to contribute to its implementation. In addition, the Strategy also tries to review the "globality" of the problems to be solved to attain "health for all". It is clearly understood that for a revolutionary goal there is a need for a revolutionary policy and strategy in all fields of health development, health manpower not excluded.

Considering health manpower, the Strategy states that "in many countries health personnel are not appropriately trained for the tasks they are expected to perform" [2, p. 23]. In addition, the inequalities we talked about earlier also exist in this field. For example, in the least developed countries, of which there are now 31, one health worker of all categories, including practitioners of traditional medicine, serves on average 2400 people, while in the developed countries this one health worker serves 130 people, that is, 18 times less. In addition, there are often further extreme inequalities within the *same* country; for example, there are sometimes 20 times more people for every doctor in rural areas than there are in the metropolitan ones. At the same time, more and more countries in Europe, and not only in Europe, are facing the serious problems of overproduction of health personnel, especially physicians.

It is evident that to achieve the goal set for the year 2000 there is a need to plan, train and deploy health manpower in response to specific needs of people as an integral part of the health infrastructure, both from the point of view of quality and of quantity.

The Strategy stipulates that a policy should be introduced whereby health manpower will be prepared "to perform functions that are highly relevant to the country's priority health problems, in contrast to accepted practice in many countries ... (and countries) will review the functions of health personnel throughout the health system, and will take the necessary measures to ensure their reorientation as necessary" [2, p. 44].

The process described as integrated *h*ealth *s*ervices and health *m*anpower *d*evelopment (HSMD), that has so actively been promoted in the past few years, has now to gather new strength. This means that the quality *and* quantity of health manpower has to be planned in response to the specific needs of the national health system and, through this, to the health needs and demands of the population. Then health personnel should be trained according to these plans with a view to "placing at the disposal of the system the right kind of manpower in the right numbers at the right time in the right place". This training should also "ensure that health workers are socially motivated and provided with the necessary incentives to serve communities" [2, p. 45].

Management of health personnel should thus ensure that personnel planned and trained in view of *needs* will be most efficiently deployed to meet those needs, and obtain job satisfaction by satisfying the health needs and demands of people they are meant to serve. An effective monitoring system would provide feedback data on which to base the adjustment of planning and "production" of health personnel.

Within the framework of the HSMD concept it is understood that health manpower has no meaning in isolation; it is but an instrument to effect health care. Therefore, the self-directing, cybernetic circle of the health manpower development process (planning, "production" and management of health personnel) has to be entirely geared to, and in fact integrated with, the process of health services development (Fig. 1).

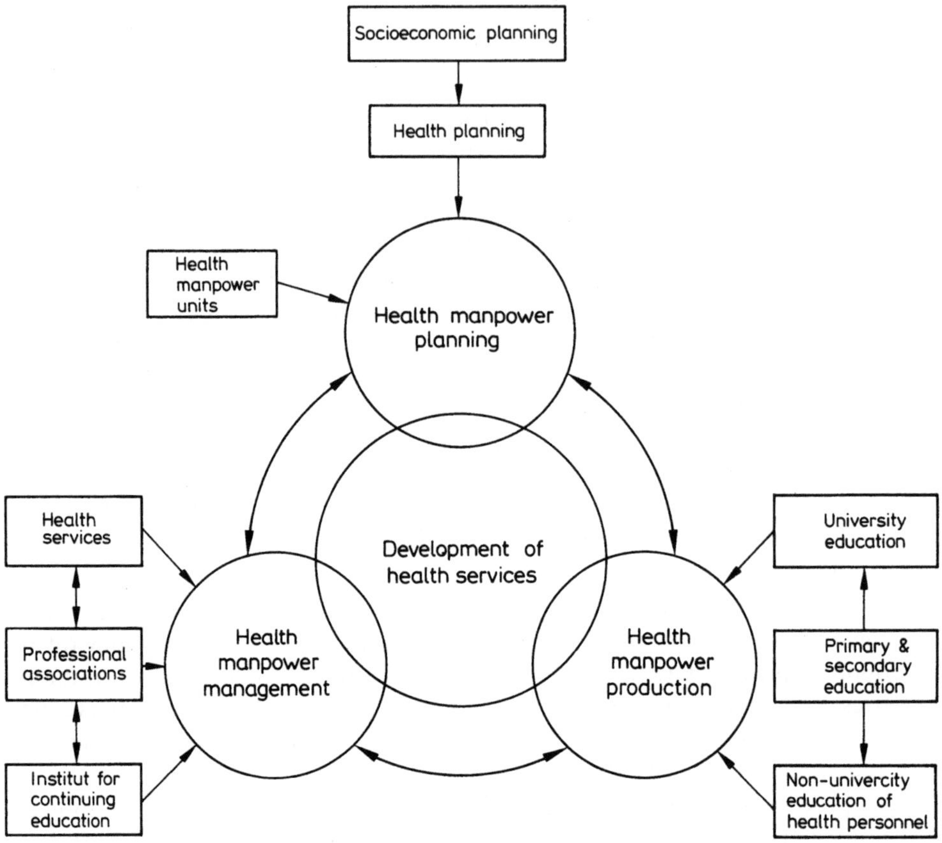

National bodies involved:
- Ministry of Health (or equivalent)
- Ministry of Social Welfare (or equivalent)
- Ministry of Education (or equivalent)
- Ministry of Socioeconomic Development (or equivalent)
- Ministry of Planning (or equivalent)
- Ministry of Labour (or equivalent)
- National Research Institutes

etc., etc.

Fig. 1. National activities in health services and manpower development (HSMD) and some of their interrelationships

To effect this type of integrated HSMD process, a permanent national mechanisms is needed. This will, of course, take different forms in different countries. However, the national health councils together with the national health development networks seem to be appropriate vehicles to carry out the functions of such permanent HSMD mechanisms.

This discussion of what "health for all by the year 2000 through primary health care" means and what it involves in the health manpower field provides in a nutshell a basis for judging on what basis and how curricula for different types of health workers, and among them for physicians, are to be defined.

It seems to be obvious that if we accept that health workers, and thus physicians too, should be socially highly motivated to be able and willing to serve where they are needed, in such a way as they are needed, then the learning experience provided for all of them should be planned not only to *let* them acquire the necessary knowledge, skills and especially attitude, but to *stimulate* them to do so. If graduates of our programmes are assumed to be going to meet the real health needs and demands of people and obtain job satisfaction through this type of service, then we have to revise most of our present programmes, which certainly were not devised with such objectives in mind.

Graduates of our programmes, in this concept, should certainly be able to
- respond to health needs and expressed demands of the community, and
- work with the community, so as to
- stimulate healthy life-style and self-care
- educate the community as well as their co-workers
- solve, and stimulate the solution of, both individual and community health problems
- orient their own as well as community efforts to health promotion and to the prevention of diseases, unnecessary suffering, disability and death
- work in, and with, health teams, and if necessary
- provide leadership to such teams
- continue learning life-long so as to keep their competence up-to-date and even improve it as much as possible.

An educational programme designed to develop such competences, including the necessary awareness, attitudes, values and sense of responsibilities, would certainly rely, in addition to experience provided in the so-called "disease palaces", i.e. in teaching hospitals, in tertiary care also and, last but certainly not least, on experience to be gained in the community, in primary health care. Community oriented, and especially community-based[1] education with emphasis on health promotion and prevention should evidently be one of the characteristics of such education and multiprofessional, i.e. team character the other. If we want our graduates to be able to work in the community, in and with teams, obviously the learning experience which we provide them with should give them ample opportunity to do so. Equally, if we expect them to be able to solve, and stimulate the solution of, problems relevant to the health of individuals *and* of smaller and bigger collectives, their learning experience should provide them with ample opportunity to practise the solution of individual and community health problems. In this sense, a programme built on *problem-based* integration is far more preferable than a programme based on teaching of individual and hardly related disciplines. Also, graduates can be expected to continue learning life-long only if, instead of being spoon-fed in their student days, they are given the full responsibility for their own learning.

---

[1] Community-oriented education is defined here as one focussed on both population groups and individual persons, which takes into account the health needs and demands of the community concerned. Community-based education, on the other hand, is defined here as one that involves the use of the community throughout the entire educational experience as an important environment in which learning takes place

Thus, it seems that the "health for all" movement gives clear guidance for those planning curricula for health workers, physicians included. Programmes that are planned with this most important social target in mind, aiming at competencies relevant to its achievement, will tend to be

- competency based
- community oriented
- community based
- multiprofessional
- integrated on a problem-basis
- student-centred (self-learning oriented)

The Global Strategy itself turns directly to curriculum planners and expresses the hope that all efforts will be made "to introduce the necessary reforms in faculties of medicine, health sciences and other relevant training institutions so that in addition to their technical training, health personnel will become imbued with the philosophy of health development as defined in the Declaration and Report of Alma Ata and in this Strategy" [2, p. 45]. It then speaks about stimuli to be given "to medical, nursing and other health-science schools, to include in their educational programmes the philosophy of health for all, the principles of primary health care, and the essentials of the managerial process for national health development, and to provide appropriate practical training in these areas" [2, pp. 58, 59].

It is quite evident from this brief discussion that the Health for All movement represents the greatest challenge ever to those who deal with planning, training and managing health personnel. This whole process of health manpower development (planning, training, management) will have to be reoriented to become relevant to this most noble social goal of Health for All. Non-governmental organizations, like ours here, have a major role to play in this reorientation process as well as in the promotion of the whole Health for All movement.

The Strategy constantly refers to the important role nongovernmental organizations can and certainly should play in the implementation process. It stresses that "*at the international level,* all technical nongovernmental organizations whose activities could contribute to the acceptance and promotion of health for all through primary health care will be provided with information concerning the health for all movement. They will be requested to incorporate in their programmes activities aimed at influencing their members to become deeply involved in this movement in their own countries. Such activities might consists of general progress reports, the review of specific technical issues from the perspective of the needs of countries to implement their strategies, the pursuit of research that is relevant to health for all, and the retraining of their members" [2, p. 59].

It is also clear that prevention is one of the leading concepts that runs right through both the Alma Ata Report and the Strategy. It should not be forgotten that when we clarified what health for all means, we insisted that it means, inter alia, preventing disease and alleviating unavoidable disease and disability. Also, the list of the eight essential elements of primary health care contains five which are purely or basically of a preventive character (health education, nutrition, water supply and sanitation, maternal and child health, immunization), while a sixth is of largely preventive character (prevention and control of endemic diseases). In developed countries much ill-health results from abundance and consumerism: oversmoking, overeating, overdrinking, overdriving, overuse and abuse of drugs, overpollution of the environment, etc. Therefore, for example, in the European Region the health-for-all strategy includes measures to prevent disease and promote health inter alia by the promotion of life-styles conducive to health, by programmes reducing exposure to self-imposed risks such as alcohol and other drug abuse, smoking, lack of exercise, careless driving, sexual promiscuity, etc.

There is therefore abundant justification for the conclusion that a non-governmental organization devoted primarily to the problems of prevention, such as the International Federation for Hygiene, Preventive Medicine and Social Medicine, should play a role of the greatest importance in the implementation of the Strategy, i.e. in the noble fight for health for all by the year 2000 through primary health care, inter alia, through promoting the reorientation of the whole health manpower development process to become relevant to Health for All.

It is to be hoped that an action plan will be worked out as to how our Federation intends to fight for that main social target in collaboration with other non-governmental organizations and with WHO. Some evident areas of action, in addition to those listed by the Strategy, come to mind such as promoting the development of, and collecting and distributing information on, appropriate preventive technologies, especially for primary health care; promoting the learning of preventive aspects of medicine by all categories of health personnel, especially by primary health workers and their supervisors; promoting research into the preventive aspects of medicine and health care, especially of primary health care; being instrumental in bringing about political commitment of governments to distribute resources for health more evenly; and first and foremost mobilizing the membership and sympathizers to become the flag-bearers in their respective countries, as well as internationally, of this great movement of health for all. When the Federation works out its own plan of action, it will certainly find the best ways to contribute actively and significantly to the achievement of the main social target of health for all.

References

1. WHO (1983) Handbook of resolutions and decisions of the World Health Assembly and the Executive Board, vol 2, 5th edn (1973–1982). WHO, Geneva, p 1
2. WHO (1981) Global strategy for health for all by the year 2000. WHO, Geneva (Health for all series, no 3)
3. WHO (1978) Primary health care. WHO, Geneva (Health for all series, no 1, p 3)

Primary Health Care: The Challenge of Participation

J. McEwen

Introduction

'Self-help', 'consumer participation' and 'demystification' are terms now found regularly in both professional and lay literature. They are part of an amorphous and yet manifest social phenomenon which embraces such notions as self-care, alternative medicine, consumer satisfaction, holistic medicine and patient power. Many of these terms mean different things to different peoples and have special implications in certain types of health care and in some countries. The simple words 'participation' or 'involvement' seem to be most useful to describe the process whereby a person can function on his or her own behalf in the maintenance and promotion of health, the prevention of disease, the detection, treatment and care of illness and adaptation to continuing disability. This may occur both independently of, or within, the existing system of care. Participation also includes activities performed by individuals on behalf of others in areas of health care similar to those just outlined and in the planning, management and evaluation of health care provision.

The main concepts involved in this participation are:

1. An active involvement by the individual in all aspects of his or her own health care rather than the traditional passive role normally associated with being a patient – *self-help.*
2. A process of substitution and/or complementation whereby tasks normally thought to fall within the medical or professional sphere are taken on by the individual – *demedicalisation* or *deprofessionalisation.*
3. A desire to assume responsibility for decision-making with regard to the wider aspects of social policy and health care provision – *democratisation.*

Participation: Who Is Involved?

In the past, individuals had a responsibility for their own health care usually as a result of necessity (only the wealthy or educated made use of professional services). Within a community people helped each other and some individuals became accepted as having special skills, but there was little participation by the majority of people in the development of policy. Today, individuals

Primary Health Care in the Making
Ed. by U. Laaser, R. Senault, H. Viefhues

(sometimes grouping together), professionals and government are all seen to be exponents of the principle of participation.

Government

In Britain, the government has sought to encourage individual responsibility for individual health, particularly prevention. In documents such as *Prevention and Health: Everybody's Business,* the well known practical steps that an individual can take to reduce the risks of illness – not smoking, suitable diet, exercise, restriction of alcohol consumption etc. – are emphasised but there has been little encouragement for active participation in policy and indeed the administrative structure of the health service is such that only limited participation is possible.

Although there is government support for health education directed at the individual, campaigning organisations which seek to tackle alcohol abuse, advertising, cigarette sponsorship of sports or powerful industrial groups get no support from the health department at government.

Professionals

Doctors are split on participation. Some consider that active participation will lead to an unacceptable doctor-patient relationship, destroying the authority of the doctor and leading to a profusion of alternative therapies and dangerous self-care. Other doctors feel that they should assume an active role in helping the public to accept more responsibility and seek to work with them in providing information, advice and support. Such doctors welcome the new role that this involves and argue that such a partnership will improve health and health care, resulting in greater satisfaction for both professionals and the public.

Patients

Some patients are happy to be the passive recipients of individual care and have no desire to be involved in policies, while others desire an active role. It is probably easier for the individual patient to achieve this new relationship with a general practitioner, who provides comprehensive and continuing care, than with the staff in a hospital.

Participation in Primary Care: Some Examples

Self-medication

Self-medication has three main divisions:

1. Health promotion or health maintenance
2. Treatment of trivial, self-correcting conditions or early stages of more serious illness

3. Additional care to that provided by health services in more serious illness and in chronic conditions

Generally, the first two occur with no reference to the doctor or other health personnel and the largest category is the second one, which is related to the widespread and frequent occurrence of symptoms. Self-medication is a normal and appropriate part of the overall provision of health care. This is recognised by professionals who equally recognise that the general practitioner could not cope if self-care was to be abolished. Considering the amount and significance of self-medication, there appears to be a paucity of educational material associated with it.

A key role lies with professionals and in particular with the pharmacist in the chemist shop. In 1983 the British Pharmaceutical Society launched an advertising campaign to encourage the public 'to ask the pharmacist' and at the same time through professional education, the pharmacist is being encouraged to develop a broader educational function, providing a key role in primary care.

Primary Care

Starting with a few enthusiastic general practitioners in the mid-1970s, the concept of patient participation in primary care has been translated into practice in a number of health centres throughout Britain. The individual groups in practices made up of respresentatives selected by patients now have a national organisation which provides for exchange of ideas and support to individual groups. As yet these exist in only a minority of general practices and are found mainly in health centres. The overall aim is simple – "to open a channel of communication between patients and doctors".

The following are the aims of one practice association:

1. To participate with the doctors and other members of the health team in the running of the primary care service
2. To consider complaints and improvements in the service
3. To provide health education lectures and discussions, to teach positive and preventive health, including the early signs and symptoms of disease
4. To communicate the opinions of the patients to other bodies such as the community health council, the health authority and local authorities
5. To improve the levels of care available
6. To set up subcommittees to deal with the various aspects of patients' needs

Patient groups have received the support of the Royal College of General Practitioners, and indeed the Royal College of General Practitioners has been the first college to establish a formal patient liaison group.

Such innovations may well act as a stimulus to other doctors and patients to establish groups and these in turn may enable better communication and participation at the level of individual care in general practice.

Community Health Councils

During the reorganisation of the Health Service in 1974, lay members were appointed to health authorities to provide managerial responsibilities, rather than provide a consumer monitoring function (as they were supposed to have done previously). Accordingly, new bodies, community health councils, were established whose tasks were to represent the views of local users of the health services to the district health authorities.

Each council is made up of members with a particular interest in health services. Half are appointed by local authorities, one-third by voluntary organisations and one-sixth by the Regional Health Authority. Generally, each CHC has two full-time staff – the secretary and an assistant. Expenses and salaries for full-time staff come from the health authority. The power of the CHCs is limited since they have no managerial responsibility for the provision of any services. They have the right to ask for and receive information from the administration, they have the right to visit National Health Service premises and they have the right to be consulted about development plans. Consultation with them on hospital closures and substantial change of use is obligatory.

Although not directly involved with individual complaints, they do tend to act as the official watchdog for the local community and inevitably receive criticism and complaints about all aspects of health care. They can provide support and help on such issues and they can help the individual through the complex procedures of the health service and make constructive comments to health authorities.

Although there is a national association, inevitably, due to the diverse composition of the CHCs, there is great variation in their role and function. Some have emphasised the watchdog role while others have sought to work constructively with all aspects of health service provision to achieve overall improvement in care.

Self-help Groups

It is important to differentiate between "self-help" groups and "voluntary organisations". Generally, self-help groups are run by, and composed of, the sufferers themselves (sometimes parents and immediate family), whereas helpers in voluntary organisations are not usually victims of the disease or problem.

Two of the main features of self-help groups are firstly that the problems or illness concerned be of some gravity and secondly that the group has the potential to help overcome some of the isolation, anxiety, uncertainty or frustration caused by that problem. A further characterstic closely linked to these is that those who have passed through the crisis period and are back on an even keel, or have learned to cope with the chronic problems of a condition, still feel sufficiently strongly about their period of suffering that they are motivated to help others in the same situation. This may be either a feeling of bonding together against a common enemy or a sort of parental protective attitude. Those who have suffered in the past often have a desire to turn a potentially negative experience into something positive by building on their experience and doing something constructive for others in the same position. They feel that their contribution is unique, that it constitutes an expertise, one which is outside the scope of professionals. This means that although all members have the same problem, they are at different stages and this lends optimism, some expectation of progress, to those in deepest difficulty.

It is difficult to categorise groups since many have overlapping functions but a group will tend to emphasise one or more of the following:

1. Provision of support, comfort and "therapy" for members
2. Practical provision of care, courses, education etc. not elsewhere available
3. Pressure group activities which seek change in national or social policy

Directories of these organisations are available, nationally and locally, but they are often not well known to either health professionals or members of the public. Many produce excellent educational publications and some of the material has been used to influence professionals in training as well as altering professional attitudes to participation.

Implications

Developments in participation inevitably are not comprehensive or organised since they are frequently the result of individual enthusiasm or concern and perhaps if participation is to be effective it should continue to be founded on such attributes although it may gain from co-operation and the dissemination of ideas.

We have noted new developments in participation, new educational initiatives and a new professional and public awareness, yet we are not making full use of these and professionals are slow to accept new responsibilities and challenges or to revise their training and education to meet new needs.

Clearly there is a need for:

- further examination of existing activities, possibly examining components of this large topic area in greater detail
- development of a sound theoretical base
- evaluation studies of ongoing activities
- setting up of well planned controlled studies to test new ideas and to determine the benefits and the hazards of different aspects of participation
- determination of health needs and assessment of the tasks required to meet these needs
- review of the roles of different health personnel
- development, testing and evaluation of educational materials and methods
- creation of new models for a more participatory health service

There is much discussion on the role of the primary health care team and the need to integrate preventive and curative health care. An exciting proposal for a Primary Health Care Unit for Continuing Education within the Open University which would combine the educational expertise of the Open University with existing professional networks might do much to enhance teamwork, highlight changing health needs and improve and encourage public participation in health.

Participation is too large and too important a subject for it to continue to mushroom without efforts at evaluation and attempts to relate it to the health and social needs of individuals and communities or to existing services. Now is an appropriate time to begin this.

Acknowledgements. This paper is based on the book *Participation in Health* by J. McEwen, C. J. M. Martini and N. Wilkins, Croom Helm, London, 1983, and I would like to express my appreciation to the colleagues involved.

The Promotion of Health Through Changes in Life-style: Epidemiological, Psychosocial and Ethical Aspects

E. A. Sand

Introduction

Those persons responsible for health education have for several years been re-orientating their efforts towards a more global, and probably in some respects more promising approach, i.e. changes in life-style. This concept has followed a certain disillusionment about the efficiency of trying to modify behavioural traits considered or demonstrated to involve risks to health. But the extent of this new orientation moves us to critically investigate its advantages and the risks it might involve. This criticism is meant to be constructive.

The reasons for this investigation are of at least five kinds:

1. The reduction in the resources available for health education requires a choice between projects and activities; it is easy to prove that a programme aimed at modifying life-styles may be more expensive than a programme focussed on a behavioural trait or on a restricted group of symptoms (e.g. consumption of food, alcohol, tobacco).
2. The power of the means available to health education is impressive: books, scientific articles, mass media, teaching systems etc. Moreover, particularly competent authors in health education have clearly expressed the need to extend interventions [1].
3. Results have already been achieved in health education through programmes that concern life-styles (treatment of alcoholics and drug addicts, intervention aimed at reducing cardiovascular morbidity etc.)
4. It appears that on the whole, neither adult nor youth populations assign high priority to health and to its improvement with respect to, for example, economic, social or simply hedonist interests.
5. Definition of health promotion is not easy. In a simplified form, one might consider that it means, in keeping with the definition of health proposed by the World Health Organisation, a reduction in the different forms of disease but also better access to well-being at the levels of community and individual. It should be noted that this latter aspect is at the level of life-style.

Life-styles

Here again, definitions are not always clear, nor are they in harmony with one another. Style of life and behaviour are not to be mixed up. Behaviour is in fact

Primary Health Care in the Making
Ed. by U. Laaser, R. Senault, H. Viefhues

only the visible manifestation of life-style, which itself belongs to a deeper level of the personality, or, when related to groups or communities, to a kind of set of options.

It is possible to define the abstract concept of "life-style" as a dynamic pattern of attitudes, beliefs (convictions) and knowledge which, by defining priorities, leads to acts and behavioural traits. These acts may concern a large range of life situations: work, leisure, food, sleep, love, sex, religion.

Life-styles develop throughout life under the influence of numerous factors. Notice has to be taken of the fact that retroactive effects can, in their turn, exert an influence on the variables that determine new priorities.

Changes in Life-style

It is clear that life-styles alter in a spontaneous way, particularly during certain periods of life: youth, retirement, crisis etc. They also change on the level of the community. A deliberate external intervention aimed at changing them will undoubtedly have to clash, at the level of the individual and, even more, at the level of the group, with the original elements of the system represented in Fig. 1, i.e. with deeply rooted motivations that have long been accepted without argument and to a large extent unconsciously.

This imposes on educators obligations of a scientific and ethical order. In scientific matters, we are convinced that only interventions based on solid psychological, epidemiological and sociological findings are acceptable. However, the methods of analysis of epidemiologists, and even the statistical approaches, pose a problem, mainly because of the multivariate nature of the foreseen phenomena and of the dynamic group of variables that constitute real systems (Fig. 1). Accuracy is essential, but not an obsession with perfection; the latter would no doubt lead to abstention from any interventions at all.

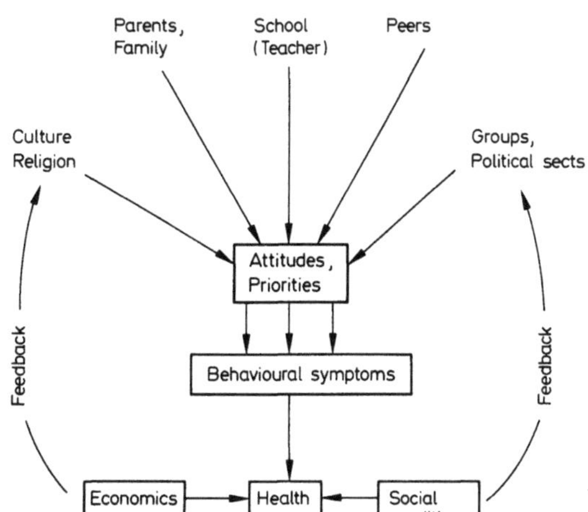

Fig. 1. The development of life-style

The ethical restraints on intervention have already been the object of numerous thoughts. Let us recall some aspects of them. The choice or the constitution of a life-style results from social and psychological but also from moral, philosophical and religious, in short, ethical factors that often take precedence over technical and rational (e.g. medical and sanitary) considerations.

A second ethical restraint results from the possible use of information and educational methods that are inspired by subtle psychological approaches and aim to affect people at a pre- or unconscious level. Such methods are used in advertising and certain forms of political propaganda. In health education, these methods give rise to sharp discussions. At the present time, we can foresee the ethical problems connected with them only in part.

Moreover, another point, both epidemiological and ethical, cannot be left unconsidered: Information on health and health education requires, to my mind, provision of complete and honest information to the public, i.e. balanced information that reflects the uncertainties of research (limits of confidence of the statistical tests, for example). However, such information inevitably loses in impact what it gains in honesty and accuracy, and we are thus faced with an uneasy choice! It goes without saying that the suggested life-styles can in no case involve risks to health. The sincerity of the educators cannot be questioned here, but again, one must sometimes be able to prove the harmlessness of the proposals.

As Doxiadis has pointed out in a personal communication, no proposition should be accepted that does not include the cost and benefit that it will represent to the population. And let us not forget that it is precisely this population which provides the resources for action regarding health education, i.e.

1. The life-styles we are aiming to change
2. The change itself (health education)
3. The new life-styles

One should not forget that between stages (1) and (3) elapses a waiting period that can be extended.

Presuppositions Behind Intervention to Change Life-styles

Recalling the view of C. Rogers, we believe that the large majority of human beings have a deep craving for life and hence for good and better health, linked with a fear of death, suffering etc. The efforts in health education should therefore aim at fortifying this desire, so that it has more impact on behaviour. If this desire is lacking or is weighed down by contrary feelings (suicidal, neurotic, some cases of depression), health education will not be easy, even though it must bear these possibilities in mind.

Conclusion

As a conclusion to these few considerations, which no doubt give rise to more questions than they answer, I have three proposals to make:

1. Interventions aimed at changing life-styles are all the more effective when they answer a demand, explicit or implicit, of a population group motivated by a (some) health problem(s). In this case the educator offers, within a frame of dialog based upon equality, his scientific knowledge but also his human conviction in a common effort towards "problem solving". Co-operation with self-help groups is an example of this approach.
2. Some serious aspects of health problems (high incidence, serious after-effects, duration, precocity of risks, e.g. during early childhood) justify action by the health education teams, based on complete and balanced information. It seems to me that it is also essential to work closely with the population concerned, having a full dialogue with them. This may relate to the health of schoolboys, (young) families or retired people.
3. Let us remember that, due to the scarcity of epidemiological studies in health education, an estimation of the efforts to be undertaken will always have to be included in the programme.

Reference

1. Kickbusch I (1981) Un concept social pour l'éducation pour la santé. Rev Int Educ Sante 2414:140–153

Social Support and Coronary Risk Factors

K. Orth-Gomér, B.-M. Wallin, and A.-L. Undén

Kristina Orth-Gomér, Britt-Marie Wallin and Anna-Lena Undén, National Institute for Psychosocial Factors and Health, Box 60210, S-104 01 Stockholm, Sweden,

Much research has been devoted to the identification of unhealthy stressors, e.g. within working life. Much work has also been done to demonstrate that certain behavioural patterns, such as type A behaviour, do contribute to the development of coronary heart disease (CHD). Not everybody exposed to stressors, nor every man exhibiting type A behaviour, gets CHD. Some manage to cope quite well both with stressors and behaviour. Successful coping seems to be one of the vital health-preserving mechanisms of modern society.

One possible buffer against the effect of stressors seems to be a well functioning social network providing good social support. In a number of studies a lack of social support or a lack of capability to utilize the social support system has been associated with psychiatric disorders, but less work has been devoted to social support systems and somatic disease.

In some studies, socio-demographic indicators of social support have been associated with CHD. In California, Berkman et al. found that a combination of four social network characteristics predicted both total mortality and mortality from CHD. Men and women with a low network index had a 2–4.5 times higher mortality than those with a high network index. In Sweden, as in many other countries, marriage seems to protect against premature coronary death. Married men have a lower CHD mortality than unmarried men, divorced men and widowers (Fig. 1).

We wanted to examine the psychological aspects of the social support system, rather than socio-demographic characteristics. What does social support mean to people? Who provides it? Is it generally felt to be adequate? Which are the associations with disease or precursors of disease?

We used an instrument which in our opinion quite extensively describes the emotional and psychological aspects of the social network system: the Interview Schedule for Social Interaction. This instrument was developed by S. Henderson and D. Byrne, Canberra, Australia. After lengthy theoretical and experimental work, the authors were able to identify two main dimensions of social support:

1. Attachment, including close affectional relationships
2. Social integration, including relationships which provide possibilities for

Primary Health Care in the Making
Ed. by U. Laaser, R. Senault, H. Viefhues

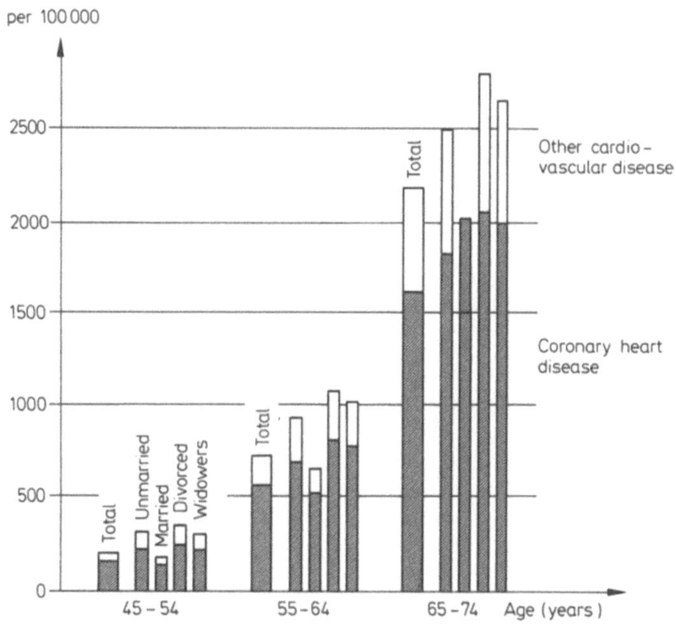

Fig. 1. Mortality rates for cardiovascular disease among Swedish men by marital status, 1974–1978

a) shared interests and values,
b) reassurance of personal worth, and
c) a sense of reliable alliance giving instrumental and other types of support.

For each of the two dimensions the availability of relationships and the adequacy of the existing relationships were described.

This instrument was translated into Swedish and used in a study of 83 Swedish men, aged 45–70 (mean age 62 years). About half of the men were retired; 92% were married; 36% had signs or symptoms of CHD, 32% were healthy and 32% had other chronic disorders, such as hypertension, diabetes or hyperlipidaemia.

The interview procedure was two-fold. After a thorough explanation of the aim of the study and the structure of the questions, each man filled out the questionnaire alone. Then each question was discussed with a trained interviewer and comments and reactions were noted. All men were also examined for coronary risk factors and for symptoms and signs of CHD.

Results

The two attachment scales – availability and adequacy – were distributed in a very similar way in the sample (Figs. 2, 3). Both were quite skewed. It is con-

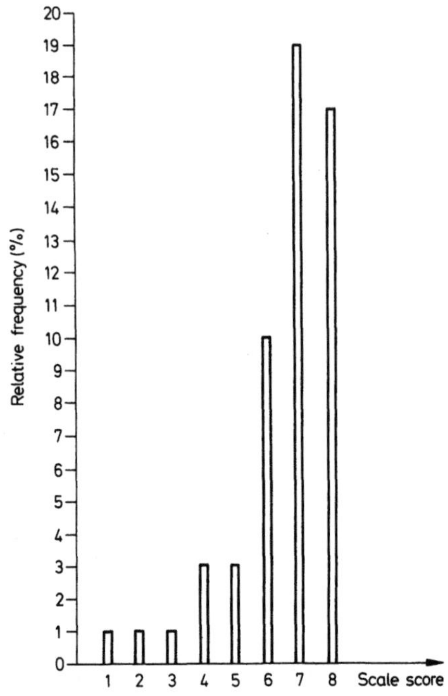

Fig. 2. Availability of attachment

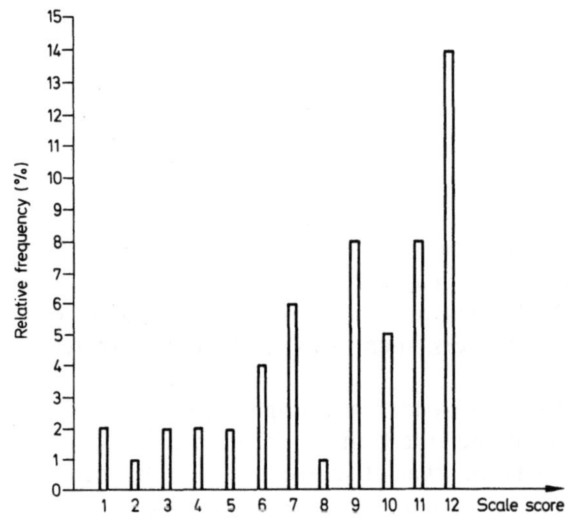

Fig. 3. Adequacy of attachment

ceivable that the way of answering these rather threatening questions may be governed by social desirability and that people therefore tend to have very high scores.

Men with high scores differed from men with low scores in only two ways: they were married and they were overweight. None of the other risk factors was associated with these scales.

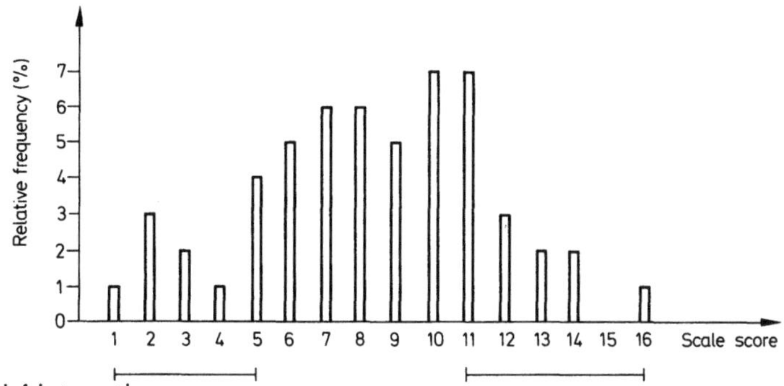

Fig. 4. Availability of social integration

Table 1. Availability of social integration

	Low score ($n=18$)	High score ($n=23$)	t-value
Occupational grade (1–7)	4.0	3.1	2.57 ($P<0.05$)
Social class (1–5)	3.4	2.7	2.33 ($P<0.05$)
Smoking	8.6	1.8	3.39 ($P<0.001$)
Complaints about own health (1–4)	2.1	1.5	1.88 ($P<0.10$)
Exhaustion after work (1–5)	2.8	2.4	1.71 ($P<0.10$)

Table 2. Availability of social integration

	Low score	High score	t-value
Age	61.8	61.9	0.05 NS
Systolic BP (mmHg)	131.9	138.1	0.94 NS
Diastolic BP (mmHg)	82.5	85.3	0.78 NS
Alcohol consumption (g/week)	214	130	1.25 NS
Pressure at work (1–5)	3.2	3.0	0.55 NS
Type A behaviour (yes = 1, no = 2)	1.6	1.6	0.06 NS
Retirement (yes = 1, no = 2)	1.6	1.7	0.61 NS

The questions of the third scale, availability of social integration, are less threatening. The distribution of scale scores was more like a normal distribution (Fig. 4). When comparing men with low scores with men with high scores, they differed in the ways shown in Table 1. They had a lower occupational grade, belonged to a lower social class and were more often smokers. They also had had more symptoms of ill health – mainly cardiovascular – during the past 5 years. On the other hand, there was no association with age or with retirement. Neither did systolic and diastolic blood pressure, or pressure at work or type A behaviour, differ between high and low score groups (Table 2).

The fourth scale, adequacy of social integration, was distributed in the same skewed way as the first two – and did not yield any differences between high and low scorers (Fig. 5).

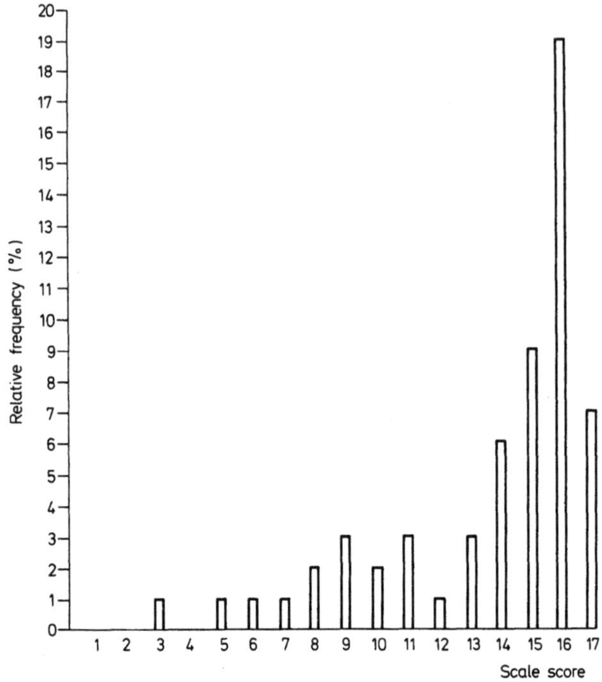

Fig. 5. Adequacy of social integration

It seems to us that social support is rather difficult to measure and that the influence of social desirability may be quite pronounced. At least the social interaction dimension, however, should be included in prospective studies of CHD. It is also possible that it may be important for the success of primary prevention. Anti-smoking programmes, for example, might be more efficient if combined with social skill training.

B. Learning from the Third World Experience

Maternal and Perinatal Death in Indonesian University Obstetrics: Risk Display for Selected Social and Biological Determinants *

R. P. Bernard and S. Sastrawinata

Introduction

The Government of Indonesia is desirous to promote across the entire reproductive health care system a spirit of service that is nurtured by continuous monitoring of the current status of health in order to *identify unmet needs.* The monitoring of the unmet needs by the service providers cannot but mobilize programmatic determination to improve and better specify the services to be rendered both by medical and paramedical personnel. In essence, an endogenous school of thought is wanted.

The 12 departments of obstetrics and gynecology – cognizant of the important contribution they would be able to make – associated into the Coordinating Board of Indonesian Fertility Research (BKS PENFIN) to initiate a process of "working together" and radiating this spirit to the more peripheral reproductive health care structure. The rationale was that such cooperation may lead to a new kind of perception on priority needs to *accelerate the reduction in all mortalities related to birth* (late fetal death, neonatal death, and maternal death).

The first action was to develop and deploy a monitoring system across the entire top referral/teaching structure, that is the 12 university hospitals in Jakarta, Bandung, Yogjakarta, Semarang, Surabaya, Malang, Denpasar, Medan, Padang, Palembang, Ujung Pandang, and Manado. The goal was to first get sufficient experience at the top referral level so that the deployment at more peripheral levels would become a vertically linked system for learning, teaching, and evaluation. Since future directors of peripheral clinics are trained at the top, it was considered essential to initiate the new spirit there as well. Top responsibles would be diffusors.

Many reports have been developed from the findings so far [1–4]. By spring 1982 it had become obvious that a *genuine information gap* came to impede the meaningful feedback to the clinics. While standard computer outputs were feeding the clinics, the statistical tables could not really be read by the service professions. Therefore we resolved to experiment with a new approach. Statistical information was transformed into two kinds of table: (1) risk tables and (2)

* This report is derived from a new Risk Atlas: Risk of Death at Birth for Mother and Infant, 76 Panels and 2 Diagrams. Geneva, July 1983, MCM-28. The results are discussed in the Appendix

Primary Health Care in the Making
Ed. by U. Laaser, R. Senault, H. Viefhues

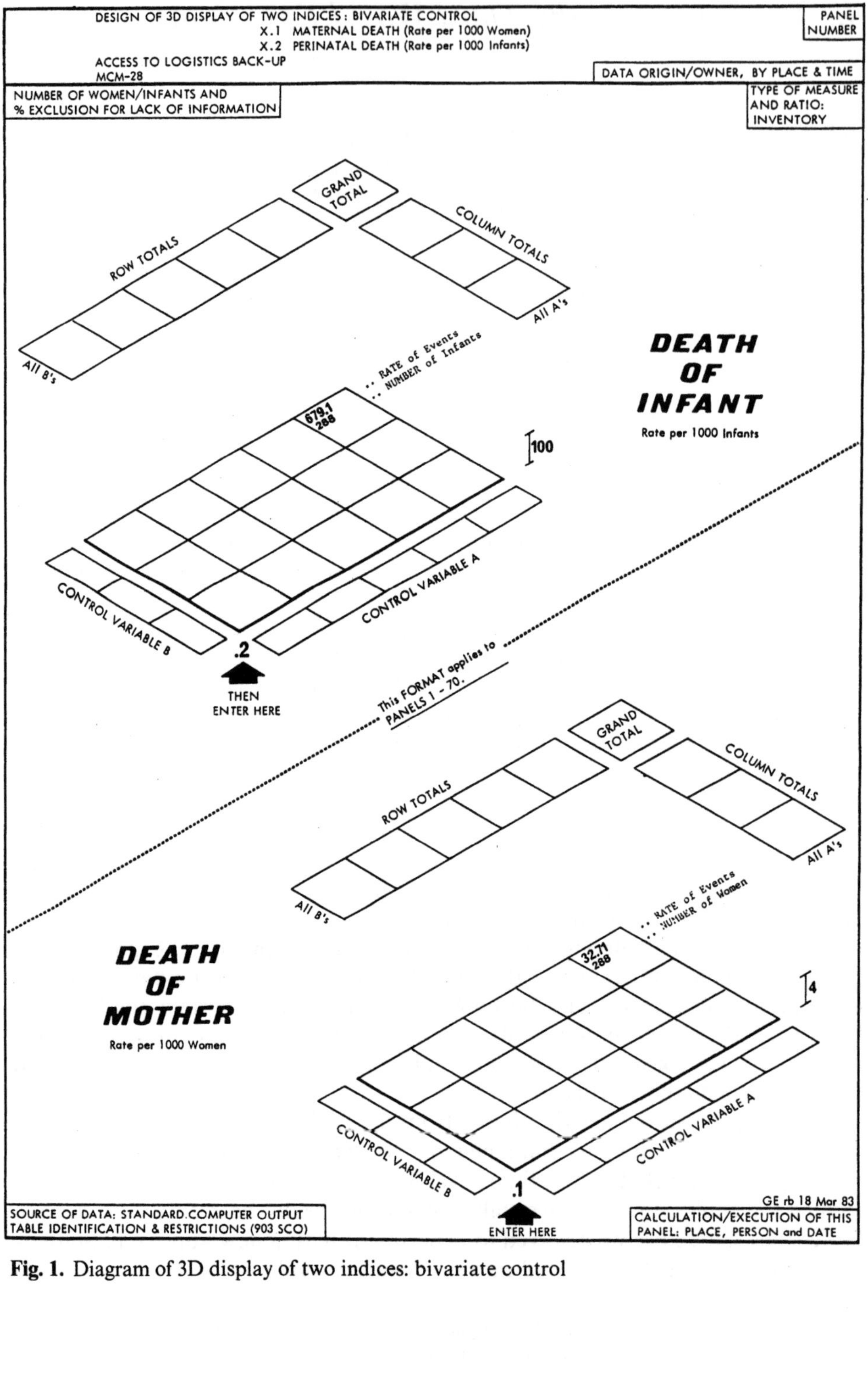

Fig. 1. Diagram of 3D display of two indices: bivariate control

prevalence tables. Unfortunately, these tables still did not "pass the message." Hence we experimented with developing a *holistic presentation* that would give these tables in *three dimensions*.

The messages in the tables passed instantly and the "charts" soon became "standard panels," i.e., an inalienable cross-sectional document with built-in controls and proper identification by place and time. The 3D panels were soon "linked together" into a focussed "pathway of analysis," as given in a *diagrammatic strategy of analysis*. Collating these "panel sequences" led to the "risk atlases" or "prevalence atlases." What had occurred?

Without ever planning the current status of sophisticated and fully accessible detailed feedback, we had simply tried to meet a serious need: to communicate on risks and prevalences without sacrificing scientific desiderata. The impact across the 12 university centers of obstetrics and gynecology is considerable. A genuine esprit de corps is emerging and professors, assistants and students, together with midwives, now have a new vocabulary of "incidence," "prevalence," "excess risk," "base risk," "peak risk," "relative risk," "prevalence ratio," "anemia baseline," and "controlled for." Probably never has an entire medical profession sharpened up its professional language in such a short time. And this simply by providing the information in the form of *holographic pictures*.

By May 1983, it had become obvious that the *two* most important unfavorable end-points in obstetrics – maternal and perinatal death – could be presented together: in each panel one could show the risk of maternal and perinatal death controlled for two selected variables (Fig. 1). In addition, a pointed "strategy of analysis" might be designed so that multivariate control systems would be part of the result feedback in 3D display. Upon this would start discussions.

This paper proposes to show and briefly discuss selected panels (Figs. 3–13) from a now terminated atlas of 76 panels on the risk of death at birth for mother and infant as it prevailed across the top referral/teaching system of a nation of 150 million people from 1978 to 1980. Apparently, for the first time the Indonesian profession now knows about factors affecting both end-points: to what extent, in what kind of interactions, etc.

Materials and Methods

All risk panels were developed without "dialoguing" a single time with the computer's console. The sole source were unrestricted and restricted standard computer outputs of the 11-center pool of December 1980, which contains 36 802 singleton birth deliveries and on which various analyses have been performed in Bandung, Geneva and Research Triangle Park (USA) (Fig. 2).

The information was collected from 1978 to 1980 with the 903-Maternity Record developed in cooperation between the International Fertility Research Program (IFRP) and the International Federation of Gynaecology and Obstetrics (FIGO) from 1975 to 1977 [5]. Headquarters of the World Health Organi-

DIAGRAM 1: STRATEGY OF ANALYSIS with STANDARD COMPUTER OUTPUTS (SCO's). FOCUS ON AGE/PARITY AND OUTCOMES. ACCESS TO 3D DISPLAY FOR BOTH FORMAT AND FINDINGS IN 11 CONSECUTIVE PANELS. BKS PENFIN, INDONESIA, 1978-1980. 11-CENTER POOL WITH 36,802 WOMEN WITH SINGLE BIRTH.

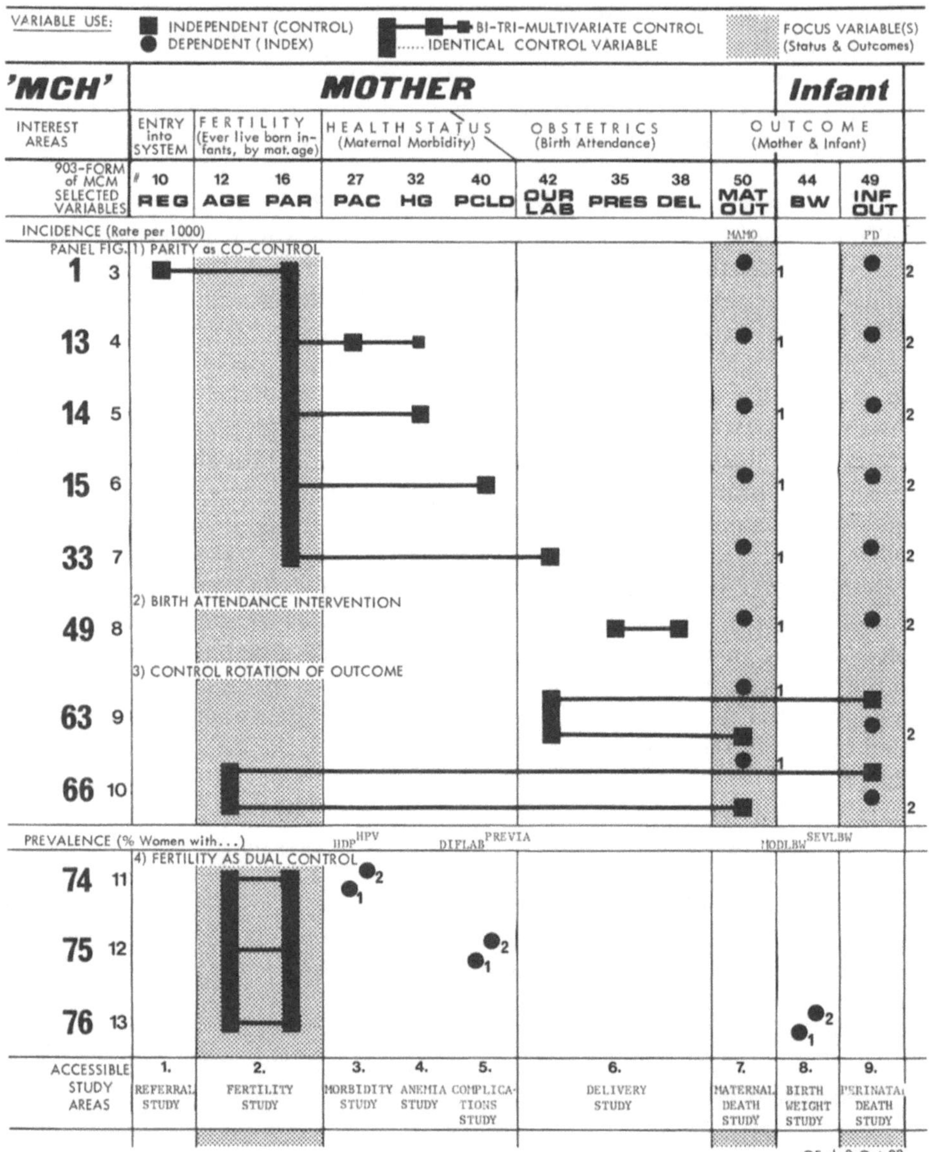

NOTE: The 11 selected PANELS here assembled into a "PATHWAY OF ANALYSIS" are borrowed from a new RISK ATLAS: RISK OF DEATH AT BIRTH FOR MOTHER AND INFANT (BKS PENFIN, INDONESIA, 1983). PANELS of 3D-Displays are selfcontained information modules that may be linked with one another according to specific research focuses. The current report focuses on age/parity as control of outcomes.

Fig. 2. Strategy of analysis with standard computer outputs (SCOs). Focus on age/parity and outcomes. Access to 3D display for both format and findings in 11 consecutive panels. BKS PENFIN, Indonesia, 1978–1980. 11-center pool with 36 802 women with single birth

zation (WHO) in Geneva had been helpful with an overall review and the development of a two-digit code system for the most important morbidity conditions to be reported and linked with the four-digit International Classification of Diseases activated in mid-1977 (ICD-9).

Each university center had received several times an updated standard computer output. Studies of variation among centers were performed centrally and fed back to the centers. National seminars and peer reviews then focussed on these differences and solicited common recommendations on standards and necessary improvements. Only then were the data pooled into the 11-center national pool, eliminating one center from that final exercise for technical reasons. The question arose: How would the Indonesian Ministry of Health wish to study the data on Maternal and Child Mortality (MCM)?

An important money-saving device was used to produce the dual control risk tables of two end-points. The unrestricted standard computer output with its more than 60 detailed cross-tabulations was considered as the denominator. The restricted pool of perinatal deaths (PD) and the one restricted to maternal death (MAMO) were the two indispensable numerators. Desk calculator divisions then generated an extraordinarily rich matrix of risks of the two end-points at virtually no computer time costs but labor-intensive work.

In order to secure continuity and technical proficiency, the rhythm of a panel-a-day was adhered to. All the production steps (some 25) were handled in one day, inclusive of final checking of the drawing. Isometric paper was used to produce the 3D displays of the risk tables. Chartopack, Letraline, and Letraset were used for the artwork.

The basic concept of the 3D display is to "render the entire statistical information of the dual control risk table in the third dimension." This means that each specificity (block) needs to have inscribed two informations: the cell size and the rate. This information is also needed for the row and column totals, as well as for the grand total. Since the origin of the graph is on the base, the row and column totals appear at the top as a roof that ends in the grand total. The roofs then provide additional 3D perspective, together with summary statements on risks and relative risks (RRs).

Any panel contains programmed information on the risks, the cell sizes, relative risks, logistical information pertaining to quality (percent exclusion), source [SCO table number(s)], type of measure (incidence or prevalence), institution (BKS PENFIN, Indonesia) and calendar time. In short, the document is inalienable and gains in value with time, since it becomes part of a serial cross-sectional evaluation system that will be critically used over the decades to measure progress and basic differences along the vertical chain of referral.

A cautionary point needs to be made, as well as one of expectation. The data are, of course, only representative of the university centers. And we do not know *how* different they are from the periphery. As soon as the monitoring is enacted at the peripheral centers it will be possible to learn about the differences. Hence the current exercise is the first necessary step to a *national monitoring scheme.* The current findings may help to accelerate the diffusion of the monitoring approach. On the other hand, great expectations are currently being nurtured for the mobilization of the profession of birth attendance, medi-

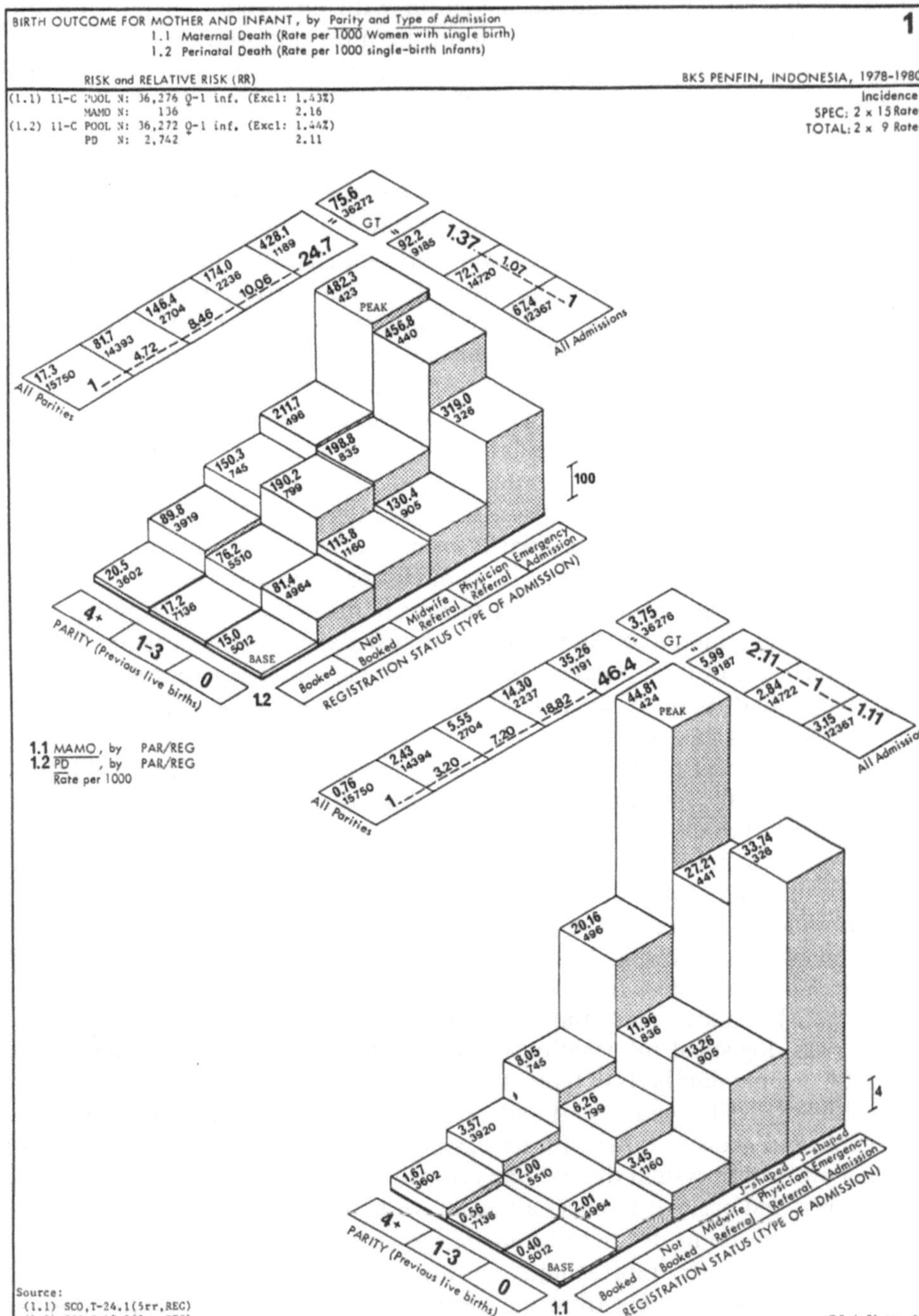

Fig. 3 (Panel 1). Risk of MAMO and PD, by parity and registration status

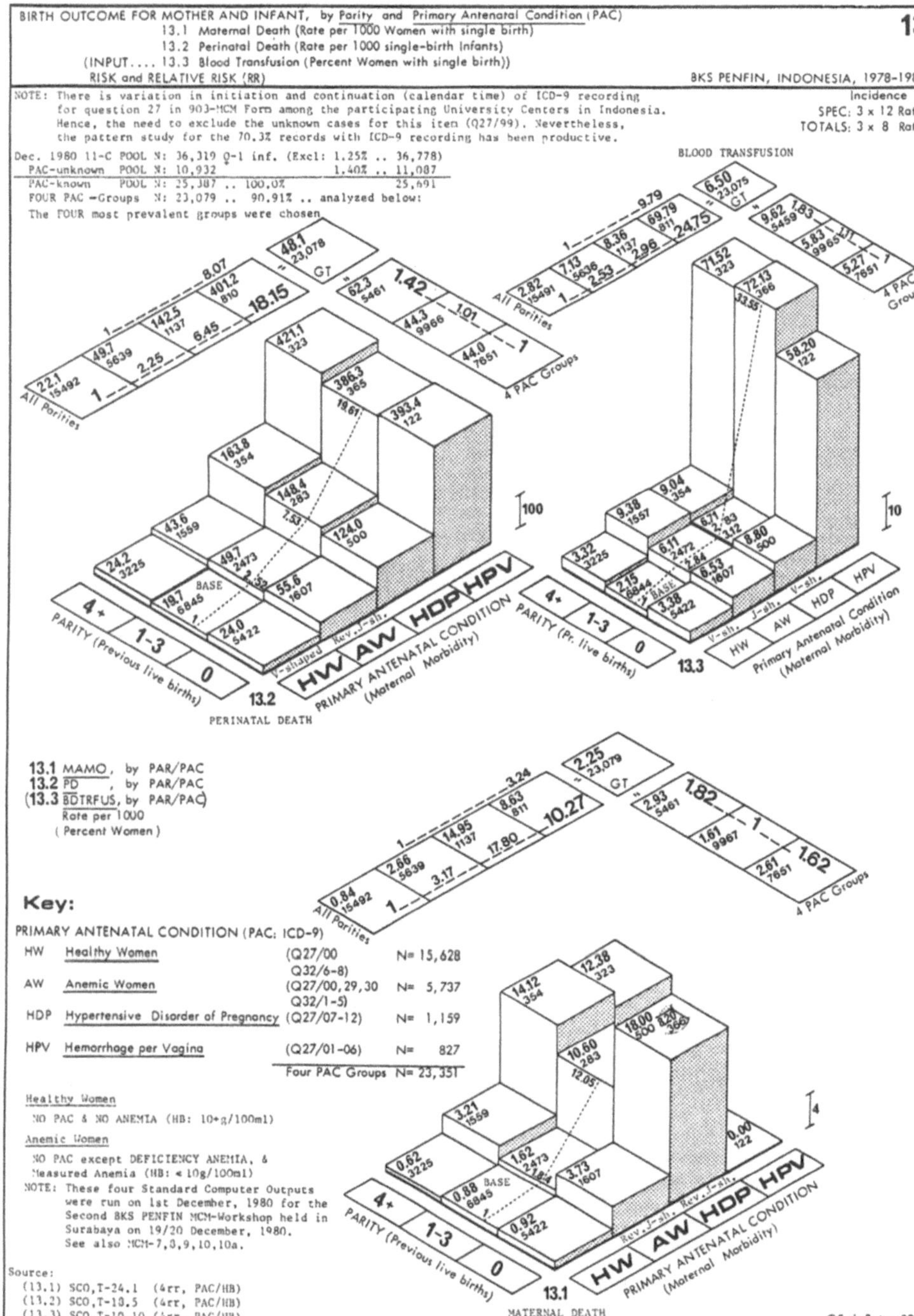

Fig. 4 (Panel 13). Risk of MAMO and PD, by parity and maternal health

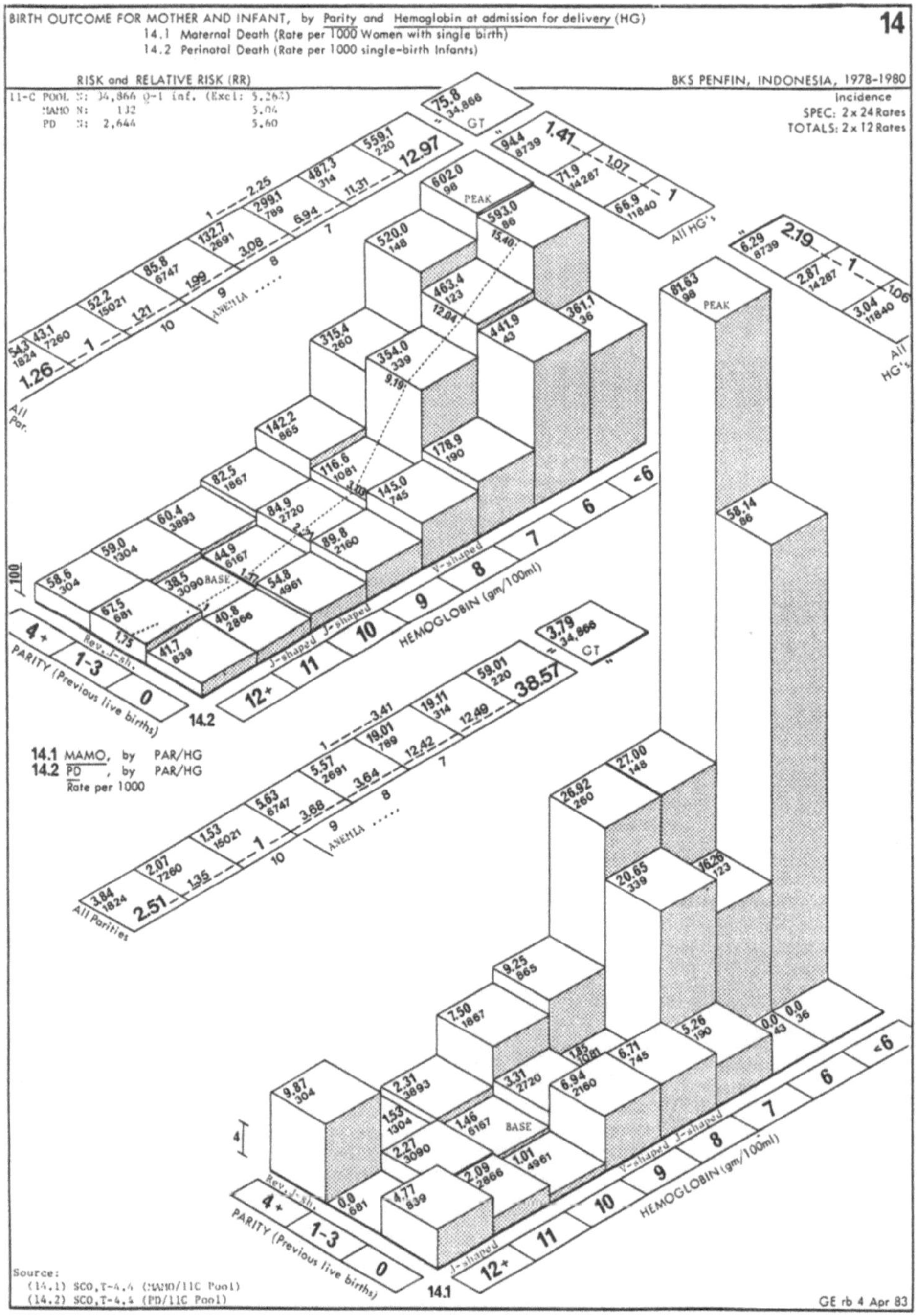

Fig. 5 (Panel 14). Risk of MAMO and PD, by parity and hemoglobin (g/100 ml)

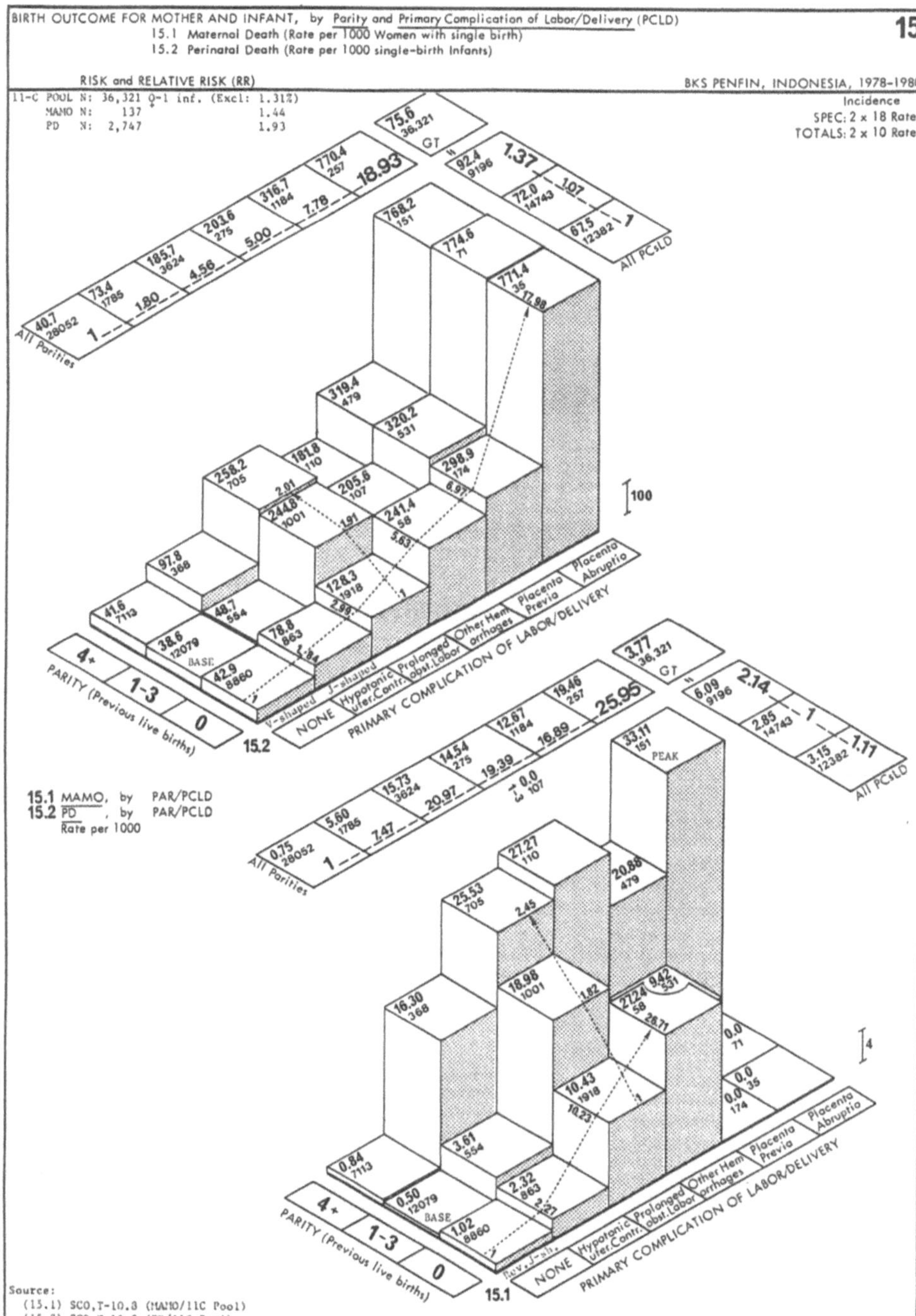

Fig. 6 (Panel 15). Risk of MAMO and PD, by parity and primary complications of labor/delivery

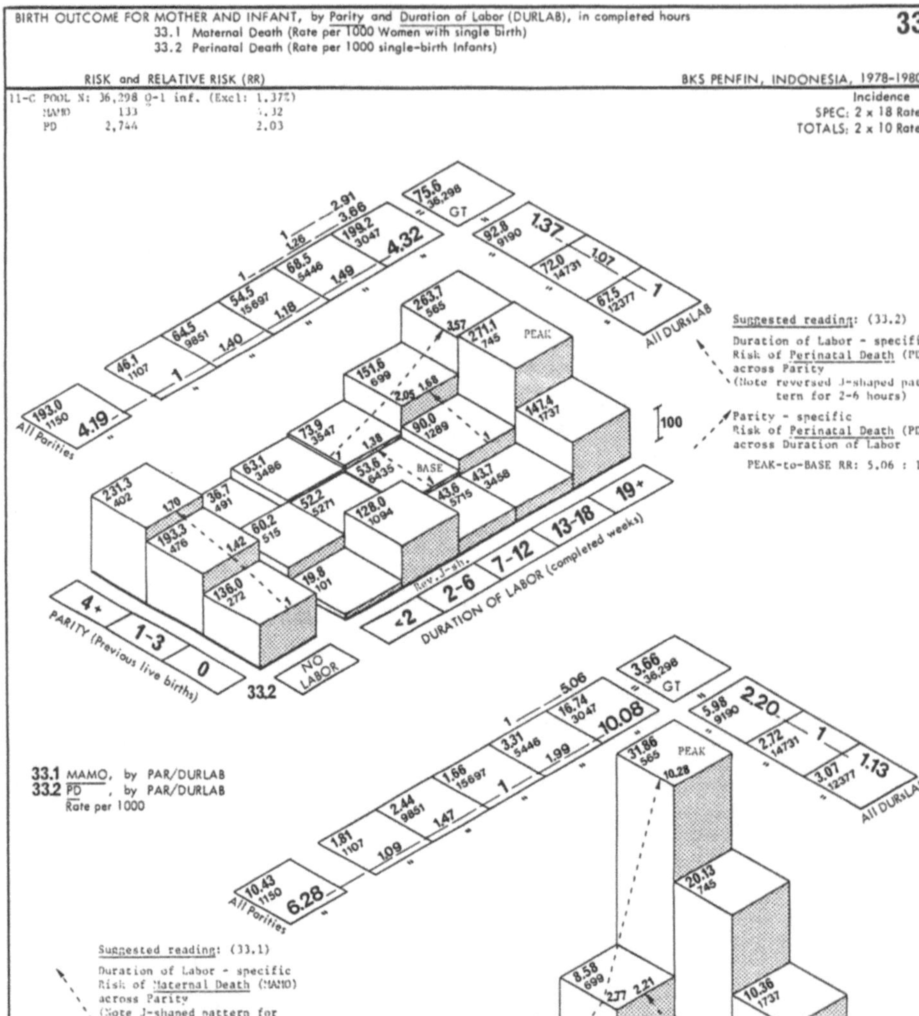

Fig. 7 (Panel 33). Risk of MAMO and PD, by parity and duration of labor

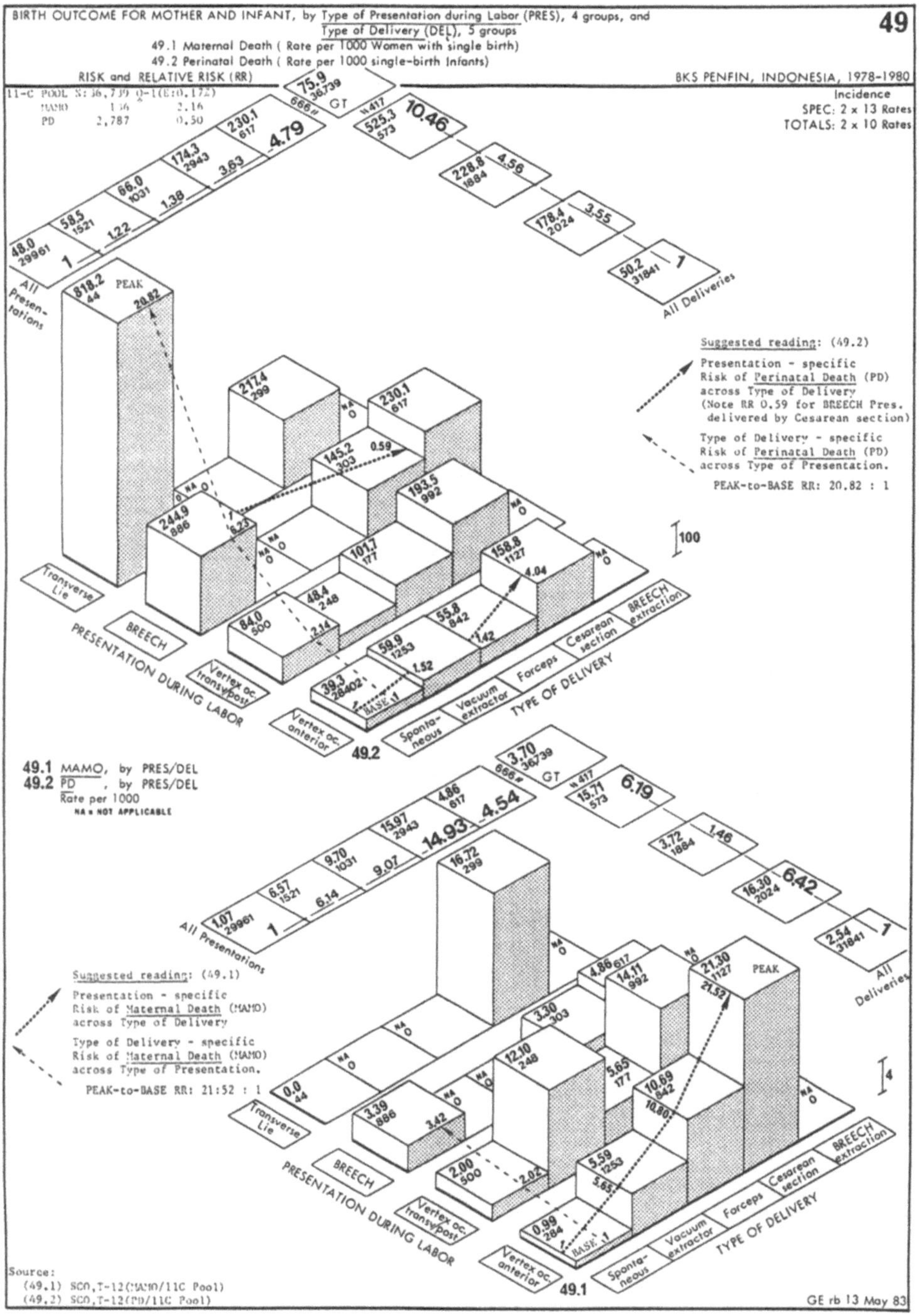

Fig. 8 (Panel 49). Risk of MAMO and PD, by presentation during delivery and type of delivery

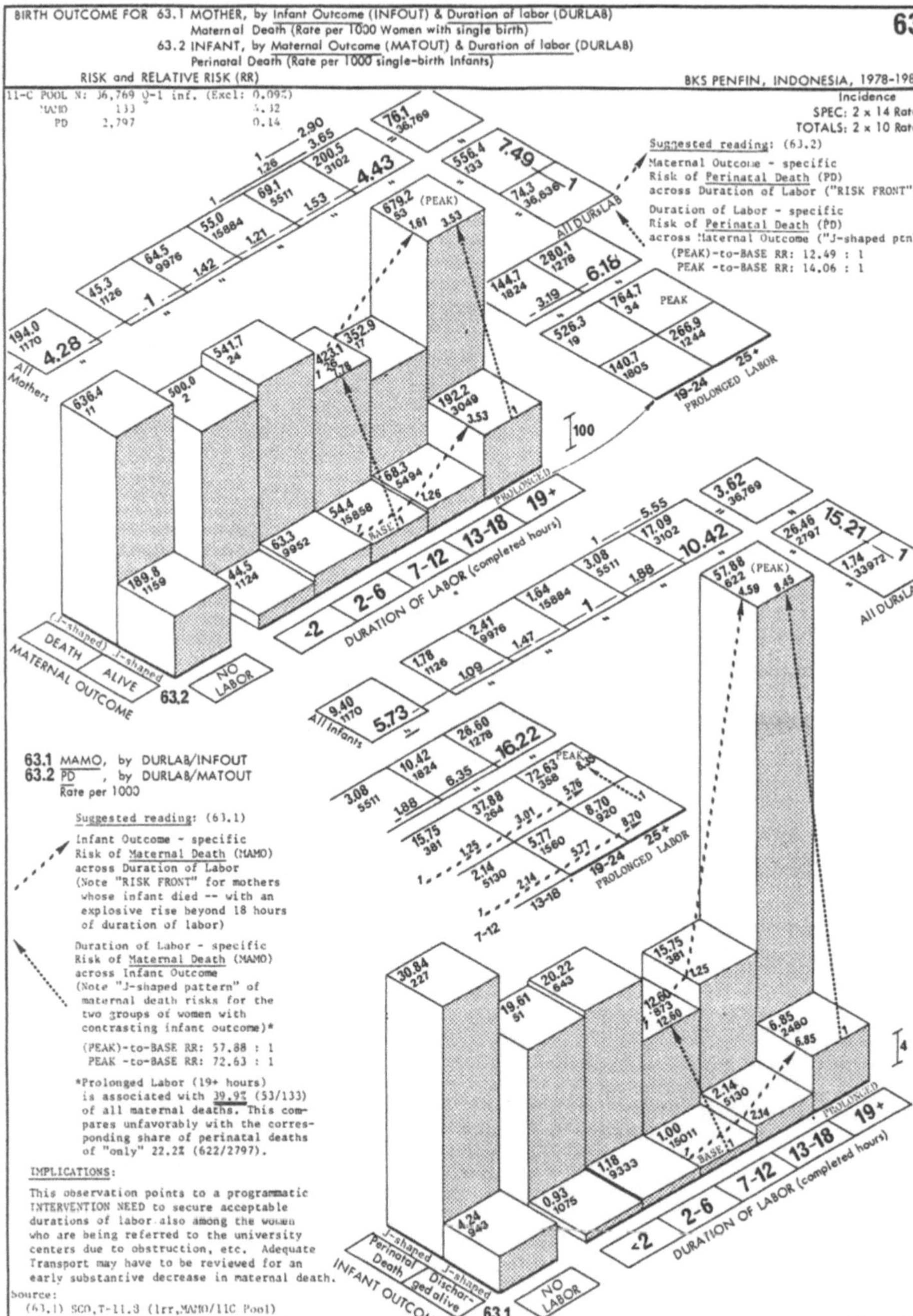

Fig. 9 (Panel 63). Risk of MAMO, by infant outcome and duration of labor, and risk of PD, by maternal outcome and duration of labor

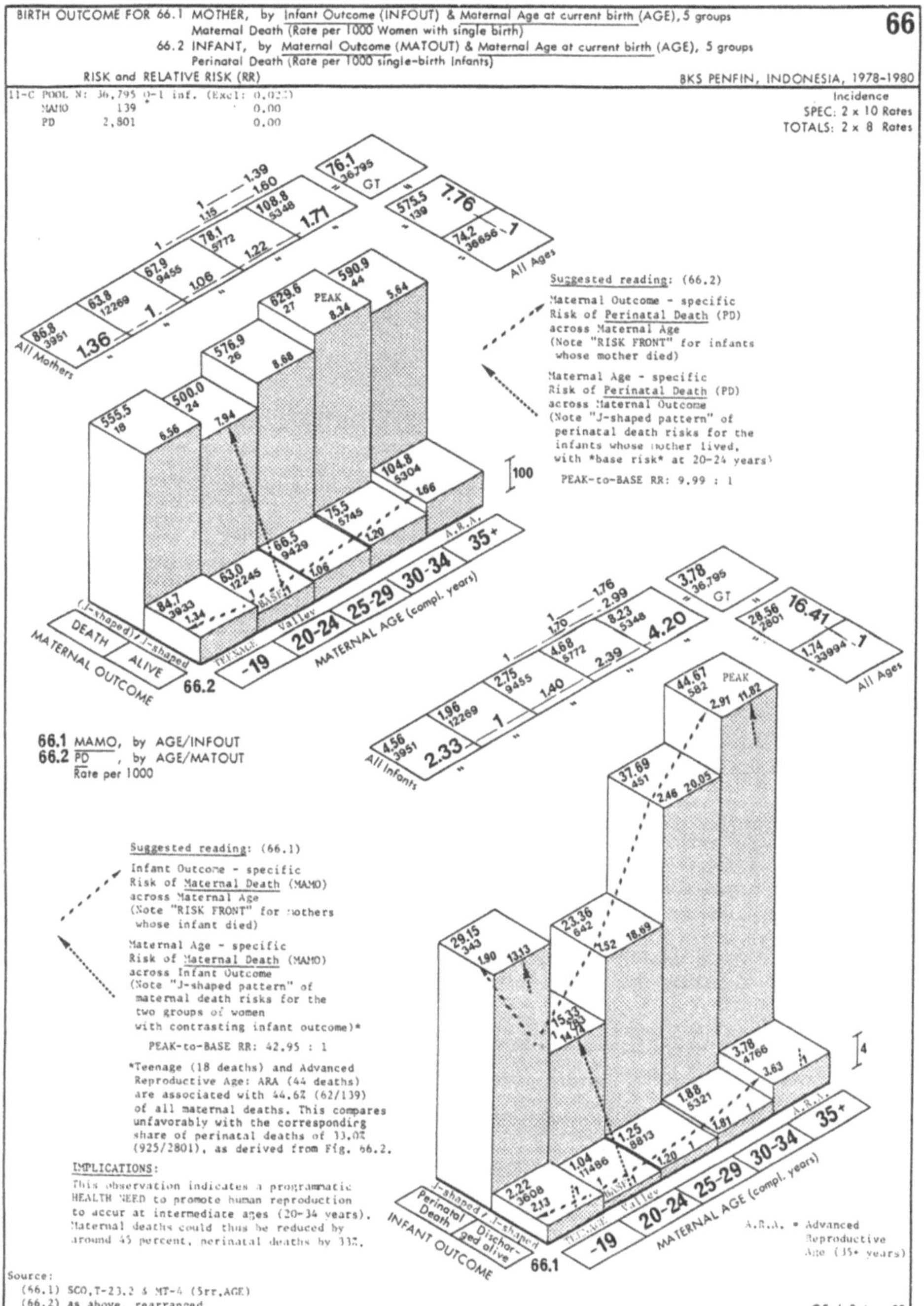

Fig. 10 (Panel 66). Risk of MAMO, by infant outcome and maternal age, and risk or PD, by maternal outcome and maternal age

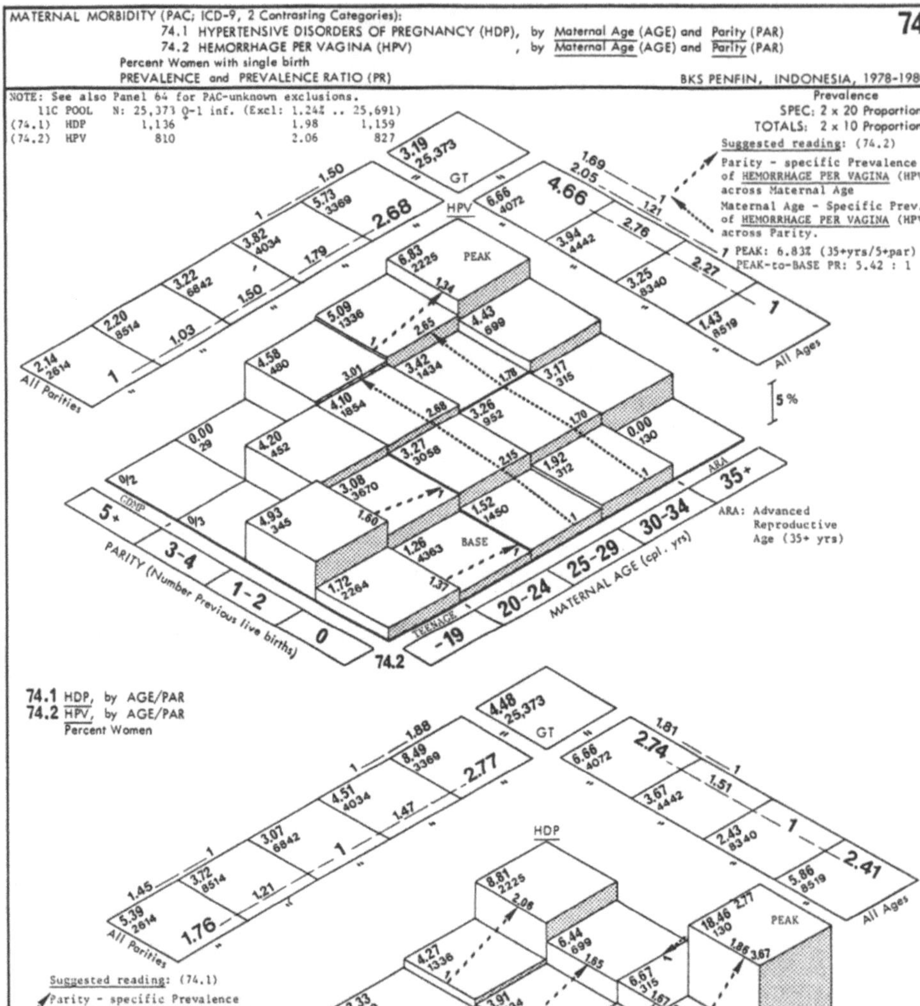

Fig. 11 (Panel 74). Hypertensive disorders of pregnancy (HDP), by age and parity, and hemorrhage per vagina, by age and parity

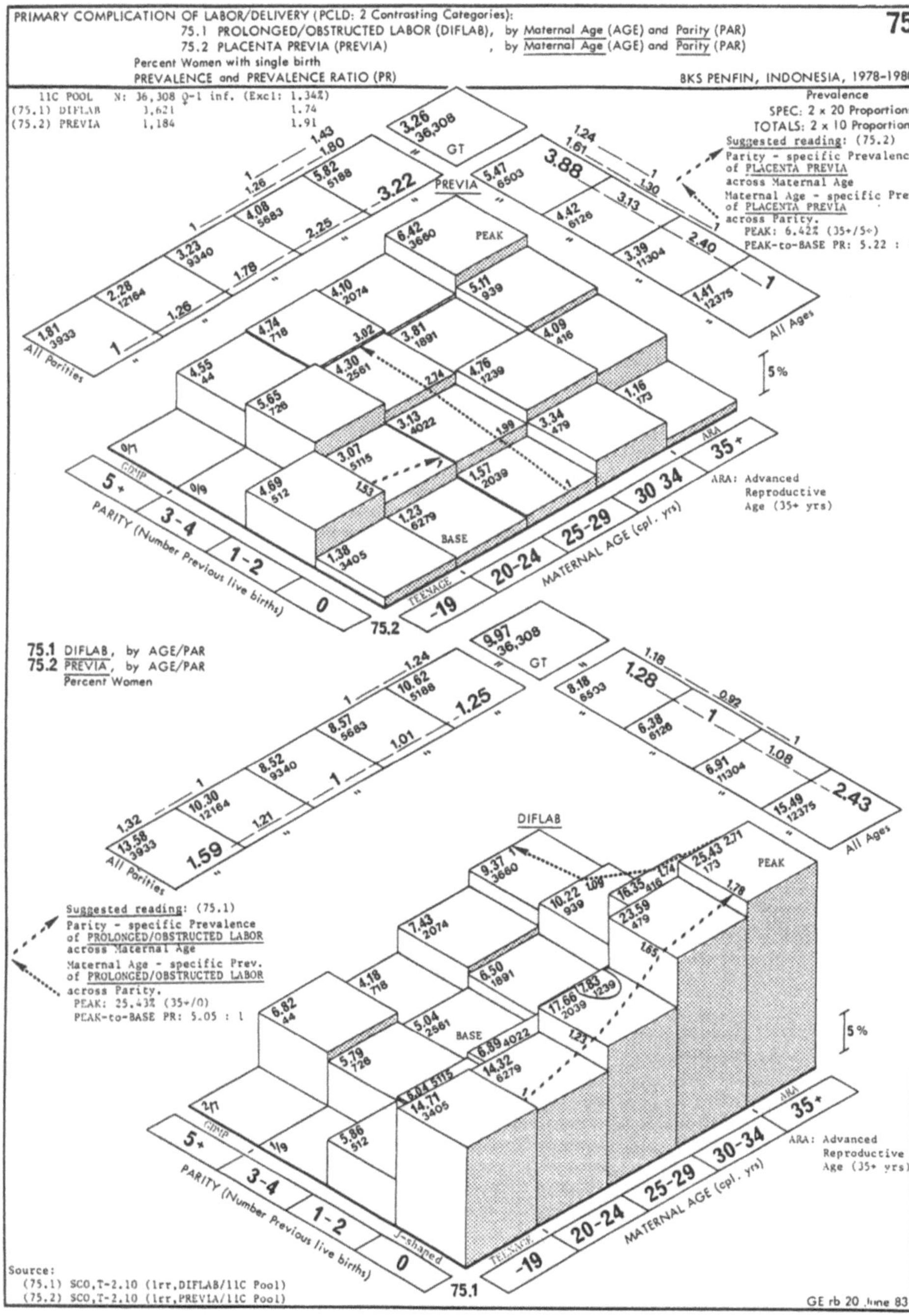

Fig. 12 (Panel 75). Prolonged/obstructed labor, by age and parity, and placenta previa (PREVIA), by age and parity

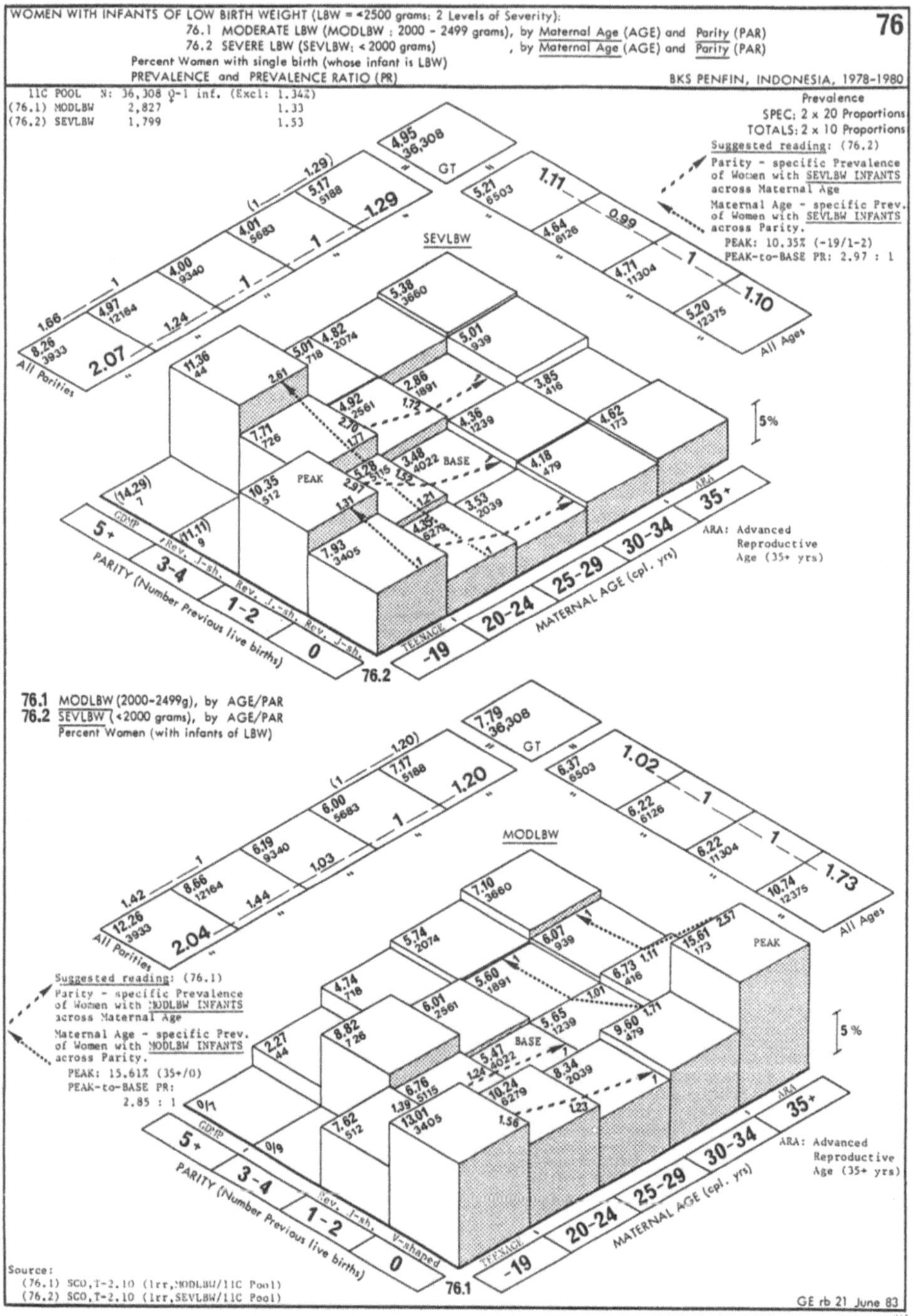

Fig. 13 (Panel 76). Moderately low birth weight (MODLBW), by age and parity, and severely low birth weight (SEVLBW), by age and parity

cal and paramedical, for a better understanding and selection of priorities in *primary reproductive health care provision.*

References

1. Bernard RP (1977) Maternity care monitoring: a new opportunity in service statistics. Population reports, Series J 17:338–339
2. Bernard RP, De Watteville H, Kessel E, et al. (1979) International maternity care monitoring: results of a pretest. Int J Gnaecol Obstet 17:24–39
3. Bernard RP, Kendall EM, Peng JY, et al. (1979) Maternity care monitoring (MCM): where next? In: Sodhy LS (ed) Proceedings, IGCC/IFRP East and South East Asia seminar on regional fertility research, Bangkok, Thailand, 18–20 July 1979. Available from IGCC, PO box 550, Kuala Lumpur, Malaysia, pp 1–24
4. Bernard RP, Kendall EM, Manton KG (1980) International maternity care monitoring: a beginning. In: Aladjem S, Brown AK (eds) Clinical perinatology, 2nd edn. Mosby, St. Louis, chap 23, pp 521–559
5. Bernard RP, Sulaiman S, Agoestina T, et al. (1980) Maternity care monitoring (MCM) in Indonesia: early findings and implications for the 1980's. Indonesian J Obstet Gynaecol, 6:191–290

Additional Reading

Backett EM, Davies AM, Petros-Barvazian A (1984) The risk approach in health care. WHO Public Health Papers, No 76. World Health Organization, Geneva

Bernard RP, Sulaiman S (1983) Maternity care and perinatal mortality in Indonesia. In: Mundo FD, Ines-Cuyegkeng E, Aviado DM (eds) Primary maternal and neonatal health: a global concern. Proceedings of the 1st int. congress of IAMANEH, Manila, Philippines, 2–7 Nov, 1981. Plenum, New York, pp 265–305

Bernard RP, Sulaiman S (1983) Risk of death at birth for mother and infant: 3D display for a multivariate control system (MCM-28). RISK ATLAS with 76 panels. In preparation. BKS PENFIN/IFFH/IAMANEH

Bernard RP, Kendall EM, Potts DM (1980) Promotion of postpartum contraception using MCM as a tool of management. In: Schima ME & Lubell I (eds) Voluntary sterilization: a decade of achievement. Available from AVS, 708 Third Av., New York, 10017, USA, pp 197–205

FIGO NEWS (1980) Int J Gyn Obstet 15:476–477

Freedman R (1980) The future of the world fertility survey. Work paper No 9, plenary session. World Fertility Survey conference. Wembley conference centre, London, 7–11 July 1980. Available at WFS, 35–37 Grosvenor Gardens, London SW1W OBS

Omran AR (1983) Interrelations between maternal and neonatal health and family planning: conceptualization of the theme. In: Mundo FD, Ines-Cuyegkeng E, Aviado DM (eds) Primary maternal and neonatal health: a global concern. Plenum, New York, pp 23–42

Sulaiman S, Agoestina T, Bernard RP (1981) Maternity care monitoring in Indonesia (MCM-14): surveillance research tabulations (SR TABLES) assembled from standard computer outputs (SCOs). Findings presented at the 3rd Annual Meeting of BKS PENFIN, Bandung, November 1981. Available from BKS PENFIN, Bandung, Indonesia

WHO/GE (1977) International classification of diseases, vol 1, 2. Available from World Health Organization, Geneva

Maternal Transmission of Hepatitis B and Its Prevention

C.-L. Chen, Y.-M. Chang, C.-C. Lin, and J.-Y. Lin

Introduction

It is well established that hepatitis B virus (HBV) plays an important role as the cause of liver cirrhosis and/or heaptocellular carcinoma. It has been estimated that there are approximately 200 million HBV carriers throughout the world and perhaps 25% of them die from liver cirrhosis and/or hepatocellular carcinoma. Maternal transmission of HBV to the newborn is one of the most important routes because the newborn is vulnerable and high frequency of transmission occurs during perinatal period.

In Taiwan approximately 15%–20% of the population are HBV carriers and at least 40% were infected by their own mothers. Among the HBs antigen (HBsAg) carriers, 40%–50% are HBe antigen (HBeAg) positive. When the mothers are HBeAg-positive HBsAg carriers, more than 90% of their babies are infected with HBV. Most of the newborns infected with HBV are asymptomatic but have a tendency to become chronic HBsAg carriers. Eighty percent of infected babies in Taiwan remained HBsAg positive for 6 months or more; by contrast a chronic carrier state results in only 5%–10% of cases when infection occurs at a later age.

The route of transmission from mother to baby remains uncertain; however, several possible routes have been suggested, including:

1. Leakage of virus across the placenta in late pregnancy or during delivery
2. Swallowing of amniotic fluid or maternal blood
3. Close contact with the mother through the mother's saliva
4. Early breast-feeding through the mother's milk

Study of Sources of HBV Transmission

For the study of the sources of HBV transmission from the mother, maternal blood, cord blood, maternal colostrum and saliva were examined for HBsAg and HBeAg. 3286 women who attended prenatal clinics of the Taipei Municipal Women's and Children's Hospital between 5 January and 19 July 1983 were routinely screened for HBsAg and HBeAg by radioimmunoassay (Abbott). Of

Primary Health Care in the Making
Ed. by U. Laaser, R. Senault, H. Viefhues

them, 544 (16.6%) were HBsAg positive. Of 535 cases of HBsAg-positive maternal blood, 211 were also HBeAg positive, while none of 863 cases of HBsAg-negative maternal blood was HBeAg positive. Cord blood, colostrum and saliva of the HBsAg-positive mothers were also tested for HBsAg and HBeAg. Cord blood was taken by venipuncture to avoid contamination of maternal blood, and colostrum was collected by milking the breast at the 3rd or 4th day after delivery. Saliva was collected at the 2nd or 3rd day after delivery.

Results

In only 9.9% of cases did the cord blood reveal HBsAg positivity, while in 71% of cases it was HBeAg positive. The molecular weight of HBeAg is lower than that of HBsAg, and it is thus easier for it to cross the placenta.

In 38.6% of cases the colostrum was HBsAg positive and in 57.7% it was HBeAg positive. Apparently it is easier for HBeAg to cross the breast. Maternal saliva was HBsAg positive in 62.3%, and HBeAg positive in 48.1%.

Cord blood from the HBeAg-positive mothers was HBeAg positive in 88%; this again shows the ease of passage across the placenta. HBeAg in the cord blood implicates the possibility of congenital infection with HBV.

In 75.7% of cases, colostrum from HBeAg-positive mothers was HBeAg positive. Although Beasley et al. (1975) reported no evidence for a relationship between breast feeding and the subsequent development of antigenaemia in a follow-up study of 147 babies born to mothers who were HBsAg carriers in Taiwan, colostrum from the HBeAg-positive mother cannot be excluded as the possible source of HBV infection. Saliva from the mothers of HBeAg carriers was HBeAg positive in 58%. Close contact of the baby to the HBeAg-positive mother is another possible route of HBV transmission from the mother to the baby through the maternal saliva.

The actual roles of these possible routes of transmission have not been determined. A follow-up study of the babies born to these mothers with positive HBsAg and/or HBeAg is now being undertaken.

Hepatitis B Immune Globulin (HBIG)

One approach to treatment of maternal transmission is the use of HBIG. Beasley et al. (1975) reported trial of HBIG in babies born to mothers with high HBsAg titres in Taiwan. The babies received injection of HBIG or placebo immediately after birth. All infants were followed for 15 months or more. Among 35 placebo-treated infants, the carrier rate of HBsAg was 91%; this compared with a carrier rate of only 23% among 40 infants who received 0.5 ml HBIG at birth, 3 months and 6 months, and a 45% carrier rate among 42 infants receiving a single 1.0 ml dose of HBIG at birth only. Efficacy was 75% and 45% respectively for the two treatment schedules.

HBV Vaccine

HBsAg vaccine is highly immunogenic in young children and infants as well as in adults. Even the presence of passive antibodies does not interfere with the development of an active response to vaccine.

Recently, Beasley and co-workers studied the prevention of perinatally transmitted HBV infections with HBIG in combination with HB vaccine. All 17 570 women attending prenatal clinics at our hospital and the McKay Memorial Hospital between 16 November 1981 and 31 December 1982 were routinely screened for HBsAg by reverse passive haemagglutination. 2561 were found to be positive (14.6%). Each HBsAg-positive specimen was tested for HBeAg and 1026 were positive (40.1%). Infants of these women who were delivered at the hospital with a birth weight of at least 3000 g and a 1-min Apgar score of at least 9 were included in the study on a voluntary basis. The study concerns the 159 infants who received HBIG and vaccine and 84 controls, all 243 of whom were at least 9 months of age at the time of this analysis.

Immunization Schedule

All infants except controls received 0.5 ml HBIG (Abbott Laboratory) shortly after birth (2.1 ± 4.8 h) and vaccine in different temporal combinations thereafter. Twenty micrograms of vaccine provided by Merck, Sharp and Dohme Laboratory was used.

Group A infants received HBIG at birth and a second dose at 3 months of age, at which time vaccination was initiated (88.6 ± 14.5 days). Group B infants received HBIG at birth only, and vaccination was initiated at 4–7 days of age (6.3 ± 1.5 days). Group C infants received HBIG at birth only, and vaccination was initiated at approximately 1 month of age (30.2 ± 4.3 days). In all three groups the initial vaccination was followed by boosters at 1 month and 6 months. Follow-up visits were scheduled at 3-monthly intervals following birth. At each visit, blood specimens were obtained. Of the 159 infants, 136 completed all follow-up visits.

Results

Only 9 of 159 (5.7%) infants treated with any of the three HBIG vaccine schedules developed the chronic HBsAg carrier state, in contrast to 74 of 84 (88.1%) of the control infants who received no prophylaxis. Thus the overall protective efficacy of HBV vaccine was 93.6%. The HBsAg carrier rate was 2.0%, 6.0% and 8.6% among infants in the three prophylaxis schedules: differences which were not statistically significant.

All 150 infants who did not become HBsAg carriers developed anti-HBs antibodies, usually with very high levels.

An active nationwide control programme against hepatitis B, including vaccination, has been launched recently.

References

1. Beasley RP, Steven CE, Shiao IS, Meng HC (1975) Evidence against breast-feeding as a mechanism for vertical transmission of hepatitis B. Lancet 740
2. Beasley RP, Hwang LY, Lin CC, Leu ML, Stevens CE, Szmuness W, Chen KP (1982) Incidence of hepatitis B virus infections in preschool children in Taiwan. J Infect Dis 146:198–204
3. Beasley RP, Hwang LY, Stevens CE, Lin CC, Hsieh FJ, Wang KY, Sun TS, Szmuness W (1983) Efficacy of Hepatitis B Immune Globulin (HBIG) for prevention of perinatal transmission of the HBV carrier state: Final report of a randomized double-blind placebo-controlled trial. Hepatology 3:135–141
4. Beasley RP, Hwang LY, Lee CY, Chen CL, Hwang FY, Wu CL, Lan CC, Roan CH (1983) Efficacy of HBV vaccine for the interruption of the perinatally transmitted hepatitis B virus carrier state. N Engl J Med (in press)
5. Beasley RP, Hwang LY, Lee GCY, Lan CC, Roan CH, Huang F, Chen CL (Nov. 1983) Prevention of Perinatally Transmitted Hepatitis B Virus Infections with Hepatitis B Immune Globulin and Hepatitis B Vaccine. Lancet No. 8359, 1099–1102

Psychosocial Factors in Childhood Diseases in Nigeria: A Preliminary Study

L. V. Adekunle and O. S. Oduntan

Introduction

Stress in sociological terms usually implies distress, that is, any situation that produces disturbances or disrupts the normal flow of social activities. Several researchers have observed that disruption of the social system, e.g. economic depressions, social change or the breakdown of law and order, often create severe psychological damage or threats to individuals in the social system. These threats were found to have profound effects on physical and mental ability, especially in the form of disturbances related to 'emotion or coping' [9]. As defined by psychologists, therefore, stress 'is any system in which organization or individual are taxed by stimulus conditions beyond the demands of individual ability to adapt or cope' [8].

Few researchers have tried to study the close association between disease and stress. According to Hass [6], for the individual, things just seem to get tougher. He is of the opinion that though we need to be successful, to be liberated and to be loved, fulfilment of these needs always seems just beyond our grasp. Our craving for more self-assurance and self-knowledge is coupled with more and more self-doubt. In short, we are living through an age of stressful change caused by convulsive waves of shifting values on every front. The first series of problems in the hierarchy of social changes are those that produce stress. These are drug abuse, alcoholism, mental illness, teenage pregnancy, venereal disease, divorce, child beating, wife abuse, inflation, unemployment and so on. Thus, Homes et al. [7] concluded, "the more charges you have, the more likely you are to get sick". He and his colleagues, in their study of stress and disease, remarked that one of the by-products of rapid diverse changes in our lives was increased susceptibility to illness; this is especially so when it requires much efforts to cope with our environment, in which case we have less to spare for preventing disease.

Several other researchers have also observed a close association between social changes and occurence of illness. For example, Haggart et al. [5] found that a common crisis such as death of an important member of the family, change in residence or loss of job reduced some groups of children's susceptibility to infection. Such groups of children often exhibit streptococcal infection 2 weeks after the crisis.

Primary Health Care in the Making
Ed. by U. Laaser, R. Senault, H. Viefhues

Groern's [4] studies on the influence of psychosocial factors on bronchial asthma found that the sociocultural root of bronchial asthma lies in the psychological structure of the family. Much better results were achieved by transferring patients, especically children, from the parental or family environment to specific asthma institutions. The large majority of the patients were noted not to have an attack even without any special anti-allergic measures, and in the majority of the cases attacks reoccurred sooner or later after the patient returned to his family environment. Hence, she concluded that asthma started as a disturbed pattern in reaction to frustration of the individual by a beloved but domineering authority figure. The disease was said to be responsible for a good deal of absenteeism from school and industry, thereby causing economic loss to the society.

However, as important as this area of research is, relatively few if any attempts have been made in Nigeria to study closely the interrelationship between social stress and childhood illness. Hence, this investigation examines the effect of psychosocial factors, if any, on childhood patterns of disease severity and outcome. We hope the result will be useful in the treatment, rehabilitation and prevention of some childhood diseases.

Methodology

A sample of 1500 mothers whose children were either admitted to hospital or were attending the out-patient unit of the hospital were selected for interview. The selection was made on a proportional basis from children seen at the general out-patient department, those seen in the emergency room, and those admitted to the hospital wards of the three urban hospitals, namely University College Hospital, Adeoyo State Hospital, and Catholic Hospital, all of which are in Ibadan, Nigeria. Data were obtained from mothers whose children were below 5 years old. Information obtained included the pattern of the child's disease and its severity based on the doctor's diagnosis on contact or on admission, complications (if any) since admission and outcome of the disease. Other information obtained included the family structure and social conditions, the mother's reaction to the disease, and the treatment given prior to hospital contact, when there was a delay in treatment or the presence of social stress prior to child's illness. Also recorded were the respondents' social characteristics. In the case of motherless babies, the person in charge of the child was interviewed.

Results

Socio-economic Characteristics of the Respondents

Age. About 69.2% of the respondents were below the age of 30 years, while 28.3% were aged 30–50 and only 2.5% were 50 years or above (Table 1).

Table 1. Age of respondents

	No.	%
Below 20	346	23.1
20–29	691	46.1
30–39	396	26.4
40–49	29	1.9
50+	38	2.5
Total	1500	100

Table 2. Religion of respondents

1. Moslem	1022	68.1
2. Christian	336	22.4
3. Other (Traditionalist)	142	9.5
4. Total	1500	100

Religion. A large proportion were Moslem, i.e. 68.1%; 22.4% were Christians, and the rest – 9.5% – professed traditional faith (Table 2).

Education. Over 90% of the fathers were either illiterate or had only some elementary education, while 8.9% had post-primary training (Table 3).

Occupation and Social Class. A large proportion of the children's fathers belonged to the labouring class; 21.1% were drivers, 32.7% were traders and only 3.3% had upper and middle level occupations (Table 4).

Table 3. Educational level of father

	No.	%
1. Illiterate	3631	42.0
2. Primary	689	45.9
3. Arabic training	19	1.2
4. Adult education	18	1.2
5. Modern school	77	5.1
6. Secondary school	53	3.5
7. University	15	0.3
Total	1500	100

Table 4. Social class based on father's occupation

I.	Professional, businessman etc.	9	0.6
II.	Middle level manpower (e.g. civil servants)	40	2.7
III.	Drivers	317	21.1
IV.	Traders	491	32.7
V.	Farmers	329	21.9
VI.	Labourers	166	11.1
VII.	Unemployed	111	7.4
VIII.	Students	37	2.5
	Total	1500	100

Table 5. Sex of the children

	No.	%
Male	837	56
Female	663	44
Total	1500	100

Table 6. Age of the children

	No.	%
Under 3 months	158	10.5
4–7 months	194	12.9
8–11 months	208	13.8
1–2 years	504	33.6
3–4 years	239	15.9
5+	193	13.3
Total	1500	100

Table 7. Birth rank of children (by mother)

	No.	%
1st child	318	21.2
2nd child	348	23.2
3rd Child	443	29.5
4th child	217	14.5
5th child and above	174	11.6
Total	1500	100

Socio-economic Characteristics of the Child

Sex. The vulnerability of the male sex as against that of the female was confirmed: 56% of the sick children were male (Table 5).

Age. A third of the sick children were aged 1 – 2 years; of the rest, approximately equal numbers were below 1 year or above 2 years old (Table 6).

Birth Rank. Almost 30% of the sick children were the third child in the hierarchy by mothers; 21% were the first child, and 23.2% were the second child (Table 7).

Pattern of Illness

Measles and diarrhoea accounted for over 80% of the child hospitalization and 84% of the child illness. Among other illnesses, bronchopneumonia accounted for 3.8% and 1.5% of out-patients and in-patients respectively, convulsions for only 1.4% and 1.5%, and tetanus for 1.4% and 0.2% (Table 8).

Severity. Only 14.9% of the illnesses were very severe; 72% were mild, and 13.1% moderate (Table 9).

Outcome. Over 63% of the children were discharged alive and well, while 25.6% had some residual damage and 11.1% died (Table 10).

Table 8. Pattern of disease

	Out-patient		In-patient	
	No.	%	No.	%
Measles	442	40.9	186	44.3
Bronchopneumonia	20	1.8	16	3.8
Diarrhoea	580	53.6	161	28.3
Meningitis	7	0.6	10	2.4
Convulsions	16	1.5	6	1.4
Malaria	6	0.6	31	7.4
Tetanus	4	0.4	8	1.2
Polio	5	0.5	2	0.5
Malnutrition	2	0.2	0	
Total	1082	100	420	100

Table 9. Severity of disease

1. Very severe	224	14.9
2. Moderate	196	13.1
3. Mild	1080	72.0
Total	1500	100

Table 10. Outcome of disease

	No.	%
i. Discharged well and alive	940	63.3
ii. Discharged with residual damage	384	25.6
iii. Dead	176	11.1
Total	1500	100

Family Social Conditions (Tables 11–14)

Thirty-two percent of the children had no father while 7.7% were motherless. The rest – 59.5% – had both parents alive. A large proportion of the families were polygamous – 87.3% – and over 61% had between one and four children. With regard to family stability, 47.7% of the children's parents were either divorced, separated or dead (Table 13). Over 48% lived with a grandmother, and 44.7% were being maintained economically by this grandmother (Tables 14 and 15).

Table 11. Family social conditions

	No.	%
1. Both parents alive	892	59.5
2. Father alive	489	32.6
3. Mother alive	116	7.7
4. None	3	0.2
Total	1500	100

Table 12. Type of family

	No.	%
1. Monogamous	190	12.7
2. Polygamous	1310	87.3
Total	1500	100

Table 13. Marital status of the parents

	No.	%
(i) Still living together	784	52.3
(ii) Separated	149	9.9
(iii) Divorced	275	18.3
(iv) Dead	292	19.5
Total	1500	100

Table 14. Person(s) with whom the child lives

	No.	%
(1) Paternal grandmother	633	42.2
(2) Maternal grandmother	92	6.1
(3) Father's relative	15	1.0
(4) Mother's relative	33	2.2
(5) Mother alone	39	2.6
(6) Father alone	142	9.5
(7) Both parents	546	36.4
Total	1500	100

Table 15. Person(s) economically responsible for the child

	No.	%
(1) Father alone	183	12.2
(2) Mother alone	140	9.4
(3) Both parents	476	31.7
(4) A grandmother	670	44.7
(5) Other relatives of father	20	1.3
(6) Other relatives of mother	11	0.7
Total	1500	100

Psychosocial Factors

Of the 1500 respondents only 9.2% confessed that there had been a sad occasion in the family prior to the child's illness, and of these 9.2%, over 52.2% responded that the event happened nearly 4 days before the illness (Tables 16 and 17 respectively).

However, on further probing on specific events that occurred 1 or 2 weeks prior to the child's illness, many respondents recalled events such as loss of job or lack of employment (46.5%), absence of financial support from the father or other relative of the child (13.7%), constant quarreling and nagging from husband (4.5%), alcoholism (2.6%) or the death of an important member in the family (1.6%). Only 26% stated that no such event had occurred in the family during the 2 weeks prior to the child's illness (Table 18).

Table 16. Had there been any sad event prior to the child's illness?

	No.	%
(1) Yes	138	9.2
(2) No	1362	90.8
Total	1500	100

Table 17. When did the sad event happen?

	No.	%
(1) A day later	27	19.6
(2) 1–2 days later	18	13.0
(3) 3–4 days later	72	15.2
(4) 4+days later	21	15.2
Total	138	100

Table 18. Did any of these events occur 1–2 weeks prior to your child's illness?

	No.	%
1) Quarrel with husband/wife	68	4.5
2) Death of an important member of the family	24	1.6
3) Separation or divorce	18	1.2
4) Loss of income	205	13.7
5) Loss of job/lack of employment	697	46.5
6) Imprisonment	12	0.8
7) Parents-in-law problems	20	1.4
8) Mental illness	2	0.1
9) Personal disaster	3	0.2
10) Movement from rural to urban area	2	0.1
11) Movement from urban to rural area	–	–
12) Sickness of a family member	10	0.7
13) Alcoholism	40	2.7
14) Unplanned pregnancies	7	0.5
15) None	390	26.0
Total	1500	100

Table 19. How long was the child ill before hospital contact?

	No.	%
Less than 1 day	877	58.5
1–2 days	189	12.6
3–4 days	119	7.9
5–7 days	284	18.9
Over 1 week	3	2.1
Total	1500	100

Table 20. If the child's illness existed for more than 1 day before hospital contact, why was contact not made sooner?

	No.	%
1) Thought the illness would soon go off	262	17.5
2) Gave child care personally, because there was other social pressure	1039	69.3
3) Thought illness was minor	73	4.9
4) Thought it was teething problem	87	5.8
5) Due to transport difficulties	12	0.8
6) Because of personal illness	13	0.9
7) Others	14	0.8
Total	1500	100

Effect of Psychosocial Factors on Childhood Illness

Over 20% of respondents waited more than 1 week before making hospital contact (Table 19). More than 60% confessed to having given the child medication themselves because of social pressure. About 5% thought the illness was minor, while 17.5% thought that the child would recuperate (Table 20).

Effect of the Illness on the Life Patterns of the Family

Of the mothers, 35.1% stated that the child's illness made it impossible for them to carry on other family and domestic responsibilities. 25.6% were unable to work as a result of the illness, while 22.1% fell ill themselves; 17.2% reported having depression (Table 21).

When asked how they had been coping, 69.7% stated through prayer, 28.3% elder's advice and 0.6% family support (Table 22).

Table 21. How has the child's illness affected your life?

	No.	%
1) Unable to work	384	25.6
2) Can not take care of the family properly	526	35.1
3) Feel sick	332	22.1
4) Feel depressed	258	17.2
Total	1500	100

Table 22. How do you cope with the situation?

	No.	%
1) Prayer	1045	69.7
2) Elder's advice	424	28.3
3) Support from family	10	0.6
4) Others (specify)	21	1.4
Total	1500	100

Chi-Square Significant Results (Tables 23–25)

Test of significance showed that there was a significant association between social pressure, pattern of disease, severity and outcome.

Table 23. Chi-square significant result: social pressure pattern of disease

Social pres-sure[a]	Pattern of disease[b]									
	1	2	3	4	5	6	7	8	9	
1	0	30	14	6	0	0	15	0	0	65
	0.0	8.3	2.8	0.9	0.0	0.0	8.3	0.0	0.0	4.5
	0.0	23.8	16.2	36.4	0.0	0.0	23.8	0.0	0.0	
	0.0	2.3	0.8	0.3	0.0	0.0	2.3	0.0	0.0	
2	0	18	1	2	1	0	5	0	0	24
	0.0	9.0	6.3	10.2	16.7	0.0	20.0	0.0	0.0	1.6
	0.0	27.2	0.7	1.0	0.7	0.0	1.9	0.0	0.0	
	0.0	2.7	0.1	0.1	0.1	0.0	0.3	0.0	0.0	
3	0	9	1	3	2	1	1	0	0	18
	0.0	2.0	14.3	0.5	0.5	14.3	0.2	0.0	0.0	1.2
	0.0	34.6	0.4	27.3	25.0	0.7	100.0	0.0	0.0	
	0.0	0.6	0.1	0.2	0.2	0.1	0.1	0.0	0.0	
4	13	240	0	0	0	1	20	3	1	265
	61.9	45.2	0.0	0.0	0.0	14.3	45.2	0.7	14.3	13.7
	2.0	80.7	0.0	0.0	0.0	0.6	5.8	18.9	0.7	
	0.9	35.5	0.0	0.0	0.0	0.1	2.5	0.5	0.1	
5	14	634	0	4	0	0	37	1	1	697
	13.1	14.9	0.0	8.8	0.0	0.0	6.3	0.1	6.3	46.5
	5.7	73.2	0.0	5.4	0.0	0.0	0.6	100.0	0.7	
	0.7	11.7	0.0	0.5	0.0	0.0	0.1	0.1	0.1	
6	1	3	7	0	0	0	2	0	1	12
	0.2	19.0	8.8	0.0	0.0	0.0	4.8	0.0	1.1	0.8
	100.0	2.1	5.4	0.0	0.0	0.0	0.7	0.0	8.3	
	0.1	0.3	0.5	0.0	0.0	0.0	0.1	0.0	0.1	
7	2	10	4	0	1	0	5	0	0	20
	11.0	38.1	19.0	0.0	0.1	0.0	8.8	0.0	0.0	1.3
	4.8	1.0	2.1	0.0	100.0	0.0	5.4	0.0	0.0	
	0.7	0.5	0.3	0.0	0.1	0.0	0.5	0.0	0.0	
8, 9,	0	7	0	0	0	0	2	0	0	9
10, 14	0.0	11.0	0.0	0.0	0.0	0.0	1.1	0.0	0.0	0.5
	0.0	5.2	0.0	0.0	0.0	0.0	9.1	0.0	0.0	
	0.0	0.7	0.0	0.0	0.0	0.0	0.1	0.0	0.0	
11	0	1	0	9	0	0	0	0	0	10
	0.0	0.1	0.0	11.9	0.0	0.0	0.0	0.0	0.0	0.6
	0.0	100.0	0.0	6.3	0.0	0.0	0.0	0.0	0.0	
	0.0	0.1	0.0	0.7	0.0	0.0	0.0	0.0	0.0	
13	0	30	0	5	0	2	0	3	0	40
	0.0	1.9	0.0	25.0	0.0	12.5	0.0	26.7	0.0	2.6
	0.0	34.6	0.0	0.4	0.0	0.7	0.0	3.3	0.0	
	0.0	1.5	0.0	0.1	0.0	0.1	0.0	0.5	0.0	
15	10	315	0	5	1	15	0	10	0	390
	17.9	34.4	0.0	16.7	0.4	16.7	0.0	0.9	0.0	26.0
	6.3	80.2	0.0	2.6	100.0	6.7	0.0	90.0	0.0	
	1.0	26.9	0.0	2.3	0.1	0.9	0.0	0.7	0.0	
Total	45	1303	28	16	9	17	77	13	3	1500
	3.0	86.9	1.9	1.1	0.6	5.1	0.9	0.2	0.2	100

$\chi^2 = 513.30835$; $df = 135$; significance < 0.001

[a] According to Table 18 [b] According to Table 8

Table 24. Chi-square significant result: social pressure/severity of disease

Social pressure[a]	Severity of disease[b]			
	1	2	3	
1	11	9	45	65
	33.0	45.0	9.0	4.5
	1.3	1.4	27.2	
	0.7	0.6	2.7	
2	10	6	8	24
	62.5	2.8	12.0	1.6
	1.2	16.2	25.5	
	0.7	0.8	3.5	
3	1	3	14	18
	0.2	75.0	13.6	1.2
	100.0	0.4	38.0	
	0.1	0.2	4.0	
4	32	35	178	265
	16.0	11.6	45.7	13.7
	38.9	34.5	307	
	6.2	4.5	13.5	
5	154	63	480	697
	33.8	10.0	38.4	46.5
	28.7	36.7	34.8	
	15.9	3.9	21.2	
6	0	1	11	12
	0.0	0.2	62.5	0.8
	0.0	100.0	1.2	
	0.0	0.1	1.7	
7	4	4	13	20
	42.9	57.1	62.5	1.3
	0.4	0.6	1.2	
	0.2	0.3	0.7	
8, 9,	0	0	9	9
10, 14	0.0	0.0	0.5	0.5
	0.0	0.0	53.6	
	0.0	0.0	0.3	
11	1	1	8	10
	16.7	33.3	50.0	0.6
	100.0	0.3	0.4	
	0.1	0.1	0.2	
13	10	5	25	40
	62.5	37.5	7.8	2.6
	1.2	0.9	20.9	
	0.7	0.4	2.2	
15	40	70	280	390
	11.6	13.4	44.0	26.0
	34.5	37.5	38.7	
	4.5	5.2	17.0	
Total	224	196	1080	1500
	14.9	13.1	72	100

$\chi^2 = 340.31738$; $df = 45$; significance < 0.001 [a] According to Table 18 [b] According to Table 9

Table 25. Chi-square significant result: social pressure/outcome of disease

Social pressure[a]	Outcome of disease[b]			
1	35	29	1	65
	53.5	51.6	0.1	4.5
	11.0	1.9	50.0	
	6.1	1.1	0.1	
2	12	12	0	24
	48.4	51.6	0.0	1.6
	2.3	1.9	0.0	
	1.0	1.1	0.0	
3	1	8	9	18
	6.3	37.5	56.3	1.2
	100.0	0.9	1.1	
	0.1	0.4	0.0	
4	153	105	7	265
	58.2	41.8	43.8	13.7
	17.1	15.5	1.1	
	9.5	6.8	0.5	
5	442	164	91	697
	46.1	61.8	53.5	46.4
	57.5	13.9	6.1	
	25.3	7.7	11.0	
6	7	5	0	12
	0.5	71.4	0.0	0.8
	11.1	0.6	0.0	
	0.1	0.3	0.0	
7	10	10	0	20
	37.5	51.6	0.0	1.3
	0.9	1.9	0.0	
	0.4	1.1	0.0	
8, 9,	0	9	0	9
10, 14	0.0	56.3	0.0	0.5
	0.0	1.1	0.0	
	0.0	0.6	0.0	
11	9	1	0	10
	56.3	6.3	0.0	0.6
	1.6	100.0	0.0	
	0.6	0.1	0.0	
13	30	10	0	40
	48.4	1.0	0.0	2.6
	1.9	38.9	0.0	
	0.6	0.5	0.0	
15	250	62	78	390
	52.8	45.9	45.9	26.0
	52.4	11.8	11.8	
	28.9	5.2	5.2	
Total	949	384	176	1500
	63.3	25.6	11.1	100

$\chi^2 = 368.6384$; $df = 45$; significance < 0.001

[a] According to Table 18

[b] According to Table 10

Discussion

The results of this research tend to confirm the observations of many psychologists [2, 13] who have perceived health as a function of the harmony which an individual is able to achieve in a social, physical and cultural environment. There is no doubt that social pressure and cultural factors played an important part in the severity and outcome of the diseases of the children studied. Thus the study also tends to confirm Zbronwski's [14] statement that "When considering actual exposure to a disease and subsequent contracting of it, the traditional factors such as filth, overcrowding, and other class related variables may be important; *however, of more importance is the feedback concerning rates of illness and reaction to disease rather than more exposure to it.*"

In this study it has been shown that people's positive or negative reaction to childhood disease depended on the state of mind of the mothers or guardians of the children. This may also be a reflection of the enormous social pressure that preoccupied their mind during the initial stage of the child's illness.

The effect of social pressure on the preventive health behaviour of mothers in general was highlighted in an earlier investigation [1].

Many lives might have been saved if only mothers had appreciated the immense dangers facing their children when they reacted poorly to preventive health services or failed to report to the hospital at the appropriate time. It is obvious that early detection, early diagnosis and early treatment are essential for good recovery from diseases, especially those of noted high morbidity. This phenomenon may be illustrated as follows:

1. It was observed during the course of this study that many babies died of neonatal jaundice because the parents were preoccupied with the 8th-day naming ceremony. By the time they were ready to bring the child to the hospital, it was usually too late to save the child.
2. A 9-month-old girl was first seen at the children's ward. At that time, she had already been admitted to the hospital for gastro-enteritis on at least four occasions. The mother was a businesswoman, while the father was a civil servant of intermediate rank. The child was febrile, pale and malnourished. According to the father, the girl was plump and healthy until about 3 months previously, when the mother was jailed for helping a taxis-driver to assault the chauffeur of a high court judge. The father was depressed, and nobody would take care of the child until an elderly aunt of the father who was about 69 years old assumed responsibility for the child. The child had suffered so much that she died 3 days after the interview with her parents.
3. A middle-aged mother of a boy who at the time of the interview was about 1½ years old confessed that prior to the child's illness, she had a big quarrel with the child's father about his failure to support her financially when she lost her father. To her this was a big disgrace, since all the other members of her family had their husband's support. She felt depressed and lonely to the extent that when the child's illness first started she paid little attention to it until it became severe.

References

1. Adekunle AV (1977) Child immunization – What are the impediments for reaching desired goals in a traditional society? Soc Sci Med 12:353–357
2. Dubos RJ (1959) Mirage of health. Herper, p 180
3. Gans B (1961) Pediatric problems in Lagos. West Afr Med J
4. Groen J (1971) Psychosocial influences in bronchial asthma. In: Levi L (ed) Society, stress and diseases. New York, pp 352–361
5. Haggert RJ (1975) Family diagnosis: Research methods and their reliability for studies of medical social unit in the family. Am J Paedr Health 55:1521
6. Hass DA (1978) The exhilarating age of stressful change. Amsassador 23–25
7. Holmes TH, Hawkins NG, Bowomen CE, Clerk ER, Jofte RR (1957) Psychosocial and psychophysiologic studies of tuberculosis. Psychosom Med 19:134–143
8. Lazarus RS (1966) Psychological stress and the coping process. New York
9. Lazarus RS, Averil JR, Opton EM (1970) Towards a cognition theory of emotion. In: Arnold M (ed) Feelings and emotion. New York, pp 207–320
10. Morley DC (1963) A medical service for children under five years of age in West Africa. Trans R Soc J Med 57:79–88
11. Oduntan SO (1971) The effect of environmental factors on intellectual behavior of Nigerian children of school age. J Trop Pediatr Environ Child Health 17:67–70
12. Ogbiede MI (1968) The influence of protein calorie malnutrition in patterns of pre-school childhood disease. Clin Pediatr 425
13. Wolff HG (1958) Disease and pattern of behavior. In: Jaco EC (ed) Patients physicians and illness. Glencoe, Ill
14. Zbronwski M (1955) Cultural components in response to pain. In: Jaco EG (ed) Patients, physicians and illness. Free Press, New York

Primary Health Care and Feasibility of Yaws Eradication in India

V. B. Saxena

Because of the marvellous success achieved by yaws control programmes, there was a great temptation to try to achieve the eradication of yaws, but the problem of case detection and surveillance in primitive people in geographically cut-off areas was so difficult that the idea was abandoned, and by 1966–1967 the word 'eradication' had been dropped in connection with anti-yaws activities in most of the reports and documents of WHO [5]. However, the present global drive to strengthen primary health care services in all countries and particularly in developing countries has enhanced the prospects for eradicating yaws. The present paper deals with the feasibility of yaws eradication with special reference to India, where it is being contemplated (NICD 1983, Meeting on yaws, unpublished).

Present Status of the Yaws Problem in India

Yaws in India was mostly a tribal disease of primitive tribal communities living in hilly and forest areas of peripheral regions of Madhya Pradesh, Maharashtra, Andhra Pradesh and Orissa, with some additional pockets in Tamilnadu, Assam, Bihar and Utter Pradesh (see Fig. 1). According to the 1981 Census, there are about 50 million tribes in India and of these, about 9 million are exposed to the risk of yaws because they live in areas where yaws is known to be present. About 0.2 million cases of active yaws were treated under the various yaws control programmes in the country between 1952 and 1964. The prevalence of yaws as detected in these control programmes varied from 15% to 3% during initial surveys and it was less than 1% in most re-surveys. After 1964, control programmes in some states were rounded up into a consolidation phase where the responsibility for detecting and treating residual cases was handed over to the medical and paramedical workers of the newly started network of primary health centres. The number of cases reported officially dwindled very quickly, and in maps prepared by WHO [3] it appears that India is already yaws-free (see Figs. 2, 3).

Auto-eradication of a disease after suspending a control programme is theoretically possible, especially if this is accompanied by simultaneous socio-economic development in the community with regard to roads, schools, cloth-

Primary Health Care in the Making
Ed. by U. Laaser, R. Senault, H. Viefhues

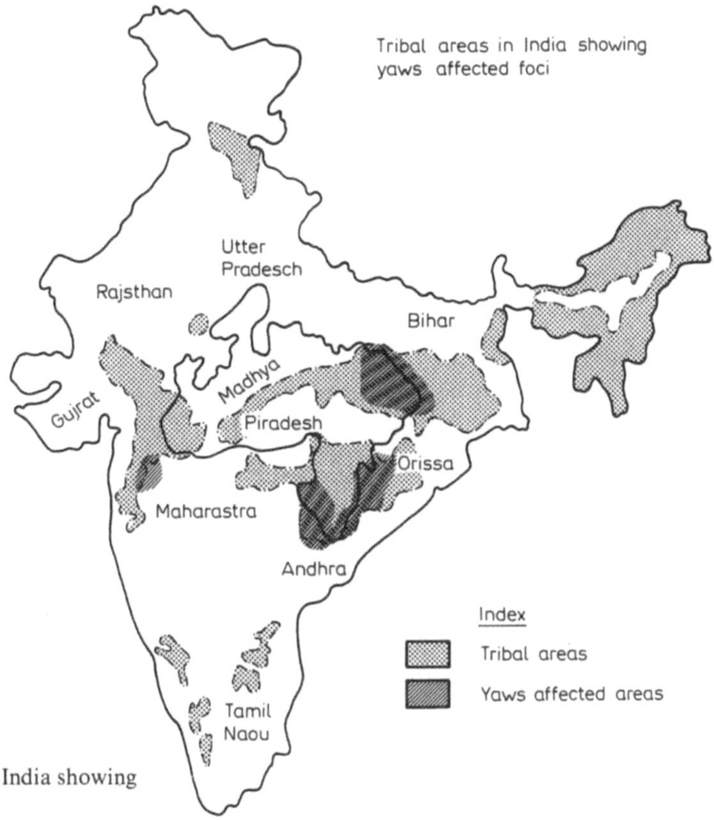

Fig. 1. Tribal areas in India showing yaws-affected foci

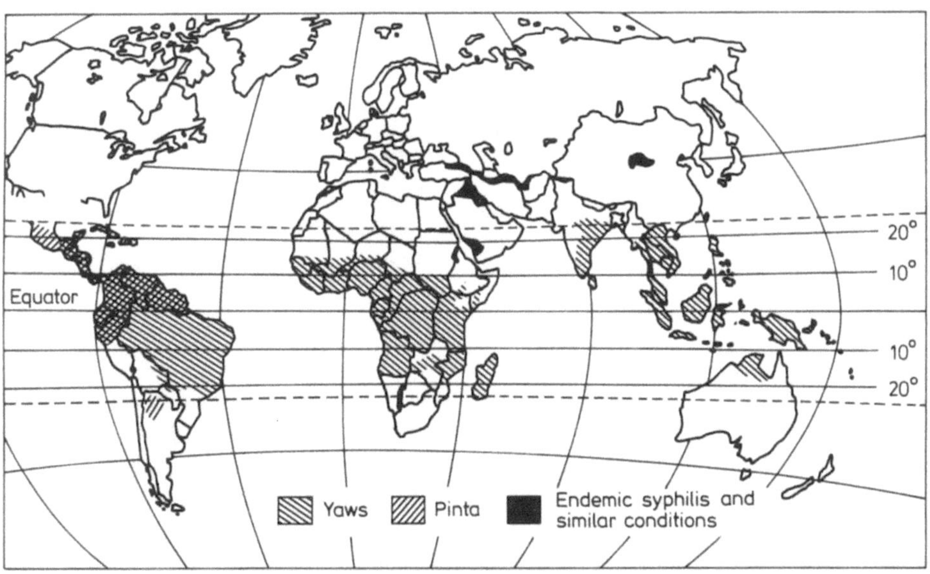

Fig. 2. Geographical distribution of the endemic treponematoses in the early 1950s

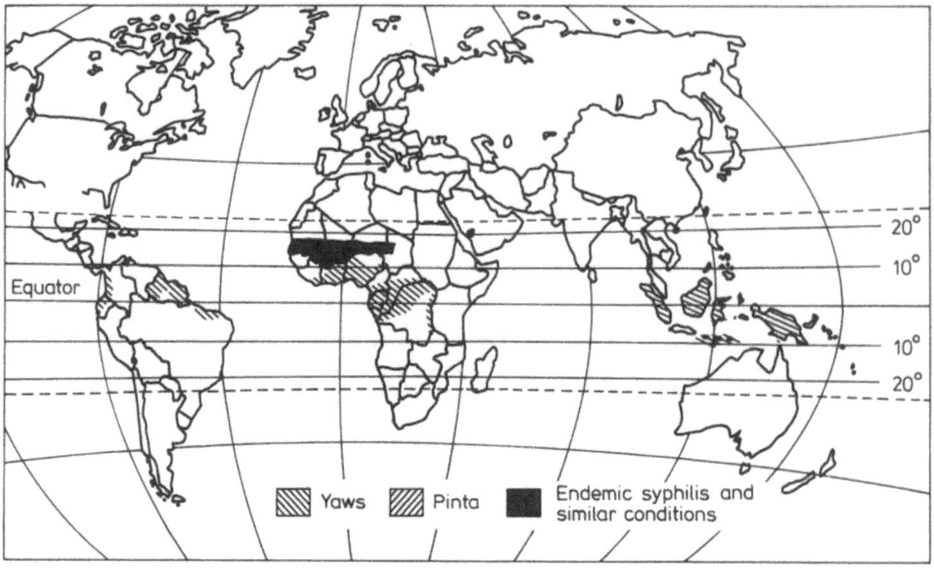

Fig. 3. Geographical distribution of the endemic treponematoses in the early 1980s

Table 1. Recent cases of yaws reported in India (A. N. Raichowdhuri, personal communication)

State	Area	Cases reported		Reporting agency
		Year	Number	
Madhya Pradesh	Baster district (nine villages)	1977	21	Saxena et al. [2]
Orissa	Six tribal districts	1980–82	1222	Four yaws teams in Orissa
Andhra pradesh	Bhadra giri block of Vijaya nagar district	1980	41	Anti-yaws unit Bhadragiri
Andhra pradesh	Bhadrachalam area of Khamman district	1977	150	Anti-yaws unit Bhadrachalan
		1978	136	
		1979	241	
		1980	65	
		1981	229	
Gujrat state	Dang district	1982	3	Dept. of Dermatology, Medical College Baroda

ing etc. However, detailed probing into the yaws reports of India revealed that, as shown in Table 1, cases of yaws continued to occur throughout the period in most of the affected states. The nil report at the WHO level appears to be only a block in the reporting channel and a dampening of the surveillance system. The decline of yaws due to control programme is very likely to have caused a decline of yaws consciousness and a consequent slackness in surveillance. It would not be wise to believe that yaws would be eradicated so quickly without much effort. Even if the problem is that of receding yaws, action is needed in respect of the left over pockets of the disease. If the eradication of yaws is to be expedited, special efforts will be needed to maintain proper yaws consciousness and yaws surveillance in the community.

Problem of Yaws Surveillance

Surveillance is a system of activities originating from mental alertness at various levels to ensure the accurate observation of factors relevant for guiding necessary remedial measures. Surveillance is necessary at both the peripheral and the central level.

For peripheral surveillance, it is important to remember that the resurgence of yaws will take place mostly in cut-off areas, away from roads and during the rainy season, when visits by medical workers are least frequent. Therefore, the active support of the people is very essential for any surveillance in these areas. The primary health care programme will be very useful for this anti-yaws activity because it also envisages involving the people through a network of health guides and volunteers (one for each 500 – 1000 population). Saxena et al. [2], in their report on the resurgence of yaws in the Baster district of Madhya Pradesh, observed that the tribal people have not forgotten the miracle of PAM injection for chronic ulcers and during market days queue up in large numbers before the health centres for their injection. The primary health care programme can easily use these people's co-operation for yaws and guide them towards a continuous linkage with the professional system.

The greater barrier in surveillance is, in fact, from the medical profession itself, and it was observed that though the profession was treating chronic ulcers and late yaws by penicillin, it was not recognising them as yaws [2]. Only papillomatous eruptions were faintly recognized as yaws but even these were not usually reported and no efforts were made to identify contacts who required treatment. Consciousness of yaws needs to be reinforced by special teams who will look after the reports, maintain the supply of drugs, data and educational material, and evaluate the situation continuously. One team cannot cover more than four contiguous primary health centres.

Surveillance at central level also requires attention. In most directorates in India, yaws is bracketed with sexually transmitted diseases (STD). It is likely that microbiologically the same treponema is responsible for both yaws and syphilis. However, epidemiologically the diseases have different characteristics and require a different strategy. Nobody even thinks of eradicating STD, but the possibility of eradicating yaws is just visible. Therefore, establishment of effective yaws cells in various health directorates is essential for proper surveillance. If reports on yaws are responded to with adequate action, the eradication of yaws will be a natural by-product of surveillance.

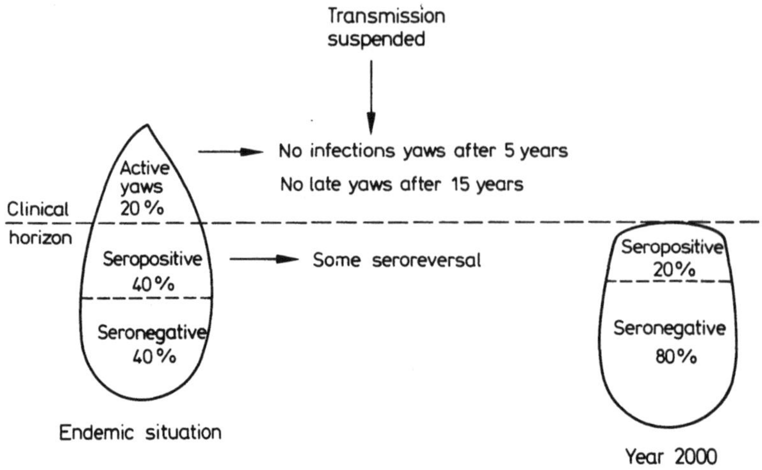

Fig. 4. Clinico-serological changes visualised

Concept of Eradication

Epidemiologically, all the seropositive cases in previously endemic areas should be considered as yaws or tribal treponematoses. However, for the present discussion, eradication does not mean the total disappearance of seropositivity from the community but only cessation of transmission. Theoretically, if yaws transmission is effectively stopped by treatment of all infectious cases, then no indigenous cases of early yaws would be left after 5 years and all children under 5 years of age would be seronegative. Late cases of palmar and plantar hyperkeratosis, bone and joint pains and late yaws ulcers will, however, continue for some years to come. These late cases will also disappear slowly, and by the year 2000 only some weak seropositivity in the older population will persist (Fig. 4). However, the most important issue demanding attention at this juncture is the practical aspect of the feasibility of this cessation of transmission.

Considerations Regarding Feasibility

The various issues that need to be considered are epidemiological, geographical, sociopolitical and administrative factors relevant to the eradication of yaws.

The *epidemiological* outcomes of all yaws control programmes indicate the effectiveness of long-acting penicillin in lowering the incidence of the disease. However, one obvious defect of these programmes was that the interval between two visits by yaws teams was not tuned to the incubation period of yaws, which is about 3–5 weeks. Thus a revisit to the village after 6 months might permit about nine transmission cycles from residual cases, resulting in a rebuilding of the infectious reservoir, especially when the population coverage during the initial survey was poor. With the establishment of an infrastructure of community health guides and multipurpose workers, the programme of diagnosis and treatment of yaws can be changed from a vertical one to a horizontal one by giving suitable training to the workers concerned. It is rational to believe that such a network of treatment centres in endemic areas will be able to nip in the bud all cases of yaws. The eradication of yaws will thus be a by-product of the primary health care programme, and the success in its eradication will be a measure of the effectiveness of the primary health care programme in tribal areas. The yaws programme is also bound to increase the prestige and status of the workers involved in primary health care programmes by providing for a liberal use of a potent and long-acting drug (penicillin).

Geographical considerations regarding the feasibility of eradicating yaws highlight some important features for yaws strategy in India. The present residual foci (Fig. 1) in India are so few and so localized that the problem appears to be well within the grip of an eradication programme. However, since most of the previous epidemic areas of yaws are located in the peripheral areas of adjoining states like Madhya Pradesh, Maharastra, Andhra Pradesh, Orissa etc., to ensure that efforts are co-ordinated it is obligatory that the entire eradication programme be launched centrally, under the full control of the central Government. It may also be pointed out that with the resurgence of yaws in Burma, a careful eye is needed for the adjoining Indian border.

Sociopolitical considerations are very important when undertaking any eradication programme. The disease must be of recognized socio-economic importance to bring out the desired financial and other support for eradication activities. Yaws is mostly a tribal tragedy in India and like leprosy, it seldom kills but often cripples and disfigures the victim. Nitsen [1] has said that in highly endemic areas, yaws is responsible for more suffering and misery than all other diseases put together. There is no social stigma attached to yaws among tribes, but it is definitely associated with a national stigma. Any country having children affected with preventable yaws can never aspire to be called a humanly developed country. Fortunately for India, the new 20-point programme has given high priority to tribal problems in the country, and special inputs have been granted to the primary health care programme in the tribal areas. It is now left to technical planners and academicians to decide upon a feasible and suitable strategy for achieving the desired success.

Administrative considerations deserve special attention. One is likely to think that, because of the development of the primary health care programme, yaws eradication will require little input apart from drugs. Fears have, however, been expressed [4] that the categorical nature of an intensive yaws programme makes it difficult to integrate it into a system based on the current concept of primary health care. The staff, resources and attention required for the yaws eradication programme are not likely to be less than those required for the control programme.

Though reporting and treatment of yaws will be decentralized to primary health care workers, special teams will be needed for supervising and yaws surveillance. These teams will have to keep a continuous watch on the changing yaws map of India, which will have to be prepared block-wise (and not district-wise). As mentioned above, roughly one team will be needed to enforce anti-yaws activities in four contiguous blocks. For proper monitoring of the programme, creation of yaws cells at central and state level will be obligatory. Special efforts will be needed to maintain the consciousness of yaws among the medical profession, and involvement of medical colleges in the region will be very useful in this respect.

Conclusion

It can be said that geographical and sociopolitical factors are very favourable for the eradication of yaws in India. It should, however, be mentioned that it is a challenging job which will test the adequacy of the primary health care programme in tribal areas. Many yaws programmes have failed because of low population coverage due to inadequate planning, deficient public notification or education and failure to treat the contacts of reported cases. Therefore the achievement of our objective requires proper attention from national and international authorities.

References

1. Nitsen RVN (1944) Man Inst R Colon Belge Sect Sci Nat Med 13
2. Saxena VB, Darbari BS, Jain MK (1978) Resurgence of yaws, a preliminary report from Jagdalpur district, Madhya Pradesh India, Indian J Prev Soc Med 9/2:41–46
3. WHO (1981) Endemic treponematoses, weekly Epidemiol Rec 56:241–248
4. WHO (1982) Treponemal infectious. WHO Tech Rep Ser 674
5. Yekutial P (1981) Lesson from the big eradication campaigns. World Health Forum 2/4:465–490

Human Resources for Primary Health Care in Developing Countries

G. Lachenmann

Introduction

The present paper tries to analyse the problems faced by a primary health care (PHC) approach as conceived in Alma Ata in the field of human resources development. It is mainly based on three case studies carried out in countries with very different economic and social background as well as health care approach: the Dominican Republic, Egypt and Malawi.

As far as personnel for the institutional health system are concerned, the most important aspect is that human resources for PHC must not only be developed for peripheral services, but that all categories of health personnel must be trained to support this approach. PHC does not only concern those "barefoot doctors" working at the grass-root level, and not only those providing primary medical care (including first referral system), but all personnel of the health sector. Human resources should also not be reduced to formal categories and training for the institutional health system, but the "productive resource" which constitutes the "patient" and the population in general should be tapped for health. This mobilization concerns self-help through village health workers, integration of traditional medical knowledge and personnel and community involvement for planning, decision-making and execution of health activities.

As the roots of bad health are those of underdevelopment and the social organization of health care can be effective only if the large gap existing between people, their concepts of illness and health, and their living conditions on the one hand, and the "modern health institutions" on the other hand can be overcome, not only other sectors and their human resources should be activated for health policy, but an overall interdisciplinary approach to PHC development is needed.

Integration into the Institutional Health System

A growing dualism is encountered in health care systems as the overall structure, which is not directed towards the periphery and the middle level to form the necessary link between primary care and other services, is deficient. Underlying this process is one of inadequate human development by which a

Primary Health Care in the Making
Ed. by U. Laaser, R. Senault, H. Viefhues

polarization takes place between professionals and lower-level auxiliaries or volunteer health workers. The PHC workers lack the support of the other levels of the health care system and thereby are, on the one hand, overburdened with tasks they cannot meet adequately and, on the other hand, abandoned and discouraged, so that the tasks they could perform are not effectively fulfilled. The thesis of the paper is that the PHC approach as found in reality, i.e. consisting mainly of utilizing a cheap labour force for primary care, not only does not succeed in providing effective care at the peripheral level but contributes to perpetuate the former system by preventing structural changes in training, personnel careers and management.

Training in the health professions continues to be as clinically oriented as before with regard to the subjects taught and the learning environment; there is no link between training and services. In order to avoid serious conflicts with the professional and academic establishment, additional community- and PHC-oriented training is provided to those health workers who are going to enter public health institutions. Thereby the basic health education remains unchanged and the PHC system does not gain high esteem. The introduction of an obligatory social service for doctors in the most peripheral health units might be counter-productive due to the lack of support from the other health institutions and difficult working conditions. Also, the training and role of paramedicals and medium level auxiliaries who might be more able to fulfill the needs of PHC at the peripheral level is not adapted accordingly.

Rural primary health care in Dominican Republic can be taken as an example. Health promoters only receive a monthly compensation, and it is unavoidable that with the high unemployment rate this income is very essential to them and the notion of voluntariness cannot be strictly maintained. The network is vertically integrated through shortly trained supervisors attached to rural clinics, and area and regional supervisors who report directly to the central level. Links with the formal health care structure at all levels are insufficient. The medical personnel have not yet assumed the role of health team leader; also, the nursing sector is not involved to a very large extent with regard to special fields such as MCH, and no perspectives of future development are perceived such as introducing a community outreach programme or transfering certain services back to the institutionalized system (such as immunizations).

Informal Sector and Community Involvement

Due to the transfer of more and more tasks to the community health workers, they tend to become professionalized as far as their own conception of their activities is concerned and thereby are no longer part of the community, or, put the other way around, communities are required to contribute beyond their own ability. On the other hand, the health system tends to be oriented towards the delivery of services, e.g. in community medicine and outreach programmes, instead of towards the mobilization and participation of the population. Thereby, the potential constituted by the communities and the population as a whole is not tapped for PHC. This is especially obvious with regard to traditional resources, knowledge and manpower. The PHC system is often even used to justify neglect, ignoring the fact that sometimes the major part of deliveries still take place with the help of traditional birth attendants or that people still recur to traditional healers.

An example is the rural health care system in Egypt. On the one hand, the activities of the traditional health sector are neglected; on the other hand, an overqualification of professional groups takes place. Although in some regions the majority of the deliveries are attended by traditional birth attendants, the training and licensing of these "dayas" has been abandoned as they are supposed to be replaced by nurses in outreach programmes. As they often continue to work uncontrolled and unsupervised by professionals, their factual activity is not as high quality as possible, and their important social role which is inherent to home deliveries and which will never be taken over by the health system in its totality is not recognized. Decentralization efforts mobilizing labour and human resources of the communities have not yet been applied in the health field, and there are problems of overlapping competence of volunteers recruited through different programmes of the Ministry of Social Affairs and Family Planning.

Intersectoral Co-operation and Interdisciplinary Approach

In PHC development, many similarities are overlooked in other fields which have a longer tradition of community involvement, decentralization, integration of services etc. It is not realized that community development as a concept, and often as an administrative sector, is based on the same idea as PHC, which could be paraphrased as "community development for health". Therefore, the community development resources existing in many countries are not tapped for community mobilization, recruitment of volunteer health workers, organization of water supply and sanitation, health education and training of health personnel. The same applies to social sciences, which are neither utilized for conceptual purposes of policy and programme formulation, needs assessment, research on health care potential in the communities, evaluation etc., nor for the training of professionals. Also, the health sector does not take the initiative to advise and impose its criteria on the sector of agriculture, infrastructure etc., although these are the only ones where decisive progress can be made with regard to nutrition, water and sanitation.

An example is the primary health care programme in Malawi, which is oriented towards mobilizing people to better utilize services and become responsible for their own health. However, the community health component and PHC orientation in the training institutions of para-medical personnel is still very limited. They, as well as the PHC programme, could make use of teaching and service staff in community development and rural development, the faculty of social sciences as well as the Centre for Social Research. Also the human resources allocated to the priority sector agriculture could be actively involved.

At present, the main emphasis is on production in the case of male agricultural extension workers, on home economics in the case of farm home instructresses, and on self-help efforts for school construction and similar activities in the case of community development assistants. The sectoral integration should not be sought by establishing a separate interdisciplinary structure in the Ministry of Health, but by trying to mobilize these other resources so that they assume the responsibility for the aim "health for all by the year 2000".

Evaluation of Polyclinic Services Run by Primary Health Care (PHC) Nurses in Soweto

T. D. Wilson, L. M. Irwig, and L. D. Saunders

Soweto and Its Polyclinic Services

Soweto is a relatively poor urban area situated about 20 km from the centre of Johannesburg. It has a population of between 1 and 2 million people, about one-third of whom are under the age of 15 years. Most of the housing consists of four-roomed, single-story detached units that are drab and uniform, but solid. A programme of electrification is in progress, but most people still use coal stoves for both heating and cooking with the result that, particularly in winter, the whole township is often covered by a thick blanket of smog. The houses are also very overcrowded, estimates of the average number of people per four-roomed house varying from 7 to 14, and respiratory infections are common. (General information on Soweto: [1])

Health care services for Soweto are divided into preventive and curative services, the curative services being provided by the Transvaal Provincial Administration, through Baragwanath Hospital. The hospital itself is on the edge of Soweto, and it also staffs and runs nine polyclinics within the township, and one at the hospital. Up until 1976 all patients attending these polyclinics were seen and treated by doctors. As in most Western countries, these doctors had been trained almost exclusively in academic hospitals where they had been taught to recognize and treat serious organic disease. They had, however, had little or no training in the skills needed by a general or family practitioner. In addition, most of the doctors were white and relatively rich, and were unable to speak the languages of their patients, who were black and mostly poor. Interpreters were available, but the barriers to communication were formidable. Yet because of the large numbers of patients needing to be seen, the average consultation lasted less than 5 minutes.

Four of the polyclinics are still run entirely by doctors, but since 1976 increasing use has been made of specially trained "primary health care" (PHC) nurses to help staff the other six [2, 3]. Usually there is one referral doctor for about every six PHC nurses. The nurses selected for training were all black nurses with considerable hospital nursing experience. Most of them live in Soweto and speak at least the most commonly used languages in the township – Zulu, Sotho and Tswana – as well as English, which is used for all patient records. These nurses have been trained to take complete histories, to examine all patients fully, to diagnose and manage common conditions, to issue antibiotics

Primary Health Care in the Making
Ed. by U. Laaser, R. Senault, H. Viefhues

and other medication as indicated, and if in doubt or if faced with a patient with a serious illness, to refer that patient to a doctor. Patient management is set out in protocols which depend upon the signs and symptoms elicited by the nurse. In practice the PHC nurses can manage about 80% of the patients on their own, and of the remaining 20% most are referred for a second opinion. Because emphasis has been laid to listening to patients, on explaining the use of any medication issued and on giving appropriate health education, the average consultation with one of these PHC nurses takes about 20 minutes. This is four times as long as the doctor consultations used to take and is expensive; it can only be justified if the service can be shown to be good.

Evaluation

Measuring how good a health service is, is often difficult. All those who have worked closely with the PHC nurses in Soweto, and many who have merely visited the polyclinics, believe that these nurses are very competent and do an extremely good job, but this is really just a clinical impression. Clinical impressions may well be valid, particularly if the same impression is shared by a wide range of people, but they may also be misleading. In many health services the most influential evaluation is the clinical impression formed by those responsible for running the service, but this is far from ideal. Particularly for a relatively new service like that provided in Soweto by the teams of PHC nurses and their referral doctors, more solid data are needed.

To decide if the polyclinic service is effective, data are needed on three separate questions. We need to know firstly whether the service is necessary at all, secondly whether it reaches the people who need it, and thirdly whether the health care that is provided to those patients who do come to the service is good. Routinely collected statistics can help to answer the first two questions, and the results of a number of studies of the PHC nurses can help to answer the third.

A curative service for Soweto certainly is necessary. Despite the existence of the polyclinics and of about 20 general practitioners with consulting rooms in the township, a number of eminently treatable conditions are still very prevalent. Hypertension, gastro-enteritis, pneumonia, and other acute and chronic bacterial infections still cause considerable morbidity and mortality in the community [4].

The extent to which the second requirement for an effective service is met, is less certain. A great many people attend the polyclinics, but they do not necessarily represent a large proportion of the total population. Although there were 779 955 attendances at the polyclinics in 1982 (personal communication), for a population of 1.5 million this gives an average of only 0.5 visits per person per year. Even this figure gives a falsely high impression because many of the patients who do come, come repeatedly for treatment of chronic conditions. A small study done among adult patients attending one polyclinic on one day, revealed that nearly 30% had attended within the previous 5 weeks, and only 25%

of the attenders were new patients [5]. It seems likely, therefore, that many people in Soweto with treatable conditions do not attend the polyclinics. One possible reason for this is that the polyclinics are usually crowded, and the average visit may take 3 hours [5].

The third question posed about the effectiveness of the polyclinic service concerns the quality of care offered to the patients with treatable conditions who do attend. The main aim of the PHC nurses is to reduce morbidity and mortality in these patients. For them to achieve this goal, at least six criteria must be met:

1. The PHC nurses must have the training and the resources to treat common conditions effectively.
2. The PHC nurses must examine the patients and elicit the correct symptoms and signs.
3. The management protocols must be appropriate.
4. The PHC nurses must follow the protocols.
5. The patients must understand the instructions given.
6. The patients must comply with the instructions.

The available evidence on each of these criteria will now be reviewed:

1. Most of the training of the PHC nurses is done in a polyclinic setting, and is very practical. The emphasis is always on the management of common conditions, appropriate drugs are freely available, and during training the competence of the nurses is continually re-assessed. The first of the six criteria listed is therefore met.
2. The second criterion suggested for good care is that the PHC nurses must examine the patients and elicit the correct symptoms and signs. Two studies have looked at aspects of this. In the first study the records of nearly 2000 new patients aged 15 years and over were reviewed, and it was found that the PHC nurses had recorded the blood pressures of 87% of them at the first consultation [6]. In the second study, the PHC nurses were compared with experienced paediatricians for their competence in detecting clinical signs in children [7]. The whole group of 31 PHC nurses seeing children in Soweto at the time was studied, and the inter-observer variability that is known to exist whenever two clinicians examine the same patient was taken into account. The study again demonstrated the extent to which doctors may disagree with each other, and showed that the PHC nurses were just as competent as paediatricians in detecting important signs. The nurses were found to over-diagnose to a significant extent one important sign, namely follicular tonsilitis, and this could possibly be explained by the fact that the high prevalence in Soweto of post-streptococcal rheumatic fever and rheumatic carditis has been stressed in their training.
3. The management protocols used by the PHC nurses have not been formally evaluated in Soweto. However, they are based on generally accepted medical practice, and most of them have in fact been drawn up in consultation with senior members of the teaching staff of the University of the Witwatersrand medical school.
4. Evidence that the PHC nurses follow the protocols comes both from the study of their management of hypertension [6] and from unpublished data

collected in the assessment of the clinical competence of the nurses seeing children [7]. In the first study the nurses were found to follow the hypertension management protocol in 98% of all patients.

5. Two studies have reported on the degree to which patients understand the instructions given to them by the PHC nurses. Wagstaff et al. [8] interviewed the mothers on other escorts of children leaving the polyclinics, and compared those who had seen a doctor with those who had seen a PHC nurse. They found that those who had consulted a PHC nurse had a much better knowledge of how and when to give the medication issued. The other study which reflects on this criterion was one in which patients who had failed to re-attend regularly for treatment of hypertension were interviewed at home, and asked why they had not re-attended regularly [9]. Apart from those who had been away from Soweto, the commonest reason given was that they did not know that they needed to come back. Further studies are obviously indicated to clarify the extent to which any instructions given by the PHC nurses are understood.
6. The compliance of patients who have consulted the PHC nurses has only been studied in terms of the attendance compliance of hypertensive patients. This has been found on two occasions to be of the order of only 20% [6, 9]. Attendance compliance of hypertensives is often very poor in any health service, but the fact that the problem is common to other services does not make this service any better.

Finally, instead of looking at the process of care as has been done in terms of the six criteria listed, one can evaluate the quality of care by looking at the outcome. This is easiest to do in a specific group of patients with a treatable disease. Again, the only direct evidence available at present is on hypertensive patients, but here, apart from the problem of non-compliance, care does seem to be effective. Those patients who did attend regularly in the study already quoted [6] had a mean drop in diastolic blood pressure of 21 mmHg over a 1-year period.

Conclusions

The question is frequently asked, "How good is the service provided by the PHC nurses in Soweto?" What is often meant, however, is, "How does it compare to a more traditional service where all patients are examined by doctors?" What little evidence there is on this point [6–8], apart from clinical impressions, suggests that the nurses provide a service that is at least as good as a more traditional one, and that in some ways it may be better.

More important, however, is the question "How effective is the service in promoting the health of the community?" One aspect of promoting health is the significant reduction of the morbidity and mortality that would otherwise be caused by treatable disease. When the PHC service is examined in this light it is apparent that there are still problems to be overcome.

The first is the extent of the coverage. Until the polyclinic service is reasonably accessible to, and is consulted by, most of those who need it, it cannot claim to provide the whole community with an effective curative service.

The second aspect of the service that needs to be investigated further is the extent to which patients really understand and accept the instructions given to them. The fact that they appear to understand the nurses better than they understand doctors is no excuse for complacency.

The third problem area may well be related, at least in part, to the other two. This is the problem of poor patient compliance. Again, the fact that poor patient compliance is a world-wide problem, particularly in the management of chronic conditions, is not relevant to the question being asked. What is relevant, however, is that recognition of the problem of non-compliance has been found elsewhere to be an important step in improving the situation [10].

Hopefully, recognition of the limitations of the present PHC service in Soweto will in the same way help those running it, and the PHC nurses themselves, to build on its undoubted strengths and to make it even more effective in promoting the health of the community.

References

1. Morris P (1980) A review of existing conditions and some guidelines for change. Urban Foundation, Johannesburg
2. Wagstaff LA, Beukes PJ (1977) The paediatric primary health care nurse project in soweto. S Afr Med J 52:1086–1088
3. Duncan MO, Gear JSS (1980) Training the primary health care nurse. The Baragwanath experience. S Afr Med J 58:207–210
4. Johannesburg City Health Department (1977/1978) Annual report, pp 96–98, 149
5. Berger M, Wilson TD, Saunders LD (1982) Queueing and patient flow at a Soweto polyclinic. S Afr Med J 61:547–550
6. Saunders LD, Irwig LM, Wilson TD (1982) Hypertension management and patient compliance at a Soweto polyclinic. S Afr Med J 61:147–151
7. Irwig LM, Porter BA, Wilson TD, et al. (to be published) Clinical competence of paediatric primary health care nurses in Soweto.
8. Wagstaff LA, Shuenyane EN, Mkhasibe CM, et al. (1982) Comparisons in the therapeutic management of black paediatric outpatients by primary health care nurses and doctors. S Afr Med J 62:654–657
9. Saunders LD, Ntoane C, Wilson TD (1983) Why don't patients return for antihypertensive treatment in Soweto? S Afr Med J 64:208–210
10. Sackett DL, Haynes RB (eds) (1976) Compliance with therapeutic regimens. Johns Hopkins University Press, Baltimore

Primary Health Care – A New Strategy? Lessons to Learn from Community Participation

W. Bichmann

Primary health care (PHC) originally meant first-contact care of patients. In contrast, the expanded meaning of PHC, as promoted by WHO, has been referred to as the "PHC approach" [17]. This front-line, first-contact care is being related to five principles: (1) equitable distribution, (2) community involvement, (3) focus on prevention, (4) appropriate technology and (5) a multisectorial approach. The emergence of PHC strategy coincided with the broad acceptance of an interrelatedness of health and economic development at the beginning of the 1970s – as underlined with regard to the changing World Bank's health sector policy [8, 13]. Furthermore, the official adoption of the PHC approach by international organizations was paralleled by the promotion of the "basic needs" concept in international development funding at the end of the 1970s [3, 10, 16]. PHC has three main fields: (1) basic health services, (2) community involvement and (3) intersectorial development. Each of these main components has been stressed within development policies ever since colonial times with changing emphasis: the concept of basic health services has been focused on since the early years of WHO, whereas intersectorial development and community involvement are notions which were already considered as constitutent elements of community development (CD) in the early 1950s. What is really new is the combination of these concepts within one overall strategy.

In the People's Republic of Benin, German technical co-operation with the Ministry of Health to develop the basic health services has taken place since 1968. When government priorities in health shifted to PHC, a new programme was designed jointly to implement the national PHC policy, to build up a functional referral system and to support the integrated curative and preventive services on the district, commune and village levels. The programme is now being operated in seven medical districts in different rural regions. The programme provides primary curative and preventive services, mother and child health services (including family planning), staff training activities and technical assistance in the construction of wells. One of the priority tasks of the programme has been the recruitment, training and supervision of village health workers and traditional birth attendants and the creation of village health posts. An evaluation of the programme's achievements in its first 3-year phase is presently being prepared by external experts. Simultaneously an ongoing participatory evaluation exercise has been started. On the basis of a qualitative analysis of programme documentation, in this paper we present a typology of problems en-

Primary Health Care in the Making
Ed. by U. Laaser, R. Senault, H. Viefhues

countered in this PHC programme. We can discern three categories of problems: (1) resources and logistics, (2) operation and process and (3) perceived needs and politics.

The first category of problems (resources and logistics) is related to the effectiveness of the programme. It includes problems of insufficient materials, supplies, funds, facilities and personnel as well as infrastructure and transport. These problems are related to the overall economic situation of the country. The project intervened by three means: (a) conceptual planning on the local level within the national planning framework, (b) the provision of appropriate equipment and essential drugs, as well as teaching simple and acceptable diagnostic and treatment procedures, and (c) financing the upgrading of existing facilities without providing for running costs.

The second category of problems (operation and process) encompasses problems related to programme efficiency, i.e. the functioning of services. This concerns the attitudes and competence of staff, including the organizing capacities, attitudes and belief systems of the patients and the community and of village health workers. These problems are mainly behavioural ones and can ideally be influenced by training, health education and other means of inducing behavioural changes. As Foster [6] stresses, whereas "almost all assume that effective health care can be achieved only when members of traditional communities change their health behaviour", the question of how to change "bureaucratic behaviour that inhibits the design and operation of the best possible health care systems" has rarely been asked by professionals. This set of problems requires a careful but complete "community diagnosis". Furthermore, it demands that the health team is continually being retrained and supervised, not only with regard to their professional skills but also with regard to their attitudes vis-à-vis community members. In our project we attempted to solve the health team part of the problem through regular team sessions, meetings and on-the-job advice, whereas a systematic community diagnosis was not carried out during the programme's starting phase – an omission that seriously affected village health work. Therefore a special community diagnosis exercise was prepared in each project area for the programme's fourth year.

The third category of problems (perceived needs and politics) is the most delicate. It is made up of differences in the assessment of health priorities between health officials, politicians and the population and emphasizes the basic problems of health planning philosophy. These problems are related to individual and collective value choices and are influenced by the existing economic, social and political status quo. Instead of opposing needs felt by community and discouraging community actions controversial in respect of the professionals' priorities, PHC programmes have to be oriented according to these priorities. Problems related to perceived needs and politics are of an entirely different character to those mentioned above. Health planning experiences in general have shown for a long time that the outcome of non-personal health measures is closely related to community motivation and participation. Where health services are just delivered to the clients, this will result in the phenomenon of under-use. PHC cannot just be imposed; rather it needs active participation by an informed population. If the objectives of programmes do not coincide with the perceived needs of the target population, programmes are likely to fail [5, 12].

In practice, all three sets of problems are inter-related. However, whereas problem solving with regard to the first two categories is of a more technical character, though in reality difficult enough to perform, problem solving with regard to community involvement finds its limitations in its political character. David Werner [18] discerned "community-supportive" and "community-oppressive" approaches with regard to community involvement. Susan Rifkin [15] presented a four-fold typology of approaches in this regard: (1) the public health approach, (2) the health planning approach, (3) the community development approach and (4) the self-care approach. This series reflects a shifting spectrum from "top-down" to "bottom-up" approaches, paralleled by a decreasing influence of professionalism.

There are surprising analogies between the PHC and the CD approach. This has been highlighted by several authors [1, 2, 4, 7], but in the documents promoting PHC strategy no clear reference to this fact is made. One may wonder whether the CD strategy in rural agricultural development had been fully worked up before a similar strategy was launched in the health sector. As PHC, with its comprehensive approach, encompasses sector-external health-related subjects like agricultural development, road infrastructure and education, so did the CD programmes of the 1950s and 1960s aim at integrated rural development, including health-related activities, as a means of improving agricultural production. Generally speaking, CD did not yield the expected results on a nationwide scale, though there have been extraordinary local achievements. Why, then, should PHC produce a better outcome than CD? One of the main failures of CD programmes has been the complete neglect of existing political and power structures within communities and between the community and the national level [11, 14]. The same is now being experienced in PHC programmes.

Now, what are the elements of community participation in most PHC programmes? (1) Village health committees, and (2) participation in money, material and labour in the construction of village health posts and in remunerating village health workers. Communities cannot express their felt needs in programme planning, nor are they generally involved in programme evaluation [9, 19]. There are no major technical obstacles to including these two elements in PHC programmes as further steps towards increasing community involvement. But there seem to be major reservations and rejection from the administrative bodies and the medical professions.

With regard to the three types of problems discussed above, the success of the various PHC schemes actually under way on a worldwide scale will depend on:

1. Sufficient central budget allocations to implement PHC as well as to provide for running costs
2. Strong committment of governments to social change
3. Realization of decentralization of administrative power together with democratization

Communities cannot develop if they cannot participate in – or even control – decision making upon what matters to themselves. Today's PHC as compared with the earlier CD programmes may have – as Foster [7] suggests – better conditions at the outset. But unless the political implications of decentralization and democratization are accepted by governments, thus favouring community participation in decision making, it is doubtful whether the health status of a population can improve.

Returning to our example of a PHC programme in Bénin, the national policy options were clearly in favour of decentralization and community involvement. And the implementation of a permanent participatory evaluation mechanism will constitute a built-in element for ongoing community participation.

There do exist such favourable factors contributing to PHC outcome, but there will never exist a set of factors warranting the success of PHC programmes, which are, after all, dependent on the socio-economic, cultural and political conditions of the very local setting.

References

1. Bichmann W (1978) Theses on the relevance of traditional medicine in the context of the "primary health care"-strategy in Africa. Curare 1:99–106
2. Bichmann W (1979) Primary health care and traditional medicine – considering the background of changing health care concepts in Africa. Soc Sci Med [B] 13:175–182
3. Diesfeld HJ (1982) "Grundbedürfnisstrategie" – "Health for all by the year 2000" und "Primary Health Care". Utopie oder Lösung des Problems der Armut. In: Wagner N, Rieger HC (eds) Grundbedürfnisse als Gegenstand der Entwicklungspolitik. Steiner, Wiesbaden, pp 135–151
4. Feuerstein M, Lovel H (1983) Introduction: Community development and the emergence of primary health care. Community Dev J 18:98–103
5. Foster GM, Anderson BG (1978) Medical anthropology. Wiley and Sons, New York Chichester Brisbane Toronto Singapore, p 225
6. Foster GM (1982) Applied anthropology and international health: Retrospect and prospect. Hum Org 41:189–197
7. Foster GM (1982) Community development and primary health care: their conceptual similarities. Med Anthropol 6:183–195
8. Gish O (1979) The political economy of primary care and "health by the people": an historical explanation. Soc Sci Med [C] 13:203–211
9. Kroeger A (1982) Participatory evaluation of primary health care programmes: an experience with four Indian populations in Ecuador. Trop Doct 12:38–43
10. Lachenmann G (1982) Entkolonisierung der Gesundheit. Theorie und Praxis der Gesundheitsversorgung in Namibia und Bénin. Rüegger, Diessenhofen (Konkrete Fremde. Interkulturell vergleichende Studien der Arbeitsgruppe Entwicklungsländer an der Universität Konstanz, vol 4)
11. MacCormack CP (1983) Community participation in primary health care. Trop Doct 13:51–54
12. Mackey DM (1982) Primary health care may be needed, but is it wanted? World Health Forum 3:88–89
13. McEvers NC (1980) Health and the assault on poverty in low income countries. Soc Sci Med [C] 14:41–57
14. Mott BJF (1969) The politics of health planning. II. The myth of planning without politics. Am J Public Health 59:797–803
15. Rifkin SB (1981) The role of the public in the planning, management and evaluation of health activities and programmes, including self-care. Soc Sci Med [A] 15:377–386

16. Schwefel D (1978) Grundbedürfnisse und Entwicklungspolitik. Nomos, Baden-Baden
17. Walt G, Vaughan P (1981) An introduction to the primary health care approach in developing countries. Ross Institute, London (Ross Institute Publication, no 13)
18. Werner D (1981) The village health worker: lackey or liberator? World Health Forum 2:46–68
19. White A (1983) Obstacles to full community participation in water supply programmes. Community Dev J 18:182–186

C. Modification of at Risk Behaviours

The Relation of Pattern of Support for Smoking and Achievement Motive in Young Women

B. Mausner and D. Brandspiegel

The fact that the level of cigarette smoking in young women is either not decreasing or actually rising has serious implications for health. The traditional view of smoking in girls is that it occurs among those who press for early emancipation, are socially and sexually active, and are inadequate in academic work. This view, based on work from the fifties and sixties, is probably inadequate. An ecological model for smoking behavior developed by the senior author suggests that sources of support for smoking would differ depending on the life circumstances and motivations of the person. To test this concept it was proposed that female college students high in need for achievement would report different sources of support for smoking than those low in this motive.

Thirty female students at a small liveral arts college, randomly selected from among dormitory residents who smoke cigarettes regularly, were given the Mehrabian Test for need achievement (nAch) and a measure of sources of support for smoking (Mausner and Platt) (Table 1[1]). Subjects high in nAch were significantly more likely than those low in nAch to resport smoking for tension release and to support the self-image. They were more likely to exhibit a pattern of psychological addiction (Table 2[1]). An analysis using the Mehrabian nAch score as a continuous variable gave four significant correlations with the subscales on the measure of Patterns of Support for Smoking out of eight possible relations (Table 3[1]).

The hypothesis is advanced that smoking serves different functions for women high and low in nAch. For the former it is used to mitigate the tensions caused by striving. In the latter the functions of smoking are less related to tension release and self-concept, more tied in with social and hedonic factors. The implications of this difference for measures to prevent the onset of smoking in women will be discussed elsewhere.

Reference

Mausner B, Platt ES (1971) Smoking: A behavorial analysis. Pergamon, Elmsford, NY

[1] Tables 1–3 see pages 392 and 393

Primary Health Care in the Making
Ed. by U. Laaser, R. Senault, H. Viefhues

Table 1. Summary of test of patterns of support for smoking [1]

Factor 1:	Tension reduction – 14% of total variance
	Feeling "blue" or wanting to take my mind off cares and worries
	Feeling uncomfortable or upset about something
	Feeling angry about something
	Feeling ashamed or embarrassed about something
	Feeling upset
Factor 2:	Pleasure – 9% of total variance
	Finding cigarettes pleasurable
	Smoking cigarettes is pleasant and relaxing
Factor 3:	Social/self-image – 13% of total variance
	Feeling closer in a crowd to those who smoke
	Smokers are basically different kinds of people than non-smokers
	Feeling more like "myself" when I smoke
	Enjoying the steps I take to light up
	Enjoying lighting up and smoking with someone I like
	Enjoying a cigarette more if offered by someone I like
Factor 4:	Habit/self-image – 11% of total variance
	Finding a cigarette in mouth and not remembering putting it there
	Smoking automatically without even being aware of it
	Lighting up without realizing I still have one burning in ashtray
	If I suddenly stopped smoking, people wouldn't recognize me
	When thinking of myself, picturing myself with a cigarette in hand
	When other people think of me, they think of me as a smoker
Factor 5:	Social stimulus to smoking – 7% of total variance
	With friends who aren't smoking, tend to smoke less than usual
	With friends who are smoking, tend to smoke more than usual
	When some place others are not smoking, I don't smoke
Factor 6:	Psychological addiction – 15% of total variance
	Get a gnawing hunger for a cigarette when I haven't smoked for a while
	Between cigarettes, I get a craving only a cigarette can satisfy
	When out of cigarettes, it's unbearable until I can get them
	Not feeling content for long unless smoking a cigarette
Factor 7:	Stimulation – 10% of total variance
	Smoking to stimulate me, to perk myself up
	Smoking in order to keep myself from slowing down
	Smoking to give me a "lift"
Factor 8:	Sensory Motor – 9% of total variance
	Having a different brand recommended than one smoking and trying it
	Part of enjoyment of smoking is watching the smoke as I exhale it
	Part of enjoyment of smoking is handling a cigarette
	Part of enjoyment comes from the steps I take to light up

Table 2. Comparison of subjects high and low on need for achievement (Mehrabian scale) on patterns of support for cigarette smoking (30 female college students)

Pattern of support	Need for achievement		*t*	*df*	*P*
	Mean high	Mean low			
Tension release	9.8	8.4	2.21	28	<0.05
Pleasure	7.7	8.0	1.11	28	NS
Psychological addiction	9.0	7.7	1.96	28	<0.10
Habit/self-image	6.7	5.6	2.08	28	<0.05
Social-self-image	8.5	5.9	2.4	28	<0.5

Table 3. Correlations of scores on patterns of support for smoking with need for achievement (Mehrabian scale) (30 female college students)

Psychological addiction	0.35*
Social stimulation	0.07
Pleasure	0.27
Habit/self-image	0.31*
Social/self-image	0.46***
Sensory motor	0.26
Stimulation	0.26
Tension release	0.42**

* $P<0.10$; ** $P<0.05$; *** $P<0.01$

On the Effectiveness of Smoking Cessation Treatment Methods

M. F. Schuntermann

Introduction

It is well known that smoking and earning capacity are at least indirectly interrelated. In order to find out whether smoking cessation treatment methods can effectively change attitudes towards smoking and which method is most effective, the Association of German Pension Insurance Agencies (VDR) conducted a model trial in cooperation with the Gemeinnütziges Institut für Therapieforschung, Munich (Prof. Dr. J. C. Brengelmann), the Institut für Sozialmedizin, Prävention und Rehabilitation, Tutzing (Prof. Dr. U. Stocksmeier) and Dr. O. Hammer, Bad Nauheim, in the years 1977–1982.

Three different methods of smoking cessation treatment were used: self-control (Brengelmann), group therapy (a special kind of Roger's non-directive method, Stocksmeier) and the Bad Nauheim method (Hammer). In selected rehabilitation facilities, smokers consuming at least ten cigarettes a day, suffering from chronic bronchitis, cardiovascular or rheumatic diseases, and undergoing therapeutic treatment (usually for 4 weeks) participated in the programme. Actually, patients suffering from other diseases could not be excluded from the programme for obvious reasons. In addition, medical, psychological and sociological data were obtained by means of questionnaires at the beginning, during and at the end of treatment, and three times during a 2-year follow-up period.

At the end of the investigation 5400 data sets of persons who had finished the smoking cessation therapies or had belonged to the control group were available, together with about 3600 data sets of those persons who had responded to each of the three questionnaires during the follow-up period. A detailed analysis showed that there is no reason to assume a dependence between attitude towards smoking and attitude towards responding.

Concepts and Methods

This paper is concerned with the main questions of the model trial. All patients who did not suffer from coronary heart disease, hypertension, chronic bronchitis or rheumatic diseases were excluded from this analysis. Moreover, only the

Primary Health Care in the Making
Ed. by U. Laaser, R. Senault, H. Viefhues

more homogeneous and largest subsets of cardiovascular diseases, i.e. coronary heart disease and hypertension, were considered.

The effectiveness of a form of smoking cessation therapy can be evaluated in different ways. However, one of the most important aspects is its capability to generate non-smokers. Therefore, it is reasonable to compare the different percentages of non-smokers at the end of the different types of treatment in order to evaluate their short-term effectiveness. Their long-term effectiveness could be analysed in a similar way by comparing the different percentages of non-smokers after the complete follow-up period. However, this would not allow a clear-cut epidemiological interpretation because of the strong dependency of the two percentages. Rather, long-term efficiency is defined as an additional effect of the smoking cessation treatment methods. It refers to the change of attitude towards smoking. There are positive changes (i.e. from smoking at the end of treatment to non-smoking in the follow-up period), and negative ones (i.e. from non-smoking at the end of treatment to smoking at least once in the follow-up period). If there were any long-term effectiveness, the proportion of positive changes to negative changes within the therapy groups should be significantly greater than those within the control groups.

In the primary analysis the following factors were introduced simultaneously: medical indication, treatment (including the control group), sex and insurance branch [workers' pension insurance (LVA), social insurance for employees (BfA)]. Unfortunately the rehabilitation facilities in general could not be introduced as an original factor, because the patients are fairly strongly concentrated on the facilities. Consequently it was only possible to take the percentages of non-smokers as indicators of the effectiveness of treatment.

Log-linear models were applied to describe the effects of the factors and their interactions on the "non-smokers odds" (i.e. the ratio of non-smokers to smokers).

Results

In order to develop an appropriate model for explaining the variation (of the logarithm) of the non-smoker odds (with respect to the independence model) by means of the four factors, Goodman's method of forward selection was used. All of the factors proved highly significant and explained 56.8% of the variation. The most important of the factors was treatment, which explained 27.4% of the variation. Indication explained a further 19.9% and sex another 6.8%. Moreover, there were strong interaction effects on the non-smoker odds. The interaction between treatment and indication was most important, explaining a further 21.5% of the variation. The interaction between treatment and insurance branch was important, too (6.1%). All the other interactions were statistically and empirically insignificant. The model containing all the main factors and both significant interactions fitted the data appropriately (likelihood ratio $\chi^2 = 40.09$ with 43 degrees of freedom, significance > 0.5).

Table 1. Percentages of non-smokers at the end of treatment according to sex (sample size in parentheses)

Male	27.7% (2584)
Female	17.5% (1148)

Table 2. Percentages of non-smokers at the end of treatment according to insurance branch (sample sizes in parentheses)

Treatment	Insurance branch	
	LVA	BfA
Selfcontrol	33.9% (431)	27.0% (820)
Group therapy	30.4% (138)	19.0% (179)
Bad Nauheim	25.9% (424)	27.7% (676)
Control group	19.7% (198)	16.7% (866)

Table 3. Percentages of non-smokers at the end of treatment according to medical indication (sample sizes in parentheses)

Treatment	Medical indication			
	Coronary heart disease	Hypertension	Chronic bronchitis	Rheumatic diseases
Selfcontrol	41.9% (227)	29.9% (137)	15.6% (173)	28.6% (714)
Group therapy	59.5% (42)	33.3% (24)	17.1% (105)	17.1% (146)
Bad Nauheim	28.0% (75)	16.7% (54)	32.2% (398)	24.3% (573)
Control group	36.2% (47)	20.0% (75)	19.9% (397)	9.5% (545)

Tables 1–3 show the results by means of the percentages of non-smokers at the end of treatment. As Table 1 indicates, men clearly give up smoking more easily than women. Table 2 shows that the self-control method was significantly (5% level, adjusted and two-tailed) more effective within the group of LVA patients than within the group of BfA patients, while neither the effectiveness of the Bad Nauheim method nor the results in the control groups showed significant differences between the two groups. The results of group therapy were clearly better in the LVA patients, but the difference in effectiveness just missed the critical value on the 5% level of significance.

Again using two-tailed and adjusted tests on the 5% and the 1% levels of significance in order to explore which treatments were effective (as measured against the control groups) and to ascertain differences in the effectiveness of treatments, the only effective smoking cessation treatment methods were the Bad Nauheim method and self-control therapy for rheumatic diseases (both of the 1% level), and the Bad Nauheim method for chronic bronchitis (1% level). For rheumatic diseases the effectiveness of both methods differed at the 8.3% level of significance. Thus there was no substantial evidence to support the hy-

Table 4. Percentages of positive changes within the various treatment groups (sample sizes in parentheses)

Selfcontrol	Group therapy	Bad Nauheim	Control group
33.8% (195)	46.7% (45)	31.6% (171)	38.7% (119)

Overall $\chi^2 = 4.35$ with 3 degrees of freedom, significance = 0.23

pothesis that the two methods differ in their effectiveness. Concerning coronary heart disease and hypertension, no smoking cessation treatment method showed a significant effect as compared with the control groups.

With regard to long-term effectiveness, we found that 530 patients had changed their attitude towards smoking in the period from the end of the treatment to the end of the 2-year follow-up period. In order to analyse the "change odds" (i.e. the ratio of positive changes to negative changes) by means of the four factors introduced above, log-linear models were again applied.

The independence model already described the change odds satisfactorily with respect to the fit (likelihood ratio $\chi^2 = 47.02$ with 63 degrees of freedom, significance over 0.5). But, in addition, two of the four factors had a statistically significant (5% level) effect: sex and insurance branch. The other factors and interactions between them were statistically insignificant ($P > 0.1$). This result shows that there is no evidence that the cessation treatment methods under considation have a long-term effect. However, this result might have been inadequate due to too many sampling zeros within the data set for the four-factor model. In order to overcome this problem, the analysis was repeated, excluding medical indication.

The results were similar to those of the previous analysis. The model containing both sex and insurance branch fit the change odds satisfactorily ($\chi^2 = 16.65$ with 13 degrees of freedom, significance = 0.216). Incorporating treatment into the model results in no additional significance ($\chi^2 = 4.62$ with 3 degrees of freedom). Analysing the interactions of treatment with the other factors, only the interaction of treatment with sex is worth mentioning ($\chi^2 = 6.39$ with 3 degrees of freedom, significance nearly 0.1). But this interaction is of no empirical relevance. Thus a long-term effectiveness is not traceable from the data (see Table 4, original data).

A detailed discussion of these rather formal results will be given elsewhere after including the psychological and social variables in the analysis.

Acknowledgements. I wish to thank Dipl.-Psych. H.-D. Kijanski, M.Sc., BfA, and Dr. W. F. Kaufmann, VDR, for numerous discussions and helpful comments.

Cigarette Smoking, COHb Level and Physical Fitness

V. Milošević

Introduction

Many authors are of the opinion that tobacco smoking represents a very significant factor in the appearance of coronary diseases, lung cancer and some other disorders. In his recent comprehensive study, Hammond [1] has proved that the death rate due to cardiovascular insults is 5–10 times greater among smokers than among non-smokers. Doll and Hill [2] and Goldsmith and Ladaw [3] have also indicated the important role of tobacco smoking in the incidence and mortality of coronary disease.

It is well known that the CO concentration in tobacco smoke is relatively high [4], and so is the COHb level of blood [5]. One can believe that the oxygen debt during exercise is probably higher in smokers than in non-smokers, which may be of great importance for physical fitness. These studies have induced us to examine the relationship between smoking habits and some cardiovascular effects of exercise.

Methods

The best indicator of physical fitness is, according to many authors [6], maximal oxygen consumption (MOC). In this study, MOC was determined by the Astrand–Rhyming method. The test work consisted of exercise on a bicycle ergometer (mechanical type). The intensity of effort was the same for all examinees (100 Watts). The test lasted 6 min in a steady state. During the last minute of testing, pulse rate and blood pressure were registered, and MOC was then predicted using a nomogram by Astrand–Rhyming.

The COHb level of blood was determined by the Commins–Lawther method [7], and blood lactate by the Burker–Summerson method. The blood sample was taken 8–10 min after the end of testing.

The study included 90 male volunteers aged between 20 and 50. The examined persons were either students of medicine, industrial workers or white-collar employees.

All examinees were categorized into three groups: heavy smokers (more than 20 cigarettes per day), moderate smokers (10–20 cigarettes per day) and

Primary Health Care in the Making
Ed. by U. Laaser, R. Senault, H. Viefhues

non-smokers. The information concerning smoking habits was considered in relation to the following parameters: COHb level of blood, MOC, pulse rate, blood pressure and lactate concentration. All the data were statistically processed.

Results

The results obtained may be summarized as follows: The majority of examined persons were heavy smokers (63.3%) who had been smokers for a long period (80.0% for longer than 8 years).

The COHb level of blood was found to be higher in smokers than in non-smokers, while MOC was far lower among smokers than among non-smokers (Table 1). In the 20–30 year age group, for instance, the COHb level in the

Table 1. Cigarette smoking in relation to COH[b] level (MG%) and maximal oxygen consumption (ML)

	Non-smokers	Moderate smokers	Heavy smokers	*t*-test[a] $P<0.01$
COHb level				
$\bar{x}$	2.0	7.5	13.0	14.1
SD	+0.6	+1.6	+1.7	
MOC $\bar{x}$	44.5	33.5	29.5	14.0
No. of persons	14	19	57	

[a] *t*-test = heavy smokers : non-smokers

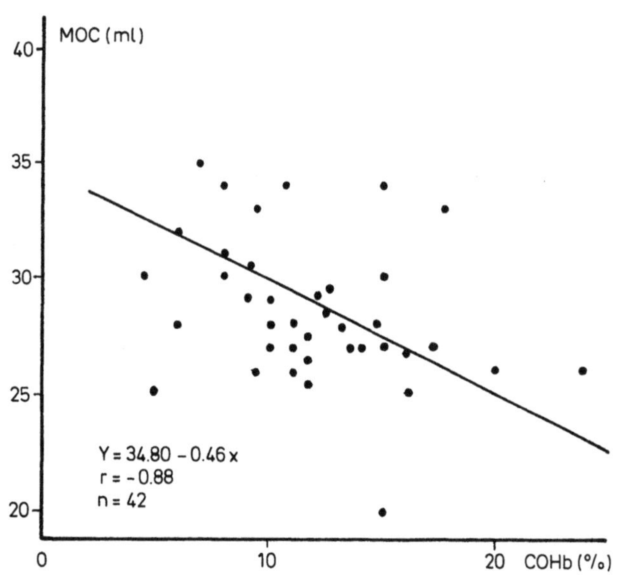

Fig. 1. Correlation between MOC and COHb

Table 2. Cigarette smoking in relation to pulse rate and systolic blood pressure (kPa)

	Non-smokers	Moderate smokers	Heavy smokers	*t*-test[a] $P<0.01$
Pulse rate				
x̄	128	152	166	12.0
SD	+6.0	+5.2	+5.0	
Blood pressure (systolic)				
x̄	18.7	20.0	24.0	6.6
SD	+1.0	+1.2	+1.3	
No. of persons	14	19	57	

[a] *t*-test = heavy smokers : non-smokers

Table 3. Cigarette smoking in relation to lactate concentration (mg%)

	Non-smokers	Moderate smokers	Heavy smokers	*t*-test[a] $P<0.01$
Lactate concentration				
x̄	27.0	48.9	61.3	5.5
SD	+3.0	+5.0	+5.1	
No. of persons	14	19	57	

[a] *t*-test = heavy smokers : non-smokers

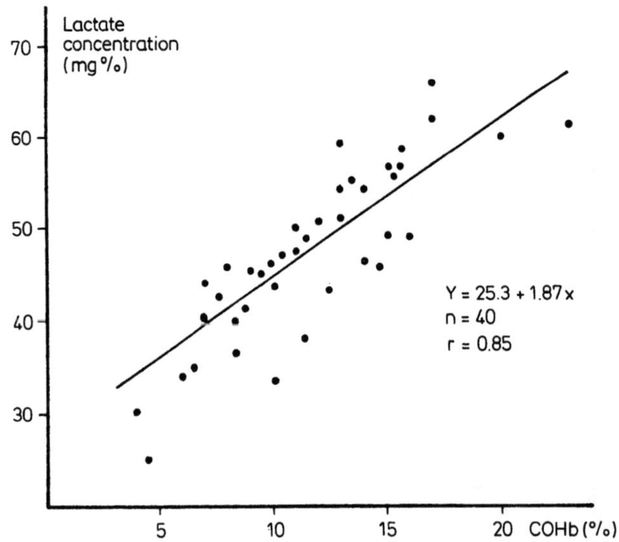

Fig. 2. Correlation between lactate concentration and COHb

blood of heavy smokers was six times higher than that in non-smokers, while MOC was statistically significantly lower in heavy smokers than in non-smokers. A significant negative correlation was found between COHb level and MOC ($r = -0.88$) (Fig. 1).

The pulse rate during the last minute of testing (the "work pulse") was significantly higher in heavy smokers than in non-smokers (x = 166 : 128), as was systolic blood pressure (x = 24.0 : 18.7 kPa) (Table 2). A positive significant correlation was found between COHb level and pulse rate ($r = +0.7$) and between COHb level and blood pressure ($r = +0.8$).

The lactate concentration of blood in heavy smokers was also significantly higher than in non-smokers (Table 3). There was a positive significant correlation between COHb level and lactate concentration in the blood of heavy smokers ($r = +0.85$) (Fig. 2); in non-smokers such a correlation was not found.

Discussion

Investigation of the relationship between smoking habits and physical fitness showed that heavy smokers have a very bad aerobic capacity. By contrast, non-smokers have a good aerobic capacity.

It may be pointed out that there were high COHb and lactate concentrations in the blood of heavy smokers. These findings are connected with low MOC in heavy smokers, and also with a high pulse rate and high blood pressure.

All these factors indicate that the COHb level in the blood of heavy smokers is of great importance for physical fitness.

References

1. Hammond EC (1972) The relationship between human smoking habits and death rates. Arch Environ Health 1316:166
2. Doll R, Hill AB (1964) Mortality in relation to smoking: ten years observation of British doctors. Br Med J 1:1399
3. Goldsmith J, Landaw AS (1968) Carbon monoxide and human health. Science 162:1352
4. Guillerm R (1978) La fumée du tabac. Composition et effets physiologiques. Rev Prat 28:1403
5. Goldsmith JR (1970) Contribution of motor vehicle exhaust industry and cigarette smoking to comminuty carbon monoxide exposure. Ann NY Acad Sci 174:122
6. Astrand PO, Rodhal K (1970) Textbook of work capacity physiology. McGraw-Hill, New York
7. Commins BT, Lawther PJ (1965) A sensitive method for the determination of carboxyhemoglobin in a finger prick sample of blood. Br J Ind Med 22:139

Reduction of Cigarette Consumption as the Most Important Task of Preventive Medicine and Health Policy

F. Schmidt

Smoking has become one of the most important single causes of disease and death. This has been documented in a previous publication [1]. What has been done up to now to deal with this evident threat to national health in our country? The answer is shattering: practically nothing! Without intervention, constantly rising advertising expenditure has been allowed to win new customers for tobacco, specifically amongst adolescents and women, although in a press release the Federal Health Ministry already observed years ago that 40% of all cases of cancer in men could be prevented by not smoking. In men and women together, according to a report by Doll and Peto [2] for the American Congress, 30% of all cancer deaths are due to smoking. Besides numerous further smokers' cancers, 90% of all bronchial carcinomas are due to smoking. In this connection, I do not hesitate to speak of a bankruptcy declaration of our health policy in the field of smoking. A convincing example of this is the description of the situation and review of the second major cancer conference in 1982 which I recently published [3]. In the meantime, this conference convened by the Federal government in 1979 has held countless sessions in numerous working groups. Despite my constant admonitions as chairman of the medical study group on smoking and health and as a member of the expert advisory panel Smoking and Health of the WHO, the topic of smoking was not put on the agenda in a single session in the last 3 years. What should be done has been known for a long time. Five world conferences on smoking and health have made numerous suggestions on this. The Scandinavian countries have shown a good example by practical measures which have already produced clearly recognizable successes. For years, the medical study group on smoking and health at the spearhead of the struggle against smoking in the Federal Republic of Germany has endeavored in vain to prompt the responsible authorities, especially the Committee on Youth, Family and Health of the Federal Parliament and the responsible Health Ministry to institute the forceful countermeasures.

You will doubtless understand that I cannot discuss in detail a program of action against smoking in the time available here. Our suggestions and demands have been available for scrutiny for a long time. There is no doubt that the most urgent task of lowering cigarette consumption cannot be solved by a single measure, but only by an entire bundle of measures. Activities should be focused on those who do not yet smoke, i.e. schoolchildren and adolescents in order to motivate as large a proportion of them as possible to remain non-

Primary Health Care in the Making
Ed. by U. Laaser, R. Senault, H. Viefhues

smokers. Worldwide experience has shown that only modest partial successes can be achieved in habitual adult smokers who are already nicotine dependent.

I should like to restrict myself here to two suggestions or demands from which positive results can be expected with a comparatively small effort.

Demand No. 1

Since it is understandably not interested in lowering consumption, the cigarette industry should attempt to reduce the health damage from smoking in another way, primarily by reduction of the content of toxic substances in their products. However, the attempt to ward off the serious threat to national health by "light smoking" has in the meantime proved to be on the wrong track. This has just been proved in an extensive review of the world literature on this topic which I have published elsewhere [4]. Here are only the most important facts:

The tar and nicotine content of cigarettes which must be printed on every pack and on every advertising poster is determined under standardized conditions with a smoking machine. However, the smoker does not orientate himself according to the measurement values of a machine, but according to his individual needs and habits. Here, the nicotine content of the tobacco is the primary determining factor, as has been shown by numerous investigations, e.g. by Jonston, Finnegan et al., Lucchesi et al., Ague, Ashton et al., Knapp et al., Frith, Kirsch, Russell et al. (see [4]). The fact that smokers do not smoke dried lettuce leaves etc., but dried tobacco because of its nicotine content should be sufficient evidence.

If one recognizes this basic fact, then a simple logical deduction results from it: reduction of the nicotine content below a certain level will not be accepted by the smoker. The disappearance of the "nicotine-free cigarettes" from the market is a clear proof of this. The smoker either switches to another cigarette brand or attempts to ingest the usual amount of nicotine in another way. Above all, two possibilities are available here: raised consumption or increased inhalations. Both means of raising nicotine intake are practiced. The rise in cigarette consumption from year to year, e.g. in the Federal Republic of Germany is not attributable to an increased number of smokers, but to a raised average consumption of the individual smoker. The most obvious explanation for this phenomenon is that the market share of filter cigarettes in West Germany has risen to more than 87% in the meantime. Nevertheless, numerous investigations (not the least from the research institute of the German cigarette industry itself) leave no doubt that the (unconscious) increase of the depth of inhalation, which can vary by 2 powers of ten, and the increased number of draws on the cigarette to take up nicotine are very much more important than the content of toxic substances (Harke, Benowitz et al., Jarvik et al., Russel et al., Kirsch, Jaffe et al., Ashton et al., Wald, Lundh et al., Lynn and Kozlowski et al.; see [4]). This means that even a halving of the content of toxic substances can be readily compensated or even overcompensated by a more intensive inhalation of only 1%.

Accordingly, the 1981 report of Surgeon General of the USA "The Changing Cigarette" was summarized as follows (see [4]): Indications are that there is no safe cigarette and no safe level of consumption. Smoking cigarettes with lower yields of tar and nicotine reduces the risk of lung cancer and, to some extent, improves the smoker's chance for a longer life, provided there is no compensatory increase in the amount smoked. However the benefits are minimal in comparison with giving up cigarettes entirely ... Compensatory behavior may negate any advantage of the lower yield product or even increase the health risk....

This observation is also underscored by epidemiological studies, e.g. by the development of the lung cancer mortality in the Federal Republic of Germany. Although the content of toxic substances in the cigarettes on the market in Germany was reduced to less than half from 1961 to 1975 according to data from the industry and has fallen since then by a further 36% according to analysis carried out by the Consumer Goods Testing Foundation, the number of lung cancer deaths has risen continuously since 1961 and reached a new absolute record in the last year evaluated with 25.000 lung cancer deaths according to the data of the Federal Office of Statistics. Even if one takes into account the long latency period of bronchial carcinoma, the incidence of lung cancer in West Germany should not have increased, but should have decreased if a lowered tar content had indeed entailed a lowered risk of cancer.

Convincing proof of this is the large decrease of lung cancer incidence in former smokers. According to Doll and Pike (see [4]), 3 500 out of 35 000. British doctors gave up smoking in the period from 1951 to 1966. The proportion of cigarette smokers fell from 44.1% to 22%. In parallel with this, the age-corrected incidence of lung cancer of British doctors fell by around one quarter from 1951 to 1965, whereas it continued to rise sharply in the same period in the rest of the British population.

In California, the proportion of smokers among doctors decreased dramatically according to Enstrom from 53% in 1950 to 10% in 1980. The standardized lung cancer mortality accordingly sank from 62 to 30 up to 1979, i.e. to less than one half. The age-corrected mortality for other smoker's diseases fell from 100 to 63, e.g. from 106 to 71 for myocardial infarction and from 62 to 35 for chronic bronchitis, emphysema and asthma.

On the other hand, in the Framingham study, it was shown that the rate of myocardial infarction and angina pectoris cases among filter cigarette smokers is not less than amongst smokers of unfiltered cigarettes, even if the age, systolic blood pressure and the serum cholesterol levels of the two groups are also considered.

The same applies to the lung function and respiratory symptoms which may indeed even be intensified by deeper inhalation of filter cigarettes. The same applies to the fetus in mothers who smoke in pregnancy.

According to Miller, the life expectancy of filter cigarette smokers is shortened by an average of 2–3 years compared to smokers of unfiltered cigarettes (see [4]).

Although initially I was also skeptical with regard to this result, I considered it prudent to include the survival time in a study on the epidemiology of lung cancer in the Mannheim-Ludwigshafen-Heidelberg region at our research department: among 792 bronchial cancer patients of whom 97.3% were smokers, the average age of death of the smokers of filter cigarettes was significantly lower by 1.6 years than in smokers of cigarettes without filters. This shortening of life expectancy of the filter smokers was especially remarkable since their average daily consumption was 4.6 cigarettes less than in smokers of nonfilter cigarettes and because the total number of cigarettes smoked was about 20% less in the smokers of filter cigarettes. A total duration of smoking was also very much shorter than in the smokers of cigarettes without filters (40.5 years as compared to 43.1 years) and not vice versa as would have been to be expected with a lower carcinogenic activity of the smoke from filter cigarettes.

The incidence of gastric and duodenal ulcer is also not reduced by smoking filter cigarettes. The same applies to cancer of the oral cavity, the esophagus, the pancreas, the kidney and bladder. All these results are clear evidence that an evaluation of the harmfulness of cigarettes merely on the basis of the content of toxic substances is inadmissible and misleads the smoker.

There are individual studies which indicate a lower rate of lung cancer in smokers of filter cigarettes. However, even in these investigations the reduction in cancer incidence did not exceed 20% in any case. Even if one were to regard these results as substantiated, then there is no question that a lowering of the content of toxic substances does not make smoking a cigarette brand "safe", especially since it cannot be excluded that smokers of filter cigarettes constitute a selection of smokers. For example, they are likely to smoke less on average, and according to a natural health survey in the USA have also attempted to stop smoking more often than smokers of unfiltered cigarettes.

The slight lowering of the mortality rate from lung cancer in men less than 60 years of age, above all in the USA, also cannot be recognized as evidence for the reduced harmfulness of raised consumption of filter cigarettes, as alleged by the cigarette industry. It is likely to be attributable to the considerable number of smokers who have stopped smoking.

Conclusions

If the nicotine content of tobacco is decisive for smoking and as has been described its reduction can be compensated without difficulties either by increased inhalation and/or by raised consumption, there is the following logical consequence:

If one wishes to reduce the harmfulness of smoking to health, then the content of tar and other toxic substances (e.g. the highly toxic CO of the gas phase, notification of which is mandatory so far only in a few countries such as Sweden) should be lowered as far as possible, but not the nicotine concentration. On the contrary, the nicotine content should if anything be raised, in order to give the smoker the possibility of satisfying his individually different requirement for nicotine with a smaller number of cigarettes. In this way, at least the uptake of other toxic substances will be reduced. This expectation is also encouraged by the fact that nicotine can be degraded and detoxified relatively easily in chronic incorporation of subtoxic doses, in contrast e.g. to carcinogenic substances. If this were not so, many chain smokers who ingest more than fatal nicotine dose (if taken at once) in the course of a single day would very rapidly suffer an acute intoxication. It appears that the rapid breakdown of nicotine is also the reason why there are practically no results on the health damage from chronic small doses of nicotine. I therefore already advised the German cigarette industry in 1977 that they should by no means lower the nicotine content in cigarettes but should raise it. In view of the results described, I should like to raise this recommendation to a demand.

Demand No. 2

However, as an even better alternative I should like to repeat here the demand I already presented in 1980 that, in order to reduce the health damage from smoking, natural untreated tobacco, which does not tempt the smoker to inhale, should also be prescribed for cigarettes.

The "main killer" in smoking is known to be the cigarette. Cigar and pipe smokers are endangered less than cigarette smokers because pipe and cigarette smoke is as a rule not inhaled due to its alkaline reaction. It is beyond comprehension that for example in Germany in the tobacco regulation the use of foreign substances, including such harmless additives as liquorice and logwood extract is laid down as far as the smallest detail, but that incomparably more important and more dangerous processing by fermentation, addition of dressings, etc., which make tobacco smoke inhalable has been completely ignored so far here and in other countries.

Such a regulation would have at least four advantages:

1. It would not cost a penny.
2. It could be put into practice without technical difficulties.
3. It would probably prevent more disease and (at least in the long term) save more human lives than all measures together instituted so far against smoking.
4. The health minister in his own responsibility can institute such a regulation without a new law, that must first pass numerous parliamentary obstacles.
   In Germany, the health minister is empowered by § 21 of the Foodstuffs and Utility Goods Law to restrict or prohibit completely the use of certain techniques in the manufacture and treatment of tobacco goods by the legal statute when this is necessary to protect the consumer from health damage. This is doubtless the case here.

There is no question that the lowering of consumption probably connected with this will meet the resistance of industry. However, it is unacceptable that cigarette consumption continues to increase and that ever new classes of buyers, e.g. young girls and women, are caught in the vortex of unscrupulous advertising, not in the least due to an enormous rise in advertising expenditure.

Similar to the introduction of a warning notice on cigarette packs, increased pressure should be placed on the cigarette industry to use natural untreated tobacco in the manufacture of cigarettes in the future (as used for cigars) and if necessary to enforce this by statute. The switch could be made easier both for cigarette companies and for smokers by giving a transition deadline of 6 to a maximum of 12 months. It should be left to the cigarette companies themselves to determine the stages by which they wish to effect the transition by mixture of the cigarette tobaccos used so far with natural untreated tobacco.

Summary

1. Analytical determination of the toxic substances in cigarette smoke does not permit any assessment of the practical health damage to the smoker.
2. The large-scale advertising for "light smoking" is therefore misleading and is of more value to the health of the industry than of the consumer.
3. The only healthy cigarette is the cigarette which is not smoked.
4. Two alternatives are suggested in order to make cigarette smoking less dangerous to health:
   a) Voluntary agreement with the industry or if necessary a statutory regulation to permit in the future only cigarettes with natural untreated tobacco on the Federal German market and to prohibit all processing measures which favour the inhalation of tobacco smoke
   b) The demand on industry to lower only the content of tar and other toxic substances in the cigarette smoke as far as possible, but to raise the nicotine content

References

1. Schmidt F (1982) Der öffentl. Dienst 35:97–120, 122–129
2. Doll R, Peto R (1982) J Nat Cancer Inst 66:1191
3. Schmidt F (1983) Mitteilungsdienst Ges. Bekämpfung d. Krebskrankh. Nordrhein-Westfalen 11:39–40
4. Schmidt F (in press) Suchtgefahren

A New Approach to Diet Counseling of Overweight Patients and Diabetics

E. Poetter, L. P. Krall, K. Huth, F. W. Schmahl

Summary

Health education and diet counseling are essential elements in the treatment of overweight patients and diabetics. In the past, physicians and nutritionists have developed a variety of highly sophisticated methods for formulating diabetic diets. In the Federal Republic of Germany, diabetic diet prescriptions either focus on carbohydrates or recommend calculations based on nutrient value tables that are too academic and impractical for everyday nutrition or patient education. The practical result of such calculations is often a monotonous meal plan.

In the United States and Switzerland, a more pragmatic system utilizing an exchange plan for six food groups is preferred. There are plans in which the portions of these six food groups contain different nutrient amounts (USA) or 10 g of carbohydrates, protein, or fat in each of the exchange portions (Switzerland). In the Federal Republic, one single exchange portion containing 12 g of carbohydrate, i.e., the "Broteinheit," is recommended.

A basic food exchange system is presented which is based on familiar measures and portions and combines the different national approaches in order to establish a more international exchange system based on the six food groups and the "Broteinheit" (12 g carbohydrate exchange unit) with exchanges that have the same energy value.

The nutritional values are characterized by three colored symbols which encourage visual comprehension. This basis of diet counseling is well suited for the less educated patient, since it does not require calculation of food values for energy, carbohydrate, fat, and protein contents.

The nutrition counselor will appreciate the quick, thorough meal planning which can be closely adapted to individual eating habits. With this approach, any kind of energy-, carbohydrate-, protein-, and fat-defined diet can be taught in mixed groups of overweight patients and diabetics.

It is unfortunate that diets do not come in pill form. Such a diet would be "easy to prescribe, easy to take, and easy to adjust to the patient's needs." In reality, however, the diet is the most difficult aspect of therapy, both for the physician and for the patient. Setting up a diet prescription involves a considerable investment of time for the physician and the nutritionist, and the patient usually finds the prescribed diet difficult to follow. Patient compliance therefore is poor.

Why is the diabetic diet so difficult to follow? Maintenance of a balanced diet usually requires a great deal of self-discipline as well as meticulous planning, calculating, and weighing. In the German diabetic diet schedule, a certain nutritional content, particularly a defined amount of carbohydrate, is prescribed for each meal. The patient must be capable of evaluating and calculating all

Primary Health Care in the Making
Ed. by U. Laaser, R. Senault, H. Viefhues

foods according to their nutritional value. Like the caloric value, the nutritional value is a scientific, abstract calculation that can be neither seen nor tasted. Most people have no idea how many grams of carbohydrate there are in a slice of bread or a small apple or what these two foods weigh. The problem, however, becomes increasingly more complicated when the amount of fat and, perhaps, protein as well as the number of calories in different kinds of luncheon meats or dairy products, for example, must also be taken into consideration.

Planning and calculating a complete meal made up of a variety of foods in different portions using nutrient tables is virtually impossible without a calculator and complicated calculations. For everyday use, such nutrient calculations are impractical and the patient does not have the necessary knowledge. The German Nutrition Report of 1980 states: "The average person is not in a position to associate calories with nutrients or amounts such as 100 g. These are abstract concepts for the average person who is familiar with the food itself and practical portions, such as teaspoons, bottles, and slices [1]."

The housewife plans meals with different portions of food: a bowl of soup, a glass of milk, a slice of bread. The selection and amount are dictated by habit and experience, without knowledge of the caloric value or nutritional content of each food.

A didactic revision of dietetic terminology, which contains concepts such as "caloric value" and "absorbable carbohydrate," is imperative. The diet plan must be expressed in a language the layman can understand and facilitate meal planning with food portions that can be varied.

To fill this need, exchange systems were developed. In Germany, the calculation of carbohydrate-rich foods with "Broteinheiten" was adopted. In this diabetic diet prescription, each meal is assigned a certain number of Broteinheiten. The exchange table then lists amounts of food that contain 12 g of digestible carbohydrate. Since the portions are easy to remember, constancy of carbohydrate intake from day to day is ensured.

Calculating the diabetic diet with Broteinheiten, however, also has its share of problems (Table 1): Diabetics often slice their bread extremely thin, so that it weighs no more than 25 g and represents 1 Broteinheit. An average slice of bread, however, weighs 50 g! This thin slice is then spread thickly with butter. Lunch consists of a small helping of potatoes swimming in butter and a large

Table 1. Diabetic diet calculated according to "Broteinheiten" (carbohydrate exchanges) and alternative concepts

Diabetic diet calculated according to "Broteinheiten" (carbohydrate exchanges)	Alternative concepts
Energy is not limited	Calculation of fat (e.g., 10 g portions)
Carbohydrate-rich foods have a different "blood sugar effect"	Subgroups of carbohydrate-rich foods (e.g., A, B, C)
Patient attitude: "Carbohydrate-rich foods are bad"	Complete exchange system for all foods

steak. Even whipped cream on a piece of cake does not upset the Broteinheit calculation.

The problem is that the Broteinheit system does not limit calories, a serious problem given the fact that most diabetics are overweight and should be consuming low-calorie foods.

The diabetic must also calculate calories, or at least fat. Precisely here most errors are made, since fat is hidden in many foods. Even though 10-g fat

Table 2. Exchange lists

● = ca. 12 g carbohydrate (1 Broteinheit) 1.5 g protein 50 calories (210 Joules)	▲ = ca. 7 g protein 2 g fat 50 calories (210 Joules)	■ = ca. 5 g fat 50 calories (210 Joules)

● Bread

Kaiser roll	1/2	20 g
White bread	1/2 slice	20 g
Rye bread	1/2 slice	25 g
Whole wheat bread	1/2 slice	25 g
Ryvita	2	15 g
Pretzelsticks	15	15 g
Crackers	6	15 g
Rolled oats	1 Tbsp	20 g
Flour	1 Tbsp	15 g
Cornstarch	1 Tbsp	15 g
Farina	1 Tbsp	15 g
Pudding powder (without sugar)	1 Tbsp	15 g
Potato	1/2 medium-sized	60 g
Potato dumpling		
Mashed potatoes	1/2 portion	90 g
Rice, boiled	1/2 cup	50 g
Nudels, boiled	1/2 cup	50 g
Thickened soups (can or package)	1 cup	1/4 liter

Clear bouillon (without fat) may be used as desired

● ■

Potato pancake	1 small	40 g
French fried potatoes	6	35 g
Cookies (diabetic)	4	20 g

● Fruit

Apple Orange Pear Peach Fruit, canned (unsweetenend)	1 small	100 g
Tangerines	2	100 g
Apricots		100 g
Plums		80 g
Plums, sweet		50 g
Blackberries Strawberries Raspberries Honeydew melon	1 cup	150 g
Watermelon	2 cups	250 g
Grapefruit	1/2	120 g
Banana	1/4	50 g
Currants, red Gooseberries Blueberries	2/3 cup	120 g
Cherries, sour Currants, black Pineapple, fresh	1/2 cup	100 g
Cherries, sweet Mirabelles Grapes	10	80 g
Fruit juice	1 small glass	0.1 liter
Vegetable juice	1 large glass	0.2 liter
Fructose Sorbitol	1 Tbsp	12 g
Jam		
diabetic	1 Tbsp	25 g
with saccharin	2 Tbsp	50 g

Table 2 (continued)

● Vegetables			Leek		ca. 100 g
Cauliflower		ca. 200 g	Brussel sprouts		
Green beans			Red beets		
Brocolli			Black salsify		
Endive			Celery root		
Eggplant			Turnips		
Fennel			Onions		
Cabbage			Green peas		
Kohlrabi			Peas, canned		
Greenpepper			Legumes, dried:		
Sauerkraut			Beans, lentils, peas		ca. 20 g
Asparagus					
Spinach			Cucumbers, lettuce,		may be
Mushrooms			Cress, pumpkin,		used as
Artichoke		ca. 100 g	Radish, rhubarb,		desired
Carrots			Celery leaves,		
Rutabaga			Chicory		
●▲ Milk			**●▲■**		
			Whole milk	1 glass	0.2
Milk, skim	1 glass	0.2	Kefir		liter
Buttermilk		liter	Milk, sour		
Joghurt, low fat	1 cup	200 g	Joghurt, whole milk	1 cup	200 g
▲ Meat			**▲■**		
Veal, very lean	1/4		Beaf, lean	1/4	
Beef, very lean	portion	30 g	Pork, lean	portion	30 g
Pork, very lean			Luncheon meat	1 slice	25 g
Poultry, very lean			Cheese	1 slice	25 g
Game, very lean			(30–50% fat)		
Bacon, very lean	1/2		Frankfurter	1/3	40 g
Corned beef	slice	30 g		portion	
Cheese (30% fat or lower)	1 slice	25 g	Herring	1/2	
Cottage cheese, low fat	1 Tbsp	50 g	Bückling	portion	50 g
Fish: cod, pollock,	1/4		Fish, smoked		
halibut, mackerel,	portion	50 g	Sardines, tuna fish		
ocean perch, carp,			in oil, drained		
trout, tuna fish in water			Egg	1	60 g
■ Fat					
Butter	1 tsp	5 g	Cream cheese	1 Tbsp	15 g
Margarine[a]	1 tsp	5 g	Pork belly	1 thin slice	8 g
Lard	1 tsp	5 g	Salami	1 thin slice	8 g
Coconut oil	1 tsp	5 g	Saveloy	1 thin slice	10 g
Vegetable oil[a]	1 tsp	5 g	Olives, green	6	20 g
Mayonnaise[a]	1 tsp	5 g	Almonds[a]	10	8 g
Salad dressing[a]	1 Tbsp	15 g	Peanuts[a]	15	8 g
Whipped cream	1 Tbsp	15 g	Walnuts[a]	6	8 g
Sour cream	3 Tbsp	50 g	Other nuts[a]		8 g

[a] Contains polyunsaturated fatty acids and therefore is well suited for individuals on a fat-modified diet

exchange tables are available, the diet calculation is further complicated by the additional calculation of fat or calories.

In addition, carbohydrate-rich foods are metabolized differently. Jenkins, comparing the effect of various foods on blood sugar level with that of glucose, demonstrated that when the rise of blood sugar under pure glucose loading is taken as 100%, the rise for foods high in starch, such as bread, potatoes, and rice, is 70%; for fruit, 50%; and for dairy products, approximately 35% [2]. Some diabetes centers therefore have divided their diet plans into subgroups of carbohydrate-rich foods.

The third criticism concerns the psychological aspect: The calculation of carbohydrates gives the diabetic the idea that carbohydrate-rich foods are bad and, because the diabetic wants to follow the diet rigorously, he or she begins to reduce the prescribed carbohydrate intake, especially a few days before the next doctor's appointment. The meals therefore are not well balanced and the physician has no basis for making therapeutic decisions about, for example, an adjustment of the insulin dose.

These errors can be avoided with a diet schedule that lists all foods in portions and in food groups. Exchange tables and meal plan of such a diet schedule are presented in Tables 2 and 3. US and Swiss diets have been calculated with these six food groups for years [3, 4]. The number of portions from the six groups is given for each meal.

Bread, fruit, vegetable, and milk groups composed of carbohydrate-rich food are designated by a green circle; meat and milk groups with protein-rich

Table 3. Meal plan

Meal plan	___ calories ___ g carbohydrate ___ g protein ___ joules ___ Broteinheiten ___ g fat					
	Bread ●	Meat ▲ ■	Fruit ●	Milk ● ▲ ■	Vege-tables ●	Fat ■
Breakfast time: ___						
Midmorning snack time: ___						
Lunch time: ___						
Midafternoon snack time: ___						
Supper time: ___						
Bedtime snack time: ___						

Table 4. Carbohydrate and energy value of exchange portions

Exchanges	Standardized exchanges lists			Exchange lists USA	
	Symbol	Carbo-hydrate (g)	Energy (kcal)	Carbo-hydrate (g)	Energy (kcal)
Bread	●	12	50	15	70
Fruit	●	12	50	10	40
Vegetable	●	12	50	5	25
Milk[a]	● ▲	12	100	12	103
Meat	▲	–	50	–	55
Fat	■	–	50	–	45

[a] Low fat milk

food and a relatively high fat content, by a red triangle for protein and, when appropriate, a yellow square for fat; and the fat group with predominantly fat-rich food, by a yellow square.

The foods in the six groups are listed in their own exchange table and, in the cited portions, have about the same nutritional and caloric value. Slight differences arise due to grouping and listing of the most practical portions. Good metabolic adjustment, however, is ensured with a nutrient constancy for the meals of +/− 10% to 20%.

The carbohydrate amounts and caloric values of portions for the six exchange groups as used in the United States and then in the standardized form that seems most feasible for Germany are presented in Table 4.

Each carbohydrate-rich portion in the standardized model has 12 g carbohydrate, which corresponds to the calculation with Broteinheiten. The amounts of carbohydrate and the caloric value differ in the US exchange plan. The caloric value of the standardized exchange portions is 50 calories (210 KJ) per symbol. The symbols represent the nutritional content for each food group with about the same caloric content.

The number of symbols per meal or per day multiplied by 50 yields the caloric value, which simplifies adherence to a calorie-defined diet. The calculation therefore is well suited for diabetic and low-calorie diets for overweight diabetics and nondiabetics. Both diabetic and overweight patients therefore can be counseled together, a factor which is extremely important for smaller hospitals and for the practicing physician (see Table 5). Calculation is also simplified for the nutritionist: It can be made while the nutrition history is being taken and then discussed immediately with the patient. Tables 6–8 show the steps of a specific diet calculation [for more detailed information, see 5]. Some of the aspects supporting this simple, standardized schedule are shown in Table 9.

Carbohydrate, protein, and fat, represented by three variously colored symbols, are listed in a common exchange system that allows simple calculation of calories and ensures constancy of nutrients and calories at each meal with a widely varied selection of foods.

Table 5. Curriculum plan for instruction of diabetics and overweight patients in the clinical setting

	Lecture (60 min) (group teaching)	Counseling (20–30 min) (individual teaching)
Monday		Patient is encouraged to attend course "Nutrition at home and in the hospital"; nutrition history is taken (nutritionist)
Tuesday	"Medical aspects of nutrition-related diseases" (physician)	Normal values for weight, blood sugar, cholesterol, triglycerides; comparison with patient values (nutritionist)
Wednesday	"Fundamentals of nutrition and diet calculation (nutritionist)	Practice arranging food into groups; analysis of nutrition history (nutritionist)
Thursday (diabetics only)	"Self-responsibility and self-control" (nurse)	Practice carrying out urinalysis, insulin injection, response to hypoglycemia and hyperglycemia, sports, diabetic ID, foot care, and general hygiene (nurse)
Friday		Setting up plan (diet prescription) based on nutrition history (nutritionist)

Table 6. Calculation of diet in exchange portions, using the example of a low-calorie diet (1000 calories: 50% carbohydrate, 20% protein, 30% fat)

	%	Calories	g	Exchanges
		1000		
Carbohydrate	50	500:4[a]	125 :12[b]	10 ●
Protein	20	200:4[a]	50–[b] (10×1.5)=35: 7[b]	5 ▲
Fat	30	300:9[a]	33–[b] (5×2)= : 5[b]	5 ■

[a] Approximate caloric value per gram nutrient
[b] ● 12 g carbohydrate + 1.5 g protein
▲ 7 g protein + 2 g fat
■ 5 g fat

Table 7. Simplified calculation of exchange portions in nutrient proportions of 50% carbohydrate, 20% protein, 30% fat

Prescribed amount of energy (calories) : Energy content of 1 exchange portion (50 calories) = Number of exchange portions

1/2 carbohydrate exchanges ● | 1/4 protein exchanges ▲ | 1/4 fat exchanges ■

Table 8. Standard diets in exchange portions

Energy (calories)	Carbohydrate ●	g	Protein ▲	g	Fat ■	g
800	8	96	4	40	4	28
1000	10	120	5	50	5	35
1200	12	144	6	60	6	42
1400	14	168	7	70	7	49
1600	16	192	8	80	8	56
1800	18	216	9	90	9	63
2000	20	240	10	100	10	70
2200	22	264	11	110	11	77
2400	24	288	12	120	12	84
2600	26	312	13	130	13	91
2800	28	326	14	140	14	98
3000	30	360	15	150	15	105

Table 9. Diet calculated according to six food groups

Constancy of nutrients and energy per meal through integrated exchange system for carbohydrate, protein, fat, and caloric value
12 g carbohydrate exchanges (BE) in four different food groups: bread, fruit, vegetables, milk (foods in any one group have a similar "blood sugar effect")
Patient attitude: "Diet is well-balanced nutrition"

Carbohydrate-rich foods, in 12-g carbohydrate portions corresponding to the adopted Broteinheit calculation, are exchanged in four different food groups: bread, fruit, vegetable, and milk (i.e., groups with about the same "blood sugar effect").

The patient develops the attitude that "a well-balanced diet consists of a certain number of food portions from different food groups" and that diet is well-planned and well-balanced nutrition.

References

1. Deutsche Gesellschaft für Ernährung (1980) Ernährungsbericht 1980. Frankfurt
2. Jenkins DJA, Wolever TMS, Taylor RH, Barker H, Fielden H, Baldwin JM, Bowling AC, Newman HC, Jenkins A, Goff DV (1981) Glycemic index of foods: a physiological basis for carbohydrate exchange. Am J Clin Nutr 34:362–366
3. American Diabetes Association and American Dietetic Association (1976) Exchange lists for meal planning.
4. Teuscher A (1976) Diabetes Diät-Schema. Aldepha, Zurich
5. Poetter E (1981) Ernährungsberatung und Gesundheitserziehung im Krankenhaus. Ein Schulungsmodell für Diabetiker. Dissertation, Justus Liebig University, Giessen

Adiposity – A Challenge to the General Practitioner in Therapy and Prevention

I. Cleres-Kaiser

Motivation

During my 14 years' activity as a general practitioner in a rural environment, the failure of therapies for adiposity, such as appetite depressants, diets (including the so-called computer diet) and zero calories, has become evident. This is why I am convinced of the necessity to find another way that will lead to more lasting success.

In general, adiposity is an important factor predisposing to angiocardiopathy, which accounted for 47.2% of deaths in the Federal Republic of Germany in 1977. Adiposity also predisposes one to the following diseases: (1) diabetes mellitus, (2) hypertonia, (3) gouty arthritis, (4) arthroses of the spine and the larger joints, (5) obstipation, (6) cholelithiasis and (7) nephrolithiasis.

In the Federal Republic of Germany, probably one out of every five inhabitants is overweight. This is why the medical profession dare not neglect this field.

Practical Measures

We were fortunate in obtaining the cooperation of a female group-leader with personal experience in the field for a course open to all the citizens of Monschau, a town in the Eifel with 11 000 inhabitants. Meetings were held on a regular basis, for ca. 1 h once weekly, in the general practitioner's waiting room, which has independent access. In dietary counselling, the Weight Watchers' method was largely followed, which, for the first time, sets up a logical behavioural therapy through weekly meetings on a voluntary and cost-sharing basis. Activities comprise weighing, information, discussion, diet plans with indication of the quantity and quality of permitted foods (mainly reduced carbohydrate intake and protein-rich foods) and abstention from alcohol, sweets and sugar-containing drinks. This programme has been carried out in the Federal Republic of Germany since 1970.

Anti-adiposity training – along with dietary counselling – must take into consideration all aspects of the personality, as the symptom adiposity is the

Primary Health Care in the Making
Ed. by U. Laaser, R. Senault, H. Viefhues

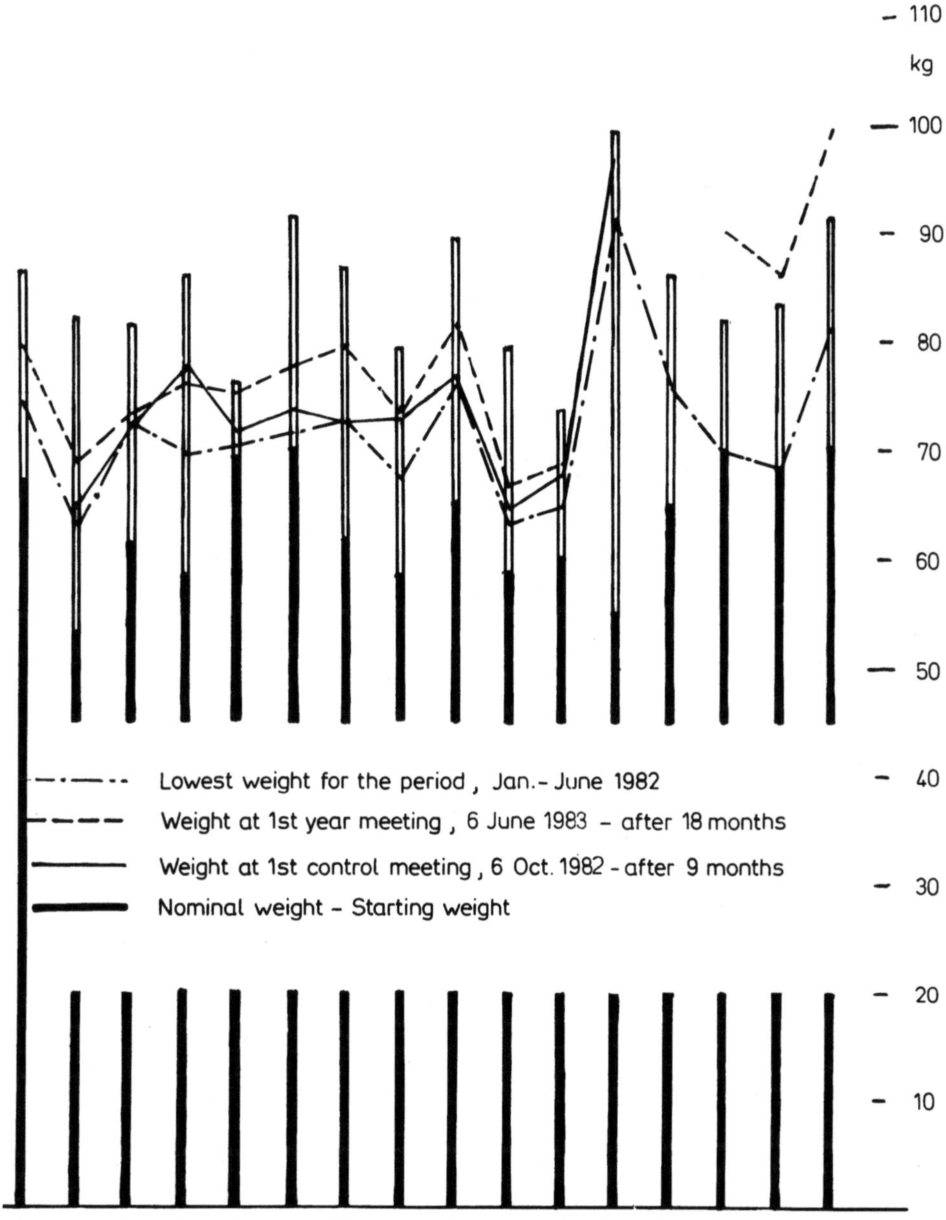

Fig. 1. Results of the anti-adiposity programme in Monschau (16 patients)

compensation phenomenon indicating a psychosocial deficiency. In order to guarantee long-term success of the *dietary therapy, personal training* is also indicated. This will consist, inter alia, of a revision of past life-styles and habits as well as a positive auto-suggestion achieved by daily training aimed at developing the individual's own abilities. Supporting the daily diet, simple *physical exercise* combined with breathing exercise has proved beneficial. Ideally, two or three yoga exercises are chosen for and in cooperation with each individual participant. *Suggestion by words* will reinforce the effect, such as: "plump is numb", "weight makes empty", "light weight is high paid", "my mind is at rest – my food was the best" and "I like to eat what's good for me – that keeps excess weight away from me" (Fig. 1).

Results of 1 1/2 Years of Anti-adiposity Measures in Monschau

All of 16 participants (aged between 14 and 59 years) had reached a maximum loss of weight: 18%–22% of their initial weight. Nine months later, at the first motivation meeting, a weight increase from 0 to a maximum of 5% was found; and another increase averaging 6% of the initial weight had occurred after 18 months. Only one participant had regained her initial weight. Four participants had left the group after 6 or 9 months; two of these were adolescents who had exceede their initial weight after 18 months.

Future Developments

In the near future, we may envisage a *medical practice with a wider range of curative, preventive, health advisory and health-promoting functions.* This could take the form of a group practice where practitioners work in these directions, each with a different point of emphasis. It might also take the form of cooperation amongst the practitioners in a larger residential area. The aim is a long-term reduction of extreme risk factors such as adiposity, alcoholism, nicotine addiction and possibly also the so-called civilisation diseases, where feasible with the participation of the nearest hospital or university clinic. The most effective way of achieving this aim appears to be a *patient-oriented local group* run by a group-leader and assisted by lay people and medical supervision, because it provides opportunities for personal relationships and mutual support beyond the group meetings.

Part IV

Cooperative Prevention Programmes in Primary Health Care

A. *The Control of Elevated Blood Pressure in the Community*

1. *Presuppositions for Community-Wide Blood Pressure Control*

High Blood Pressure Control in the Community

D. Ganten

Blood pressure is the major risk factor for cardiovascular morbidity and mortality and is therefore an important topic in the community. As will be discussed later hypertension can be classified in different ways, e.g. by aetiology as primary or secondary hypertension or by classifications according to severity as mild, moderate, labile, stable or malignant hypertension.

When looking at hypertension as a chronic disease in the population, mild hypertension, is more frequent than severe hypertension. This is the reason why a joint meeting of the International Society of Hypertension (ISH) and the World Health Organisation (WHO) was convened under the leitmotiv: "Mild hypertension is the problem."

This is certainly true, because most people who have raised blood pressure fall into this category, the percentage varying between 75% and 85%. Hence with respect to community health care, mild hypertension is of major significance and also presents a substantial financial burden to the community. For the individual, severe hypertension poses the greater problem, which, however, may be solved more easily by conventional therapeutic medical approaches.

For the purpose of this discussion I would like to rephrase the leitmotiv of the above-mentioned ISH/WHO meeting into: "Mild hypertension represents a unique opportunity", and Fig. 1 explains why this may be so: It is common knowledge that excess of salt, physical inactivity, alcohol, overweight, smoking and high fat nutrition can all lead to hypertension. The cardiovascular disease prevention programmes are all aimed at reducing these risk factors in the population. On the other hand, we know that not everybody, but only a portion of those obese, inactive salt-eating smokers develop hypertension, stroke and heart attack. This makes it difficult to impose strict cardiovascular prevention methods upon the population in general. The individual person will not understand why he should give up his old habits if he cannot be assured that he himself will benefit from the risk factor reduction. This is the point where mild hypertension plays an important role and may indeed represent an opportunity for the prevention programmes from a medical and psychological point of view.

Primary Health Care in the Making
Ed. by U. Laaser, R. Senault, H. Viefhues

It can be assumed that subjects with one or several of the above-mentioned risk factors who present with mild to moderate hypertension are in a majority of cases the ones who are sensitive to these civilisation-specific risks for genetic or whatever reasons and in whom, therefore, preventive measures are particularly meaningful and probably effective. Detection of and care for mildly hypertensive subjects thus provides us with a unique opportunity to reach about 20%–30% of the adult population at a time, when preventive measures are readily understood. Prevention at this point will be particularly meaningful because there is already the beginning of a disease but organ damage has probably not yet occurred or is still reversible. In such a situation the doctor will be more persuasive and the patient more easily convinced that certain curative or preventive measures are meaningful. The detection of these persons at risk is easy: blood pressure measurement can be done not only in the physician's office but also at home, in schools and at other places.

An obese physically inactive smoker and drinker who presents with elevated blood pressure on such an occasion can probably more easily persuaded to do something for his health and reduce such risk factors than can a person who does not have high blood pressure and who does not believe that the so-called risk factors "represent a risk for him individually". In addition, since one blood pressure measurement does not classify the person in question as a hypertensive subject, repeated measurements according to the guidelines of WHO will have to be performed. This is an excellent opportunity for the physician to test whether the patient is willing and able to do something against his risk factors and reduce overweight, salt, fat, smoking and physical inactivity.

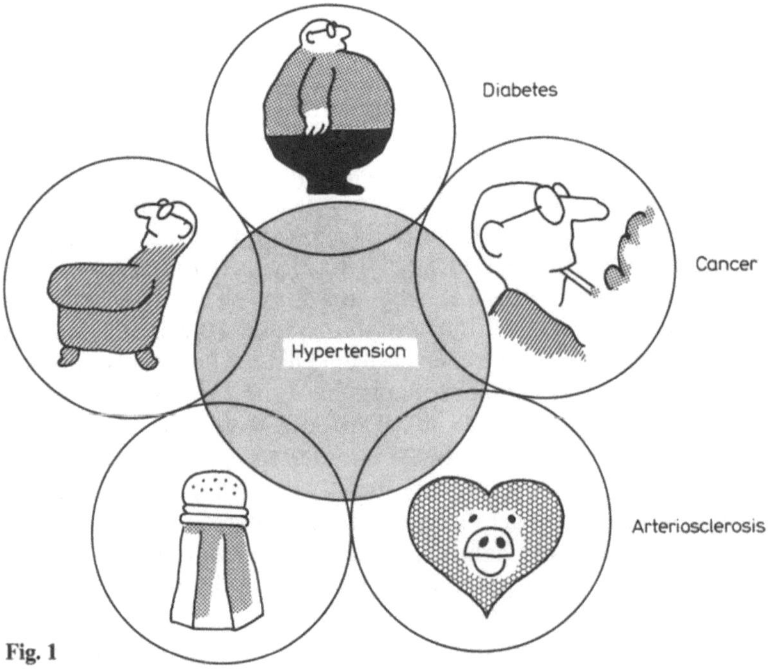

Fig. 1

The reduction of blood pressure together with the reduction of those risk factors which can be monitored and controlled by the patient himself will then be a convincing argument for the effectiveness of such health measures for the patient himself and for his surroundings.

Figure 1 also indicates that as a "side-effect", a mild hypertension programme will, without additional efforts, be effective with respect to the reduction of other diseases, such as cancer and diabetes, if we are successful in reducing obesity, physical inactivity and smoking.

It is clear that much more research is necessary to support some of the above statements and these introductory remarks may sound too optimistic for many and will hopefully provoke discussion. It is my firm belief, however, that blood pressure does represent a risk factor which gives us a unique opportunity to demonstrate the value and the success of more comprehensive cardiovascular prevention programmes to the physician and to the population. Comprehensive general health programmes are certainly needed in our countries and are to be preferred to programmes attacking just one risk factor. Since the hypertensive patient frequently, however, presents with several risk factors, the psychological approach to the patient (and the doctor) may be facilitated by artificially singling out hypertension as a starter.

Epidemiological Study of Hypertension and Stroke in Taiwan

W.-P. Tseng

Cardiovascular disease is an important problem in Taiwan and accounts for a large proportion of both morbidity and mortality after middle age [1]. Moreover, since 1963 cerebrovascular disease has been the leading cause of death in Taiwan. The purpose of this study is to show how prevalent hypertension and stroke are in our community, and to explain what has been done at the community level to control hypertension. The sources of our study are as follows: first, hypertension in the Taiwan population in 1976 and 1982; second, the outcome in untreated hypertensives in the general population during the 19-year period 1963–1982; and third, a stroke survey in 1975 and 1982.

Prevalence of Hypertension

An arterial blood pressure survey was carried out on the general population of Taiwan in 1976 and 1982. The measurements were made on 6485 subjects in 1976 and 11 967 subjects in 1982. The mean blood pressures for adults aged 18 and over were 125/80 mmHg in 1976 and 123/77 mmHg in 1982. Hypertension, as defined by the World Health Organization [2], was present in 14.1% in 1976 and in 10.0% in 1982 with a random selection of geographical location and population density. A comparison of various door-to-door hypertension surveys in Taiwan by WHO criteria is shown in Table 1. It is apparent that the prevalence of hypertension in the 1976 survey, 14.1%, is the same as that in the Taiwan

Table 1. Comparison of door-to-door hypertension surveys in Taiwan

Population group	Year	Number examined	Age	Prevalence (%)
Agricultural population in southern Taiwan	1963–1964	14 304	15+	11.4
Taiwan aborigines	1965	1 296	20+	14.1
Taipei urban population	1971	5 320	15+	10.7
Taiwan general population	1976	6 485	18+	14.1
Taiwan general population	1982	11 967	18+	10.0

Primary Health Care in the Making
Ed. by U. Laaser, R. Senault, H. Viefhues

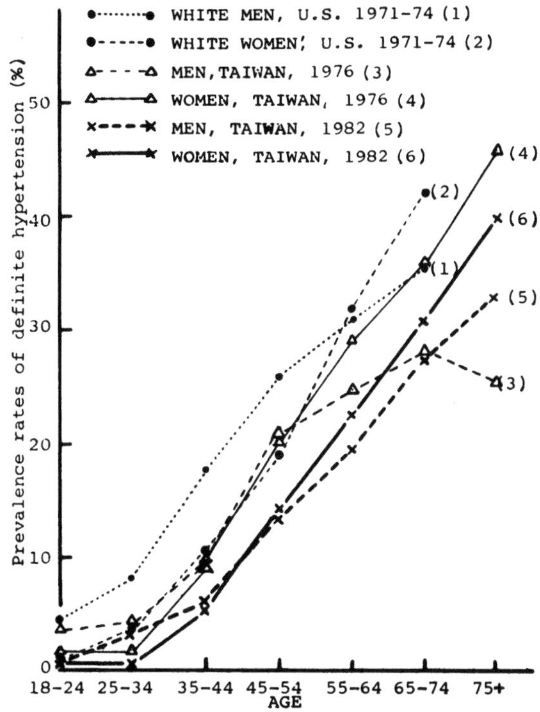

Fig. 1. The prevalence of hypertension in Taiwan (from nationwide general population surveys in 1976 and 1982)

aborigine survey [3]; however, the 1982 result, 10.0%, is considerably lower than the values in the other surveys listed [4, 5]. The frequency by age and sex is shown in Fig. 1. After 45 years of age the prevalence of hypertension was higher in women than in men; however, the reverse held true before 44 years of age. The two nationwide Taiwan general population surveys also showed a lower prevalence of hypertension by age and sex than did the U.S. Public Health Service Health and Nutrition Examination Survey, performed from 1971 to 1974, in which a representative sample of the American population, a total of 17 796 persons, was examined [6].

The Detection and Control of Hypertension in the Population

Community hypertensive surveys carried out in various parts of Taiwan (Taiwan general population survey, Taipei population survey) have shown that the majority of people with elevated blood pressure levels are either undetected, untreated or inadequately treated (Table 2). In 1976 4.5% of hypertensives were under control, and in 1982 this figure was still only 4.9%. Other hypertension surveys were also conducted in Taipei city in 1972 [5] and 1982 (Tseng, unpublished data); however, only one in eight of hypertensives aged 40 and over were under control. Obviously, there has been no improvement of treatment of hypertension under good control during the past 10 years in Taiwan.

Table 2. Findings of four hypertension surveys

	Taipei randomized population		Taiwan general population	
	1972	1981	1976	1982
No. of people examined	1061	1011	6485	11 967
Age	40+	40+	18+	18+
% with hypertension	23.8	16.0	14.1	10.0
% unknown	40.9	36.9	67.7	25.7
% of hypertensives being treated	48.0	46.9	26.4	42.4
% of hypertensives under control	12.2	12.3	4.5	4.9

Outcome Among Untreated Hypertensives in the General Population

A blood pressure survey was conducted in 17 953 members of the rural population in southern Taiwan in 1963 [4]. Hypertension was present in 11.4% (10.5% of the men and 12.2% of the women) above the age of 15 years. Of the survey group, 3272 (18.2%) died in the 19-year follow-up period. The 19-year mortality showed that while 11.9% of untreated hypertensives died from stroke, only 0.8% of normotensives did so (Table 3). Therefore, the relative risk of mortality from stroke during the 19-year period could be summarized as being 15 times higher in untreated hypertensives than in normotensives. Causes of death in 1046 hypertensives in this general population survey revealed that 26.0% died from stroke, 18.1% from cancer, 17.9% from cardiovascular diseases, 12.1% from respiratory diseases, and 25.9% from other causes. Therefore, the key to the prevention of stroke would appear to be the early detection and control of hypertension.

Stroke Survey

A stroke register among Chinese was conducted in the Yen-Ping precinct of Taipei city, population 50 160. The percentage of subjects aged over 65 was 4%. The methods used in this study were similar to those suggested by WHO in

Table 3. Mortality from cerebrovascular disease (CVD) in persons aged 15 and over during 19-year period according to the level of blood pressure at entry

	Male			Female			Total		
	Total	CVD		Total	CVD		Total	CVD	
		No.	%		No.	%		No.	%
Normotensive	5923	71	1.2	7 282	41	0.6	13 205	112	0.8
Borderline	1179	42	3.6	1 603	35	2.2	2 782	77	2.8
Hypertensive	738	126	17.1	1 228	108	8.8	1 966	234	11.9
Total	7840	239	3.0	10 113	184	1.8	17 953	423	2.4

Table 4. Comparison of incidence of cerebrovascular disease

Area	Population	65+ yrs in pop. (%)	Incidence per annum per 1000	
			Male 55–64	Male 65+
Göteborg, Sweden	450 860	13	2.3	0.2
Copenhagen, Denmark	101 970	21	4.3	13.3
Dublin, Ireland	142 255	7	1.7	8.1
Espoo, Finland	103 508	5	5.5	11.5
Zagreb, Yugoslavia	182 531	13	2.6	9.1
Zerifin, Israel	84 858	7	4.5	12.4
Akita, Japan	36 112	6	13.4	23.1
Saku, Japan	108 517	9	9.2	22.8
Ulan Bator, Mongolia	64 733	4	9.2	8.3
Taipei, Taiwan, ROC, 1975	50 160	4	11.6	25.8
San-Chih, Taiwan, 1982	16 652	6	7.1	12.7
San-Chih, Taiwan, 1982		female	8.2	26.8

1972 [7]. During a 2-year surveillance period, 194 cases of stroke, including 83 new ones, were found. Of the 83 new patients, 62 sustained initial stroke and 21 had a recurrent stroke (25.3%). The incidence per year is shown in Table 4. The incidence per 1000 from stroke was 11.6 in men aged 55–64 and 25.8 in men aged over 65. In 1982 another stroke register was conducted in San-Chih village in Taipei county, a total of 16 152 persons. During a 1-year surveillance period, 57 cases of stroke occurred; they included 30 new cases, of which 7 represented recurrent stroke (23.3%). The incidence per 1000 from stroke was 12.7 in men and 26.8 in women aged over 65. A simple comparison of data from the WHO register [7] and the Taipei and San-Chih studies is provided in Table 4. Considerable variation is noted between the registers; the data suggest that the incidence of stroke in Taiwan is extremely high and that it is indeed a serious problem.

References

1. Health Statistics (1980) National Health Administration, Taipei, Taiwan, Republic of China
2. World Health Organization (1959) Hypertension and coronary heart disease: Classification and criteria for epidemiological studies. WHO Tech Rep Ser 168
3. Tsai HC, Tseng WP, Yen TS, Cheng JT, Wang LT, Hsieh YY, Wu TL, Chen JS (1967) Coronary heart disease and hypertension in Taiwan aborigines. Am J Epidemiol 86:253–263
4. Tseng WP (1967) Blood pressure and hypertension in an agricultural and fishing population in Taiwan. Am J Epidemiol 86:513–525
5. Chen CM, Tseng WP, Tseng YZ, Huang PJ, Lin CC, Wang YT, Yang HC (1972) Prevalence of heart disease in Taipei urban population. 5th Asian Pacific Congress of Cardiology, free Communication. Singapore Cardiac Society, Singapore, pp 271–272
6. Robert J (1977) Blood pressure levels of persons 6–74 years. DHEW Publ no (HRA) 78-1648 203, Washington, DC
7. World Health Organization (1973) Community control of stroke and hypertension. Report of a WHO meeting, part 1: Stroke. WHO, Geneva

Home Blood Pressure Measurement – A Useful Tool in the Management of High Blood Pressure?

M. Maiwald

Introduction

Ideally, the preventive treatment of hypertension is initiated upon detection of increased blood pressure readings. This procedure is based on cross-sectional studies of normo- and hypertensive populations which identify high blood pressure as a risk factor for cardiovascular disease mortality and morbidity. The subsequent drug treatment of hypertension is usually coupled with adverse side-effects for the otherwise asymptomatic patient. Lack of compliance with therapeutic measures is hence a common problem for the attending physician. Excessive death rates have recently been reported in certain subgroups of a study in which risk factors, including high blood pressure, had been treated vigorously [7]. High blood pressure is a symptom which may be caused by a multitude of mechanisms, including stress from life events and working conditions. Single case studies are necessary to study more closely factors governing the course of the disease in individuals.

Self-monitoring of blood pressure at home or at the site of work is a recommended measure to ensure adherence to a physician's prescriptions. Home monitoring is an easily applicable technique to ascertain the diagnosis in borderline hypertension. Blood pressure is often reported to be lower at home than in the doctor's office [1, 2, 8]. Home monitoring of physiological variables is introduced into the management of a variety of diseases. Diabetics are trained to monitor their blood glucose concentration and thereby are able to optimize insulin consumption [4, 5]. Asthma patients learn to measure the peak expiratory flow rate to assess the airway resistance. In contrast, self-monitoring of blood pressure is only rarely employed for extended periods of time and few papers deal with observation periods exceeding 4 weeks.

The purpose of this study is to investigate in a preliminary way the long-term behaviour of patient-kept blood pressure records. The readings have been obtained from two male hypertensive patients who both started to write down their daily blood pressure readings on their own initiative. The patients represent different types of aetiology, i.e. primary vs. secondary hypertension.

Primary Health Care in the Making
Ed. by U. Laaser, R. Senault, H. Viefhues

Patients and Methods

Patient A is a master mason almost 60 years of age. He had to retire early because of his disease. Hypertension had been diagnosed at the age of 26. Ever since then he has been under medication involving many different drugs; those currently in use are minoxidil, captopril, nifedipine, sotalol and furosemide. As a result of clinical assessment, involvement of vascular abnormalities is presumed, although attempts to correct this condition have apparently failed. There are no relatives in the patient's family known to have high blood pressure. This case is considered to represent secondary hypertension. Records of blood pressure readings have been kept as plots for most of the observation period by the patient. This was abandoned only recently, when a form for numerical record keeping was provided to the patient. A standard mercury sphygmomanometer is used, which is repeatedly gauged by the bureau of standards during the observation period.

Patient B is a white-collar worker in his early 40s. Elevated blood pressure readings have been known for 19 years. Initially, office readings were around 160/120 mmHg. Glomerulonephritis was at one time suspected and treated. A reserpine/diuretic combination was applied for half a year. Later the blood pressure was left unattended by the patient for 16 years. An intensive drug regime has been in effect only for the last 3 years of the observation period. Drugs used successively are clonidine, dihydralazine, prazosin, urapidil, reserpine and various diuretics. The side-effects of the drugs have been considerable, and only prazosin and reserpine have so far been tolerated by the patient for extended periods of time. This case is regarded to represent essential hypertension. No target organ damage has been detectable with standard diagnostic techniques. Records of blood pressure readings in this case are listed only numerically in diary form. They are thus easy to transfer into a computer file. All readings are taken in the morning after rise.

The mean systolic and diastolic pressures have been calculated per month from the patient-read data together with the standard deviation. The peak values have been sorted out and plotted together with mean and standard deviation against time for both cases (Figs. 1 and 2).

Results

Patient A: The record of blood pressure readings spans a period of 5777 days. This corresponds to 190 month or 15 years and 10 months. Data are missing from a total of 84 days. This is mainly due to two extended periods of hospitalization required for treatment of a myocardial infarction in 1973. Two-thirds of the recorded values are multiples of ten, while one-third represent multiples of five. Other terminal digits occur only occasionally, thus indicating a strong digit bias.

Morphologically three periods may be distinguished in the mean blood pressure readings calculated on a monthly basis (Fig. 1). These periods differ in

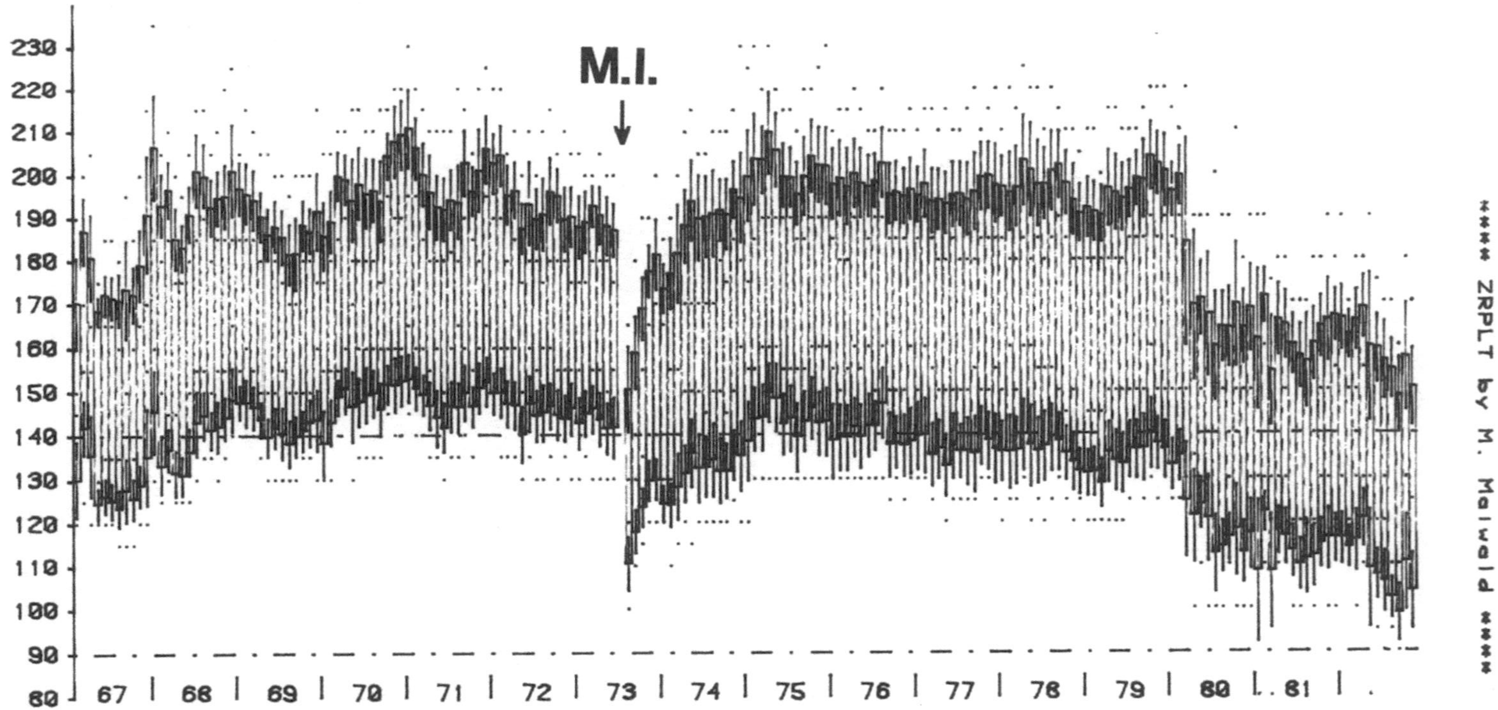

Fig. 1. Graph of monthly statistics of systolic and diastolic pressures collected once daily by patient A (secondary hypertension) for a period of 190 months. The mean pressures are represented as *columns* with the standard deviation protruding as a *line*. The accompanying peak values are depicted as *dots*. The numbers on the horizontal axis represent years. The unit on the vertical axis is mm Hg. The occurrence of the myocardial infarction is marked by an *arrow* and *M.I.*

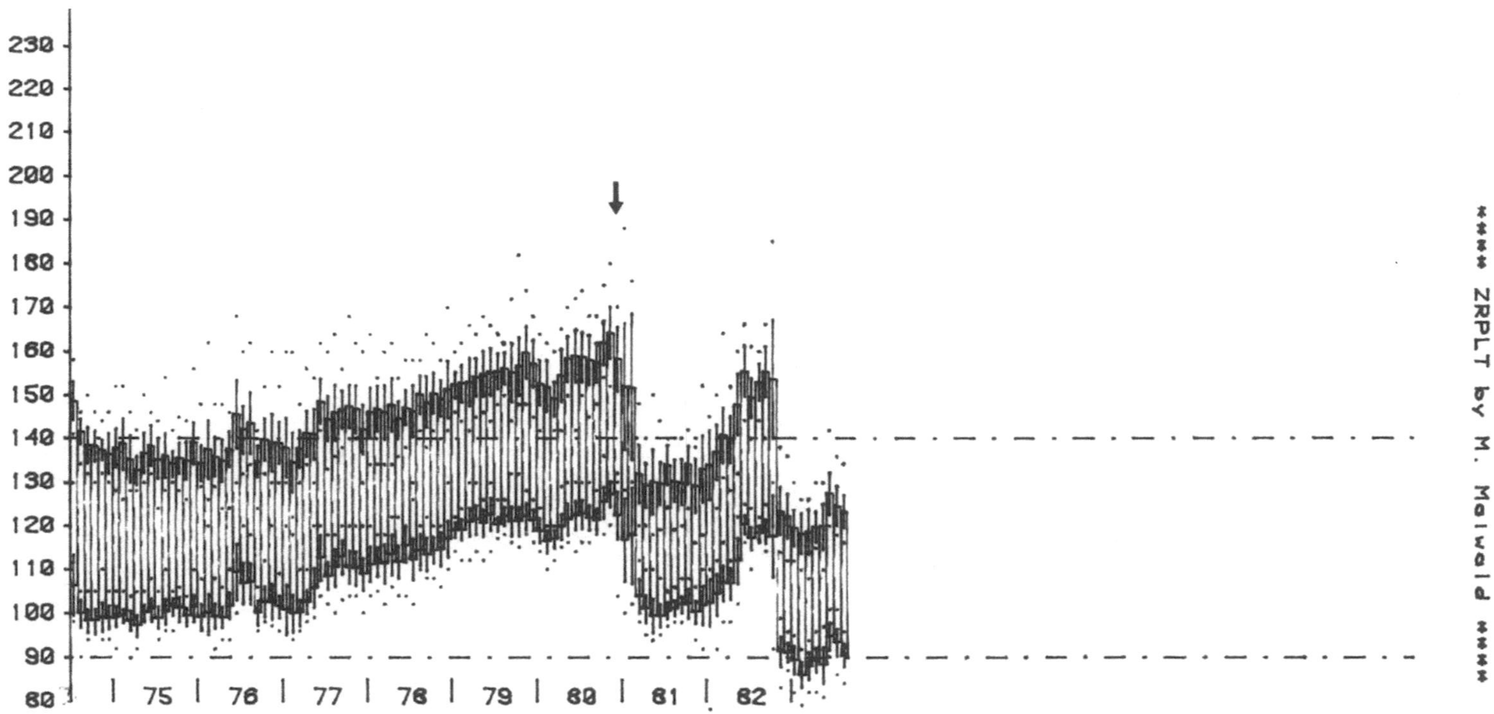

Fig. 2. Graph of monthly mean systolic and diastolic pressure readings collected by patient B (essential hypertension) over a period of 110 months. The *arrow* indicates the introduction of medication following the period without drugs. The graph is plotted to the same scale as Fig. 1

the level of blood pressure, pressure amplitude and variability of systolic and diastolic readings. The first period lasted from 1967 to 1973. It contains diastolic pressures exceeding 140 mmHg and amplitudes of 45 mmHg. This period ended when the patient suffered a myocardial infarction (marked MI) in 1973. Following this cardiac event, blood pressure fell temporarily. This apparently indicates the decreased contractility of the heart muscle. Diastolic pressures as high as before were reached within 21 months, possibly reflecting the restored contractility. The amplitude was then increased to 60 mmHg. The variability of the diastolic pressure was also increased. In the last 3 years of the observation period the blood pressure has fallen markedly, whereas the variability has increased further. This is not attributable to a specific therapeutic measure.

Patient B: The record of blood pressure readings has been kept for 3352 days, corresponding to 9 years and 2 months. Data have been lost on 105 days. This occurred mainly in the initial 2 years of the observation period, when the patient was occasionally away from home. A test for the preference of the terminal digit exhibits an increased frequency of selection for even numbers over odd ones in both blood pressure readings.

Morphologically the blood pressure curve (Fig. 2) may be segmented into three periods, as in case A. Initially the blood pressure remained at borderline level (137/100 mmHg) with only a brief period with increased readings in 1976. The latter occurred parallel with the patient's decision to change his place of work. In 1977 the pressure began to rise steadily until the end of 1980, with blood pressure readings of 164/127 mmHg. The arrow in the plot indicates the beginning of the period with drug application. The highest observed readings result from a withdrawal syndrome following cessation of a 4-week clonidine course at the beginning of the period with medication. The blood pressure fell conspicuously upon introduction of prazosin and in the later period of reserpine. Both drugs were combined with diuretics. The 5-month period with markedly increased blood pressures indicates a drug-free period necessary to conduct further diagnostic measures. The drugs produce distinctly different response patterns with respect to level of blood pressure and variability.

Conclusions

The investigation demonstrates that long-term records of home blood pressure readings can be collected with a tolerable number of missing data. To facilitate data processing, a diary form of record keeping is better suited than plots drawn by the patient. Development of a data acquisition program for pocket calculators with continuous memory would speed up the data handling. Raw data could then be transferred directly into a computer via a standard interface.

Long-term trends or periodicities are identifiable even in data sets with readings which are rounded off to zero or five as terminal digits. Patients should be encouraged to read the sphygmomanometer scale with precision.

No prodromal signs of an imminent cardiac event show up in the blood pressure readings; however, the restitution phase following a myocardial infarction is clearly recognizable. Furthermore, the efficiency of drug-free treatment procedures can be controlled. The impact of drugs on blood pressure regulation can be assessed and overmedication is avoidable. Observation periods without treatment provide an opportunity for investigations of the role of psychological stress [6] and recurring stress as experienced in places of work [3].

Further studies are necessary to elucidate the information content of patient-monitored parameters.

References

1. Ayman D, Goldshine AD (1940) Blood pressure determinations by patients with essential hypertension. I. Difference between clinic and home readings before treatment. Am J Med Sci 200:465–474
2. Cottier C, Julius S, Gajendragadkar SV, Schork MA (1982) Usefulness of home BP determination in treating borderline hypertension. JAMA 248:555–558
3. Devereux RB, Pickering TG, Harshfield GA, Kleinert HD, Denby L, Clark L, Pregibon D, Jason M, Kleiner B, Borer JS, Laragh JH (1983) Left ventricular hypertrophy in patients with hypertension: importance of blood pressure response to regularly recurring stress. Circulation 68:470–476
4. Fagin Ja, Litwak L, Gutman RA (1983) Economic realities of home blood glucose monitoring. Lancet 8351:682–683
5. Gibbins RL, Saunder J, Rowland CJ, Harding-Dempster J, Carenagh AJM (1983) Does home monitoring of blood glucose work in general practice? Br Med J 287:801
6. Light KC, Koepke JP, Obrist PA, Willis PW (1983) Psychological stress induces sodium and fluid retention in men at high risk for hypertension. Science 220:429–431
7. Multiple Risk Factor Intervention Trial Research Group (1982) Multiple risk factor intervention trial. Risk factor changes and mortality results. JAMA 248:1465–1477
8. Silverberg DS, Rosenfeld JB (1980) Comparison of clinic and home blood pressure measurements. Isr J Med Sci 16:22–24

An Education Program for Instruction in Self Blood Pressure Measurement

V. R. Coleman

Background and Rationale

Self blood pressure measurement manometers have become increasingly available to the general public. In an effort to make the use of these machines a quality experience in self-responsibility for one's own health care, the following educational program was developed. It was designed to provide health professionals with an educational module to instruct patients and other interested individuals with information regarding hypertension and information on technique of blood pressure measurement.

Curriculum

The curriculum addressed the following issues:

a) Who can benefit from self blood pressure measurements?
b) Hypertension: definition and guidelines
c) Anatomy and physiology of the circulatory system
d) How and when to measure and record blood pressure
e) Factors associated with hypertension
f) Instructions to aid clients in controlling their blood pressure

Discussion

Categories of hypertensives who can benefit from self blood pressure measurement and the rationale for their selection were identified.

Diagnosed hypertensives under treatment by their physician were cited for blood pressure measurement when multiple measurements are requested to aid in establishing the efficacy of a specific drug regimen.

Multiple measurements also can reinforce the patient's adherence to his of her treatment regimen as active participation by the patient seems to favor successful blood pressure control, and also may be requested by the physician to determine the efficacy of non-pharmacologic treatment regimens. Borderline

Primary Health Care in the Making
Ed. by U. Laaser, R. Senault, H. Viefhues

hypertensives may find it beneficial or be instructed by their physician to record multiple measurements of their blood pressure at specific intervals to aid in confirming if and when they have sustained elevated readings, as may labile hypertensives to aid in determining if and when sustained elevations exist. Some individuals only have elevations in a clinical setting and multiple measurements at home can be beneficial to their physician in making treatment decisions. Also, physicians and patients in rural areas can find self blood pressure measurements useful in avoiding travel over long distances when a blood pressure measurement alone is needed by the physician in his or her ongoing assessment of the patient; and finally, unaware hypertensives can be detected by an easily available method of periodic blood pressure measurement.

There is a brief definition of hypertension as high blood pressure and not "nervous" tension, and the fact is stressed that it usually has no symptoms. Blood pressure itself is described and the unfortunate sequelae of sustained elevated blood pressure explained.

Criteria established by the Joint National Committee Guidelines for what constitutes elevated readings are stated. Information is provided describing the function of the heart and blood vessels. Instruction is given on self blood pressure measurement technique and when to measure blood pressure, and a sample record keeping method is provided.

Finally, factors associated with hypertension are reviewed: sodium, obesity, alcohol, smoking, cholesterol, and stress. Participants are urged to control their blood pressure by keeping appointments and taking medication as ordered by their physician, to eat a healthy diet, and to keep a written record of blood pressure measurements.

Serum Insulin and Glucose Tolerance in Obese Patients with or Without Associated Arterial Hypertension

P. Strazzullo, F. Contaldo, F. P. Cappuccio, A. Fischetti, P. R. A. Soda, A. De Leo, C. Iovine, and M. Mancini

Introduction

A statistical association between body weight and blood pressure in man has been clearly shown by cross-sectional [3, 8, 14] and longitudinal [7, 14] epidemiological observations. Moreover it has been demonstrated that in obese hypertensive patients a better control of blood pressure can be achieved by a programme of weight reduction, either associated with salt restriction [4, 13] or not [11]. Nevertheless, the pathophysiological link between overweight and arterial hypertension is far from clear, and a number of working hypoteses are nowadays the subject of intensive research by interested investigators.

One of the factors which has been advocated as a possible *trait d'union* between these two common abnormalities is an excess circulating plasma insulin concentration: it is recognized that obesity is most often associated with hyperinsulinaemia and resistance to metabolic effects of insulin [1, 9]. Berglund et al. [2] have also found higher levels of plasma insulin and a reduced glucose tolerance in hypertensive as compared with normotensive subjects randomly selected from a clinically healthy population.

It has been proposed that insulin might influence blood pressure by altering the renal handling of sodium or through an effect on the sympathetic nervous system [12]. In an attempt to obtain more information on a possibly intermediary role of the hormone in the association between obesity and hypertension, we decided to compare the fasting plasma insulin levels as well as the insulin response to a standard oral glucose load in two comparable groups of obese subjects with normal or elevated blood pressure: the hypothesis was that obese hypertensive patients would have higher circulating insulin levels under fasting conditions and/or in response to a standard glucose load as compared with their normotensive counterparts. Preliminary results of this work are presented in this communication.

Patients and Methods

Twenty obese normotensive and 20 obese hypertensive patients were selected from among those attending the Obesity Out-patient Clinic according to the

Primary Health Care in the Making
Ed. by U. Laaser, R. Senault, H. Viefhues

following criteria: age between 20 and 55 years; body mass index, weight (kg)/height (m)^2, above 28; blood pressure either below 140/80 or above 150/95 mmHg on two different occasions; fasting serum glucose below 120 mg/dl; absence of any other concomitant serious pathological condition.

After the first clinic visit, the patients were invited to come back after 7–10 days to undergo an oral glucose tolerance test. They were recommended to stay on their habitual diet and to maintain a liberal carbohydrate intake.

On the day of the test they provided a urine collection of the last 24 h, from which a sample was taken for determination of the C-peptide concentration by a radioimmunological technique (RIA-mat C-peptide by Byrk Mallinckrodt).

All the patients received a standard oral load of 75 g glucose, as 33% glucose solution in water. Blood samples were drawn at 0, 30, 60, 90, 120, 180 and 240 min. A 4-h urine collection was started together with the administration of glucose, and a specimen was used for determination of the C-peptide. Blood glucose was determined by means of a glucose oxidase method using commercially available reagents with perchloric acid as protein precipitating agent. The serum insulin concentration was determined by radioimmunoassay, using the commercially available kit by Sorin Biomedica.

The statistical evaluation of the data was carried out by two-sided Student's *t*-test for unpaired observations. Logarithmis transformation was used for comparison of the fasting serum insulin levels whose distribution disclosed marked variation from normality.

The glucose and insulin response to glucose load was evaluated by estimation and comparison of the areas under the curve using the unpaired Student's *t*-test.

Results

Table 1 describes the most relevant characteristics of the obese patients participating in the study. The normotensive and the hypertensive groups were comparable for sex, age and body mass index. Systolic and diastolic blood pressures were markedly and significantly higher in the hypertensive group.

Table 2 gives the fasting serum glucose and insulin levels, the insulin–glucose ratio and the C-peptide content in the 24-h urine collection. While the

Table 1. Characteristics of the two groups of obese patients (mean ± SE)

	Normotensive	Hypertensive
No.	20 (11 M, 9 F)	20 (12 M, 8 F)
Age (yrs)	39.0 ± 2.01	41.0 ± 1.85
BMI	40.3 ± 1.36	42.8 ± 2.23
SBP (mmHg)	125.5 ± 2.52	168.4 ± 4.20 ($P < 0.001$)
DBP	82.6 ± 1.34	101.1 ± 2.01 ($P < 0.001$)

Table 2. Baseline biochemical findings in obese hypertensive and normotensive patients (mean ± SE)

	Normotensive (11 M, 9 F)	Hypertensive (12 M, 9 F)	*P*
Fasting serum glucose (mg/dl)	78.7 ±2.21	77.9 ±3.54	NS
Fasting serum insulin (log μU/ml)	1.294 ±0.03	1.438 ±0.04	<0.01
I/G ratio (log)	−0.607 ±0.03	−0.462 ±0.04	<0.01
Urinary C-peptide (nmol/24 h)	26.8 ±2.78	31.7 ±4.19	NS

serum glucose concentration was similar in the two groups, the hypertensive patients had a significantly higher average serum insulin concentration ($P < 0.01$). The actual insulin concentrations in the hypertensive and normotensive groups were 32.6 ± 4.8 and 20.9 ± 1.7 μU/ml respectively. As a consequence, the serum insulin–glucose ratio was also significantly higher in the hypertensive patients ($P < 0.01$).

The 24-h urinary C-peptide was on average 15% higher in the hypertensive group, but the difference was not statistically significant.

Figure 1 shows the average serum glucose and serum insulin curves obtained for the 20 normotensive and the 20 hypertensive patients in response to the oral glucose load.

A difference significant at the 5% level of probability was found only for the mean serum glucose concentration at 120 min (hypertensive group 123.1 ± 11.2, normotensive group 90.2 ± 6.6 mg/dl).

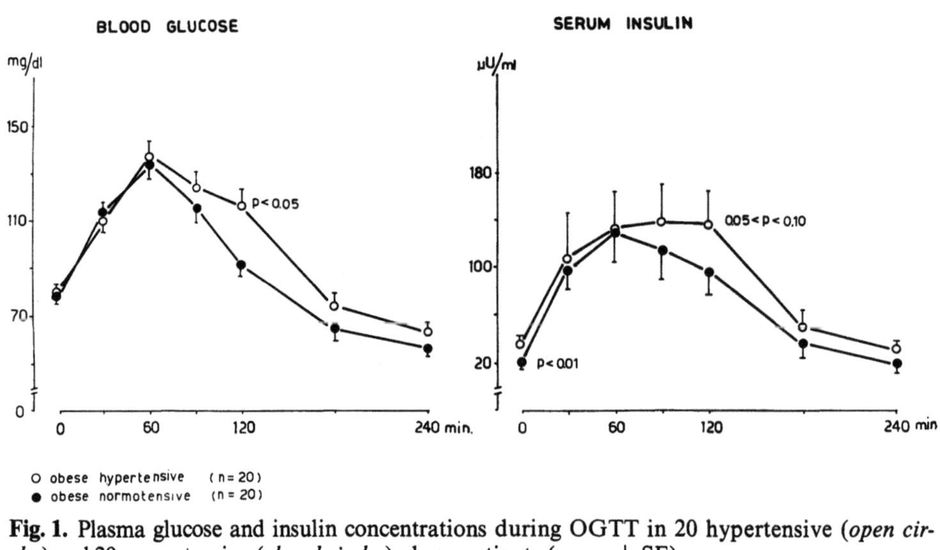

Fig. 1. Plasma glucose and insulin concentrations during OGTT in 20 hypertensive (*open circles*) and 20 normotensive (*closed circles*) obese patients (mean ± SE)

Table 3. Serum glucose and insulin (area under the curve, AUC) and urinary C-peptide during the oral glucose tolerance test (mean ± SE)

	Normotensive (11 M, 9 F)	Hypertensive (12 M, 8 F)	% difference	*P*
Insulin AUC	17 111.5 ± 1 922.5	20 732.7 ± 2 148.4	+ 17.5%	NS
Glucose AUC	21 450.8 ± 781.5	24 125.0 ± 1 754.1	+ 11.1%	NS
Urinary C-peptide (nmol/4 h)	4.72 ± 0.23	6.37 ± 0.18	+ 34.8%	NS

The values of the areas under the insulin and the glucose curve as well as the 4-h urinary C-peptide excretion in the two groups are reported in Table 3. The mean values found for the hypertensive and the normotensive patients were not significantly different: however a trend towards higher insulin and C-peptide levels was observed in the hypertensives.

Discussion

The main objective of the present study was to detect a possible difference in the fasting serum insulin concentration and/or in the insulin response to an oral glucose load between two groups of hypertensive or normotensive obese patients comparable by sex, age and degree of body excess. The selection of the patients for participation in the study was successful in as much as the two groups were almost perfectly comparable with regard to the three most relevant parameters considered to be critical. The data presented in this preliminary report indicate an appreciably higher fasting serum insulin concentration in obese patients with arterial hypertension than in normotensive controls. On the other hand, a similar difference in the blood glucose and insulin response to the standard glucose load could not be demonstrated, although a trend to reduced glucose tolerance was observed in the hypertensive group. These findings are in agreement with those reported by Hedstrand [6], who found increased fasting serum insulin levels, but no difference in the glucose tolerance of hypertensive men compared with weight-matched normotensive controls. His observation, however, was not limited to obese patients, but included subjects over a wide range of body weight.

Berglund et al. [2] studied the problem by comparing randomly selected hypertensive and normotensive men grouped according to different levels of body mass index. Their data show significantly higher serum fasting insulin levels as well as reduced glucose tolerance in "normal weight" hypertensives; nevertheless, they found no difference between hypertensive and normotensive "obese" subjects. They concluded that hyperinsulinaemia and reduced glucose tolerance might be a consequence of increased sympathetic tone, often present in hypertensive patients and causing increased insulin release and possibly decreased peripheral uptake of glucose. Their attractive interpretation, however, was not applicable in the markedly overweight group. In this regard perhaps one should remember that some degree of hyperinsulinaemia is present in the majority of obese patients. The data from the present and previous studies could therefore suggest that is probably just too difficult to detect a statistically significant difference in the stimulated serum insulin levels between various groups of obese individuals. At variance with the study of Berglund and co-workers, anyway, we were able to detect an appreciable difference in the fasting serum insulin levels of hypertensive and normotensive subjects, which was obviously independent of body weight. Whether the increased insulin concentrations are a simple accompaniment of high blood pressure or a factor playing a contributory role in this regard is a question that cannot be answered by this study.

We wish to mention that insulin has been convincingly shown to reduce the renal distal tubular sodium reabsorption in acute experiments in animals [10] as well as in man [5], within the physiological range of concentrations found in human plasma. Accordingly, the hypothesis has been advanced that chronic hyperinsulinaemia could contribute to a stable increase in blood pressure in susceptible obese individuals by a mechanism which includes a trend towards extracellular volume expansion and increase in cardiac output, followed by regional autoregulation of blood flow, with an ultimate increase in the systemic peripheral resistance and arterial pressure. In addition it has been suggested that insulin may also increase the adrenergic nerve discharge by affecting an insulin-sensitive area in the ventromedial nucleus of the hypothalamus [12].

In summary, the data provided in this preliminary report show a higher degree of hyperinsulinaemia and somehow lower gluocse tolerance in obese hypertensive than in normotensive patients. They also indicate, however, the difficulty of demonstrating a significant difference in the insulin response to a standard glucose load between groups of markedly overweight subjects.

Clearly other approaches should be tried to obtain more evidence for or against a contributory role of insulin in the association between obesity and arterial hypertension.

References

1. Bagdade EJ, Biermen EL, Parte D Jr (1967) The significance of basal insulin levels in the evaluation of the insulin response to glucose in diabetic and non-diabetic subjects. J Clin Invest 46:1549–1557
2. Berglund G, Lanson B, Andersson O, Lanson O, Svädsudd K, Björntorp P, Wilhelmsen L (1976) Body composition and glucose metabolism in hypertensive middle-aged males. Acta Med Scand 200:163–169
3. Chiang BIV, Perlman LV, Epstein FH (1969) Overweight and hypertension: a review. Circulation 39:403–421
4. Dahl L, Silver L, Christie R (1958) Role of salt in the fall of blood pressure accompanying reduction of obesity. N Engl J Med 258:1186–1192
5. De Fronzo RA, Cooke CR, Andres R, Faloona GR, Davis PJ (1975) The effect of insulin on renal handling of sodium, potassium, calcium and phosphate in man. J Clin Invest 55:845–855

6. Hedstrand H (1975) Studies in preventive medicine with particular reference to detection and treatment of risk factors for cardiovascular disease. Thesis, University of Uppsala
7. Kannel WB, Sorlie P (1975) Hypertension in Framingham. In: Paul O (ed) Epidemiology and control of hypertension. Symposia Specialists, Miami, pp 553–592
8. Kannel WB, Naphtali B, Skinner JJ, Dawber TR, McNamara PM (1967) The relation of adiposity to blood pressure and development of hypertension. The Framingham Study. Ann Intern Med 67:48–49
9. Kreisberg RA, Boshell BR, Di Placido J, Roddman RJ (1967) Insulin secretion in obesity. N Engl J Med 276:314–319
10. Nizet A, Le Febvre P, Crabbé J (1971) Control by insulin of sodium, potassium and water excretion. Pflugers Arch 232:11–20
11. Reisin E, Abel R, Modan B (1978) Effect of weight loss without salt restriction on the reduction of blood pressure in overweight hypertensive patients. N Engl J Med 298:1–5
12. Sims EAH, Berchtold P (1982) Obesity and hypertension. Mechanisms and implications for management. JAMA 247:49–52
13. Strazzullo P, Contaldo F, Trevisan M, De Campora E, Ferrara LA, Mattioli PL, Mancini M (1979) Blood pressure decrease in obese hypertensive patients during therapeutic fasting: the role of salt restriction. In: Mancini M, Lewis B, Contaldo F (eds) Medical complications of obesity. Academic, London, pp 259–262
14. Tyroler HA, Heyden S, Hames CG (1975) Weight and hypertension: Evans County studies of blacks and whites. In: Paul O (ed) Epidemiology and control of hypertension. Symposia Specialists, Miami, pp 197–204

The Treatment of High Blood Pressure: Non-Pharmacological and Pharmacological Measures

P. S. Sever

Pharmacological Treatment

The decision to treat high blood pressure must be based on the results of appropriately conducted clinical trials of therapeutic agents in hypertensive patients. Whilst such trials are essential for our understanding of the levels of blood pressure at which pharmacological intervention can be shown to be beneficial, in terms of a reduction in morbidity and mortality, the physician faced with the individual patient has many other factors to consider prior to the introduction of therapy, such as age, race, life-style and the presence or absence of coexisting disease.

Early trials clearly showed that benefit accrued to subjects with blood pressures in excess of 109 mmHg diastolic. More recently the benefits of intervention in mild hypertension have been investigated and the indications are that therapy perhaps should be initiated at lower levels of arterial pressure, for example > 100 – 105 mmHg phase V diastolic pressure [1, 2]. However, the definitive answer to this question must await the outcome of the Medical Research Council trial in mild hypertension (U.K.), from which data will also be available on whether or not lowering of blood pressure with certain agents will be associated with a reduction in the incidence of coronary deaths and morbidity from coronary artery disease, which was not apparent in earlier trials.

At the present time it is widely accepted that the first line pharmacological agents in the therapy of mild hypertension are the diuretics and the β-adrenoceptor antagonists. The choice between these two groups of drugs is, however, the subject of much debate and results from the belief (perhaps unwarranted) that cardioprotective effects of β-antagonist drugs demonstrated in recent secondary prevention trials in myocardial infarction [3] would influence myocardial morbidity and mortality when these drugs are used in the treatment of hypertension. In my opinion this view has not been convincingly substantiated. Moreover, concern has been expressed over the long-term metabolic sequelae of diuretic therapy, (namely hypokalaemia, hyperuricaemia, hyperglycaemia and effects on blood lipids). These factors, taken together with saturation marketing by the pharmaceutical industry, have led to an overwhelming shift towards the prescribing of β-antagonist drugs as first choice agents in the treatment of mild hypertension in Europe.

Primary Health Care in the Making
Ed. by U. Laaser, R. Senault, H. Viefhues

For the community this has highly important financial consequences. To provide equivalent antihypertensive effects certain β-antagonists may increase costs by as much as 40-fold compared with diuretics, and the evidence upon which this change in prescribing patterns is based is at best circumstantial.

With many diuretics available for use in hypertension, it is important to emphasise that there is no evidence to support the routine use of potent loop diuretics. Such agents have not been shown to confer any advantage over the thiazide diuretics, and electrolyte problems are more frequently encountered with these agents. The argument in favour of combining diuretics with potassium supplements, or the use of potassium sparing diuretics, has not been convincing and with the latter agents, in the elderly and in patients with impaired renal function, electrolyte imbalance may be a problem. Recent studies have shown that low doses of thiazides may be efficacious in the majority of patients and at doses of 2.5 mg bendrofluazide or 12.5 mg hydrochlorthiazide, metabolic sequelae may be minimised.

Diuretics must be considered first choice therapy in black patients and probably in patients with low renin hypertension. Failure to respond to diuretics may be associated with stimulation of the renin–angiotensin–aldosterone system and in this instance, therapy should be combined with β-adrenoceptor antagonists. There is some evidence that the hypotensive response to diuretics is enhanced in the presence of moderate dietary sodium restriction.

If β-adrenoceptor blocking drugs are used as first line therapy, there is little evidence to support the notion that additional pharmacological properties possessed by some of these drugs (e.g. partial agonist activity, cardioselectivity, membrane stabilising properties) confer any additional benefit in terms of blood pressure control. The case may be made in favour of using the less lipophilic agents which do not cross the blood–brain barrier so readily and thus are less likely to cause CNS side-effects, e.g. disturbed sleep, nightmares and impairment of concentration. Contraindications to the use of β-blocking drugs are widely known, e.g. asthma, heart failure and peripheral vascular disease, and those agents which are cardioselective do not necessarily prevent bronchospasm in susceptible subjects. Most β-antagonists can be administered on a once daily basis, for there is no evidence that plasma concentrations of these drugs correlate with their blood pressure lowering effects.

Although the mode of action of these drugs still remains elusive, these agents deservedly retain their place as first line drugs in the treatment of hypertension. Combination therapy with diuretics and β-antagonists is the logical second line approach in patients whose blood pressure is resistant to either of these agents when prescribed singly.

For those patients in whom the combination of first-line drugs fails to control the pressure, a decision has to be made as to whether methyldopa is substituted for the β-blocker, or a vasodilator is added to the diuretic and β-blocker regime. Recently the use of calcium antagonists, e.g. nifedipine, has gained favour at this stage in management.

One of the major problems with arterial vasodilator therapy is the reflex mechanisms which are brought into being as a consequence of the initial fall in blood pressure. As is well known, if vasodilators are used alone, the reflex stimulation of the heart produces tachycardia and palpitations and renin is released from the kidney in response not only to the fall in pressure but also to the sympathetic stimulation. These reflex mechanisms, including the salt and water retention occurring through aldosterone secretion, tend to limit the hypotensive efficacy of these drugs. Thus there is a rational basis for the combined use of vasodilator, β-adrenoceptor antagonists and diuretics.

Left ventricular hypertrophy is an important consequence of hypertension and is obviously dependent upon blood pressure levels. The peristence of signs of left ventricular hypertrophy despite adequate blood pressure control is at first surprising, but is not an uncommon observation either in the experimental situation or in human hypertension. Of the drugs mentioned thus far, although all would appear to lower vascular resistance with long-term treatment, in the case of diuretics and vasodilators, cardiac hypertrophy is unchanged or may, in certain cases, be increased. On the other hand, there is fairly convincing data that with methyldopa, for example, cardiac hypertrophy may be reversed, as judged by determinations of left ventricular mass.

The haemodynamic sequelae of reverse of hypertrophy are not yet fully known. It is also of interest that both diuretics and vasodilators induce secretion of renin, angiotensin and the catecholamines. It is not known at present to what extent the release of these two hormones may contribute to the development of left ventricular hypertrophy.

The choice of therapeutic regime in the more severe hypertensive may be determined by the development of side-effects. Some patients tolerate the so-called triple therapy of vasodilator, β-blocker and diuretic very well, while others will find the incidence of side-effects unacceptable. It is true that most of the unpleasant effects of hydralazine are reversed by the inclusion of a β-blocking drug in the regime. On the other hand, persistent headaches occur not uncommonly in patients on hydralazine and this may require substitution of a different regime. Methyldopa has long been incriminated as a major cause of unpleasant side-effects. It has been the experience of those physicians in hypertension clinics who use a questionnaire for the elucidation of side-effects that many complaints, such as impotence of sexual difficulties, may only be brought to light by asking the patient to fill in a questionnaire. The reluctance of discuss such problems in the clinic, often in the presence of nursing staff, is perhaps not surprising.

Other more serious side-effects of methyldopa, including the autoimmune haemolytic anaemia, drug fever and the hepatitis-like reaction are extremely uncommon.

In more resistant hypertension, the choice of therapy includes the converting enzyme inhibitors, e.g. captopril, potent vasodilators such as minoxidil and the calcium antagonists. In most instances, combination therapy with diuretics and β-antagonists is required.

A large amount of therapeutic juggling is often required with these severe hypertensives whose blood pressure is difficult to control, and it is extremely difficult to lay down any rigid rules as each case has to be judged individually.

Non-pharmacological Treatment

The suggestion that non-pharmacological methods could be effective in blood pressure reduction is not new. However, on the whole there has been a singular lack of enthusiasm in promoting such measures and this has arisen for several reasons. Firstly, epidemiological studies (often poorly controlled) may have shown associations between certain environmental influences and arterial pressure [4], but properly controlled studies have been carried out to show long-term benefits when these environmental factors are altered. Secondly, it has been a widely held belief that radical attempts to alter "life-style" by change in diet and other environmental influences would be unacceptable to the majority of subjects for whom some therapeutic measures are necessary. Thirdly, highly effective drugs are available for lowering blood pressure – so why the need for a non-pharmacological approach?

There is as yet no ideal drug for the treatment of the hypertensive individual. The pharmacological properties of modern antihypertensive drugs, although vastly superior to those of their predecessors, still lack specificity. The underlying cause of hypertension in most patients remains elusive and no drug can at present be tailored to the specific pathogenetic mechanism. Multiple unwanted side-effects occur with many agents, and in view of the fact that in the majority of cases therapy is life-long, potential benefits in terms of reduced morbidity and mortality from cardiovascular events may be offset against the sequelae of long-term drug use, e.g. hyperglycaemia, hyperuricaemia, electrolyte abnormalities, asthma, impotence and sleep disturbances.

The results of recently conducted clinical trials in mild hypertension [2] have led to the claim that physicians should be initiating treatment at lower levels of blood pressure than was previously indicated. Thus there is a drmatic increase in the number of patients for whom treatment is warranted, and the arguments outlined above apply equally to this group. Furthermore, the economic implications of these recent trials, particularly for third world countries, are considerable.

Finally, if evidence can be provided that non-pharmacological methods are successful in lowering blood pressure, consideration must be given as to whether an intervention programme at a community level, if successful, might result in an overall downwards shift in the frequency distribution of blood pressure in the population, affording considerably more overall benefit in terms of morbidity and mortality reduction than might be obtained from the concentration of efforts to develop new and specific agents for the management of the relatively small numbers of individuals at the top of the distribution curve who are at high risk.

The four major non-pharmacological approaches to the lowering of blood pressure are: the control of obesity, a reduction in excessive alcohol intake, biofeedback/meditation/yoga, and alteration in dietary electrolytes.

Weight and Obesity

In most epidemiological studies, body weight is significantly correlated with levels of arterial pressure. Several intervention studies have been carried out [5] and the results indicate that for every 1 kg weight loss, blood pressure falls by approximately 3 mmHg systolic and 2 mmHg diastolic.

In preventive programmes, weight reduction has been shown to produce a 15% or more fall in blood pressure in obese hypertensive individuals. The relationship between pressure and weight appears linear, but the slope is steeper in men than in women; thus in the markedly obese even moderate weight reduction is associated with a fall in blood pressure. In many studies it is difficult to eliminate the effects of dietary salt reduction in association with reduction in body weight. However, it is probable that the two effects are independent of each other. According to Andrews et al. [6], who compared several non-drug regimes, blood pressure lowering with weight reduction was greater than with other techniques. Thus, there is good evidence to support the proposal that in the overweight hypertensive subject, weight reduction should be an integral part of any therapeutic regime.

Alcohol

Several groups have now demonstrated a relationship between alcohol intake and arterial pressure [e.g. 7]. In these studies, subjects who regularly consumed three or more alcoholic drinks per day had significantly higher blood pressures than non-drinkers and those who drank little (1 – 2 drinks per day). Interestingly, in a prospective study of heavy drinkers abstention from alcohol was associated with a marked fall in arterial pressure over a 6-month period, compared with little or no change in a control group who maintained a high alcohol intake. Information concerning alcohol consumption (although frequently inaccurate!) should be obtained from all hypertensive subjects and recommendations given for a reduction when intake is in excess.

Relaxation, Yoga, Biofeedback

The relationship between "stress" and hypertension is a difficult one to evaluate and attempts to pursue this attractive hypothesis are fraught with problems of definition and measurement. Although to date there is no definitive proof of a causative relationship between psychosocial factors, "stress", the central nervous system and blood pressure in *essential* hypertension, there are indications that relaxation techniques, meditation, yoga and biofeedback may in certain instances lower blood pressure over a prolonged period. In an analysis of several studies, Andrews et al. [6] reported that the effects of yoga and muscle relaxation were considerably more beneficial than the effects of meditation and biofeedback. In the case of the last two techniques, these authors concluded that the effects on blood pressure were not significantly different from placebo.

However, in a recently well controlled randomised study, Patel et al. [8] have demonstrated that relaxation-based behavioural modification produced a 15 mmHg drop in systolic pressure, compared with 5 mmHg drop in the control group. Moreover, this difference was maintained at follow-up examinations 6 months after the relaxation sessions had been completed.

Diet

There is now a large body of epidemiological evidence suggesting that populations which consume small amounts of dietary sodium (< 50 mmol/day) have low blood pressures that fail to rise with age, and hypertension in these populations is virtually non-existent. At the other extreme, communities eating salt in large quantities (> 200 mmol/day) have a steep rise in blood pressure with age, and hypertension is common. In a now famous publication, Dahl has related the prevalence of hypertension in populations to their average dietary sodium intake [9] and the relationship is striking. Gleiberman [4] has extended these findings in her analysis of many populations, and the overall relationship has been confirmed. However, a cautionary note must be sounded as the data collection in many of the studies quoted was poor.

The relationship between salt and arterial pressure has been confounded by the observations that *within* populations it has seldom been possible to relate an individual's blood pressure to his/her dietary sodium intake (or urinary sodium excretion). Doubters of the salt hypothesis produce such data as support for their case. However, this apparent discrepancy must be explained: Either the cross-sectional studies were so poorly conducted that the apparent relationship between salt and blood pressure was entirely spurious and that the 'true' picture in the within-population studies is correct. Or, alternatively, the cross-sectional studies are a true representation of the facts and there must be some reason(s) why the single population studies fail to provide evidence in support of the hypothesis. In the case of the latter proposal the following factors should be considered.

The relationship between sodium and blood pressure is probably a sigmoid relationship. Thus in most within-population studies where the amounts of dietary sodium are high, the blood pressure–salt relationship is on the flat part of the curve and for large variations of dietary sodium there may be little or no effect upon blood pressure. Most within-population studies have been carried out in such high salt communities.

In many studies the number of subjects under investigation was so small that it is unlikely that any true relationship could have been found even if it did indeed exist. Watt and Foy [10] have claimed that in order to demonstrate a 0.1 mmHg rise in pressure per 10 mmol Na increase in the diet, significant at the 5% level, 5720 subjects would be needed, if each subject provided one 24-h urine specimen.

The problems of within population studies, particularly those carried out in "Westernised" societies, is that data collection may be very poor; measurements or estimates of dietary salt are notoriously inaccurate, and those of urinary salt excretion (spot samples, overnight urines, 24-h urines) no less so. Furthermore, there are marked within-individual day-to-day variations, which exceed inter-individual variations. If there was a temporal relationship between dietary or urinary sodium and blood pressure, many simultaneous readings of blood pressure and urine sodium would be required and this has seldom been performed.

It is possible that dietary potassium may influence the blood pressure response to sodium; thus future studies should include, for example, measurements of the sodium/potassium ratios in diet and urine.

Finally, there is strong evidence for a variation in the individual responses to salt. Several studies indicate that hypertensives and children of hypertensive parents differ in their handling of sodium. Thus for a given amount of dietary sodium, blood pressure responses would differ. This factor alone could account for the difficulty in arriving at a simple relationship between sodium intake and blood pressure within a population.

The effects of extreme dietary sodium restriction on blood pressure have been known for many years. Prior to the introduction of effective antihypertensive drugs, Kempner [11] demonstrated the remarkable beneficial effects of his low sodium rice diet in malignant hypertension and less severe hypertensive states.

More recently, advocates of dietary sodium restriction in the management of benign phase essential hypertension have received little support. Many hold the view that for significant pressure reduction dietary sodium intake has to be reduced to less than 70 mmol/day, at which level diets become less palatable and acceptable. Difficulties also arise in achieving this degree of salt restriction since virtually all processed and packaged foodstuffs contain substantial quantities of sodium.

Recent trials of sodium restriction show a modest fall in blood pressure in hypertensive subjects. Few trials, however, have been carried out with the rigorous attention to randomisation and control that would be expected for the assessment of a drug effect, and several authors remained sceptical of the value of dietary sodium restriction. Thus the recent report of Macgregor et al. [12] was well received. In this double blind, crossover study in patients with mild to moderate hypertension, in which dietary sodium was effectively reduced (as determined by urinary electrolyte measurements) from a mean of 162 mmol/24 h to 86 mmol/24 h, mean blood pressure fell by 7.1 mmHg (6.1%). Reviewing this and other studies it is apparent that the extent of blood pressure reduction with salt restriction is related to the initial level of arterial pressure. Thus the higher the pressure, the greater the fall. This fact may account for the failure to demonstrate significant falls in blood pressure in a group of patients with much lower initial pressures when subjected to a low sodium diet.

There are preliminary data that potassium supplementation in the diet may also have beneficial effect in the hypertensive subject by lowering blood pressure [13]. Interestingly, potassium supplements lower the blood pressure in "normotensive" subjects [14].

The magnitude of these effects of dietary manipulation on blood pressure in mild hypertensives are at least as great as those reported in the active treatment group in the Australian mild hypertension trial.

At present the available evidence suggests that dietary manipulation (reducing sodium and possibly increasing potassium) could be alternatives to drug treatment in mild hypertension. Further trials are needed to confirm these observations, and effort is required in the formulation of diets that would be acceptable to patients.

The final question concerns whether recommendations on diet should be confined to the hypertensive subjects or extended to encompass the whole population. In a number of countries, national campaigns have been launched to limit dietary salt consumption in the hope that a modest lowering of blood pressure in the population (say by 3–4 mmHg) would produce a greater overall reduction in mortality than treating those relatively few hypertensive subjects at the top of the distribution. Many stand against such proposals which, of course, are based on epidemiological data alone. What are the possible harmful effects of lowering sodium intake and/or raising potassium intake in whole populations? Answers to such questions are necessary before national campaigns are launched to radically alter the Western diet.

In the meantime, a reasonable approach is for hypertensive subjects and perhaps those subjects with a strong family history of hypertension to reduce excessive intake of dietary salt from around 200 mmol to 100 mmol per day. Furthermore, since the major source of dietary sodium is processed and preserved foods, food manufacturers should be encouraged to include information on salt content with their products.

Hopefully, large-scale intervention trials will finally resolve the question of the relationship between salt and blood pressure. If the link is confirmed by such trials, then dietary salt restriction may provide an acceptable alternative to pharmacotherapy in the treatment of mild hypertension, and the pathway is opened for studies on the prophylactic efficacy of dietary modification in the young.

References

1. The Management Committee (1979) Initial results of the Australian therapeutic trial in mild hypertension. Clin Sci 57:449s–452s
2. The Cooperative Group (1979) Five year findings of the Hypertension Detection and Follow-up Programme. JAMA 213:2562–2571
3. The Norwegian Multicenter Study Group (1981) Timolol-induced reduction in mortality and reinfarction in patients surviving acute myocardial infarction. N Engl J Med 304:801–807
4. Gleiberman L (1973) Blood pressure and dietary salt in human populations. Ecol Food Nutr 2:143–156
5. Amery A, Bulpitt C, Fagard R, Staessen J (1980) Does diet matter in hypertension? Eur Heart J 1:299–308
6. Andrews G, MacMahon SW, Austin A, Byrne DG (1982) Hypertension: comparison of drug and non-drug treatment. Br Med J 284:1523–1525
7. Beevers DG (1977) Alcohol and hypertension. Lancet 2:114–115
8. Patel C, Marmot MG, Terry DJ, Carruthers ME, Sever PS (1979) Coronary risk factor reduction through biofeedback-aided relaxation and meditation in patients with two or more risk factors. 6th Asia Pacific Congress on Diseases of the Chest, Bombay

9. Dahl LK (1961) Possible role of chronic excess salt consumption in the pathogenesis of essential hypertension. Am J Cardiol 8:571–575
10. Watt GCM, Foy CJW (1982) Dietary sodium and arterial pressure: problems of studies within a single population. J Epidemiol Community Health 36/3:197–201
11. Kempner W (1948) Treatment of hypertensive vascular disease with rice diet. Am J Med 4:545–577
12. Macgregor GA, Markandu ND, Best FE, Elder DM, Cam JM, Sagnella GA, Squires M (1982) Double-blind, randomised crossover trial of moderate sodium restriction in essential hypertension. Lancet 1:351–355
13. Macgregor GA, Smith SJ, Markandu ND, Banks RA, Sagnella GA (1982) Moderate potassium supplementation in essential hypertension. Lancet 2:567–570
14. Khaw KT, Thom S (1982) Randomised, double-blind, crossover trial of potassium on blood pressure in normal subjects. Lancet 2:1127–1129

What Can Be Learnt from the Results of the High Blood Pressure Trials?

J. Menard, G. Chatellier, and P. Corvol

The goal of the drug treatment of hypertension is to do more good than harm, which implies that an evaluation of the risk–benefit ratio of this treatment must be performed before deciding to expose an important fraction of the population to medical supervision and treatment. Indeed, the risks of the disease are well known (cardiac insufficiency, coronary artery disease, strokes, renal failure). The risk is very high in patients with the highest blood pressure levels (more than 110 mmHg, diastolic blood pressure phase V) who are not very numerous in the population, but the lower risk shown by mildly hypertensive people (90–110 mmHg) has a more important impact at the community level, because of the large number of these people. The risks of medical intervention on the other hand are not negligible, and include the side-effects of "labelling" people as patients [1], the side-effects of the drugs [2] and the cost of hypertension management to the community [3].

Therefore, both for the individual and for the group, it is of fundamental importance that a definition be provided of the exact level at which follow-up and drug prescriptions must be undertaken. The lower this threshold, the heavier will be the cost for the community of the management of the disease, and then research on the most efficient strategies becomes necessary.

The methodology used to demonstrate scientifically the benefits of treatment began in 1964, with Hamilton et al.'s trial [4]. This methodology includes the precise definition of the group under study, a randomisation process to create a control group and a treated group, and a follow-up with the registration of clearly defined terminating events. Each of these three conditions must be examined carefully if we want to learn something from the 12 trials which have attempted to contribute to solving the problem.

Definition of the Study Group. The circumstances under which blood pressure has been measured, the methodology and the number of measurements before randomisation are critical issues. So too is the source of the study group from the population: community screening, volunteers, referred patients.

Definition of the Control and Treatment Groups. The control group can be followed-up without advice or drug prescription. It can be followed-up while taking a placebo and receiving advice, or it can be referred to a system of care where no specific attention is paid to hypertension treatment in accordance with a strict protocol. The treated group is exposed to drugs available at the

Primary Health Care in the Making
Ed. by U. Laaser, R. Senault, H. Viefhues

time of the trial, and every 10 years new drugs can offer new advantages or new risks.

Definition of Terminal End-points. Total mortality is the most important end-point, since it takes account of a possible major iatrogenic factor. Cardiovascular mortality and morbidity must be analysed as carefully as possible: the definition of sudden death must be precise; its relation to the heart or to the brain has a risk of error and, among strokes, it is not always possible on clinical grounds to make the distinction between cerebral haemorrhage and cerebral infarction.

When looking at the 12 trials which have been performed (results are available for 11 of them), several general comments can be made. All trials except for the Oslo study [5] have been performed in English-speaking developed countries. The reasons for which other European countries or Japan did not provide a contribution to the problem certainly needs some explanations. From 1964 to 1984, the level of blood pressure which was investigated decreased from 135 mmHg to 90 mmHg [2, 4–17]. The incidence of terminal end-points decreased in proportion to the investigated levels of blood pressure, which led to a need for a greater and greater number of recruited patients and a longer follow-up. In Hamilton et al.'s study, 61 patients were followed-up for 24–72 months, and in the ongoing Medical Research Trial 18 000 patients will be followed-up for 60 months.

Up to 1970, the most well-known of the three trials so far completed was the Veterans Administration (VA) study. Its conclusions were that benefit from the medical treatment of hypertension can be demonstrated down to a level of 105 mmHg [8]. The severity of the disease in these patients made it impossible to extend the demonstration of these beneficial effects to mild uncomplicated hypertensive patients with blood pressure between 90 and 105 mmHg. Already at this time, the benefits of the three trials concerned a reduction in the complications of hypertension secondary to the level of blood pressure itself (vascular rupture, cardiac insufficiency); by contrast a benefit was not obtained for the reduction of coronary events, but prevention of coronary artery disease was not the specific initial objective of these trials.

Between 1970 and 1980, four trials reported results in rather small numbers of subjects; it is consequently difficult to interpret some of their negative results owing to the lack of power of these trials (beta risk). In one trial [9], the recurrence of stroke was not prevented, but antihypertensive treatment did prevent cardiac insufficiency. In another trial [10], important differences were described in favour of treated subjects on the prevention of rises in blood pressure and on electrocardiographic alterations.

The Oslo study [5] was problematic in that a non-significant higher rate of coronary events occurred in the treated patients than in the control group (20 versus 30, $P > 0.1$). Whereas nothing can be concluded from this result, it has been used to suggest, without scientific basis, a negative effect of diuretics, the first-step treatment used in this study.

In summary, from the eight trials summarized in Table 1, it can be concluded that under the conditions of these studies, the beneficial effects of hy-

Table 1. Results of the hypertension trials from 1964 to 1980

	Morbid events		Cerebrovascular events		Coronary events	
	Treated	Control	Treated	Control	Treated	Control
1964	5	16	3	7	3	3
1966	6	23	2	2	2	4
1967	2	27	1	4	0	3
1970	22	56	5	20	11	13
1974	49	61	37	42	5	7
1978	6	16	2	6	4	9
1979	8	9	0	2	8	7
1980	25	34	0	7	20	13

pertensive treatment on stroke and cardiac heart failure prevention are a reality, whereas its effects on coronary artery disease are unknown; this is a major issue, since coronary events are more frequent than strokes in the population.

Between 1979 and 1985 the results of four large-scale trials on mild hypertension performed in Australia [15, 16], Great Britain [2] and the United States [12–14, 17] have been or will be published.

The Australian Blood Pressure Study has shown that treatment of mild uncomplicated hypertension with the presently available drugs saves two lives and prevents five cardiovascular events per 1000 patient years therapy. At the present time, this result, which may concern men and women from 30 to 69 years old, is a reasonable basis for day-to-day practice. This information can always be provided to patients, even if the magnitude of these statistically significant results is not recognized in the same way by all of them. Therefore, initiation and continuation of antihypertensive treatment remains an individual problem, depending on the perception of risks, benefits and inconveniences by the individual patient. Coronary artery disease was not prevented in this trial, even if the reduction observed in the treated group was almost statistically significant.

The other results of the Australian trial concern the evolution of placebo-treated mild hypertension, which means hypertension treated by regular visits to an out-patient clinic and advice on diet and smoking habits. 48% of these placebo-treated patients had a spontaneous decline in their blood pressure after 3 years of follow-up, and 12% had an increase above 110 mmHg. This evolution could not be predicted from the initial characteristics of the patients, and therefore when it is decided to avoid drug prescription, a careful follow-up must always be provided [16].

The results of the Hypertension Detection and Follow-up Programme (HDFP) can be interpreted in different ways [12–14]. The decline in total mortality, cardiovascular mortality, strokes and coronary artery diseases in the "stepped care" group by comparison with the control group referred to community medical therapy has been attributed to the difference of 5 mmHg in diastolic blood pressure observed between the two groups. However, it could also be interpreted as demonstration that more intensive supervision of hypertensive patients, in conjunction with more active antihypertensive treatment, provides

Table 2. Results of the last three large-scale hypertension trials

	Total mortality		Cardiovascular mortality	
	Treated	Control	Treated	Control
Australian National Blood Pressure Study (intention to treat)	25	35	8	18
Hypertension Detection Follow-up Program (90–104 mmHg)	231	291	122	165
MRFIT Program (hypertensives)	174	169	80	79

general health benefits, since a decline in non-cardiovascular mortality was also observed in the treated group of this trial.

Among the hypertensive patients of the MRFIT programme, no difference at all was observed in the cardiovascular death and total mortality of the treated and control subjects. Too much emphasis has been put on whether hypertensive patients have or do not have resting ECG abnormalities, and no indeed statistically significant difference was observed between these groups.

The last trial, the MRC trial, is still in progress. So far, only the side-effects have been reported. Their incidence shows the price which has to be paid by the individual patient for being relatively protected from the risks of high blood pressure. Suspected adverse reactions to drugs necessitated the withdrawal from randomized treatment of about 17% of men and 13% of women on bendrofluazide, and of about 16% of men and 18% of women on propranolol by 5 years [2].

The magnitude of the problem of studying mild hypertension arises from the fact that a controlled study of people with blood pressure ranging from 90 to 95 mmHg, or even from 95 to 100 mmHg, is difficult to perform, since it would need still more subjects followed for a longer period of time. Nevertheless, in the HDFP, among the 2045 patients in the subgroup with diastolic pressures of 90–94 mmHg who were not receiving treatment and had no evidence of end-organ damage on entry, the 5-year cumulative mortality was reduced in the stepped care as compared with the referred care group ($P = 0.05$).

The adverse effects and the costs of drug therapy are nevertheless more acceptable in the higher risk group, defined by criteria such as blood pressure over 100 mmHg, male or black patients and associated cardiovascular risk factors. A standardized approach for hypertensive patients with blood pressure between 90 and 100 mmHg, a large fraction of the population, cannot be defined easily in the absence of the final results of the MRC trial. Moreover, the medical treatment of hypertension will progress with new drugs that should prove more effective and eventually produce less clinical and biological side-effects. They can increase the benefit/risk ratio achieved with the presently available drugs. Hopefully, the developed English-speaking countries will embark on further large-scale costly controlled clinical trials, whose results will be helpful for the worldwide community of patients and physicians.

References

1. Haynes RB, Sackett DL, Taylor DW, Gibson ES, Jonhson AL (1978) Increased absenteeism from work after detection and labeling of hypertensive patients. N Engl J Med 299:741–744
2. MRC Working Party on Mild to Moderate Hypertension (1981) Adverse reaction to bendrofluozide and propranolol used in the treatment of mild hypertension. Lancet 539–543
3. OMS, Comité d'Experts (1978) Hypertension artérielle: rapport d'un comité d'experts. Geneva OMS, (Série de rapports techniques, report no 628)
4. Hamilton M, Thompson EN, Wisniewski TKM (1964) The role of blood pressure control in preventing complications of hypertension. Lancet 1:235–238
5. Helgeland A (1980) Treatment of mild hypertension. A five-year controlled drug trial: the Oslo study. Am J Med 69:725–732
6. Wolff FW, Lindeman RD (1966) Effects of treatment in hypertension: results of a controlled study. J Chronic Dis 19:227–240
7. Veterans Administration Cooperative Study Group on Antihypertensive Agents (1967) Effects of treatment on morbidity in hypertension. Results in patients with diastolic blood pressure averaging 115 through 129 mmHg. JAMA 202:1116–1122
8. Veterans Administration Cooperative Study Group on Antihypertensive Agents (1970) Effects of treatment on morbidity in hypertension. Results in patients with diastolic blood pressure averaging 90 through 114 mmHg. JAMA 213:1143–1152
9. Hypertension-Stroke Cooperative Study Group (1974) Effect of antihypertensive treatment on stroke recurrence. JAMA 229:409–418
10. Smith McFate W (1977) Treatment of mild hypertension. Results of a ten-year intervention trial. Cric Res [Suppl 1] 40:98–105
11. Johnson HB, Pierce VR, Hamilton M (1978) Treatment of mild hypertension. An attempted controlled therapeutic trial. J Chronic Dis 31:513–519
12. Hypertension Detection and Follow-up Program Cooperative Group (1979) Five-year findings of the hypertension detection and follow-up program. 1. Reduction in mortality of persons with high blood pressure, including mild hypertension. JAMA 242:2562–2571
13. Hypertension Detection and Follow-up Program Cooperative Group (1979) Five-year findings of the hypertension detection and follow-up program. 2. Mortality by race sex and age. JAMA 242:2572–2577
14. Hypertension Detection and Follow-up Program Cooperative Group (1982) Results of the hypertension detection and follow-up program. The effect of treatment on mortality in mild hypertension. N Engl J Med 307:976–980
15. Management Committee of the Australian Hypertension Trial (1980) The Australian therapeutic trial in mild hypertension. Lancet 1:1261–1269
16. Report by the Management Committee of the Australian National Blood Pressure Study (1982) Untreated mild hypertension. Lancet 1:185–191
17. MRFIT Research Group (1982) Risk factor changes and mortality results. JAMA 248:1465–1477

Medical Care Utilization and Self-Reported Health of Hypertensives: Results of the Munich Blood Pressure Study

U. Härtel, U. Keil, V. Cairns, A, Döring, and J. Stieber

Introduction

The Munich Blood Pressure Study (MBS) is based on a random sample of the adult population of Munich. The main goal of the study was to study the prevalence, awareness, treatment and control of hypertension. Based on these data, a community-wide hypertension education and control programme has been implemented [7]. The association between the frequency of physician visits and the degree of awareness, treatment and control of hypertension in the Munich population was of particular interest and will be emphasized in this presentation.

Study Design

The Munich Blood Pressure Study is a panel study with data collected from the same subjects in 1981 and 1982. Of the 1.3 million inhabitants of Munich in 1980, 524 328 met the criteria of the study population: between 30 and 69 years of age, residents of Munich and German citizens. From these a random sample of 3400 was drawn; 2216 participated in the first study. The subjects went to one of seven examination centres for a standardized interview, three blood pressure measurements and height and weight recordings.

Blood Pressure Measurement and Categories of High Blood Pressure

The Hawksley Random Zero Sphygmomanometer was used for the blood pressure (BP) measurements. BP recording took place after the completion of the interview, which lasted on average for 30 min, so that each person had been in a sitting position for about 30 min before the first BP recording was made under the strictly standardized conditions recommended by the American Heart Association. All results in this presentation concerning blood pressure values are based on the mean of the second and third BP measurement.

The classification of normotensive, borderline and hypertensive BP levels based on WHO criteria is displayed in Table 1.

Primary Health Care in the Making
Ed. by U. Laaser, R. Senault, H. Viefhues

Table 1. Classification of normotensive, borderline and hypertensive blood pressure levels (WHO criteria). Munich Blood Pressure Study I (MBS 1980/81)

Normotension	SBP	< 140 mmHg and
	DBP	< 90 mmHg
Borderline hypertension	SBP	140 – 159 mmHg and/or
	DBP	90 – 94 mmHg
Hypertension	SBP	≧ 160 mmHg and/or
	DBP	≧ 95 mmHg

Measurement of Medical Care Utilization

In this presentation, medical care utilization refers to "physician use".Two variables are used: "whether a physician was visited in the last 4 weeks" and the "frequency of physician visits in the year preceding the examination".

No categorization according to the different medical specialists was made. However, visits to the dentist were not considered as physician visits. Each hospitalization was counted as one physician visit.

All information concerning medical care utilization is based on the subjects' answers to selected questions in the interview.

Measurement of Self-Reported Health

Two questions were asked during the interview to determine the individuals self-reported state of health: (1) "How do you rate your present state of health?" Possible answers: "excellent, good, fair, poor"; (2) "Have you ever been diagnosed or treated by a physician for any of the following diseases?" To answer this second question the participants were given the following list of chronic conditions: diabetes mellitus, hyperlipidaemia, congestive heart failure, myocardial infarction, angina pectoris, other heart diseases, stroke, chronic renal diseases, gastric ulcer, other chronic diseases.

Results

Medical Care Utilization by Hypertensives and Normotensives

The pattern of physician visits by hypertensives and normotensives is shown in Table 2. Here normotensives include borderline hypertensives.

Seventy-five percent of men with controlled hypertension reported making a physician visit during the preceding 4 weeks. 61.1% of the treated but un-

Table 2. Physician visit within the last 4 weeks by awareness, treatment, and control status of hypertensives and normotensives by sex. Munich Blood Pressure Study I (MBS 1980/81)

	Total	Physician visit within the last 4 weeks	
	n	*n*	%
Men			
Controlled hypertensives	52	39	75.0
Aware, treated, uncontr. hypert.	36	22	61.1
Aware, untreated hypertensives	59	22	37.3
Unaware hypertensives	90	28	31.1
Normotensives	805	261	32.4
Women			
Controlled hypertensives	91	73	80.2
Aware, treated, uncontr. hypert.	42	36	85.7
Aware, untreated hypertensives	50	23	67.6
Unaware hypertensives	34	14	41.2
Normotensives	957	441	46.1

Table 3. Frequency of physician visits within the last year by awareness, treatment, and control status of hypertensives and normotensives by sex. Munich Blood Pressure Study I (MBS 1980/81)

	Total	Physician visits within the last year			
		More than 10		None	
	n	*n*	%	*n*	%
Men					
Controlled hypertensives	52	27	51.9	–	0.0
Aware, treated, uncontr. hypert.	36	12	33.3	1	2.8
Aware, untreated hypertensives	59	12	20.3	11	18.6
Unaware hypertensives	90	4	4.4	32	35.6
Normotensives	805	101	12.5	176	21.9
Women					
Controlled hypertensives	91	39	42.8	1	1.1
Aware, treated, uncontr. hypert.	42	21	50.0	–	0.0
Aware, untreated hypertensives	50	14	28.0	5	10.0
Unaware hypertensives	34	5	14.7	5	14.7
Normotensives	957	165	17.5	77	8.0

controlled hypertensive men reported seeing a physician during the preceding 4 weeks. On the other hand, only 31.1% of unaware hypertensive men had seen a physician during the preceding 4 weeks. The figures for normotensive men are very similar to those for unaware hypertensive men. Twice as many treated hypertensive men than unaware hypertensive and normotensive men had seen a physician during the last 4 weeks. Among women, the groups of hypertensives and normotensives show patterns of physician visits very similar to those of men. 80.2% percent of controlled hypertensive women and 41.2% of unaware female hypertensives had seen a physician during the last 4 weeks.

Table 3 provides data on how often the different groups have seen a physician within the last year. The data are generally the same as those in Table 2. Treated hypertensives and "unaware hypertensives" – both men and women – are the extreme groups with regard to the categories "more than ten physician visits" or "no physician visit".

Thus the chance of detecting and treating elevated BP is relatively high for individuals frequently using physician services. However, there is a high percentage of treated hypertensives (33.0%) who visit their physician more than ten times a year but fail to show controlled BP values.

Number of Chronic Diseases

Table 4 shows the number of reported chronic diseases by age and sex. There were no significant differences between men and women. However, there were differences between age groups.

About 50% of the male and female participants in the age group 30–39 reported having had at least one chronic condition detected or treated, compared with 19% in the age group 60–69. Note that for those over 50, a large percentage reported three or more chronic diseases. Table 5 shows the number of chronic diseases in relationship to BP status for the age groups under and over 50 years. In the age group 30–49, 29.8% of the "aware, untreated hypertensives", 46.3% of the "unaware hypertensives" and 44.0% of the normotensives did not report a chronic condition.

In the age group over 50 there were pronounced differences between all treated hypertensives, controlled or not, and all others. For example, about 40%

Table 4. Number of self-reported chronic diseases by age and sex. Munich Blood Pressure Study I (MBS 1980/81)

Age	Total	Number of self-reported chronic diseases		
	n	None %	1–2 %	3 or more %
Men	1042	35.1	52.9	12.0
30–39	302	49.7	48.0	2.3
40–49	326	39.6	52.1	8.3
50–59	232	22.4	55.2	22.4
60–69	182	19.2	59.3	21.4
Women	1174	31.0	56.4	12.7
30–39	298	51.7	44.0	4.4
40–49	319	31.3	60.5	8.2
50–59	315	20.2	64.8	15.2
60–69	242	19.0	55.4	25.6

Table 5. Number of self-reported chronic diseases of hypertensives and normotensives by age. Munich Blood Pressure Study I (MBS 1980/81)

	Total *n*	Number of self-reported chronic diseases		
		None %	1–2 %	3 or more %
Age < 50 years	1245	42.8	51.3	5.9
Controlled hypertensives	27	18.5	59.2	22.2
Aware, treated, uncontr. hypert.	15	26.7	60.0	13.3
Aware, untreated hypertensives	47	29.8	46.8	23.4
Unaware hypertensives	67	46.3	47.8	6.0
Normotensives	1089	44.0	51.4	4.6
Age ≧ 50 years	971	20.2	59.1	20.7
Controlled hypertensives	116	9.5	54.3	36.2
Aware, treated, uncontr. hypert.	63	15.9	39.7	44.4
Aware, untreated hypertensives	62	29.0	58.1	13.0
Unaware hypertensives	57	31.6	57.9	10.5
Normotensives	673	20.7	62.0	17.4

Table 6. Self-reported health of hypertensives and normotensives by sex. Munich Blood Pressure Study I (MBS 1980/81)

	Total *n*	Self-reported health Excellent/good	
		n	%
Men	1042	801	76.9
Controlled hypertensives	52	31	59.6
Aware, treated, uncontr. hypert.	36	21	58.3
Aware, untreated hypertensives	59	46	78.0
Unaware hypertensives	90	74	82.2
Normotensives	805	629	78.1
Women	1174	772	65.8
Controlled hypertensives	91	51	56.0
Aware, treated, uncontr. hypert.	42	21	50.0
Aware, untreated hypertensives	50	27	54.0
Unaware hypertensives	34	25	73.5
Normotensives	957	648	67.7

of the treated hypertensives reported three or more chronic diseases whereas only 13% of the untreated (aware and unaware) and 17.1% of the normotensives did so.

Table 6 shows the self-reported health status of hypertensives and normotensives. Fewer women than men define their health as excellent or good. This tendency is found in all age groups. With regard to the BP status in men

Table 7. Terms in the "best-fitting" model from the log-linear analyses. Munich Blood Pressure Study I (1980/1981)

Treatment Status – Number of Chronic Diseases – Frequency of Physician Visits
Frequency of Physician Visits – Age
Treatment Status – Age
Number of Chronic Diseases – Self-Reported Health
Self-Reported Health – Frequency of Physician Visits

there are only small differences in the health status between "controlled" and "aware, treated, uncontrolled" hypertensives. However, these groups seem to feel worse than the other groups. That is, about 60% of the treated hypertensives consider their health status as excellent or good compared with about 80% of those who are untreated.

For women, the relationship between treatment status and self-reported physical condition is less clear. Among hypertensive women who are aware of their high blood pressure, those who are treated and untreated feel the same physically.

Results of Log-Linear Analyses

As we have seen, there are interrelationships among the variables mentioned: age, number of chronic diseases, self-reported health, number of physician visits and treatment status. It is therefore desirable to perform analyses that include all these variables simultaneously. We conducted log-linear analyses to investigate the interactions among these five variables.

Table 7 shows the significant interactions between the mentioned variables. The χ^2 from the "best-fitting" hierarchical model had a P value of 0.21. That is, the observed frequencies were not significantly different from the expected frequencies calculated from the model.

There was one third-order interaction term containing the variables: Treatment Status – Number of Chronic Diseases – Frequency of Physician Visits. Four second-order interaction terms were also in the model: Frequency of Physician Visits and Age; Treatment Status and Age; Number of Chronic Diseases and Self-Reported Health; and finally Self-Reported Health and Frequency of Physician Visits. The addition of other second- or third-order terms did not significantly improve the fit of the model.

Discussion

As hypothesized, the chance of detecting and treating high blood pressure increased with the frequency of physician visits. However, frequent physician visits do not guarantee an effective treatment of hypertension. A high percentage of treated hypertensives visited their physicians more than ten times in the preceding year and failed to show normotensive or borderline BP values.

The fact that treated hypertensives report more chronic diseases than untreated hypertensives and normotensives suggests that physicians are more likely to treat hypertension in patients who show further diseases or cardiovascular risk factors.

The different chronic illnesses that respondents were suffering from cannot be described here. Other analyses of the Munich Blood Pressure Study revealed that 25% of all treated hypertensives reported that they were diagnosed as "diabetic". Only 7% of the other groups reported a diagnosis of diabetes. This also suggests that the frequent physician visits of treated hypertensives is related to the treatment of other illnesses.

It appeared from log-linear analyses that the observed relationship between treatment status and self-reported health could be explained through other variables, such as the number of chronic diseases. This suggests that the treatment of high blood pressure alone does not necessarily lead to a diminished sense of well-being.

This is supported by the finding of the Munich Blood Pressure Study II (1981/82), where the hypertensives generally rated their treatment positively. More than half of the treated hypertensives said that they have felt better since they began treatment, and most of the remainder reported feeling exactly the same as before.

Drawing conclusions about the causal pathways among all these variables is not possible with cross-sectional data. The results do suggest that in the Munich population there is an association between the frequency of physician visits, the number of chronic diseases and the degree of awareness, treatment and control of hypertension. The subjects' self-reported health status, on the other hand, did not appear to be directly related to the treatment status of hypertensives.

References

1. Alderman MH, Madhavan S (1981) Management of the hypertensive patient: A continuing dilemma. Hypertension 3:192–197
2. Everitt BS (1979) The analysis of contingency tables. London
3. Hypertension Detection and Follow-up Program Cooperative Group (1979) Five-year findings of the hypertension detection and follow-up program. I. Reduction in mortality of persons with high blood pressure, including mild hypertension. JAMA 242:2563–2571
4. Hypertension Detection and Follow-up Program Cooperative Group (1979) Five-year findings of the hypertension detection and follow-up program. II. Mortality by race – sex and age. JAMA 242:2572–2577
5. Hypertension Detection and Follow-up Program Cooperative Group (1982) Five-year Findings of the hypertension detection and follow-up program. III. Reduction in stroke incidence among persons with high blood pressure. JAMA 247:633–638
6. Joint Committee on Detection, Evaluation and Treatment of High Blood Pressure (1980) The 1980 report of the Joint National Committee on Detection, Evaluation and Treatment of High Blood Pressure. US Department of Health and Human Services, Public Health Service, National Institutes of Health, Washington, DC

7. Keil U, Stieber J, Döring A, Fricke H (1982) Ergebnisse der Münchner Blutdruckstudie und Aufbau des Münchner Blutdruckprogramms. Öffentl Gesundheitswes 44:727–732
8. Keil U, Stieber J, Döring A (1983) Community studies in the Federal Republic of Germany related to mild hypertension. In: Gross F, Strasser T (eds) Recent advances in mild hypertension. Raven, New York, pp 63–83
9. Wagner EH, Warner JT, Slome C (1980) Medical care use and hypertension. Med Care 12:1241–1250

2. Blood Pressure Control Programmes and Their Effectiveness

The American National High Blood Pressure Education Program

W. T. Friedewald

About 35 million, 23% of the adult U.S. population, have blood pressures of 160/95 or higher. An additional 25 million have levels below that but greater than 140/90. High blood pressure contributes to the deaths of about 250 000 Americans each year. It causes serious complications affecting the heart, brain, and kidneys. Also, it appears to greatly accelerate the atherosclerotic process, especially in the coronary and cerebral vessels.

Most strokes, especially those before age 65, result from hypertension, the major factor leading to more than 165 000 stroke deaths and 250 000 cases of stroke-inflicted disability each year. Moreover, hypertension is a significant factor in the more than a million heart attacks that occur each year. The important epidemiological investigation known as the Framingham Heart Study, supported by our Institute, demonstrated that coronary heart disease occurs three to five times more frequently in people with blood pressures of 160/95 or higher than in people with normal blood pressure. Also, kidney failure associated with hypertension accounts for a significant number of deaths each year. Hypertension and its complications are estimated to cost the American people more than $ 8 billion in direct medical expenses and in income lost through illness, disability, premature loss of productivity, and death.

In spite of the obvious lack of knowledge about the mechanisms of most forms of hypertension, preventive measures have been remarkably successful in controlling the complications of this condition. However, since we are aware that the disease usually has no physical symptoms, many people are unaware of their condition, and if aware have little incentive to begin or maintain the level of therapy that will prevent serious complications (see Fig. 1). To address this problem, the NHLBI initiated a National High Blood Pressure Education Program (NHBPEP) in 1972 to change the attitudes, beliefs, and practices of professionals, patients, community project leaders, and government agencies, as well as the general public, in an effort to reduce death and disability through improved detection and treatment efforts.

The program was built on a consensus-building approach actively and intimately involving over the last years 15 Federal agencies, more than 150 national organizations, almost all our state health departments, and approximately 2000 local communities. The goal of this effort has been to reduce morbidity and mortality attributed to high blood pressure through an education program of health professionals and the general public. It does not fund local treatment

Primary Health Care in the Making
Ed. by U. Laaser, R. Senault, H. Viefhues

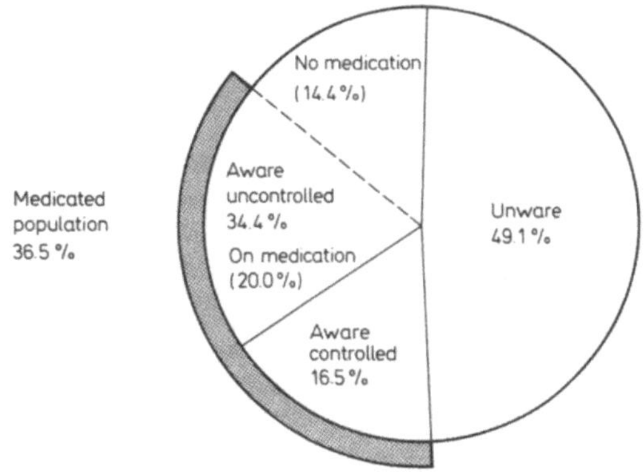

Fig. 1. National High Blood Pressure Education Program: Awareness, treatment, and control in hypertension, 1971–1972 (Source: National Health and Nutrition Examination Survey of 1971–1979 – NHANES I)

facilities. The major operating mechanism to accomplish the goals of the NHBPEP is the Coordinating Committee, a group of approximately 30 of the *key* participant units in the overall effort. The roles of the Coordinating Committee are to:

- Exchange information and views
- Examine critical issues
- Define program priorities
- Endorse strategies and activities
- Develop guidelines and standards
- Consider future opportunities
- Sponsor High Blood Pressure Month and the Bi-Annual National Conference
- Facilitate and promote collaboration

Working through the Coordinating Committee, the NHBPEP principal goals are:

- Professional and patient education
- Public education
- Information development and dissemination
- Community program development
- Standards setting and guidelines development
- Special projects

One of the key elements in this process has been the Community Program Development because it is at the local level, obviously, that care is provided. The specific objectives of this program area are to:

- Build networks and provide liaison
- Enlist key leaders
- Encourage and support cooperation and sharing
- Provide technical assistance
- Encourage use of mass media

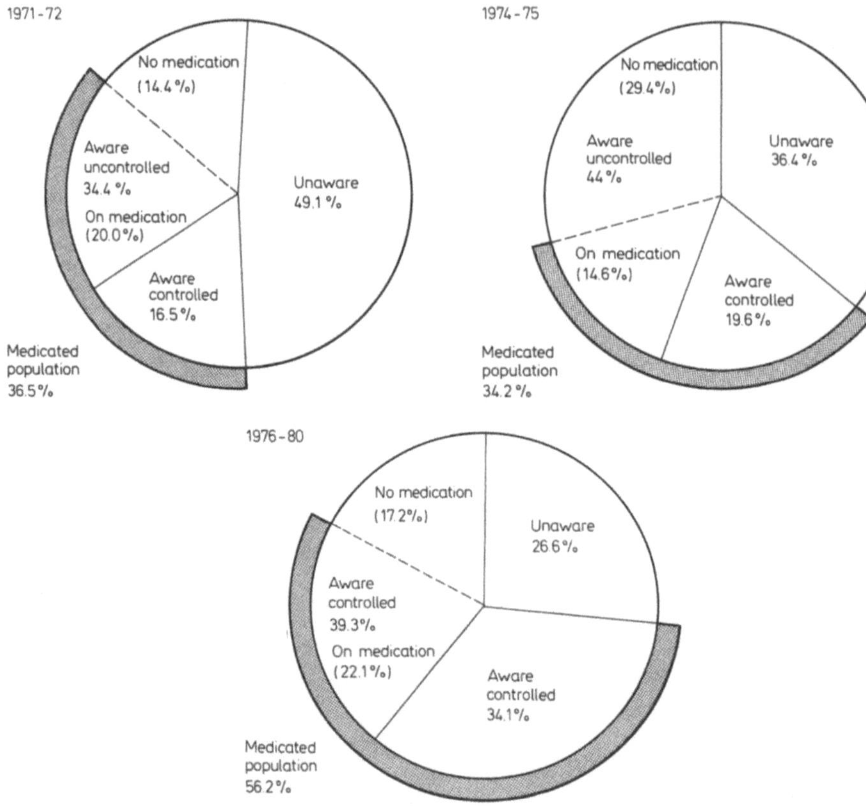

Fig. 2. National High Blood Pressure Education Program: Awareness, treatment, and control shifts in hypertensive populations, 1971–1972, 1974–1975, and 1976–1980 (Source: NHANES I and NHANES II)

- Promote conferences, workshops, and training programs
- Produce training manuals and other packages
- Integrate and coordinate educational messages

With these efforts in place to variable degrees since 1972, surveys have shown significant improvements in public knowledge and behaviors related to hypertension. We cannot know whether there is a cause and effect relationship but there have been:

- Improved knowledge about high blood pressure
- Increases in the numbers of aware hypertensives
- Increases in physician visits for hypertension (in the face of a decline in total physician visits)
- Increases in percentages of hypertensives on medication and their blood pressure controlled.

The changes in awareness, treatment, and control are shown in data in Fig. 2. But more importantly and perhaps causally related to these changes are the

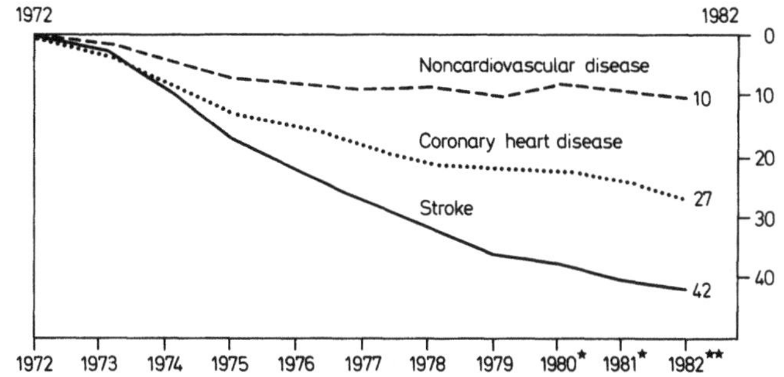

Fig. 3. National High Blood Pressure Education Program: Percent of mortality decline. * provisional rates published by NCHS; ** rates estimated by NHLBI

data from the U.S. on the decline in stroke mortality and perhaps even in mortality for coronary heart disease (Fig. 3).

We look with pride, and in truth amazement, at the level of success of this program in our country. We now must look forward to the future and in so doing we have identified the new problems of:

- Sustaining the network that has been established
- Maintaining the momentum of the last 10 years
- Continuing institutionalization of the program
- Beginning to focus messages/strategies to special populations
- Exploring new research areas, such as:
  Systolic hypertension in the elderly
  Primary prevention, including nonpharmacological approaches as the first step in treating "mild" high blood pressure

Epidemiological Situation of Cardiovascular Diseases in Slovenia and Possibilities for Prevention and Control

B. Ravnikar, N. Erzen, P. Jezersek, J, Turk, and D. Zrimsek

Introduction

It is not mere chance that the Cardiologic Section of the Medical Association of Slovenia is the most important initiator of organized action in the domain of prevention and control of cardiovascular diseases (CVDs). These conditions present our main health concern not only because of their widespread occurrence, but also because of recent research results which give us hope that we will be able to influence favourably this sort of disease in the near future.

Epidemiological Situation of CVDs

As in the 1950s, CVDs are today the seventh most frequent group of diseases diagnosed outside the hospital environment in Slovenia. Together with respir-

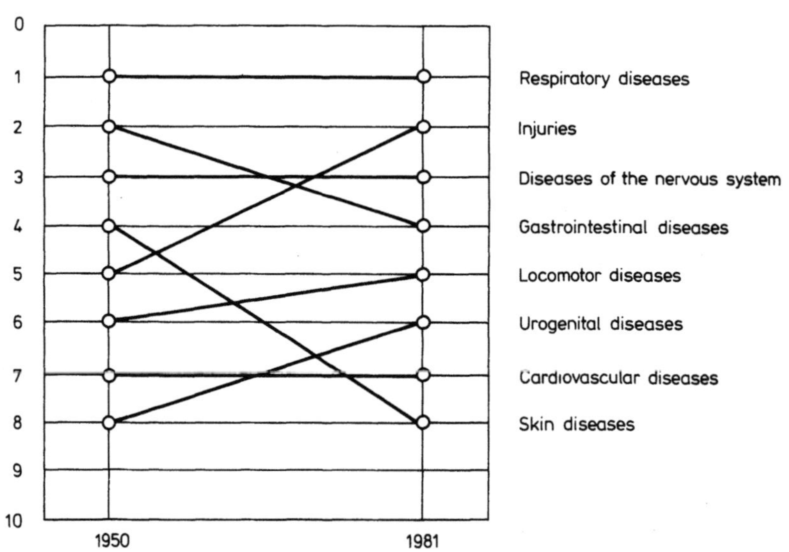

Fig. 1. Rank order of the most frequent diseases in Slovenia (according to the international Classification of Diseases), as diagnosed outside hospital

Primary Health Care in the Making
Ed. by U. Laaser, R. Senault, H. Viefhues

Table 1. Frequency of CVDs per 1000 inhabitants of Slovenia

CVDs[a]	1970	1976	1978	1980	1982
Total	91.3	157.5	155.6	131.8	143.8
Active rheumatic f.	1.7	1.3	1.2	1.1	1.1
Chronic rheumatic h.d.	6.0	4.4	3.4	3.5	3.2
Hypertensive d.	27.1	58.0	64.6	53.7	63.8
Ischaemic h.d.	4.7	9.6	9.9	9.0	10.9
Other h.d.	25.8	37.7	35.3	27.5	27.1
Cerebrovascular d.	3.0	6.5	6.3	7.2	7.6
Venous d.	5.4	7.4	5.5	4.8	4.5
Other vascular d.	17.5	32.5	29.4	25.0	25.6

[a] Cases diagnosed outside hospital, according to the International Classification of Diseases

Table 2. Hospitalization rate per 10 000 inhabitants with CVD according to age during 1981, together with the average rate during years 1969–1977

Age group	1969–1977	1981	Index 1969/77 = 100
Total	115.5	133.5	116
0– 9	7.5	6.4	85
10–19	17.9	12.7	71
20–29	25.7	23.6	92
30–39	48.1	48.0	100
40–49	95.4	107.0	112
50–59	175.5	213.4	122
60–69	338.8	381.3	113
70–79	662.4	724.1	109
80 and above	846.8	894.6	106

atory and locomotory diseases and neoplasms, they show the highest growth index over the last 10 years (Fig. 1). Most of these cases of CVD are diagnosed in general practices – 70%; nearly 22% are diagnosed in specialized medical services, 8% in departments of occupational medicine and less than 1% in out-patient departments for school children (not a negligible number) (Table 1).

Every 75th inhabitant is nowadays being treated in hospital, while in 1970 it was every 96th. The frequency of hospital treatment of CVD increases with patient age quickly and evenly. If a comparison is made between the year 1981 and the average for the period 1969–1977, a more favourable situation is noticeable only for those up to 30 years of age, which is in agreement also with the data concerning the decrease in acute rheumatic fever and chronic rheumatic heart diseases. The health situation for the 30–39 year age group remains unchanged, while the health situation of the population above 40 has worsened according to this indicator (Table 2).

A distinctive epidemiological peak and simultaneously the highest increase in hospitalization (index 122) is observed in the 50–59 year age group, the increase above this age being even and continuous. Thus 2 out of every 100 pa-

Table 3. Invalidity per 1000 insured workers

	1976	1977	1978	1979	1980	1981
Total	7.5	8.2	8.8	8.8	9.3	9.3
Locomotor diseases	1.7	1.9	2.3	2.4	2.5	2.6
Cardiovascular diseases	1.4	1.6	1.6	1.6	1.7	1.6
Mental disorders	0.8	1.0	1.1	1.2	1.3	1.3
Injuries	1.0	1.0	0.9	0.9	1.0	1.0
Respiratory diseases	0.4	0.4	0.5	0.5	0.5	0.5
Hypertension	0.4	0.5	0.5	0.5	0.6	0.5
Ischaemic heart disease	0.3	0.3	0.3	0.3	0.3	0.3

tients aged 50–59 years are hospitalized, 7 out of every 100 aged 60–69 and 9 out of every 100 in other age groups.

More males than females are hospitalized for all the CVDs with the exception of hypertension and chronic rheumatic heart diseases; in these cases one-third and almost one-half more women are hospitalized, respectively.

The hospitalization rate for hypertension is nearly even for both sexes up to 20 years of age and also in the 40–59 year age group. Between these two age groups the men prevail; above 60 years of age, however, the hospitalization rate for women increases.

Ischaemic heart disease (IHD) is epidemiologically important even in younger men, aged 30–39; however, its influence is more distinct from 40 years of age onwards, while women do not display symptoms of IHD until 60 years of age.

Among the diseases which constitute the most frequent causes of temporary absence from work (absenteeism), the share of CVD is 3%; this is an increase of 1% in comparison with the year 1970. In addition, the data concerning permanent work disability show that cardiovascular pathology together with locomotory diseases presents the greatest health problem.

Of every 1000 insured persons, each year 9 became disabled. Almost 3 per 1000 are disabled because of locomotory disease and almost 2 per 1000 because of CVDs, especially hypertension; this is therefore an area where prevention could have an important influence (Table 3).

Methodology and Conclusions

The coordination group at the Public Health Institute, which consists of primary health care physicians already dealing with this problem and of cardiologists, has completed basic guidelines for active work in the domain of CVD prevention and control. These guidelines begin with a definition of the role and viewpoints of the primary health service. Emphasis is then placed on the activities of preventive health care in the organized fight against the increase in chronic diseases.

Concrete guidelines for the prevention and control of hypertension, activities related to population-wide control, and suggestions on how to achieve early detection of hypertension are given. The standardization of diagnostic procedures and criteria is also included in the guidelines. Finally, the need to educate health personnel and motivate the population to take measures that will improve health is demonstrated.

Two phases can be differentiated. The first phase consists in the evaluation of work to date and of improvement in hypertension control in primary health care. The second phase consists in the active control of the population of a certain area. In order to normalize blood pressure among the population of a certain area – especially among the middle-aged – it is especially important:

1. To develop complex activities aimed at altering behavioural patterns in the entire community
2. To screen the population and to retain under treatment control all those with hypertension
3. To unify the diagnostic, therapeutic and rehabilitational approach
4. To ascertain the need to improve the professional knowledge of health personnel
5. To gather new information regarding the occurrence of hypertension and the effectiveness of health activities.

Summary

Analysing the epidemiological situation of cardiovascular diseases (CVDs) in Slovenia, we can ascertain that these diseases present our main health problem. Every seventh inhabitant who visits the general physician, every 40th worker in occupational medicine out-patient departments and every 30th patient in specialized medical services needs medical assistance owing to CVD.

Nowadays every 75th inhabitant is hospitalized, and hospitalization is especially frequent in cases of hypertension, ischaemic heart disease and cerebrovascular disorders. Regarding the rate of hospitalization, the health situation of the population above 40 years of age has worsened, although the epidemiological peak is not observed until 50–59 years of age. Overall more males than females suffer from CVDs, with the exception of hypertension and chronic rheumatic heart diseases, which occur most frequently in females above 60 years of age.

On the basis of these findings and recent research results which give rise to hope that successful control of CVDs will be achieved in the near future, basic guidelines for active work in the domain of prevention and control of CVDs are prepared.

Application of Epidemiology in Primary Health Care – Treatment of Hypertension

D. S. Silverberg, L. Baltuch, Y. Hermoni, and P. Eyal

Two national surveys in Israel in the 1960s and early 1970s [1, 2] showed that in the 15% of adults with hypertension (≥ 160 ± ≥ 95 mmHg) the rule of halves prevailed; about 50% of all hypertensives were aware of their condition [3], about 50% of those aware were on treatment and of those about 50% had diastolic pressures of ≥ 95 mmHg [4, 5]. Thus only about one in ten hypertensives were under control. Yet prospective studies in Israel have shown that the presence of hypertension is associated with an increased risk of cardiovascular diseases [6]. Indeed, the fraction of mortality in the community that is attributable to hypertension is 19%–23% in men [3, 7] and 36% in women [7]. The value of treating diastolic blood pressures persistently ≥ 100 mmHg has now been shown [8, 9]. Thus the detection and follow-up of hypertensives is a major health challenge.

Studies done in a random sample of family clinics in Israel showed that many patients who visited their physician did not have a blood pressure recorded [5], about one-third of patients who started medication simply stopped coming to their doctor [5, 10] and many patients taking medications were taking them irregularly [11]. Studies in Israel [12], America [8, 13, 14], Canada [15], Finland [16, 17], and elsewhere have shown that control of hypertension is much improved by activating paramedical personnel. In attempting to control hypertension in Israel, we have established a doctor–nurse team approach in an active detection and follow-up program of hypertension. In the last 5 years this program has been initiated in 400 family clinics and now involves follow-up of over 100 000 hypertensives.

Description

Kupat Holim of the Histadrut, the Health Insurance Institution of the General Federation of Labor, operates a prepaid medical scheme and runs 1230 urban and rural clinics throughout the country, with 2600 doctors and 3100 nurses. Doctors receive a capitation fee irrespective of the services they give the patient. In each clinic there are one or more nurses, and until recently their major tasks were taking blood samples, changing dressings, giving injections such as insulin, and visiting housebound patients. Since 1977 we have involved the nurse more actively in the care of hypertension.

Primary Health Care in the Making
Ed. by U. Laaser, R. Senault, H. Viefhues

The role of the nurse includes: (1) measuring the blood pressure of *all* patients who come to the clinics; (2) arranging appointments for hypertensive patients to see the nurse at times convenient to both patient and nurse; (3) accurately measuring blood pressure, weight, and pulse, and examining for leg edema; (4) inquiring about complaints, side effects, and compliance with medication and diet; (5) instructing the patient and the family about the disease, medication taking, and diet; (6) following up by telephone, letter, or home visit those patients who have not kept their appointments; (7) ensuring that the laboratory tests requested by the physician are performed; (8) in conjunction with the doctor, inviting all hypertensives and their families to attend talks given by the doctors, nurses, and dieticians (a special program, using slides, has been prepared by the Health Education Division of Kupat Holim); (9) handing out pamphlets on hypertension and diet prepared by the Health Education Division; (10) sending patients who do not comply with dietary advice to a dietician; and (11) recording all salient information on a special form included in the medical record of hypertensive patients. Furthermore, at each visit the nurse reports her findings to the doctor. If there are no problems, the doctor does not see the patient, who is told to stay on treatment and return to see the nurse in a month's time. Thereafter, the patient is seen at monthly intervals by the nurse, and once every 3 months by the doctor. However, if at any visit there are symptoms or if the physical or laboratory findings are abnormal, the patient is seen by the doctor immediately.

Results

Detection of Hypertension. This program has been associated with a large increase in the number of hypertensives detected. In general, about 5% of those people measured during routine visits have been found to have diastolic pressures of ≥ 95 mmHg on three occasions. No standard definition of hypertension was used; doctors were requested to treat patients whose diastolic pressures were consistently ≥ 100 mmHg, and to consider treatment if the pressure was 90–99 mmHg and if other cardiovascular risk factors were present.

Waiting Time. In a study of 250 hypertensives undertaken before the introduction of the program, patients waited an average of 105 min to see the doctor; they now wait an average of 7 min to see the nurse. Those patients who do have to see the doctor are then seen by him immediately.

Reduction in Visits to Physicians. With the extension of the nurse's function to the follow-up of hypertensive patients, there has been a reduction of about 20% of total visits to the physician.

Dropout. Before the program, the average dropout rate was about 30% (5). Since the start of the program, with experience of about 100 000 patients, the dropout rate averages about 1%. A dropout is defined as a patient not seen for 6 months, although still residing in the same area.

Control of Treated Patients. The records of 5541 patients who were initially being treated by their doctors alone and then by a doctor–nurse team were examined [18, 19]. At their last two visits prior to the introduction of the nurse, 2333 (42.1%) had a mean diastolic pressure of < 95 mmHg; 2 years after the introduction of the nurse, 4689 (84.6%) had a mean diastolic pressure of < 95 mmHg on their last two visits.

Weight Control. We examined the success of a doctor–nurse team (after receiving a simple course in dietary management) in getting the overweight patients to reduce their weight. In a study of 230 obese patients who had no weight loss over at least 6 months, the average weight reduction after nursing intervention over a 1-year period averaged 2.1 kg.

Effect on the Community. Recent surveys indicate that about 80% of hypertensives are now aware of their condition [20, 21], 70% of whom are on treatment [4]. Of these, about 70% are under control [4]. Thus, about 50% of hypertensives are under treatment and about 40% of all hypertensives are under control. This represents a more than fourfold increase in the proportion of hypertensives now under control.

The reduction in blood pressure in Israel parallels the reduction in the incidence of cardiovascular diseases seen in Israel in the last 5 years [22].

Effect of a Doctors' Strike. In early 1983 all Kupat Holim family physicians went on strike for 4 months. The nurses in the family clinic continued the follow-up of the hypertensive patients. In a study of 2100 patients, there was no dropout (failure to visit the family nurse) and no change in the percentage of controlled hypertensives during the 4-month period [23].

Screening for Hypertension in Industry. Kupat-Holim is also responsible for the Occupational Health Services. Up to recently the occupational health physicians and nurses were not involved in hypertensive screening. They now organize screening programs in companies and industries throughout the country [24]. Detected hypertensives are sent to their family doctor for treatment but there will be yearly follow-up of these patients at the work-site by the occupational health nurses.

Discussion

The reduction in dropouts and the 85% success rate in treating diastolic hypertension is similar to that in other countries (when a doctor–nurse team is used). When the doctor alone treats the condition this figure is generally around 40%–50% (8, 12–17). This improvement in control can probably be attributed to an increase in patient compliance [15]. The increased attention paid by the nurse to diet and medication taking, the tailoring of medication taking to regular activities, as well as the explanation of the importance of compliance, contribute to this increase. Even the slight weight reduction (average 2.1 kg) in overweight patients – achieved by the doctor–nurse team – may have a substantial effect on blood pressure [25], as may reduced salt intake [26] and a high potassium diet [27]. A controlled study in Jerusalem has shown that a program that included a concerted effort by the doctor–nurse team also caused a significant reduction in other risk factors, such as smoking, serum cholesterol, and overweight [18]. The health education sessions held with patients may also contribute to improved compliance [28, 29].

The data received from the doctor-nurse teams are now being computerized; this will facilitate studies of the treatment of hypertension in Israel.

References

1. Modan M, Modan B, Shani M, Robin D, Thurm RH (1979) Nationwide study of hypertension in Israel. In: Thurm RH (ed) Essential hypertension. Symposia Specialists, Miami, pp 21–27
2. Sive PH, Medalie JH, Kahn HA, Neufeld HN, Riss E (1971) Distribution and multiple regression analysis of blood pressure in 10 000 Israeli men. Am J Epidemiol 93:317–327
3. Holtzman E, Goldbourt U, Rosenthal T, Yaari S, Neufeld HN (1983) Hypertension in middle-aged men. Associated factors and mortality experience. Isr J Med Sci 19:25–33
4. Modan M, Halkin H, Fuchs Z, Karasyk A, Modan B (1982) Seven to ten year follow-up of blood pressure treatment of a national sample of Israeli Jews born 1912–1941. International Symposium on Hypertension Control in the Community, Tel Aviv, Israel, 7–14 November 1982
5. Silverberg DS, Rosenfeld JB, Agmon J, Regev O, Ron A (1979) Evaluation of hypertension control in general practice. Isr J Med Sci 15:817–820
6. Medalie JH, Kahn HA, Neufeld HN, Riss E (1973) Five year myocardial infarction incidence. II. Association of single variables, age and birth place. J Chronic Dis 26:329–349
7. Kark JD, Donchin M, Gofin R, et al. (1982) Blood pressure as a predictor of 10-year mortality in the Kiryat Hayovel (Jerusalem) Community Health Study. International Symposium on Hypertension Control in the Community, Tel-Aviv, Israel, 7–14 Novemer 1982
8. Hypertension Detection and Follow-up Program Cooperative Group (1979) Five year findings of the hypertension detection and follow-up program. I. Reduction in mortality of persons with high blood pressure, including mild hypertension. JAMA 242:2562–2571
9. Management Committee (1980). Report. The Australian therapeutic trial in mild hypertension. Lancet 1:1261–1267
10. Rosenfeld JB, Silverberg DS (1979) Status of hypertension treatment in Israel. Isr J Med Sci 15:1014–1016
11. Hartman B, Silverberg DS, Rosenfeld JB (1981) Long-term follow-up of a hypertension detection program in Israel (in Hebrew). Harefuah 101:102–104
12. Abramson JH, Gofin R, Hopp C, Gofin J, Donchin M, Hanin J (1981) Evaluation of a community program for the control of cardiovascular risk factors: the CHAD program in Jerusalem. Isr J Med Sci 17:201–212
13. Finnerty FA Jr, Mattie EC, Finnerty FA (1973) Hypertension in the inner city. Circulation 47:73–75
14. Wilber JA, Barrow JG (1969) Reducing elevated blood pressure. Experience found in a community. Minn Med 52:1303–1306
15. Logan AG, Milne BJ, Achber C, Campbell WP, Haynes RB (1979) Worksite treatment of hypertension by specially trained nurses. Lancet 2:1175–1178
16. Takala T, Niemela N, Rosti J, Sievers K (1979) Improving compliance with therapeutic regimens in hypertensive patients in a community health center (1975). Circulation 59:540–543
17. Tuomilehto J, Nissinen A, Solonen JT, Kottke E, Puska P (1980) Community programme for control of hypertension in Northern Karelia, Finland. Lancet 2:900–903

18. Silverberg DS, Baltuch L, Hermoni Y, Eyal P (1982) Control of hypertension in family practice by the doctor–nurse team. J R Coll Gen Pract 32:184–186
19. Silverberg DS, Baltuch L, Hermoni Y, Eyal P, Viskoper R, Paran E (1983) The role of the doctor–nurse team in control of hypertension in family practice in Israel. Isr J Med Sci 19:752–754
20. Central Bureau of Statistics (1980) Survey on use of the health services. Special series no 639, Jerusalem
21. Ben Zera Z (1976) Measurement of blood pressure: attitude of the public. Institute of Applied Social Research, no (S) ZBS/589/H, Jerusalem
22. Goldbourt U, Kark JD (1982) The epidemiology of coronary heart disease in the ethnically and culturally diverse population of Israel. A review. Isr J Med Sci 12:1079–1097
23. Adorian D, Silverberg DS, Wamoscher Z (to be published) The effect of a doctors' strike on blood pressure control in Israel
24. Mordish R, Silverberg DS (to be published) Screening for hypertension in industry
25. Reisen E, Abel R, Modan M, Silverberg DS, Modan B, Eliahou HE (1978) Effect of weight loss without salt restriction in the reduction of blood pressure in overweight hypertensive patients. N Engl J Med 298:1–6
26. MacGregor GA, Markandu ND, Best FE (1982) Double-blind randomized crossover trial of moderate sodium restriction in essential hypertension, Lancet 1:351–355
27. MacGregor GA, Markandu ND, Smith SJ, Banks RA, Sagnella GA (1982) Moderate potassium supplementation in essential hypertension. Lancet 2:567–570
28. Levine DM, Green LW, Deeds SG, Chwalow J, Russell P, Finlay J (1979) Health education for hypertensive patients. JAMA 241:1700–1703
29. Nessman DG, Carnahan JE, Nugent CA (1980) Increasing compliance. Patient operated hypertension groups. Arch Intern Med 140:1427–1430

Severity Rating of Hypertension as a Measure of Individual Rehabilitation Effects

W. Höbel, J. Stieber, P. Potthoff, and R. Thurmayr

Introduction

Every year social security funds of the Federal Republic of Germany provide about 800 000 in-patient rehabilitation courses of treatment to alleviate occupational disabilities. Hypertension is a predominant factor contributing to those disabilities.

In the light of past studies, the Association of German Security Funds (VDR) has commissioned the Institute for Medical Informatics and Health Services Research to develop a classification scheme for the severity of arterial hypertension. The main purpose of the severity rating is to assess the effectiveness of individual rehabilitation measures.

In principle there are two different ways to develop a severity classification scheme: a deductive way and an empirical way.

In the deductive method, each stage of the disease concerned and all possibly related symptoms are described, making use of the physician's experience. A severity category from a defined range is assigned to each stage or symptom. In addition there are rules that state which severity category should be chosen when more than one symptom is observed simultaneously. In this way one reaches an operationally defined severity classification scheme whose allocation algorithm corresponds to a logical decision tree.

A decision process of this type was also developed for arterial hypertension. Details of the predefined allocation are shown in Table 1.

In this paper, however, we will present some results on hypertension severity rating which were derived by empirical means. Empirical procedures essentially request medical experts to assign a patient to a severity category while evaluating the observed findings based on their experience. By means of statistical and information processing procedures, the relationship between the severity rating and the observed findings is analysed. Based on the interdependencies found, a classification algorithm is constructed.

To be an appropriate measure, each severity rating has to fulfil several criteria, whichever developing procedure has been used. These criteria are especially:

- Uniform discrimination power within the whole range
- Sensitivity to changes within its components, which means no irreversible features are decisive components

Primary Health Care in the Making
Ed. by U. Laaser, R. Senault, H. Viefhues

Table 1. Details of predefined allocation rules for operational severity rating of primary hypertension

	Severity category				
	1	2	3	4	5
Blood pressure	S: 140–159 or D: 90–94	S: < 160 and D: 95–99	S: 160–179 or D: 100–109	S: 180–199 or D: 110–119	S: ≧200 or D: ≧ 120
Heart					
Actual complaints	No	Heart trouble	Exertional dyspnoea or exertional cardiac pain	Cardiac pain	Lower leg oedema
Resting ECG	Normal	Left axis deviation	Left ventricular hypertrophy		Arrhythmia or infarction
Physical examination Chest X-ray					
Fundus of the eye	Normal	Stage I	Stage II	Stage III	Stage IV

Material and Methods

Included in our study were patients with a primary diagnosis of arterial hypertension who applied for rehabilitation. Patients in hospitals were included, too, to guarantee that cases of hypertension involving high severity stages were incorporated in adequate numbers. The sample contained 653 cases with different diagnoses (Table 2). These diagnoses were made by the examining physicians by free decision.

Besides the physician's report, data were collected by means of a form sheet developed for this study. Overall, a set of 130 features was included from each patient. These 130 variables included:
- Anthropometric features
- Anamnestic variables
- Blood pressure (taken at least three times consecutively in different positions according to the WHO recommendations)
- Organic findings of heart, lung, skin, fundus of the eye, etc.
- Chest X-ray
- Urinalysis
- The diagnosis as mentioned above, and a
- Severity category

The severity category was defined by the following question: "Given 5 categories for the severity of patient's hypertension (1 describing a moderate stage, 5 describing a very severe stage), to which category would you assign it?"

The operational severity classification as shown in Table 1 was unknown to the physicians at that time; thus "free" severity rating could be ascertained.

Table 2. Distribution of diagnoses for primary and secondary hypertension

Hypertension	N	%
Primary hypertension	528	88.3
Borderline	126	21.1
Manifest	277	46.3
Malignant	96	15.9
No specification	30	5.0
Secondary hypertension	70	11.7
Renovascular	61	10.2
Other	9	1.4
Insufficient data	55	–

The analysis and description of the association between severity categories and the variables collected was performed by stepwise logistic regression analysis. Applying this method, two aims could be achieved at the same time:

1. Those variables could be selected which are highly correlated to the severity category.
2. A classification algorithm could be constructed for assigning a severity category to a set of observed values of the selected features.

Because the "true" category is known, one may compare true and predicted categories. The usefulness of the logistic classification rule may then be evaluated by computing the proportion of correct classifications. The number of correct classifications should be high while using only few variables. The logistic regression procedure works in a stepwise manner, i.e. out of all independent features those are selected consecutively which give the best estimation.

Results

As shown in Table 2, the sample consisted of 528 patients with primary hypertension and 70 patients with secondary hypertension. Statistical analyses were restricted to the subsample of patients with primary hypertension. Out of these, six patients had no severity category, so the number of cases for statistical analysis was 522. The distribution of severity categories for these cases is shown in Table 3. Because of the too small number of cases, categories 4 and 5 had to be treated as one category.

One should note that the distribution is very skew to the left hand side. High severity categories contain only 8.7% of the cases.

To construct the classification algorithm by logistic regression, the 4-class definition was changed into three 2-class definitions: First, low categories (1 and 2) were discriminated from high categories (3 and more), followed by discrimination procedures within the low and high categories.

Table 3. Distribution of free severity ratings for primary and secondary hypertension

		Severity category					
		1	2	3	4	5	Total
Primary hypertension	N	146	204	127	40	5	522
	%	28.0	39.1	24.3	7.7	1.0	100.0
Secondary hypertension	N	10	25	17	12	2	66
	%	15.2	37.9	25.8	18.2	3.0	100.0

Variables were dropped from analysis when too many values were missing; in addition, variables had to be excluded which had very skewed distributions. Overall 86 variables fulfilled the conditions to be met in the analysis. Except for fundus of the eye, features from all organic findings could be considered.

Each of the three 2-class discriminations was processed by stepwise logistic regression. The cases were allocated to the severity category by use of the appropriate regression function. The resulting allocation matrices are shown in Table 4.

As one can see from the allocation matrices, good discrimination is not possible in any subclass. The overall correct classification rate is estimated as

		Source of findings					
Rank	Variable	Blood pressure	Age	Anamnestic variables	Clinical examination	Chest X-ray	Resting ECG
1	2nd systolic blood pressure	●					
2	1st diastolic blood pressure	●					
3	2nd diastolic blood pressure	●					
4	Age		●				
5	Heart disease			●			
6	Systolic murmur				●		
7	Antihypertensive agents			●			
8	Myocardial insufficiency			●			
9	Dilatation of the heart					●	
10	Other chronic diseases			●			
11	Cyanosis				●		
12	Aortic dilation					●	
13	Salt intake			●			
14	Peripheral blood circulation				●		
15	Left ventricular hypertrophy						●
16	Gout			●			
17	Hyperlipidemia			●			
18	1st systolic blood pressure	●					
19	Palpable carotid pulse				●		
20	Carotid murmur				●		
21	Arrhythmia						●

Fig. 1. Variables found to be most important for physicians' severity rating of primary hypertension

Table 4. Allocation matrices and classification rates derived by stepwise logistic regression procedures for discrimination of high and low severity categories (step 1), within low categories (step 2), and within high severity categories (step 3)

Step 1: Discrimination of high and low categories
11 selected variables; correct classification: 79.5%

		Physician	
		≦2	≧3
Logistic	≦2	320 91.4%	77 44.8%
Regression	≧3	30 8.6%	95 55.2%
	Total	350 100%	172 100%

Step 2: Discrimination between low categories
16 selected variables; correct classification: 80.3%

		Physician	
		1	2
Logistic	1	103 70.5%	26 12.7%
Regression	2	43 29.5%	178 87.3%
	Total	146 100%	204 100%

Step 3: Discrimination between high categories
9 selected variables; correct classification: 84.9%

		Physician	
		3	4/5
Logistic	3	115 90.6%	14 31.1%
Regression	4/5	12 9.4%	31 68.9%
	Total	127 100%	45 100%

Overall correct classification: 64.7%

64.7%. This proportion is affected adversely by the poor recognition of high severity categories in the first step. The discrimination within low categories is also poor. The error rate of 35.3% expresses the fact that the categories were not defined by operational means but by free decisions.

A certain amount of "uncertainty" had to be taken into account from the beginning.

Combining the order numbers, the variables selected in the three processing steps were ranked by their importance. The most important variables are listed in Fig. 1. From this order one can see that blood pressure was found to be most important; clinical findings rank below anamnestic variables.

The association between the variables and the severity category is positive, which means that higher categories occur when variables hold true. There is one exception: the variable "other chronic diseases" has a negative correlation. The physicians prefer low severity categories when other chronic diseases are observed.

Thus, by means of logistic regression it could be shown that a second criterion for the use of free severity rating as a measure is not fulfiled: anamnestic variables which are not reversible are an important component of the physicians' severity classification process.

Conclusion

By means of stepwise logistic regression analysis the association between the free severity categories and 86 variables was analysed and a classification algorithm was constructed. Using 31 selected features, 64.7% of the cases could be correctly classified. It should be noted here that the deductive procedure which was carried out, too, reached 100% correct classification using 40 variables and 96.5% using only 16 variables.

From the skewed distribution of the severity categories and the decisive influence of anamnestic variables for the classification, one can conclude that free severity rating is not an appropriate method for the assessment of the effectiveness of hypertension treatment rehabilitation courses. When deciding on a severity category, physicians not only consider findings specific for hypertension but also bear in mind the general state of health.

Cost-Effectiveness of Treating Hypertensives in the Federal Republic of Germany: A Model Analysis

H. Wenzel and U. Laaser

The rapid growth of expenditure is a central issue in many policy decisions concerning the medical care system of the Federal Republic of Germany. Health professionals, policymakers and consumers are seeking ways to control this growth while simultaneously improving the quality of health care. Increasingly the use of cost-effectiveness analysis (CEA) and cost-benefit analysis (CBA) is being advocated as a possible means of making the medical care system more efficient.

The principal distinction between CEA and CBA lies in the evaluation of the desirable consequences (benefits) of a decision. In a CBA all costs and benefits are evaluated in monetary terms. In a CEA the health-related effects of programmes are not valued in terms of money but rather in other units such as "years of life gained", "days of morbidity and mortality avoided" or "saved quality-adjusted years of life".

An unfortunate feature of practical economic appraisal to date is that it has concentrated on measuring the benefits to be derived from just one aspect of "being healthy": that is, the benefits in increased production of individuals being able to return to work – the human capital approach [1]. Most people think it is unethical to measure an individual's value of life in terms of money and therefore tend to reject the results of these CBAs. For this reason a CEA approach was chosen here.

In a first step the success of drug treatment is shown by the number of avoided myocardial infarctions and strokes.

The following results are based on a model analysis using data from the Munich Blood Pressure Study [3], the Framingham Study [2] and a model analysis of Weinstein and Stason [5].

Missing valid statistical data concerning the number of hypertensives in the Federal Republic of Germany, especially with respect to blood pressure categories as defined by the WHO – mild, moderate and severe hypertension –, made it necessary to compute these data.

Taking prevalence data of the Munich Blood Pressure Study as a basis, there might be 4.6 million hypertensives in Germany between the ages of 45 and 74 showing diastolic blood pressure $\geq$ 90 mmHg. The distribution of hypertensives by sex, age group and blood pressure category is shown in Fig. 1. The figure includes 2.4 million male and 2.2 million female hypertensives.

Primary Health Care in the Making
Ed. by U. Laaser, R. Senault, H. Viefhues

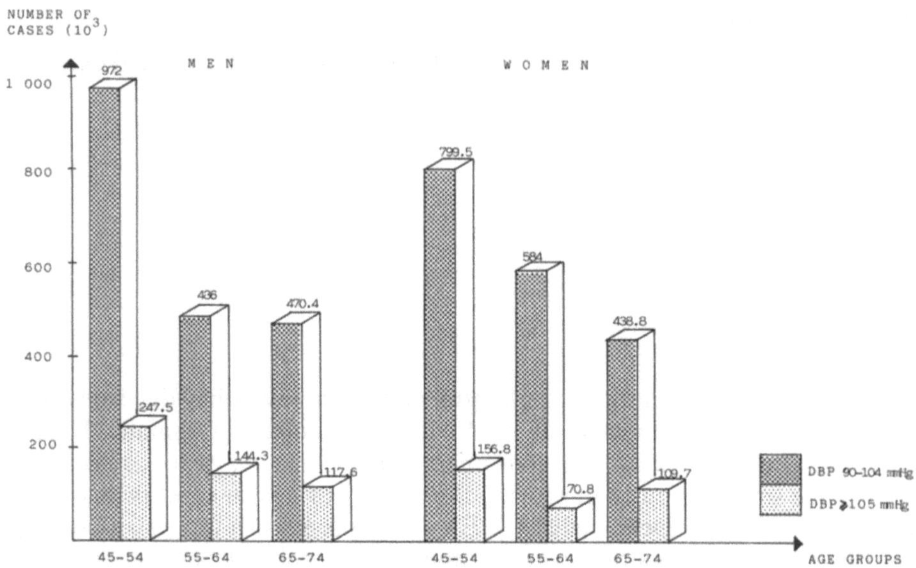

Fig. 1. Number of hypertensives with mild (DBP 90 – 104 mmHg) or moderate or severe hypertension (DBP ≥ 105 mmHg) in the Federal Republic of Germany

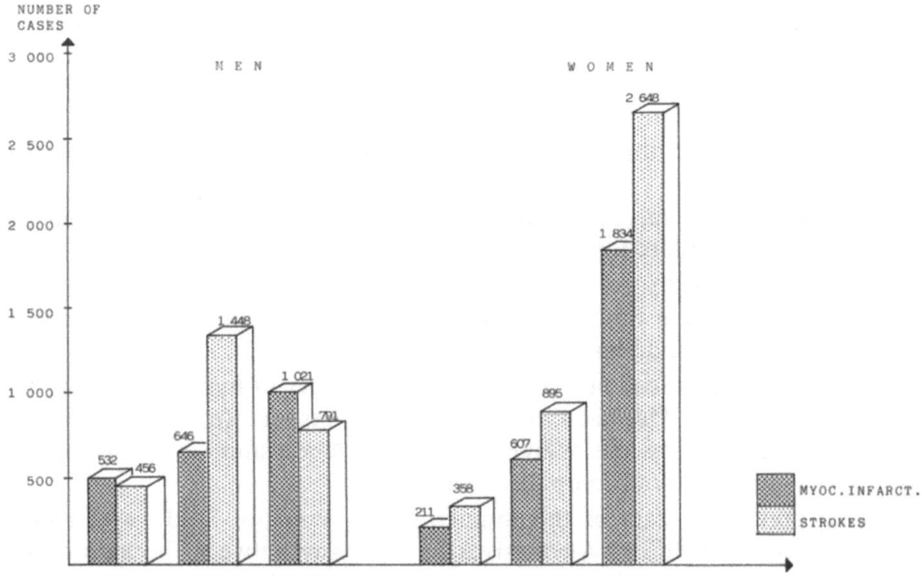

Fig. 2. Number of myocardial infarctions and strokes that would occur in a year in the population open to treatment (DBP > 90 mmHg) but without treatment

Transferring the results of the Munich Blood Pressure Study as well, of these expected hypertensives on average only 47% will be treated, i.e. approximately 900 000 men and 1.2 million women.

To show the effectiveness of drug treatment we have to know how many strokes and myocardial infarctions would occur in the group of hypertensives open to treatment and actually receiving no treatment. According to this procedure the number of strokes and myocardial infarctions in the same group must be computed assuming that it will be possible to lower blood pressure to below 90 mmHg. Comparison of morbidity data in both cases then shows the relative effectiveness of hypertension control. To estimate these probable disease rates in controlled and uncontrolled condition, the excess risk was determined according to the Framingham Study.

Figure 2 shows the number of myocardial infarctions and strokes in a year that would occur in the population open to treatment but without any treatment. There might be 4800 myocardial infarctions and 6600 strokes in a year.

If we now look closely at the group of hypertensives when treated, we have to deal with three problems that will affect the effectiveness and efficiency of treatment:

- How compliant will patients be with the regimen?
- How many of the compliant patients will be treated adequately, i.e. in how many will blood pressure be lowered?
- If patients are compliant and blood pressure is lowered below 90 mmHg, how will new excess risks of getting myocardial infarctions and strokes change as a result?

The probable benefit of lowering blood pressure depends also on how long the exposure to higher risk lasted and at which age such a lowering of blood pressure occurred. It is to be assumed that the risk of a long-term hypertensive whose blood pressure after treatment was normalized is not identical with the risk of a long-term normotensive. The risk which is actually new lies somewhere in between.

To consider these age-varying partial benefits of lowered blood pressure in the case of strokes, estimates of Weinstein and Stason were utilized. For myocardial infarctions the data of Weinstein and Stason were modified in a Delphi round-table conference which took place in the German Institute for High Blood Pressure Research in Heidelberg in 1982.

To determinate the effectively treated hypertensives, i.e. persons compliant and adequately treated, data from the Munich Blood Pressure Study about controlled hypertensives were used.

Table 1 shows the percent distribution of controlled hypertensives used in this study. The distribution of hypertensives to the two blood pressure categories – (a) mild and (b) moderate hypertension and severe hypertension – is an assumption within the framework of this study.

This study is based on an average of 57% of the persons controlled, while Taylor et al. [4], on the other hand, for a treatment interval of 6 months, list 35%.

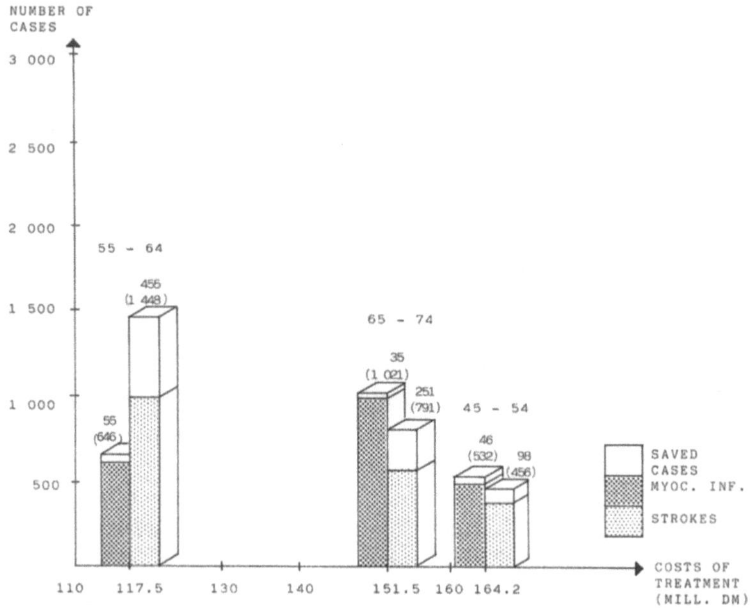

Fig. 3. Costs of treatment and avoided myocardial infarctions and strokes in male hypertensives in the 1st year. *Note:* The figures in parentheses indicate the numbers of cases without any treatment (see also Fig. 2) and are shown by the full length of the bar, i.e. stippled plus blank spaces in the bar

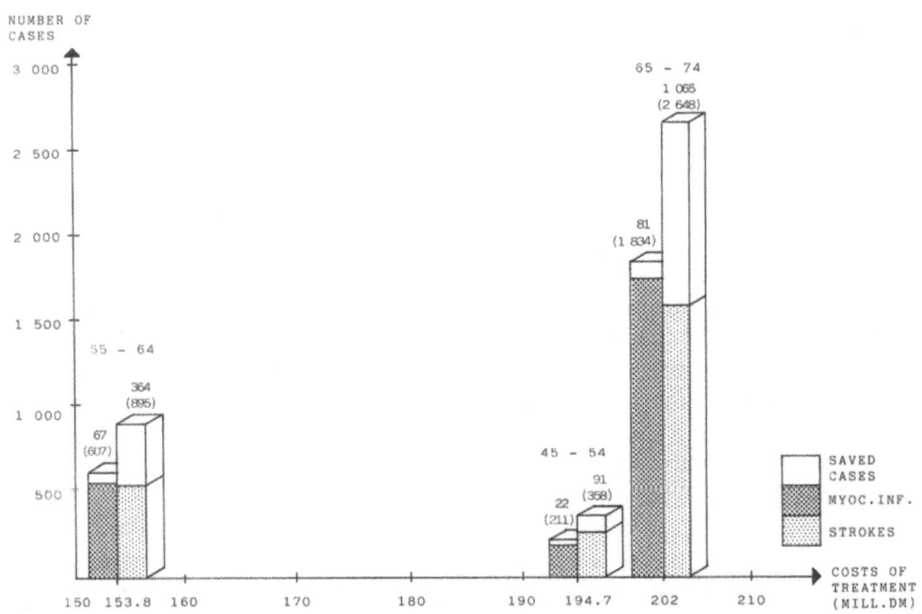

Fig. 4. Costs of treatment and avoided myocardial infarctions and strokes in female hypertensives in the 1st year. *Note:* The figures in parentheses indicate the number of cases without any treatment (see also Fig. 2) and are shown by the full length of the bar, i.e. stippled plus blank spaces in the bar

Table 1. Percent distribution of controlled hypertensives with regard to the treated population. Source: modified data from the Munich Blood Pressure Study I [3]

Age groups	Controlled Hypertensives (%)			
	DBP 90–104 mmHg		DBP ≧ 105 mmHg	
	Men	Women	Men	Women
45–54	31.6	41.2	37.5	40
55–64	56.3	70	54.6	75
65–74	63.2	76.3	60	75

Considering all these factors, 300 myocardial infarctions and 2300 strokes might be avoided in the first year. Figure 3 shows the number of events and "saved cases" for male hypertensives in the first year.

In the age group 45–54 there might be a decrease of 8.7% in myocardial infarctions and 21.5% in strokes. In the age group 55–64, 8.5% of infarctions and 31.4% of strokes could be avoided, while in the age group 65–74, 3.4% of infarctions and 31.7% of strokes might be prevented.

We can also see from the above that in the age group 55–64 117.5 million DM, in the age-group 65–74 164.2 million DM, and in the age group 45–54 151.5 million DM will possibly have to be paid in the first year.

These costs are also estimated. They include costs of anti-hypertensive drugs, laboratory fees and renumeration of the practitioner. Costs of treating side-effects could not be taken into account at this stage.

Figure 4 shows the costs and effectiveness of treating female hypertensives in the first year.

References

1. Drummond MF (1980) Principles of economic appraisal in health care. Oxford University Press, Oxford, p 12
2. Kanel WB, Tavia Gordon (eds) (1974) The Framingham study. An epidemiological investigation of cardiovascular disease. DHEW Publication no (NIH) 74–599, Washington, DC
3. Stieber J, Döring A, Keil U (1982) Häufigkeit, Bekanntheits- und Behandlungsgrad des hohen Blutdrucks in einer Großstadtbevölkerung der Bundesrepublik Deutschland: Ergebnisse der Münchner-Blutdruck-Studie I (MBS 1980/81). MMW 35:747–752
4. Taylor DW, Sackett DL, Haynes RB, Johnson AL, Gibson ES, Roberts RS (1978) Antihypertensive drug therapy. Ann NY Acad Sci 304:309–402
5. Weinstein MC, Stason WB (1976) Hypertension: A policy perspective. Harvard University Press, Cambridge, MA London

B. Community Health Promotion by Lay Involvement

Social Differences in the Long-Term Effects of Health Education in Reducing Coronary Risk

G. De Backer, M. Dramaix, M. Kornitzer, F. Kittel, and K. Vuylsteek

In prospective epidemiological surveys the relation between certain factors and the incidence of coronary heart disease (CHD) has been well documented. The reversibility of the coronary risk by intervening on the risk factors is less well documented, and the feasibility of reducing risk factors in a middle-aged population has been demonstrated [1–4] as well as refuted [5, 6].

In 1970 the Regional Office for Europe of the WHO convened a working group to consider the feasibility of multifactorial preventive trials in CHD in Europe. As a result of that meeting the Belgian Heart Disease Prevention Project was designed according to an original protocol of Rose [7]. International collaboration resulted in the WHO European Collaborative Group Trial [8].

The Belgian Prevention Project was set up to evaluate a particular programme of multifactorial prevention and to assess its ability to alter risk factor levels and the effect of such changes, if any, on the mortality and incidence of CHD. The programme was carried out in an industrial working population including various social classes.

Since the relation between social class and cardiovascular risk is a controversial issue in the literature, we analysed specifically the social determinants of the long-term effects of the multifactorial health educational programme in influencing behavioural patterns that are known to be associated with CHD. In this report results are presented concerning smoking habits and serum cholesterol.

Methods

Earlier reports focused on the design [2, 9], the baseline results [10–12] and the risk factor changes during the initial 2 years of the study [1]. In summary, 30 factories were paired off; one member of each pair was randomly allocated into the intervention group while the other was serving as a control. All men aged 40–59 years and employed by the factories were enrolled in the study. In the intervention group all subjects were invited to attend a screening visit. In the control group a 10% random sample was given the same opportunity. Using age, serum cholesterol, systolic blood pressure, smoking habits and physical activity at work, a risk score was constructed for each participant. In both the in-

Primary Health Care in the Making
Ed. by U. Laaser, R. Senault, H. Viefhues

tervention and the control group a "high-risk" subgroup was defined as those 21% of the participants with the highest risk scores.

In the intervention group a particular multifactorial preventive programme was carried out over a 6-year period. At annual intervals a 5% random sample of the total intervention group was re-examined. High-risk subjects were invited for individual counselling sessions and re-examined for risk factors every 6 months. In the control group the same 10% random sample that was invited at baseline was re-examined after 2 and 4 years. At the end of the study all subjects still at work from both the intervention and control group were invited for a final visit.

All subjects enrolled in the study were identified at entry as either blue-collar workers, white-collar workers or executives by the personnel departments of the factories.

Data on smoking behaviour were collected through self-administered questionnaires, verified and supplemented by a technician's interview. At the final screening the smoking habits were indirectly assessed by determining serum thiocyanate levels in random samples of both the intervention and the control group. Details on the good correlation between smoking behaviour assessed by questionnaire and serum thiocyanate levels were published elsewhere [13].

Throughout the study, serum cholesterol was determined in the same laboratory. An external quality control system has been operating with the WHO lipid reference centre. Annual re-examinations in the intervention and control group took place by pairs of factories.

The intervention programme aimed at a reduction of fat intake, especially of saturated fat, and at a partial replacement of saturated fat by polyunsaturated fats. Furthermore, caloric restriction was advised in cases of overweight. All smokers of five or more cigarettes a day were advised to stop smoking. The programme was further directed towards control of arterial hypertension and towards increased physical activity for sedentary subjects.

Results

Smoking and Serum Cholesterol at the Start of the Study

In the left-hand part of Fig. 1, serum cholesterol values are presented for each social class in the intervention and control group as observed at the baseline visit.

No significant differences were found between intervention and control group. As to the social class differences, serum cholesterol was significantly related with social class, the highest values being among higher grades. The percentages of subjects with a serum cholesterol value $\geq$ 260 mg% were 23, 28 and 36% in blue-collar workers, white-collar workers and executives respectively.

In the left-hand part of Fig. 2, the prevalence of ex-smokers is presented in relation to social class. In the lower risk group there was a significant relationship between percentages of ex-smokers and social class.

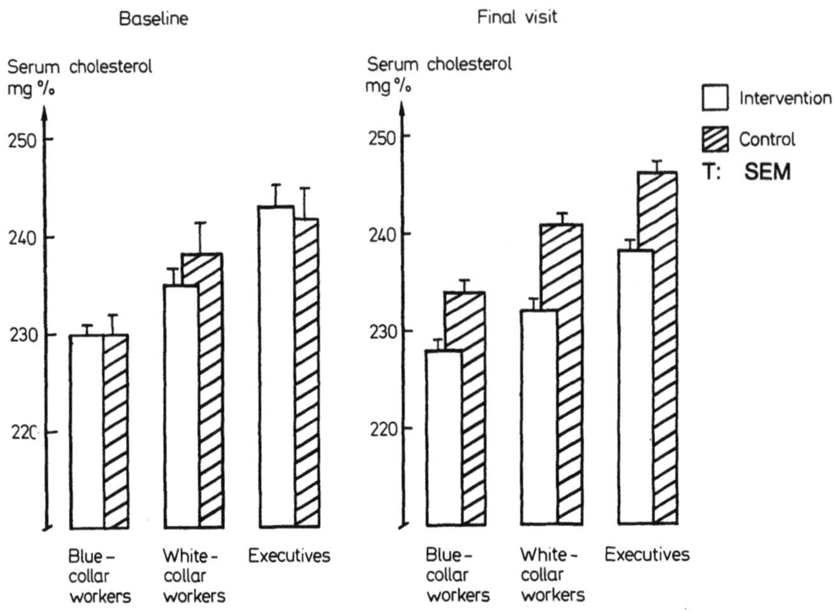

Fig. 1. Relation between serum cholesterol and social class at entry and at the final screening in the Belgian Heart Disease Prevention Project

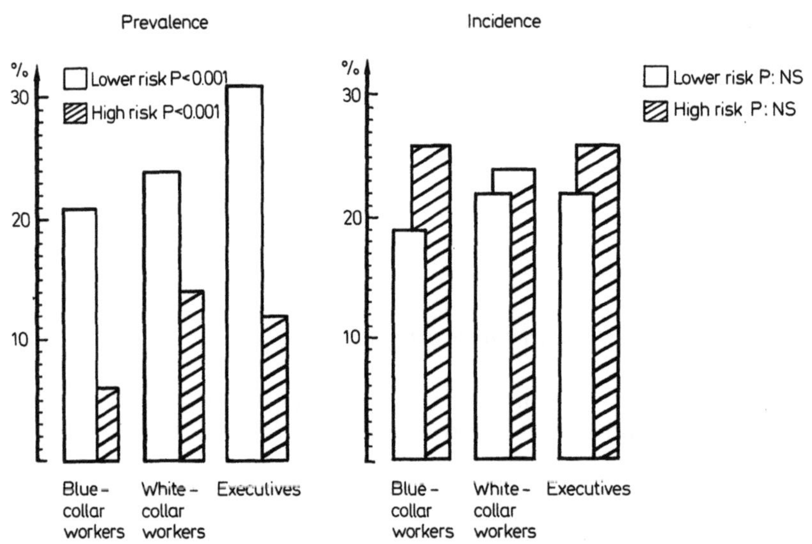

Fig. 2. Relation between percentage of ex-smokers (prevalence and incidence) and social class

Long-Term Effects of the Health Educational Programme by Social Class

Serum Cholesterol. In Table 1 the change in serum cholesterol from entry to the final visit is presented in relation to other variables for the lower-risk and the high-risk groups. For both subgroups the baseline value and the geographical area were significantly related to the change in cholesterol. The former is partially related to the regression towards the mean phenomenon, while the latter suggests a greater success of the programme in subjects living in the North-East, where the serum cholesterol was already the lowest at the start. These two variables account for 26% of the variance of the change in cholesterol. The change in the high-risk subjects was significantly greater than in the lower-risk group.

In Fig. 1 (right part) the relation between cholesterol and social class is presented at the final screening for both the total intervention and control groups. Where both groups were comparable at baseline (see left part), a significant difference between intervention and control is present in each social class at the final visit. These results indicate that the programme of health education was effective across the social classes.

Cigarette Smoking. In Fig. 2 social class is related to the incidence of ex-smokers during the trial. No difference across social classes is observed. High-risk men did somewhat better than lower-risk men, especially among the blue-collar workers.

In Table 2 results from a multiple discriminant function analysis comparing those who quit smoking with the others are presented. In the lower-risk group only marital status was related to the incidence of ex-smokers. In the high-risk men no significant discriminator was identified.

Table 1. Belgian Heart Disease Prevention Project: Change in cholesterol and sociocultural factors

Multivariate analysis – Intervention group Change in cholesterol				
	Lower risk		High risk	
	F	*P*	*F*	*P*
Baseline chol.	1210	<0.001	126	<0.001
Region	18	<0.001	13	<0.001
Age		NS		NS
Culture		NS		NS
Social class		NS		NS
Study level		NS		NS
Marital status		NS		NS
r^2 %	26.5		14.8	

NS, non-significant

Table 2. Belgian Heart Disease Prevention Project: Stopping smoking and sociocultural factors

Incidence of ex-smokers Multiple discriminant function analysis		
	Lower risk *P*	High risk *P*
Marital status	< 0.01	NS
Age	NS	NS
Social class	NS	NS
Study level	NS	NS
Region	NS	NS
Culture	NS	NS
Prediction of		
Ex-smokers %	59	–
Smokers %	49	–

NS, non-significant

Discussion

In the Belgian Heart Disease Prevention Project the random allocation of occupational units resulted in an intervention and control group, both groups being strictly comparable in all coronary risk factors studied in this trial. Within each group significant gradients were found between social class and two risk factors related to health behaviour, i.e. serum cholesterol and cigarette smoking.

The social class differences in prevalence of cigarette smoking are in accordance with other observations. A more detailed analysis of these results indicates that the low prevalence of cigarette smokers in the executives is not only due to a higher percentage of ex-smokers but also to a higher percentage of non-smokers, suggesting a social class difference in smoking habits starting in adolescence [10].

The social class difference in serum cholesterol is contrasting with results from the U.S. [14] and Norway [15], where an opposite relation was found, although earlier reports from these countries also revealed associations in the direction we found. From multivariate analyses, presented elsewhere, it was concluded that the social class–cholesterol relationship was independent from other factors as age, body mass index and job physical activity [11]. The direct association between serum cholesterol and social class is probably related to various sociocultural factors. Results from an analysis including cultural differences within our study population revealed important differences in fat consumption by cultural groups, independent of social class [16]. Data from analyses including health knowledge, attitudes, behaviour and serum cholesterol do suggest that dietary behaviour is only partially determined by rational knowledge factors but importantly influenced by non-rational factors that are induced by the cultural, aesthetic and social values of the community [17].

Against this background of prevalence data we were interested to see whether our intervention programme had different effects on the coronary risk factors by social class.

The incidence of ex-smokers was only related to marital status among lower-risk subjects – married subjects quit more – while no relation between the incidence of ex-smokers and sociocultural variables was found in high-risk subjects (Table 2).

The programme resulted in a significant reduction of serum cholesterol across social classes. A significant number of subjects quit smoking in all social classes. The extent of these changes was related to the intensity of the programme.

The results show that risk factor modification in the situation as explained, is feasible in middle-aged working men and occurs independent of social class. We still know little about the most effective means of influencing knowledge, behaviour and attitudes.

In our programme, common sense has been used as a guide. Our inability to influence the social class gradient may be related to the strong emphasis we put on what individuals should be doing. For affecting the social class gradient, values and norms of the society should be changed, not merely the behaviour of individuals. This requires more energetic public health measures by international and local governments to complement personal responses.

Acknowledgement. This work was supported by grant no. 20202 of the National Fund for Scientifc Research, Belgium.

References

1. Kornitzer M, De Backer G, Dramaix M, Thilly C (1980) The Belgian heart disease prevention project. Modification of the coronary risk profile in an industrial population. Circulation 61:18–25
2. De Backer G (1979) Studie van de omkeerbaarheid van risicofactoren voorbeschikkend tot coronaire hartziekten in een industriële bevolkingsgroep. Thesis, University of Gent
3. WHO European Collaborative Group (1982) Multifactorial trial in the prevention of coronary heart disease. 2. Risk factor changes at two and four years. Eur Heart J 3:184–190
4. Hjermann I, Holme I, Byre KV, Leren P (1981) Effect of diet and smoking intervention on the incidence of coronary heart disease. Lancet 2:1303–1310
5. Holland WW, D'Souza M, Swan AV (1978) Is mass screening justified? Tijdschr Soc Geneeskd 56:22–25
6. Maas J, Hofman A, Valkenburg HA (1982) Lotgevallen van jonge volwassenen met hypertensie (EPOZ). Tijdschr Soc Geneeskd 60:820
7. Rose GA (1970) A proposed trial of heart disease prevention in industry. Trans Soc Occup Med 20:109–111
8. WHO European Collaborative Group (1974) An international controlled trial in the multifactorial prevention of coronary heart disease. Int J Epidemiol 3:219–224
9. De Backer G, Kornitzer M, Thilly C, Depoorter AM (1977) The Belgian multifactor preventive trial in CVD. Design and methodology. Hart Bull 8:143–146
10. Kornitzer M, Dramaix M, De Backer G, Thilly C (1978) The Belgian multifactor preventive trial in CVD. Smoking habits and sociobiological variables. Hart Bull 9:7–13

11. Kornitzer M, Dramaix M, De Backer G, Thilly C (1977) The Belgian multifactor preventive trial in CVD: Cholesterolemia and psychosocio-biological variables. Hart Bull 8:147–154
12. De Backer G, Ramioul L, Kornitzer M, Thilly C (1978) The Belgian multifactor preventive trial in CVD. Epidemiology of arterial blood pressure in an industrial population. Hart Bull 7:14–19
13. Kornitzer M, Vanhemeldonck A, Bourdoux P, De Backer G (1983) The Belgian Heart Disease Prevention Project: comparison of self-reported smoking behavior with serum thiocyanate levels. J Epidemiol Community Health 37:132–136
14. Kraus JF, Borhani NO, Franti CE (1980) Socio-economic status, ethnicity and risk of coronary heart disease. Am J Epidemiol 111:407–414
15. Holme I, Helgeland A, Hjermann I, Lund-Larsen PG, Leren P (1976) Coronary risk factors and socio-economic status: the Oslo study. Lancet 2:1396–1398
16. Kornitzer M, De Backer G, Dramaix M, Thilly C (1979) Regional differences in risk factor distributions, food habits and coronary heart disease mortality and morbidity in Belgium. Int J Epidemiol 8:23–31
17. De Backer G, Kornitzer M, Dramaix M, Kittel F (1981) Socio-cultural interactions in dietary behavior and serum cholesterol. Eur Heart J [Suppl A] 2:143

The Tromsø Heart Study: The Effect of Dietary Intervention in Hyperlipaemic Men – 5-Year Follow-up

D. S. Thelle, O. H. Førde, and E. Arnesen

Background

Health education particularly aimed at promoting a more healthy daily diet is a cornerstone in today's preventive medicine in the industrialized world [1]. The Tromsø Heart Study is a population survey undertaken both to establish the basis for a longitudinal study of cardiovascular and other chronic diseases, and to institute preventive measures against groups with high risk for coronary heart disease. The study provided the opportunity to examine the effect of individual health education measures aimed at men with a high level of coronary risk factors. The theme of this paper is a description of some of the background variables which may determine the outcome of such measures, assessed as changes in total serum cholesterol.

Material and Methods

The municipality of Tromsø is located at a latitude of approximately 70 °N (400 km north of the Arctic Circle) and has a population of about 45 000 inhabitants. The study which carries the name of this town comprises two population surveys; the first was done in 1974 [2], the second in 1979/80. In 1974 all men aged 20–49 years were invited (total: 8867), whereas women aged 20–49 (total: 9906) and men aged 20–54 (total: 11 423) were invited in 1979/80. The attendance rate in 1974 was 74% and 73% in 1979/80 (Table 1).

Table 1. Population size and number examined according to age and sex. Tromsø 1974 and Tromsø 1979–80

	1974			1979–80		
	Age	Invited	Examined	Age	Invited	Examined
Males	20–49	8867	6595	20–54	11 423	8 419
Females		–	–	20–49	9 906	8 447
Total		8867	6595		21 329	16 856

Primary Health Care in the Making
Ed. by U. Laaser, R. Senault, H. Viefhues

Table 2. Total cholesterol limits for recall in 1974 and inclusion levels for controls

Age (years)	No.	Cholesterol levels (mmol/litre)	
		Recalled	Controls (not recalled)
20–29	179	>7.8	7.28–7.77
30–39	152	>9.1	8.58–9.07
40–49	89	>9.9	9.36–9.85

In 1974 420 men had total serum cholesterol levels exceeding the preset limits for recall (Table 2) and were invited to a re-examination which consisted of a single fasting blood sample for lipid analysis [3]. 390 men came to the re-examination; 152 had serum cholesterol level below the recall limits and were not examined further, only being given a brochure with dietary advice. The 238 remaining men were interviewed by a dietician and given dietary advice. They were re-examined again after 6 and 12 weeks. Of the the 420 hypercholesterolaemic men identified in 1974, 305 also took part in the 1979/80 survey.

In order to assess the effect of the intervention on the cholesterol level, a control group was established. This group comprised men who had taken part in both surveys, who had had cholesterol levels in 1974 just below the limits for recall, and who were matched with the recalled subjects for age, area of residency and date of examination.

In order to reduce the influence of age and the possible changes in laboratory methods during these 5 years, the comparison between the two groups, the controls and those recalled, has been done using standard deviation units. Standard deviation units are calculated by subtracting the observed value from the mean value of the 5-year age and sex group to which the subject belongs. The difference is divided by the standard deviation, giving the standard deviation unit (z-score). The z-score denotes the position of the actual subject in the distribution of the variable under examination. The closer the units are to zero, the closer the subject's observed value will be to the mean level of his or her age group.

Results

Cholesterol levels

From 1974 to 1979 the decrease in total cholesterol in the controls was 0.29 mmol/litre compared to 0.83 mmol/litre in the recalled group (Table 3). Part of this decrease can be ascribed the change from a Liebermann-Burchard method to an enzymatic method for total cholesterol assessment, which gives 0.30 mmol/litre lower cholesterol values. The corresponding change in z-score,

Table 3. Total cholesterol (mmol/litre and z-score) in 1974 and 1979/80 in men above and just below the limits for recall in 1974

	No.	Cholesterol 1974		Cholesterol 1979/80	
		mmol/litre	z-score	mmol/litre	z-score
Recalled	305	9.65	2.20	7.85	1.36
Not recalled	162	8.35	1.32	7.43	1.03

Table 4. Total cholesterol change (z-score) in men above and just below the limits for recall for hypercholesterolaemia according to area of residency

Area of residency	No.	Recalled	Not recalled
Town center	289	−0.65	−0.17
Suburban area	48	−0.67	+0.07
Rural area I	24	−1.23	−0.92
Rural area II	100	−1.25	−0.75

however, gives the decrease independent of the difference in laboratory methods in 1974 and 1979/80 (Table 3), and it is seen that the cholesterol level of the recalled group is much closer to the mean of their own age group than it was 5 years previously.

The municipality of Tromsø can be divided naturally into four areas; the town centre, the nearby suburban area and two more rural parts mainly inhabited by fishermen and farmers.

Table 4 shows the changes in z-score for cholesterol in the two groups according to area of residency in the municipality. The reduction in z-score was larger in the rural areas than in the urban areas. But it is also striking that the subjects who were not recalled but who were living in the rural areas were more prone to have lower cholesterol values 5 years later than the men living in the urbanized areas.

With the men classified according to length of education, those with the lowest level of education had the highest reduction in total cholesterol. Also the men with more than 13 years of schooling did not change their cholesterol level if they were not recalled.

Dietary Changes

In 1979 all participants in the survey were asked if they had changed their dietary habits with regard to the intake of meat, be it fat or lean, milk, whole or skimmed, and butter or hard margarine versus soft margarine.

The changes in dietary habits in those recalled and the controls according to their length of education are shown in Table 5. Reduction in fat meat intake

Table 5. Percentage of hyperlipaemic men ($n=467$) who changed their diets according to being recalled (R) or not (C) for hypercholesterolaemia in 1974, and length of education

Years of education	Reduced whole milk		Increased skimmed milk		Reduced margarine, butter		Increased soft marg.		Reduced fat meat		Increased lean meat	
	R	C	R	C	R	C	R	C	R	C	R	C
1–7	33%	16%	35%	18%	5%	26%	37%	20%	69%	38%	28%	18%
8–12	44%	23%	46%	24%	59%	33%	38%	22%	60%	40%	30%	17%
13+	59%	35%	50%	31%	66%	34%	52%	23%	66%	38%	44%	21%

and the consumption of hard margarine and butter were the dietary changes most frequently reported in the recalled group. Changes in milk intake were more frequent in recalled subjects of the higher educational levels. Increase in lean meat intake also showed an educational gradient, with the highest educational group reporting most changes. For all the recorded items the recalled group had a higher frequency of reported changes than the control group. The educational gradient observed in the recalled group is also reflected in the control group for changes in milk consumption, whereas the other items are more evenly distributed in the three educational classes.

Conclusions and Comments

Three main conclusions may be drawn from the present material:

- It is possible to change people's habits with regard to diet, and the results of these changes last at least 5 years.
- There are social distinctions which influence the coronary risk, especially length of education.
- It is easier to influence the whole society by intervening upon high-risk subjects in rural areas than in more urban areas.

The impact of the reported results with regard to risk for coronary heart disease is impossible to assess: the numbers are much too small. The results of the Oslo Study, however, indicate a substantial reduction in CHD morbidity in middle-aged men following dietary changes [4]. Such results, however, depend upon both our ability to identify the high-risk subjects and our knowledge about which methods to apply to induce the desirable changes. The larger effect observed in the rural areas probably suggests that closer knit societies provide a more favourable environment for inducing life-style changes. This implies that preventive efforts of this kind should be the responsibility of the local primary health care system.

References

1. Stamler J (1982) Diet and coronary heart disease. Biometrics [Supplement: Current topics in biostatistics and epidemiology] 95–114
2. Thelle DS, Førde OH, Try K, Lehmann EH (1976) The Tromsø heart study. Methods and main results of the cross-sectional study. Acta Med Scand 200:107–118
3. Thelle DS, Førde OH (1979) The Tromsø heart study: Population studies of coronary risk factors with special emphasis on high density lipoprotein and the family occurrence of myocardial infarction. Thesis, University of Tromsø, Norway
4. Hjermann I, Holme I, Velve Byre K, Leren P (1981) Effect of diet and smoking intervention on the incidence of coronary heart disease. Lancet 2/8259:1303–1310

Health Committees – A Way to Consumer Participation in Health Care Systems

A. Füller and R. Pitsch

Introduction

In the scientific and political discussion about the significance and development of health care systems in modern societies there is widespread agreement that a shift towards prevention (and rehabilitation) is necessary. Since prevention is directed at influencing everyday behaviour, life-styles and life conditions, the conditions of its effectiveness are *acceptance* and *co-operation* on the part of the addressees. Therefore preventive measures should be based on conditions and needs which are intelligible and relevant, i.e. close, to the addressees [5]. Being close to the addressees implies: Measures are performed by

- The addressees themselves
- Persons, groups, organizations and institutions
  which are important for inhabitants
  which allow for identification processes
  which are interested in the aims and questions of prevention.

Prevention at the Community Level

Preventive (and other innovative) actions can be facilitated by using already existing and active groups. This is one of the reasons for implementing preventive measures at the community level. In practice this means initiating *co-ordination* of existing (and partly active) groups. It is assumed that between them a basic consensus concerning the necessity of preventive measures either already exists or can be produced [2].

An initiative to bring together different local groups and organizations with the aim of promoting preventive measures and coordinating the measures being taken may result in the formation of a committee that will take responsibility for health and social questions at the community level.

In the initiation of such a committee some opportunities to improve social conditions may be recognized, e.g.:

1. Strengthening the autonomy and responsibility of medical lay personnel towards their own health and that of their environment
2. Activating citizens at the local level

Primary Health Care in the Making
Ed. by U. Laaser, R. Senault, H. Viefhues

3. Increasing the orientation of social measures to concrete needs
4. Supporting groups in the community
5. Reinforcing consumer participation in public life

But the initiation and establishment of a committee of social groups and the implementation of preventive measures can also have negative side effects:
1. Growth of disparities between groups in the population – because some parts of the population may use preventive measures while others do not [4].
2. Formation of a group of new "experts", which makes participation of inhabitants more difficult [7].

To avoid such side-effects, the *supplementation* of the work of such a committee by two elements would seem useful:
1. *Community work* (its function is, for example, the detection and compensation of deficiencies, and activation of inhabitants and participation).
2. Promotion of *self-organization* and self-help to develop the growing competence and self-confidence of inhabitants (e.g. by promoting meeting points, initiatives and self-organized groups).

Co-ordination of Prevention by a Local Committee

A local committee for health promotion principally represents important everyday areas relevant to health (work, housing, leisure, communication, social services, education etc.). In particular, members of the committee are representatives of:
- Schools
- VHS (adult education)
- Voluntary organizations (for sports, leisure)
- Public and voluntary social services
- Self-help organizations
- Health care (hospitals, physicians, pharmacists, health insurances, health office etc.)
- Health and welfare centres, advisory boards
- Youth organizations
- Firms, unions
- Administration

For efficient co-ordination and communication the committee should not be too large. In keeping members to an effective minimum, the health-related importance of local organizations and the advice of local peers are of paramount importance. Therefore, a selection of members seems necessary; the criteria of selection may relate to the local health-related importance of organization. In the process of selection, information from members of the local newspapers, the municipal administration and personal contacts within the community may help.

Members of the committee and other interested persons and groups may then initiate *working groups* for special tasks and target groups; the main task of these groups is to promote new ideas in the field of prevention, which especially relate to self-help, self-organization and community work. It is supposed that most of the members of the committee will be primarily oriented towards more traditional health information and education.

It should be mentioned that the formation of such a committee with health-related but also less specific tasks may provoke problems and conflicts, e.g. between on the one hand the project group and the committee and on the other, organizations of health professionals (e.g. physicians) or administrative bodies. The latter may fear, for example, the formation of public responsibility for issues in which they claim a monopol at present.

Experiences Regarding the Formation of a Committee

Based upon the considerations mentioned above and upon experiences with other community-oriented preventive programmes (e.g. Aarau, Emmendingen) [3, 6], our project group tried to stimulate the formation of a health committee in Weinheim (a town of 45 000 inhabitants, 15 km from Mannheim). The *procedure* involved in forming this committee comprised the following steps:

1. Considerations about the tasks and composition of the committee
2. Contacting (in 1981) the heads of the municipal administration and local newspapers, and checking on the possibility of co-operation; first information on the aims and tasks of the project and about the sociological structure of the municipality.
3. Collection of information on groups with whom co-operation may be possible.
4. Personal contact (spring 1982) with these groups, providing information on the prerequisites, aims and tasks of the project and acquiring information on the interests and ideas of the potentially co-operative groups and persons.
5. A first meeting of the committee; planning and performance of joint public action. At the first meeting the results of the aforementioned dialogues were considered.
6. A further meeting to appraise the realization of the programme; formation of working groups to prepare special measures (e.g. for children, young people, to promote self-help). Through these groups, which also include some who are not members of the committee, we tried to achieve the co-ordination of more traditional health informational and educational measures.

Development of Preventive Measures

As the public commencement of committee actions (in October 1982), two health weeks incorporating many measures were organized under the motto *"Aktion gesundes Weinheim"*. In particular there were:

- Informative lectures and discussions
- Exhibitions
- A so-called information market (*Informationsbörse*) involving various groups and organizations
- A festival for children (with games, the possibility of preparing a healthy meal etc.)
- A circus for children with a health-related programme
- Action to promote home baking of healthy bread
- A citizens' meeting on healthy housing
- Different sporting events
- Films about psychic health
- Tests and measurement actions (e.g. risk-factor screenings)

The actions were supported and complemented by an extensive press campaign.

In spite of these extensive programmes and the great number of participating groups and organizations, a part of the population could not be reached by most measures while more easily reachable sections were more active. This was expected by the project group.

Therefore, after these programmes were over, steps were taken to reach *underprivileged* people and those less interested in health questions in order to promote activity in health questions. These efforts involved, for example:

- Establishment of a self-help telephone service to promote self-help groups. Three groups have already been established and further groups are in preparation.
- Close co-operation with a *youth organization* (*Stadtjugendring*) which is involved in self-responsible youth work and starts initiatives for jobless young people. Together with this organization, activities are planned for the prevention of alcohol abuse in adolescents.
- Promoting leisure time offers for young people by preparing a games festival for 1984 – in contrast to the traditional school sport festivals.
- Co-operation with a local working group of social workers to promote social work in health care.

These measures represent the *first steps* in a medium-sized town towards:

- Bringing together and activating local groups, organizations and persons to partake in health promotion
- Promoting the interest of lay persons in their own health and that of the community,
- Making persons and groups aware of discrimination against social groups – vis-à-vis health and social conditions – and of the necessity of eradicating these disadvantages.

References

1. Badura B, von Ferber C (1981) Selbsthilfe und Selbstorganisation im Gesundheitswesen. Oldenbourg, Munich Vienna

2. Ferber C von (1980) Wie läßt sich die Wirtschaftlichkeit im Gesundheitswesen verbessern? In: Leistungssteigerung im Gesundheitswesen bei Nullwachstum, WIDO, Bonn, pp 103–122
3. Gutzwiller F (ed) (1982) Gesundheit lehren, Manual. Sandoz, Basel
4. McKinlay JB (1972) Some approaches and problems in the use of services. J Health Soc Behav 13:128–132
5. Trojan A, Waller H (1980) Gemeindebezogene Gesundheitssicherung. Urban und Schwarzenberg, Munich Vienna
6. Troschke J von, Füller A (1981) Gesundheitswochen in Emmendingen. GESOMED Freiburg
7. Zola IK (1979) Gesundheitsmanie und entmündigende Medikalisierung. In: Illich I (ed) Entmündigung durch Experten. Rowohlt, Reinbek

A Model for Co-ordinated and Integrated Lifelong Health Security

F. Haux

When the efficiency and effectiveness of public health services are discussed, the established system of professional medical care is criticised. Innovative aims and new organisational structures in medical care are necessary if society wants to be able to meet the subjective and objective demands of today. The following examples show the urgent need for corrections. Surveys have proved that every other person in West Germany believes health to be most important, but only every fourth is willing to lead a healthy life. It is estimated that about 70% of all persons feeling ill prefer to avoid professional medical care and either help themselves or receive help from their relatives and other non-professionals. A further aspect is the current political and economic situation, which calls for a re-examination of the structure of expenditure for medical care totalling about 200 billion DM last year.

The Hypothesis

Effective and efficient health protection is only possible if a lifelong therapeutic strategy is established in which all the professions of the public health services participate, backed by lay helpers and self-help groups. The decisive share of the therapy must take place at home, carried out by family physicians, community nurses, social workers and self-help groups, with the active involvement of lay people. Especially today self-help is the most important element of modern therapy with regard to the increasing number of chronic illnesses. Self-help requires knowledge, understanding, experience and testing, and successful therapy calls for some major adjustments in the patient's way of life; these can only be achieved within the framework of a medical security system with out-patient and in-patient phases, in which the patient can be successfully motivated within his familiar social surroundings as well as in a learning- and self-oriented situation, e.g. when on a "Kur" (cure). The cure can only be the beginning of a lifelong therapy, which is only effective and economically justifiable if the subsequent out-patient phase secures the continued achievement of the therapeutic goals. The aim of lifelong therapy is an affirmative attitude towards a healthy life-style and a responsible patient, who knows that it is his own health he is aiming at. He should also know that even a perfectly operating health service

Primary Health Care in the Making
Ed. by U. Laaser, R. Senault, H. Viefhues

system cannot exclude the personal consequences of illness. He should be aware of the fact that he can only remain healthy if he understands the functioning and structure of his body and if he accepts that risk factors are the cause of acute and chronic illness and can be traced back to defective behaviour which can only be corrected by lifelong therapy based on self-help. Below a model for co-ordinated and integrated lifelong health security system is outlined.

The Model

The In-patient Phase

The in-patient phase – the cure – of this lifelong therapy takes place in the AOK-Kurklinik Pfaffenberg in Bad Sachsa; this is a health centre for preventive and rehabilitative medicine. Under the guidance of an internal chief physician, 102 patients insured by the AOK Niedersachsen (Public Health Insurance Company of Lower Saxony) are taken care of by doctors, nurses, social workers, masseurs, physical therapists and dieticians. The programme is especially designed for patients with risk factors.

The Therapeutic Possibilities on Offer

Besides providing adequate medical treatment, the therapeutic measures offered by the AOK-Kurklinik Pfaffenberg lie in the field of interventional psychological, pedagogic and social strategies; the services on offer cover the following elements.

1. Instructions to Self-help. This is the most important part of the therapy. It consists of physical training with general and specific gymnastics, affect management, techniques to control body functions, physical treatment, first aid, diet cooking etc.

2. Health Information. Knowledge and understanding are necessary for changes in behaviour. All members of the medical staff take part in daily 1-h round table sessions, informing the patients by means of various media about general and specific aspects of health.

3. Behavioural Therapy. By way of behavioural therapy and training, new patterns of behaviour are practised and tested.

4. Life-style Analysis and Life-style Guidance. Since most chronic diseases have multiple causes, it is necessary to view the entire human being, including his social surroundings. The data collected are most essential for the therapy as a whole, particularly for the change in behaviour.

5. Organisation and Guidance of Leisure-Time Activities. The growing qualitative and quantitative significance of free time requires that this time of day receives consideration. Leisure time during the cure is organised with the help and co-operation of the patients.

6. Medical Care. Medical diagnostics and therapy are accomodated to the Kurklinik. In co-operation with health care professionals, lifelong therapy is initiated.

Cure Procedure

In accordance with their physical state of being, the patients are divided into small groups which are guided by a therapist. Every patient performs his specific cure programme adjusted to his physical state. The cure procedure is made up of the following chronological phases of behaviour. The first phase requires the patient to forget the daily routine and concentrate on himself, the second phase involves exploring the therapeutic possibilities, the third phase stabilising the new patterns of behaviour and in the fourth phase every patient has to consider how he can establish this new life-style in his everyday life, especially with regard to the personal and structural conditions at home.

The Out-patient Phase

All the cognitive, affective and physical progress made during the in-patient phase and the resulting new life-style must now be transferred into everyday life. It stands to reason and is indispensable that the family physician continues the medical treatment at home and guarantees the success of a lifelong therapy.

Apart from the family physician, it is essential that community nurses, persons in charge of rehabilitation in the health insurance companies, and social workers take part in the therapy because they are acquainted with the patient's surroundings and his home.

Methodological Procedures

To secure the progress made during the cure it is necessary that the therapeutic measures are practicable at home in the everyday life and working situation of the patients and that the therapy at home takes up and continues most parts of the cure treatment. It is the aim of this out-patient phase to secure a permanent change in life-style. Out-patient care should include the following services:

1. General Post-cure Care. By way of meetings every patient should evaluate the out-patient phase. With the help of a health care team, every patient has to test the intended new life-style. It is important to stabilise the newly learned behaviour and to take advantage of newly developed self-confidence and vitality so that the patient continues to abstain from risk-taking behaviour during the out-patient phase without embarrassment.

2. Special Post-cure Case. If necessary, these special meetings should include those in the patient's immediate social environment, e.g. family members, relatives and social workers. It is the task of the interprofessional health care team to convince the family members and friends of the necessity of lifelong maintenance of the change in life-style.

3. Health Information. Health information can be part of the service mentioned above or can be offered by itself; it is a specific task of the physician.

4. Setting up of Self-help Groups. As soon as possible, self-help groups should be initiated. Later on the health care personnel may advise the established groups.

5. Provision of Social-Therapeutic Help. In special cases consultative or other institutions should be involved in this work.

Model Experience

The co-ordinated follow-up care by the family physician is being established in Lower Saxony in cooperation with the "Kassenärztliche Vereinigung" (State Association of Doctors) and the AOKs (Public Health Insurance Companies). In special meetings the interested physicians will be informed about the out–patient care of patients who have already been through the in-patient phase with its special programme. For 2 years there has been intensive co-operation with the social workers and the persons in charge of rehabilitation at the AOKs in Lower Saxony. Apart from personal care, information days and training for patients at risk are offered, self-help groups are advised or initiated and addresses of social aid authorities are provided. Another cooperative project between the Technical University of Braunschweig-Wolfenbüttel, the AOK-Kurklinik Pfaffenberg and the AOK Braunschweig was 4 months ago. Students try to build up post-cure groups for patients seeking social aid and contact, leisure time activities or health information; furthermore the students contact family members and friends in order to reinforce the progress made during the in-patient phase. Before starting the cure, the students inform the patients about the programme which is going to face them in the AOK-Kurklinik Pfaffenberg in Bad Sachsa and take part in several therapeutic measures during the cure, so that they become familiar with their clients. The resonance is surprisingly positive; on average more than 50% of the patients came to fortnightly meetings. The out-patient phase conducted by physicians, community nurses, social workers and clerks of the health insurance companies is supported by the local AOKs. Furthermore, the AOKs in Lower Saxony plan to employ a social worker in their insurance programme.

Community Prevention: The Program of the People's Medical Society

R. Rodale

My contention is that the present system for the prevention of disease is incomplete, and faulty. It is too small. It is considered less important than the cure system. It is not growing fast enough. And not enough people are involved in disease-prevention efforts in our communities.

Looking at the problem from a planning as well as an action perspective, there are two ways we can try to remedy that situation. One is to fine tune the present health system, adding prevention components wherever and whenever possible. The alternative is to take a "zero base" approach and plan the creation of an entirely new health system, in which prevention efforts would occupy an appropriate place.

I recommend that second strategy, and suggest that we begin to undertake it, knowing at first that it is an experiment in visionary thinking. Let's start by imagining that we are creating an entirely new health system in all respects. We have a good, well-functioning society that lacks only hospitals, doctors and other health professionals, and the makers of all the products and services now used by the health industry. What we do have, however, is all the knowledge and information about health and disease that is now a part of our health resource culture.

Looking at the role of human resources within the new system, we would begin with two assumptions. First, it is not our responsibility as planners to provide work for any professional group, or for any people, as a matter of fact. We are trying to deliver health, not income. Second, the new health system is to be regenerative, in the sense that its purpose is to cause health to spring from within people, using self-generated resources to the greatest extent possible.

Next, it would be an information-intensive system. Information is by far the most powerful tool to understand and create health. Our new system would provide much information about prevention, about self-care, and would furthermore use information to cause people to need curative procedures less. It is the procedures of cure that are expensive, cause people to lose their sense of self-reliance, and lead to iatrogenic problems.

The final planning element I suggest is that we be sure from the outset that in the new system, people should perceive a certain tension between the prevention system and the cure system. The two are not one and the same. Prevention comes first, and the cure part of the system is used only when the prevention part fails to accomplish its mission. That is perhaps the most important

Primary Health Care in the Making
Ed. by U. Laaser, R. Senault, H. Viefhues

thought that is needed to assure that prevention emerges from the shadows of "soft and less-important health strategies."

A few words about doctors. How will they feel about being a part of a system which places greater emphasis on a portion of the health art that they have historically relegated to a lesser role? It is important not to worry about that point. The doctors' position within even the present system is eroding. Consider the information function of doctors. There is now so much medical and health information that no doctor can know it all. No doctor can even know where all the health information is, what it can do, and why it is needed. In order to try to understand the uses of medical information, doctors have become specialists. They now know more about smaller and smaller parts of the whole structure of health. Doctors in each speciality look at health through the colored lens of their own particular discipline. But almost no doctors can now look at health in the white and true light that is complete vision.

That failure of members of the medical profession to have a complete view of health is particularly limiting in an information age. Access to information and use of information is now exploding. Lay people, who more often see health in white light, want a way of getting information that offers every element of possible use. I see the computer eventually becoming the tool to provide broad access to information in that way.

The People's Medical Society, which we have organized in the United States, has as its primary goal the use of health and medical information in the reorganization and reorientation of the entire health system. It is not anti-doctor. We know that doctors are needed, and will always be needed. But change in the role of the doctor that has already occurred will continue and accelerate. Our goal is to organize as lay people in ways that will cause that change to be as beneficial as possible – which means primarily that the system must move more in the direction of prevention. I feel that lay people, with their capacity to see health in terms of all its components, can and will be the catalyst to cause that change to happen.

There are two main elements to the program of the PMS. First, to increase the public's access to health/medical information. People need better access to their medical history, through their records. They need to know more about self-care and mutual aid. Iatrogenic problems need to be brought out of the shadows and be discussed and understood more clearly. Facts about medical performance should become more open. "What was my doctor taught?" "What does my doctor know?" These are questions people have a right to have answered, and they want the answers. The ever-higher cost of medicine, as well as our growing sense of social justice, entitles us to that information.

Then there is the activist part of the program of the People's Medical Society. We are using our growing grasp on the information resource to show that continued expansion of the professional and physical resources of the system is reaching the limits of sensible policy. Do we need more doctors and hospitals, or more extensive resources for catalyzing the prevention capacity that people have within themselves? I think the question almost answers itself.

Community prevention is the phrase we use to encompass the expansion of prevention activity that we visualize. What is provided to the public in a community prevention system is not the service of care, but the information that will enable people to understand how both individual acts and group decisions are influencing their health future in profound ways. All the standard and well-known elements that make up prevention are included, but they are taken far more seriously. Every possible strategy to give added importance and urgency to prevention is used.

We live today in a transition period between two health ages. In our past is the period when expansion of the cure system, and cure-oriented professions were seen as the primary object of health policy. In our future is the age of total and aggressive prevention.

Where does that leave us today? With organizations like the People's Medical Society, whose prime function is to awaken us to the change that is taking place. Our goal is to announce the need for every person, not just the professions steeped in traditional philosophies and technologies, to participate in the creation of a series of new and more efficient ways to create health.

The Role of Health Insurance Companies in Primary Prevention

P. Lemke and F. Pfirrmann

Taking into consideration the expansion of costs in the field of health and above all the increase in those chronic diseases caused by civilization that has occurred within the past decade (e.g. in cancer, cardiovascular diseases, psychic disorders and metabolic diseases), primary prevention has become of decisive importance. Accordingly, there is a broad social consensus that primary preventive health services should be built up, even if various political and institutional organizations working in the field have developed diverse strategies to deal with the health and social problems involved [1]. As 90% of the West German population are members or co-members of the sickness insurance schemes, the insurance companies take a special interest in developing concepts and strategies for improving preventive health care. The fact that health insurance companies are fully aware of their obligations is proved by the large number of activities which have led to the voluntary extension of primary preventive measures on offer, the centre of interest being the extension of information through media, special actions and exhibitions, lectures, courses etc. [2].

In spite of these very expensive and intensive measures, there has been little success in changing the attitude of the insured towards their own health. This relative failure is mainly due to the fact that a mere, quantitative extension of measures on offer cannot sufficiently increase people's interest in making use of these services.

Positive changes may be expected only if the preventive measures offered are much more closely adapted to the living and working conditions of the insured. This is especially true for those with a lower social status who are exposed to disadvantageous working conditions, often accompanied by unhealthy living and leisure conditions. Such conditions result in manifeold strain for these social groups, while on the other hand subjective and objective social barriers prevent them from making use of the services offered [3] (see Fig. 1).

An essential measure which might contribute to the removal of such barriers for the insured living in unsatisfactory "Lebenslagen" [4] are preventive strategies concentrating on communities and urban districts. This would mean that spatial distance – a conclusive factor in preventing people from making use of the services offered – could be overcome, as these social groups are more intensively tied to their immediate environments. This is especially true for the population of cities.

First results confirm that these facts, proved by sociological research programmes conducted in various regions, are relevant with regard to primary pre-

Primary Health Care in the Making
Ed. by U. Laaser, R. Senault, H. Viefhues

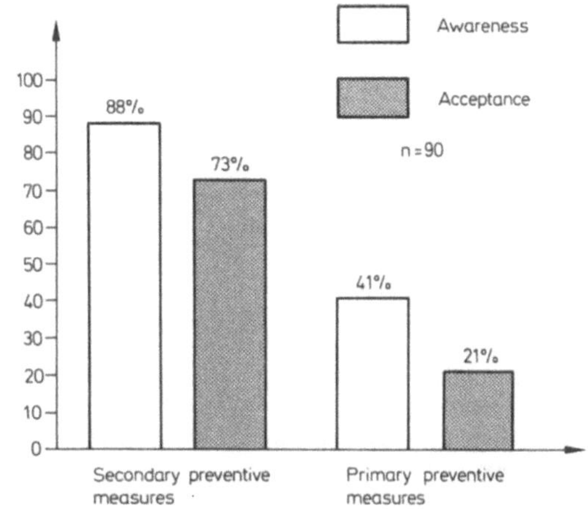

Fig. 1. Awareness and acceptance of primary preventive measures

vention. Thus 79% of people interrogated within the framework of the research project "Primary Prevention Measures by Health Services in Communities and Urban Districts" (Supported by the Bundesministerium für Arbeit und Sozialordnung) would more probably make use of primary preventive measures offered by health insurance companies if these offers were made in the neighbourhood of their homes. As a consequence, health insurance companies should avail themselves to a greater extent than hitherto of the existing decentralized organizational structures in the local areas to develop actions and measures suited to urban districts and adapt them to the specific needs of the residents in order to open up new methods of distribution and thus reduce the social selection that occurs with regard to primary preventive health services.

It will be necessary to replace the prevailing passive services by active strategies [6] in such a way that health services strongly intensify contacts with their insured. Such a modification of past strategies along these lines requires the development of personal and social alternatives at the community level. Most important would seem the development of programmes focussing on essential problems, as the measures developed by health insurance companies frequently do not correspond to the interests of their members (see Table 1). The quite considerable divergencies between those questions of health in which the insured are interested and the information offered by health insurance companies can only be overcome if the local health insurance office draws up statistics on illness which make possible insights into correlations between health disorders, working conditions, environmental factors of the district etc. and then develop specific primary preventive programmes giving special consideration to the health risks specific to certain social strata.

Moreover, it will be necessary to motivate the insured to take an active interest in these measures even at the time of planning. This can only be done effectively if the health insurance companies are ready to take up new methods of health education and health information.

Activities aimed beyond an essentially *behaviour-oriented prevention* have recently been implemented by some health insurance companies – above all

Table 1. Area of primary prevention requiring attention, in the order of importance, assessed on the basis of the responses of members of health insurance companies ($n=167$) (multiple responses possible)

Area[a]	No. of times cited
1. Alcohol and drug problems	36
2. Healthy nutrition	35
3. *Environmental problems*	30
4. *Psychic health*	27
5. Action and sports	23
6. Prevention in children	17
7. *Home and health*	16
8. *Self-help groups in the field of primary prevention*	15
9. Smoking and health	15
10. High blood pressure, diabetes mellitus	13
11. Problems of the disabled	10
12. Others	3

[a] The underlined topics have not been covered by the health insurance companies, although participants found them to be important

the Allgemeine Ortskrankenkassen (AOK). The results of these activities have not yet been evaluated; nevertheless, it is already obvious that they have had some positive results. By including the personal experience of the population concerned and discussing with them the strain resulting from working and living conditions, the companies were able to improve the utilization of their services, especially by the population in lower *social strata.*

These results have been confirmed to a certain extent by Anglo-American research groups; their findings are not, of course, completely comparable with German findings owing to the different organization of the health systems. On the whole, however, the agreement between the findings makes it seem likely that health services will be able to motivate the insured with regard to primary preventive health care if they succeed in extending the initial steps taken and forego the traditional concepts of health education. In contrast to pedagogic attempts based on the behaviour-oriented prevention concepts [7, 8], which in practice have proved insufficient, a procedure seems advisable which identifies and discusses factors detrimental to the health of different social groups at their place of work, their homes and during their leisure time; an analysis of the complex interactions as well as the inclusion of personal and social coping strategies is also required [9, 10, Lemke 1983, Die Bedeutung des Konzepts der "sozialen Prävention" für die Gesundheitssicherung von Bevölkerungsgruppen in unterschiedlichen Lebenslagen, unpublished). This kind of *condition-oriented policy of primary preventive health care* by health insurance companies must include problem selection as well as the ensuing strategies of problem solving; the efficiency of the measures applied will also have to be evaluted. Moreover, it seems necessary to carry through follow-up studies in order to check the stability of behavioural changes.

In order to develop practicable approaches, i.e. approaches which consider the needs of the insured, the autonomy of the local offices of health insurances must be increased and these bodies must endeavour to improve co-operation with other relevant local institutions. In this way, better and more extensive knowledge of those situations and conditions detrimental to health could be acquired by health insurance companies, which would serve to ensure more effective co-ordination of preventive measures at the community level [11].

Only if health insurance companies are ready to take up the initiative in these matters will they meet their obligation to contribute to the creation of healthy living and working conditions. By changing from being institutions of health administration to being institutions of health care, health insurance companies will be able to take care of the interests of the population in preventive health care and health maintenance.

References

1. Hofmann K, Huster E (1979) Präventive Sozialpolitik: Ideologie und Realität. Wirtschafts- und Sozialwissenschaftliches Institut des deutschen Gewerkschaftsbundes, Cologne (WSI-Mitteilungen 10/1979)
2. Großjohann K, Neuhaus R (1979) Die Rolle der Krankenversicherung in der präventiven Gesundheitspolitik. Gesellschaft für sozialen Fortschritt, Bonn
3. Hauß F, et al. (n.d.) Schichtspezifische Versorgungsprobleme und leistungssteuernde Strukturpolitik im Gesundheitswesen. In: Hauß F, et al. (ed) Schichtspezifische Versorgungsprobleme in der Bundesrepublik. Bundesministerium für Arbeit und Sozialordnung, Bonn (Forschungsbericht, vol 55)
4. Nahnsen I (1975) Bemerkungen zum Begriff und zur Geschichte des Arbeitsschutzes. In: Osterland M (ed) Arbeitssituation, Lebenslage und Konfliktpotential. Frankfurt
5. Müller R (1978) Lebenslage als Ziel der Politik. In: Präventive Sozialpolitik. Wirtschafts- und Sozialwissenschaftliches Institut des deutschen Gewerkschaftsbundes, Cologne (WSI-Mitteilungen 10)
6. Ferber C van (1979) Soziale Distanz zwischen Versicherten und Krankenkassen – Möglichkeiten der Gesundheitsvorsorge im Rahmen der Krankenversicherung. In: WIAD (ed) Gesundheitsvorsorge und Krankheitsfrüherkennung. Wissenschaftliches Institut der Ortskrankenkassen, Bonn
7. Freudenberg N (1981) Die Rolle der Gesundheitserziehung bei der Veränderung des sozialen Umfeldes. Int J Gesundheitserz 24/3
8. Troschke J von (1983) Präventive Gemeindestudien in der Bundesrepublik Deutschland. Dtsch Ärztebl 42
9. Jürgens U, Dohse H, Russig H (1980) Die präventive Wendung der staatlichen Sozialpolitik, Formen des Unterlaufens und der Verkehrung auf Betriebsebene. In: Grottian P (ed) Folgen reduzierten Wachstums für Politikfelder. Politische Vierteljahresschrift [Sonderheft] 19
10. Vobruba G (1983) Prävention durch Selbstkontrolle. In: Wambach M (ed) Der Mensch als Risiko. Frankfurt
11. Lemke P (1983) Bewohnerorientierte primäre Prävention durch Krankenkassen. In: Gesundheitserziehung durch Krankenkassen. Tagungsbericht der Bundeszentrale für gesundheitliche Aufklärung (BzGa), Cologne

Health Work in a Working-Class District of Mannheim

K. Becker and B. Laugsch

"... listening to a passer-by, who talks about our health and gives good advice, without knowing anything about us ..." (Sibilla Aleramo)

"... four weeks ago a self-help group for the unemployed came together. Unemployed, you know, are people who have problems and like many others cannot go to someone and say: 'Listen, I'm frightened, I have stomach ache, I cannot sleep. Tomorrow I have to go to the employment office, I am totally down, I can't face going there again ...'. One cannot go to anyone and say: 'I am unemployment sick'. The least reaction would be a shrugging of shoulders. ...
... what I wanted to say here is: an unemployed person can only be understood by another unemployed person." (Round table discussion, broadcast from the *Gesundheitstreffpunkt* by *Südwestfunk*, May 1983).

Background Considerations

What we are trying to do is to vitalize concepts like "lay involvement", "health promotion" and "community participation". Scientists and experts use these terms when discussing new approaches to health education, but all too often these discussions take place far away from the conditions in question, and usually they do not progress beyond the stage of making declarations.

We want to make a serious attempt to withdraw from this type of "expert knowledge" and turn instead towards a broader concept of health, starting from where behaviour (including at-risk behaviour) has its origins, in the area of social interaction as perceived by the individual. Our task is primarily to create a climate where people can become more aware and agree to undertake common action aimed at influencing these restrictions.

Our central term is "everyday life". For about 18 months we have been collecting the demands, ideas and wishes of people in a working-class district of Mannheim, and holding common discussions on how to take action. Through organizational work in the community and community-related media work, we support and induce the growth of self-help groups, new social networks and social action in the district.

"Ausgangspunkt der Überlegungen und Gegenstand der professionellen Aktionen ist das Gemeinwesen als politisch-ökologischer Raum. Dieser kann betrachtet werden als relativ selbständiges sozial-räumliches Gebilde, dessen Be-

Primary Health Care in the Making
Ed. by U. Laaser, R. Senault, H. Viefhues

wohner eine Anzahl von Lebensbedingungen gemeinsam unterworfen sind und sowohl von 'außen' als auch von 'innen' als relative Einheit identifiziert werden. Letzteres impliziert – wie gebrochen auch immer – eine Identifikation der Einwohner mit 'ihrem' Raum."[1]

Health in this context is understood as

- a part of the living conditions in the area concerned
- an indirect goal, which is approached by overcoming personal restrictions and extending room for action, leading to
- a process of emancipation and not of domestication (Paulo Freire).

Some Facts About Neckarstadt-West

Neckarstadt-West, situated at the perimeter of the city, is an old traditional working-class district. Gradual industrialization around the port of the Neckar at the turn of the century changed the population structure from one of gardeners and tradesmen to workers. War destruction and declining population density, primarily caused by the departure of young families to more prosperous areas, resulted in an overrespresentation of foreigners. Also the proportion of elderly people is higher than in other districts. According to the categories of town planners and social administrators, Neckarstadt is known as an "island of backwardness" and is in their view the most deficient part of the city.

Other relevant information about Neckarstadt-West is that:

- The infrastructure of services is insufficient for infants, adolescents and old people.
- Frequent inversion of the local weather leads to a high level of pollution, which is worsened by the great heat output in the area.
- Official demands for structural improvement in the Neckarstadt aim mainly at
  - changing the microclimate by introducing green areas
  - creating new public spaces
  - improving housing conditions
  - traffic-free locations for children, playgrounds

The sanitary measures undertaken so far by the city of Mannheim have not been without problems. One result was a rise in rents which the majority of inhabitants could not afford; this led to a widespread initiative against total and compulsory sanitation.

Even today, Neckarstadt-West still has many independent craftsmen, tradesmen, small shops and popular pubs. These pubs constitute a meeting point, especially for young foreigners. Hence many conflicts between foreigners and the

---

[1] The starting point of the reflections and object of professional action is the community as a political and ecological area. It can be understood as a relatively self-sufficient social unit, whose inhabitants share common experiences and life conditions, and are identified as a relatively homogeneous unit both from "without" and from "within". This implies – at least to some extent – an identification of the inhabitants with their area

original inhabitants take place. In spite of all this, many local clubs are still active and the inhabitants have retained their political working class ideals.

How We Started

We did not enter completely unknown territory in Neckarstadt-West. Some contacts to so-called important persons had been established in advance. In the beginning we wandered through the area for several weeks to gather impressions and talked to already established groups and initiatives, trying to familiarize ourselves with the quarter. In addition, we worked through official statistics and materials and looked for rooms suitable for self-help groups as well as for larger meetings.

We found a former shop near the "Mannheimer Motorenwerke", one of the big machinery factories in Mannheim, and contacted our immediate neighbours in the street. The same problems were named by all: noise, air pollution, general neglect of the quarter, almost no parks, the small number of playgrounds, problems with the housing programme of the city of Mannheim, the increasing number of immigrant workers – always the same problems.

However, we also enquired after people's personal living situations and their understanding of health, especially among those who came to our rooms during the first month. We offered some rooms and advice for the establishment of self-help groups and lay initiatives, and we used posters, handouts and public discussions to try to give people an idea of what could happen in the *"Gesundheitstreffpunkt"*.

During this first year we more or less concentrated on the work with self-help groups within our rooms, trying to build up contacts and connections with our local environment. Here an important help was our local health monthly, "Wurzelwerk", which could be printed and distributed at no cost.

Wurzelwerk

This quarter-related health monthly is an attempt to approach people, adhering to the concepts of the *"Gesundheitstreffpunkt"* and applying the principles of its work.

This means opening the monthly to all topics which are raised by people, exceeding by far the limits of classical health education. Our philosophy is to approach people in connection with their perceived needs, that is to say: everyday life should be the key theme in this paper. The goal is to identify common aspects of individual problems and to enhance social activation through their recognition.

The paper provides the people of Neckarstadt-West with:

- Information about what is happening in their area
- The experience of not being isolated with regard to personal problems

- The possibility of going beyond the private sphere and of solving common problems together.

Work in the *"Gesundheitstreffpunkt"* benefits from

- Regular presentation of all activities
- An additional opportunity for groups and initiatives to advertise and present their aims, views etc.
- A forum which reaches relevant persons of public life beyond the limits of Neckarstadt, thereby supporting the "Gesundheitstreffpunkt" by increasing general acceptance of it.

Steps Already Taken

With a Christmas action in December 1982 the *"Gesundheitstreffpunkt"* and *"Wurzelwerk"* organized their first common measure: on Christmas eve guest families were to be found for all people living alone in Neckarstadt and meetings within the city of Mannheim were to be presented. After a public advertising campaign we established a telephone service and, together with the members of self-help groups, organized an "open night" for "the people in the street". After this experience some people started an initiative to organize a weekly "Teestube" (tearoom) on Saturday afternoons. This initiative developed into a means for establishing far-reaching contacts that also involved Turkish and other foreign citizens of Neckarstadt.

Our experience with the "Christmas eve action" motivated us to move from the *Treffpunkt* rooms to the quarter in general. Together with some inhabitants of Neckarstadt and interested groups, initiatives and members of political parties, we established a working group for Neckarstadt which deals with three problems:

- Introducing greenery to public places and backyards
- Improving the playground situation
- Establishing a traffic-free area in Neckarstadt

The ideas of the working group have been brought to the attention of the public by *"Wurzelwerk"* and through public activities (street festivals, street interviews etc.). Subsequently, other groups in the area became interested in organizing related activities: e.g. a group of the "Grey Panthers" has been established, as has a women's network and a language group for Turkish women. Together with a traditional youth centre (Erlenhof), we are preparing an exhibition "Working Days" which will include a 2-week programme based around the exhibition and involves official and informal organizations and groups.

Conclusion

- In spite of our attempts not to present ourselves as experts, to create closeness and to work in a catalytic manner – in spite of all this goodwill, our relations with the inhabitants of the quarter are asymmetrical. Our salaried empathy meets their "indigence".

- In our working situation we mostly meet people during their leisure time, which determines a priori a different orientation and limitation of action. As paid actors we expect similar but unpaid motivation and involvement from the people concerned.
- The declared readiness to become really involved with the daily life of people is limited by the dependency of professionals. The expert involved comes to sit between all sorts of stools if he really wants to work "on the other side".
- The attempt to create conditions for symmetrical communication requires a "demystification of institutional mysteries" [8]. This means that our own dependency has to become transparent when we communicate with people.

References

1. Alinsky S (1973) Leidenschaft für den Nächsten. Burkhardthaus, Gelnhausen
2. Bahr, Gronemeyer (ed) (1974) Konfliktorientierte Gemeinwesenarbeit. Luchterhand, Neuwied
3. Barabas, Blanke, Sachsse, Stascheit (1975) Jahrbuch der Sozialarbeit 1976. Rowohlt, Reinbek
4. Barabas, Blanke, Sachsse, Stascheit (1977) Jahrbuch der Sozialarbeit 1978. Rowohlt, Reinbek
5. Betrifft: Erziehung; Die Methoden, Paulo Freire, Heft 7, 1973
6. Betrifft: Erziehung; Sonderdruck Nr. 4, Aktionsforschung, Weinheim 1976
7. Beier, Horn (1980) Gesundheitsverhalten und Krankheitsgewinn: Europäische Monographien zur Gesundheitserziehung, vol 2
8. Boulet, Krauss, Oelschlegel (1980) Gemeinwesenarbeit, Bielefeld
9. Freire P (1971) Pädagogik der Unterdrückten. Stuttgart
10. Freire P (1975) Erziehung als Praxis der Freiheit. Stuttgart
11. Gronemeyer M (1976) Motivation und politisches Handeln. Hamburg
12. Gronemeyer, Bahr (1977) Nachbarschaft im Neubaublock. Weinheim
13. Habermas J (1974) Können komplexe Gesellschaften eine vernünftige Identität ausbilden? Frankfurt
14. Haug F (1972) Kritik der Rollentheorie. Frankfurt
15. Karras, Hinte (1978) Grundprogramm Gemeinwesenarbeit. Wuppertal
16. Oelschlegel D (1978) Gemeinwesenarbeit als Prinzip sozialer Arbeit, in: Rundbrief 2, 1978
17. Seippel A (1976) Handbuch: Aktivierende Gemeinwesenarbeit. Gelnhausen

Health Promotion in A Large City

S. Panico, R. Landolfi, and L. Minelli

A large amount of knowledge in favour of health promotion is available. Improvement of both the quality of life and life expectancy are probably dependent on health promotion programmes. Individual and community participation has been recognized as being a prerequisite for the credibility, feasibility and success of these programmes. A life-style approach has emerged as a key component of health promotion programmes, and in the last few years extensive debate has provided diffuse support for this concept.

However, health promotion is difficult. Health and social service organization and community socio-economic features affect the feasibility and the success of health promotion programmes. Methods of elaborating and making these programmes work are needed.

In recent years attention has been paid to the Italian health system because of some peculiar characteristics:

a) It is based on Local Health Units (LHUs), which are geographically defined and cover from about 30 000 to 150 000 inhabitants;
b) LHUs are aggregates of municipalities or of city quarters (in Italy social services are managed by municipalities or city quarters – this favours integration between social and health services and allows for local intersectorial intervention);
c) LHUs are locally governed;
d) Participation of users in governing the LHUs and elaborating and controlling programmes is legitimized by law.

This system appears to favour health promotion programmes which may be locally formulated, organized and developed. However, there is a national tendency to cut social costs, thus affecting negatively intersectorial programmes which are essential to improve programme effectiveness. Furthermore, an unfavourable diffuse health professional attitude and culture – founded on the privilege of specific "technicism" and high technology – often makes it difficult to appreciate people's needs in terms of understanding and participating in decisions that affect their own bodies and everyday lives. These features are particularly negative for health promotion programmes in big cities and even more so in those characterized by depressed socio-economic conditions. Therefore it is a major challenge to promote action to develop health promotion programmes in such places; but it seems necessary for at least the following reasons:

Primary Health Care in the Making
Ed. by U. Laaser, R. Senault, H. Viefhues

- To improve the health conditions of large numbers of people
- To detect the key difficulties in order to find some clues on how to promote health
- To find original ways of stimulating community participation
- To determine the development of life-styles conducive to health

A specific action-research project is being commenced in Naples, the biggest city of the southern part of Italy, in order to implement health promotion programmes based on active community participation and oriented towards a life-style approach. Naples is a city of 1 200 000 inhabitants where one-third of the active population is unemployed or misemployed, where traditionally the welfare state has worked little and very badly; where there are low standards of health services in general and low levels of accessibility to them, where social tensions are very severe and condition everyday life, where the uneven distribution of resources is evident, and where poverty is the rule. Some other features can also be listed:

- Low average income
- Low standards of economic development
- High population density
- High level of promiscuity
- High level of infant mortality
- High level of certain infectious diseases
- 70 000 people relying on cigarette smuggling

Over the last 15 years the history of Naples has been characterized by active movements for health involving several health professionals and a large number of people. Before the new health system started, in the early 1970s several "people's health centres" were founded and many of them made a contribution to the development of community participation methods. In the last few years the interest of many health professionals and of active social groups has been concentrated on applying and experimenting with these methods diffusely in the health and social services.

The action-research project will be the local project for a large LHU in the city of Naples, including two quarters of the city with about 150 000 inhabitants.

People actually working in the health and social services in the area will be directly involved in the project, together with volunteers active in the community. Action will be directed towards forming a network of activities relating to different social and health problems (drug addiction in youth, isolation of the elderly, users' rights movements and so on).

The main objectives of the project will be:

a) Organization of districts (they are subunits of the LHU, with a population of about 30 000, aggregated according to some criteria such as the transport system in the area or some homogeneous features of several blocks).
b) Organization of work according to programmes elaborated in a participatory planning process, of which the major agents of change are:
   - Individual or associated users
   - Health and social workers

   - Active social organizations
   - LHU elected authority
c) Organization of work according to group work and multidisciplinary action.
d) Matching priorities resulting from the actual activities in the community.
e) Identification of new methodological aspects of the evaluation process with special respect to:
   - Access of individuals and groups to places or occasions where their needs can be expressed
   - Compliance of professionals with the rules of the participatory planning process
   - Critical use of techniques (epidemiological, phenomenological etc.)
   - Overall involvement of the community, intended as dialectic confrontation between its agents of change as defined above
f) Integration between the social and health services.
g) Action to implement an echological idea of health problems, based on the cultural and professional development of the life-style approach.

The project will consist of three phases:

The *first phase* will be characterized by the education and self-education of people to be involved in the project with respect to the spirit, the objectives and the methodology of the work.

The *second phase* will be characterized firstly by the analysis of the community through statistical, demographic and ad hoc data. Strategies to give people opportunities to express their own needs will be formulated in this phase, together with methodologies capable of weighting the complexity of people's needs.

In the *third phase* local health promotion programmes will be formulated. They will be oriented towards the described participatory planning process and inspired by the life-style approach.

The practical, cultural and scientific products of this action-research project in Naples will hopefully be of help to all health promotion programmes, especially those attempted in cities, where the way of life is more detrimental to health.

Lay Involvement in the Primary Prevention of Cardiovascular Disease: The Rhein-Neckar Community Study (GRN)

U. Laaser (for the project-group)

Historical Background

Since the earliest beginnings of medicine, prevention has always been the more logical and more effective approach to maintaining health and reducing the burden of disease. Nonetheless, cure forever seems to occupy pride of place in terms of social acknowledgement and resource allocation. This attitude is perilous in an epoch in which early precursors often determine the irreversible late stages of chronic disease.

For cardiovascular disease and to some degree for certain malignancies, such precursors, in the form of risk factors that at least in part play a causal role, have been identified with the help of classical epidemiological methods in a complex staged research process. However, two problems remained unsolved:

1. Many, if not all, risk factors for chronic disease relate to at-risk behaviour, which is embedded in the complex procedural patterns of daily life. What determines the formation of these patterns has so far remained obscure, but there is likely to be a strong local or cultural influence, often vaguely summarized as life-style.
2. Traditional cognitive health education succeeded only to a very limited degree in its attempt to influence at-risk behaviour, especially in disadvantaged social groups whose living conditions restrict quite rigidly the scope for behavioural adaptation. The social gradients for many indicators of health in essence remained unchanged [1]. Meanwhile what enables and motivates people to change their way of life in a way that favours disease prevention became a central issue.

Whereas the first of these two open questions led to intensified research into the so-called psychosocial determinants of health, the second created two different developments, both based upon the notion that the healthier choice has to be made the easier choice in order to attain population-wide attraction:

a) The *'provider approach'*: This approach involves the improved and co-ordinated delivery of information and skills by the preventive services, relying predominantly on professional expertise in an attempt to remove barriers to utilization.
b) The *'consumer approach'*: This approach involves the identification of perceived health needs by concerned individuals or population groups and the

Primary Health Care in the Making
Ed. by U. Laaser, R. Senault, H. Viefhues

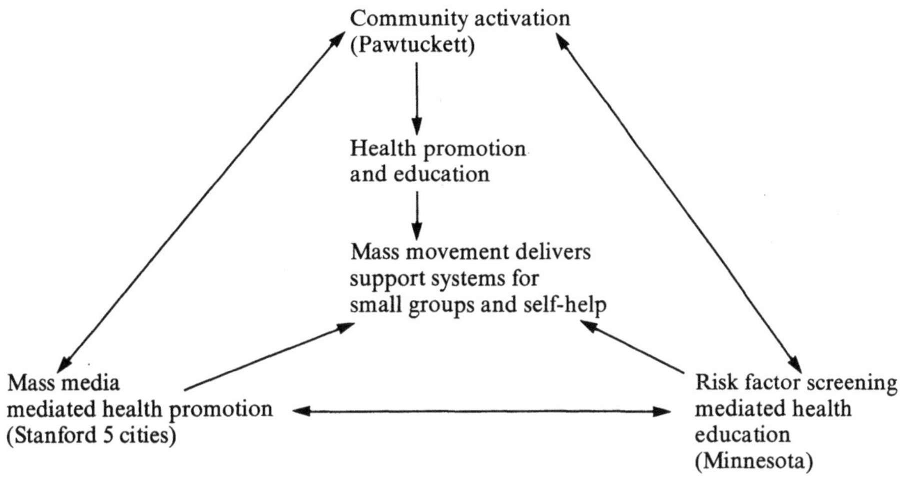

Fig. 1. Community intervention studies in the united states evaluated for a reduction of cardiovascular disease (acc. to R. Carleton/Pawtucket, Rhode Island)

pursuit of improvement through broad lay involvement, utilizing expertise only in a supportive, not in a directive, way.

The German Cardiovascular Prevention Study (DHP) [2] is the first intervention study which

- integrates both of the aforementioned approaches towards a community-wide modification of life-style,
- covers an unselected, predominantly metropolitan population of about 1 million (a population typical for the FRG),
- monitors the disease end-points in reference to the total FRG, and thus
- intends to provide a national model.

The DHP may be called a second-generation study as compared with the first project of this kind in North Karelia, Finland [3] and to three American community studies of the National Institutes of Health (Fig. 1); of these three studies, that in Stanford predominantly emphasizes a mass media strategy (based on the social learning theory of Bandura), that in Minnesota a mass screening programme (linked to the medical health belief model) and that in Pawtucket community activation work (referring to models of social change). None of these includes central urban populations; rather all compare smaller communities or suburban areas in quasi-controlled designs.

The Rhein-Neckar Community Study (GRN) Group is responsible for one of four fully monitored (i.e. including the determination of disease outcome and mortality) DHP intervention areas, namely the towns of Mannheim (310 000 inhabitants) and Weinheim (45 000) in the Rhein-Neckar region[1] (Berlin-Spandau, Bremen-Nord and the rural area of Traunstein in Bavaria being the others).

[1] Meanwhile for the main study (1984–1991) Mannheim and Weinheim have been replaced by corresponding quarters of Stuttgart

During a pilot phase (1982–1983) it was one of the main objectives of the GRN to develop an effective strategy for broad lay involvement in accordance with the declaration of Alma Ata (1978) on the strengthening of participatory elements in primary health care (PHC), taking into account the conditions in the FRG. In the main study phase (1984–1991) the Community Participation Model as developed in the GRN will be supported by an externally directed, community-centred campaign covering all the basic functions of society which are relevant to health (services and facilities, work, education, recreation, family and neighbourhood) by special programmes aiming at mutually reinforcing effects upon cardiovascular morbidity [see elsewhere 2].

The Role of Lay Involvement

So far, population-wide cardiovascular prevention studies have yielded ambiguous results, e.g.:

- The reduction of specific mortality in North Karelia [3] was accompanied by an almost similar reduction in the neighbouring reference area of Kuopio (5-year results).
- The overall reduction in mortality achieved in the European Multifactorial Risk Prevention Trial [4] was statistically inconclusive, and in one of the participating countries (England) even negative.
- The achieved risk factor reduction in almost all studies ending in the 1980s was below target level [4, 5].
- The use of drugs in primary prevention, i.e. for risk factor reduction, was associated with increased risks in subgroups [5, 6].

These results support stronger lay involvement in the decision-making processes in community-wide prevention programmes on ethical grounds (even if such programmes concern only health education) [4]; however, the limited success of all educational efforts as regards lasting risk reductions points also to an important motivational deficiency of the programmes that has restricted their approach to positive or negative recommendations regarding certain medically defined behaviour without considering subjective expectations or interest and the social context. A third argument relates to the limited capacity of the available services and professionals if primordial prevention, i.e. prevention in the total still healthy population, is taken into consideration.

Therefore in September 1981 the First Conference of European Ministers responsible for Public Health discussed "a European approach to health promotion". In the same year the WHO European Regional Committee 31 approved a Regional Programme on Health Education and Lifestyles. In 1982 the Regional Committee 32 accepted a Regional Programme on Health Promotion for the Seventh General Programme of Work. Several member states have begun to run explicit health promotion programmes. In general, the movement for promoting healthy life-styles has taken a social rather than a medical form, often without the active encouragement of governments and health professionals. On the contrary, the potential for developing health seems to lie to a considerable extent with the public and its expectations of, and demand for, better health and improved quality of life [7].

In the Federal Republic of Germany lay involvement has taken two channels:

a) Training of lay volunteers under professional direction in order to increase the limited capacity of the health care system, especially in the area of preventive services (development of curricula for 'lay experts').
b) Involvement of lay people under their own direction in self-help or mutual aid groups formed around problems of personal subjective concern.

Both categories of lay involvement may be differentiated:

1. By their organizational structure:
   a) Rather vertical for lay experts in voluntary organizations built around a specific problem/disease
   b) Rather horizontal for self-help groups and lay initiatives, organizing themselfes as regional working communities based on their common approach of mutual aid irrespective of the group-specific subject.
2. By the condition of *'Selbstbetroffenheit'* (self-concern) which does not apply to professional and only slightly to lay experts but which creates the unique motivation of a broad population based movement ('collective' self-help) [8].

The old as well as the new federal administration welcomed the apparently growing readiness of concerned people to engage themselves in self-help activities, for the area of preventive research the following quote [9] is probably the most relevant:

> The State or anonymous organizations must not take away self-determined and self-responsible activity from the individual and his family, especially with regard to health and disease. However, state and society for their part have the duty to guarantee the necessary framework for such activity. The capabilities of the single individual would be overtaxed if he had to maintain living conditions conducive to health, render possible effective treatment and secure financially reasonable protection against the economic and social consequences of disease. Only the balanced interplay of subsidies, solidarity and self-help provides the foundation for coping successfully with the problems at present and in the future. The contribution of research is mandatory in order to reflect what is medically essential, to strive more intensively for primary prevention and preventive health protection and to accentuate self-help and strengthen effective and responsible self-administration.

Self-help and Primary Prevention

Usually the limiting factor in prevention studies is not insufficient provision of relevant information and skills but the limited acceptance of the message in terms of (a) the number of persons changing their actual behaviour and (b) the degree of change they can or will effect. By contrast with curative medicine and rehabilitation, in prevention one cannot direct the message to a sick and therefore concerned individual. In fact the more primordial the character of the programme, i.e. the healthier the target group, the more difficult it is to find accessible individual interfaces for the promotion of life-style changes, because the determinants and living conditions underpinning at-risk behaviour relate to groups, not individuals. This is the background for the recent ecological concept of 'education for health' [10] and the high priority given to the self-help and mutual aid approach in the German Cardiovascular Prevention Study [2] (in addition to mass media campaigns and the improvement of preventive services/facilities), because this study is devoted to primary prevention in an almost healthy population and less to secondary prevention, based on screening procedures and early detection.

However, perceived needs or issues do not always relate directly to specific at-risk behaviour (indeed, they may rarely do so), i.e. the priority ranking of people is often different from a scientifically based expert ranking. This leads to the concept of *'general prevention'* as distinct from 'medical prevention'. In the area of cardiovascular disease prevention the latter means the transfer of information and skills related to the medically and epidemiologically defined risk factors and associated at-risk behaviour, whereas general prevention means the development of general social competence to equip, qualify and "encourage people to make decisions for themselves" [11] so that they do not simply accept/obey expertise but learn how to use this resource responsibly and effectively.

The concept of general prevention mediating skills for the improvement of social competence may be structured further by the identification and monitoring of psychosocial factors, understood, for example, by the group of Theorell [12] as being 'everything between the immediate environment and the individual mental constitution'. Another related concept is that of *'social coping'* and distinct from the classical coping concept aimed at individual adaptation to straining conditions [13]. Social coping refers to an attempt to reduce strain by the removal or modification of stressful conditions. If measures towards that end are successfully taken – usually not on an individual basis – we are witnessing a 'social coping process'. A community centred prevention programme might also be seen as a social coping process directed at impaired health.

Figure 2 delineates the complex hypothetical connections between cardiovascular disease, risk factors, at-risk modes of behaviour and their psychosocial determinants. The psychosocial dimensions most relevant to cardiovascular prevention might be:

- The gaining of social competence to make autonomous decisions and to increase decision latitude [14–16], e.g. in a social coping process.
- The rebuilding the social network with special reference to life events (uncompensated breakdown of the social network) [19] and learned helplessness [7, p. 5]. In the latter area the mutual aid approach conceivably tends to decrease learned helplessness, i.e. the dependency on the social network, and at the same time increases the stability and the outreach of thc social network.
- The development of social support as a result of the competent use of social networks [17–19].

All of these are relevant indicators for health promotion, related to cardiovascular disease [14–19] either directly or indirectly by strengthening the coping capability of individuals, groups and neighbourhoods (geographically or sociologically defined). Such is the structure required to operationalize the life-

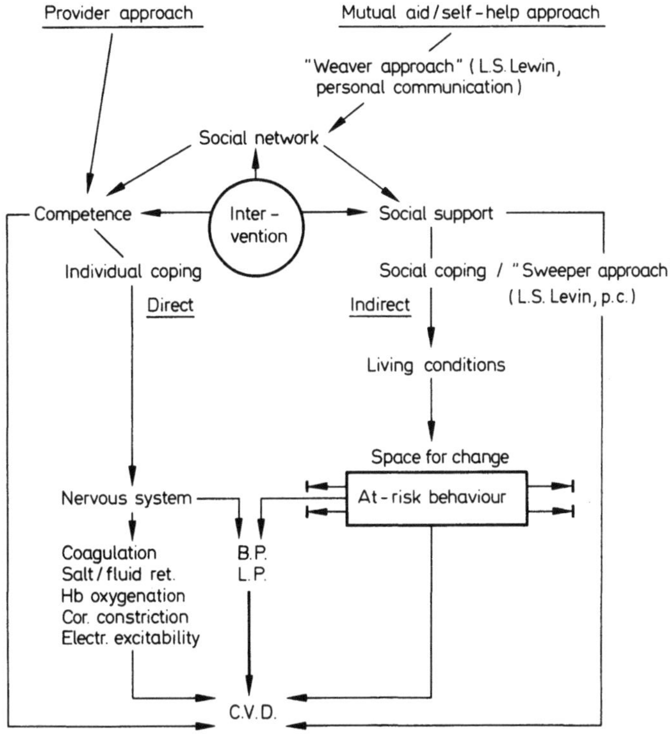

Fig. 2. Psychosocial factors and the prevention of cardiovascular disease (C.V.D.). *B.P.*, blood pressure; *L.P.*, lipoproteins

style concept as adopted by WHO for the European region: "Lifestyles are patterns of choices made from the alternatives that are available to people according to their socio-economic circumstances and to the ease with which they are able to choose certain ones over others" [7, p. 5].

Participatory Structures in the Community

The described approach – to start out at the perceived health issues of the addressees in order to support them in gaining competence for and interest in their own health and its determinants – seems especially relevant to disadvantaged (= less organized) target populations, where the effect of health messages is conditional upon the growth of a social infrastructure. As early as the last century Virchow (cited according to 20), when investigating the typhoid epidemic in Lower Silesia, surprisingly did not draw attention to a lack of knowledge or willingness of the people regarding their health but blamed the Prussian state for the great poverty, oppression and incapacitation of the Polish population.

With this in mind, two settings were chosen in the Rhein-Neckarregion to test to what extent participatory structures could be implemented: Neckarstadt-

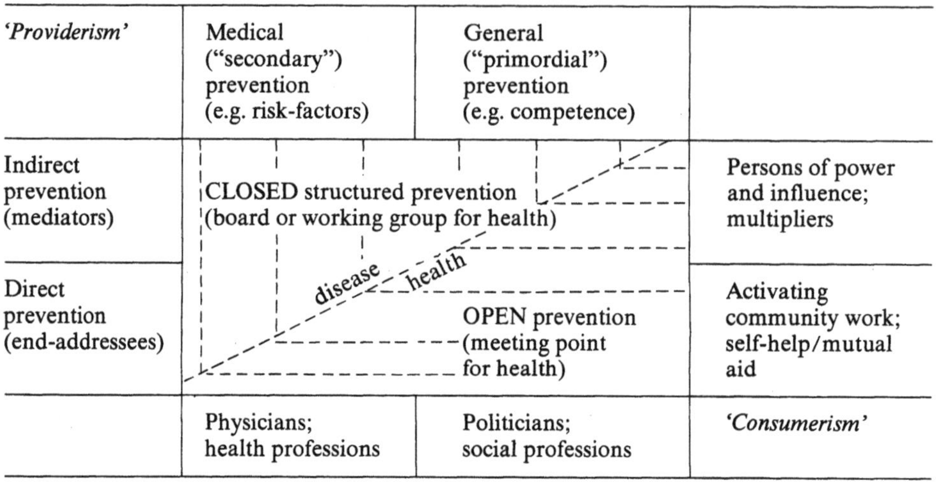

Fig. 3. The community study Rhein-Neckar (GRN) 1983

West, a lower-class quarter of the city of Mannheim with about 20 000 inhabitants, almost one-quarter of whom are guest workers, and the town of Weinheim, which has about 45 000 inhabitants, a middle/upper class population and traditionally is high ranking as regards social facilities. In Neckarstadt-West perceived needs were identified through direct contact with the end-addressees, i.e. the local population, while in Weinheim an indirect approach was used, involving mediating representatives of organizations and institutions relating to health and the social sector in general. Figure 3 tries to summarize the conceptual and terminological framework presented so far: In Neckarstadt-West the outcome of the activation process was a neighbourhood centre-like 'Meeting Point for Self-help Groups and Health Initiatives' (*Treffpunkt*), whereas in Weinheim a 'Working Group for Health' developed out of several preparatory meetings for 'Community Health Weeks' (*Gesundheitswochen*) in the autumn of 1982. The work of the Group for Health in Weinheim (*Arbeitsgemeinschaft Gesundes Weinheim*) concerns itself – due to its delegated composition – with issues of medical as well as general prevention in a more structured way, aiming at the improvement of preventive services (information, skills, screening). However, only recently the group also established telephone advice for potential self-help groups, with almost immediate success in that two self-help groups were formed. On the other hand discussion is at present taking place among the more than 20 groups in and around the Meeting Point in Neckarstadt-West (with its direct approach (of *"open prevention"*, avoiding any advance definition of health issues by experts or mediators) on whether the formation of a registered club might help to stabilize the work by involving relevant institutions and persons with power and influence. Thus it seems that both approaches show converging tendencies and merge into an integrated concept of a Community Health Board, coordinating activities to improve general as well as medical prevention of cardiovascular and other diseases by employing direct and indirect strategies. Such a Community Health Board was proposed

1) Identification of perceived health issues
   - in mediators/experts/professionals
   - in lay persons/end-addressees
2) Analysis of identified health issues according to
   - perceived importance ranking
   - scientific importance ranking
   - available know-how (intervention; evaluation)
   - available resources (personnel; finances)
   - available partners in the field
   - organizational feasibility
   - political feasibility (incl. funding policies)
3) Support for local initiatives
4) Identification of indigenous leadership
5) Development of individual and institutional networks for collaboration
6) Establishment of co-ordination
7) Provision of means for self-evaluation

Fig. 4. Community participation model (Rhein-Neckar)

by the administration of the state of Baden-Württemberg in a recent administrative act (Erlaß vom 30. 8. 82). More details with regard to the experience collected in relation to *open* and *structured prevention* in Neckarstadt-West and Weinheim are presented elsewhere (Becker and Laugsch, this volume, p. 516; Füller, this volume, p. 500). A preliminary summary of the Community Participation Model of the Rhein-Neckar Community Study is given in Fig. 4.

Evaluation of Population-Based Intervention

Population-based intervention studies have maximum generalizability and external validity, but at the price of reduced internal validity, i.e. experimental control. The most important limitations are listed in Fig. 5. For the GRN (part of the DHP study) an 8-year monitoring programme has been designed for outcome variables (total mortality and subcategories of cardiovascular mortality, information on cardiovascular morbidity in terms of analysis of curative factors

1) "Blinding" of treatment input not possible
2) Random assignment not possible (quasi-experimental design)

Therefore limitation of causal inference

3) Restricted suitability for single factor tests
4) Restricted through constraints on resources and logistics

Possible limitations:

5) Impairment of required long-term stability of setting by secular events
6) Relevance of results after completion of long-term studies

Fig. 5. Limitations of population intervention studies

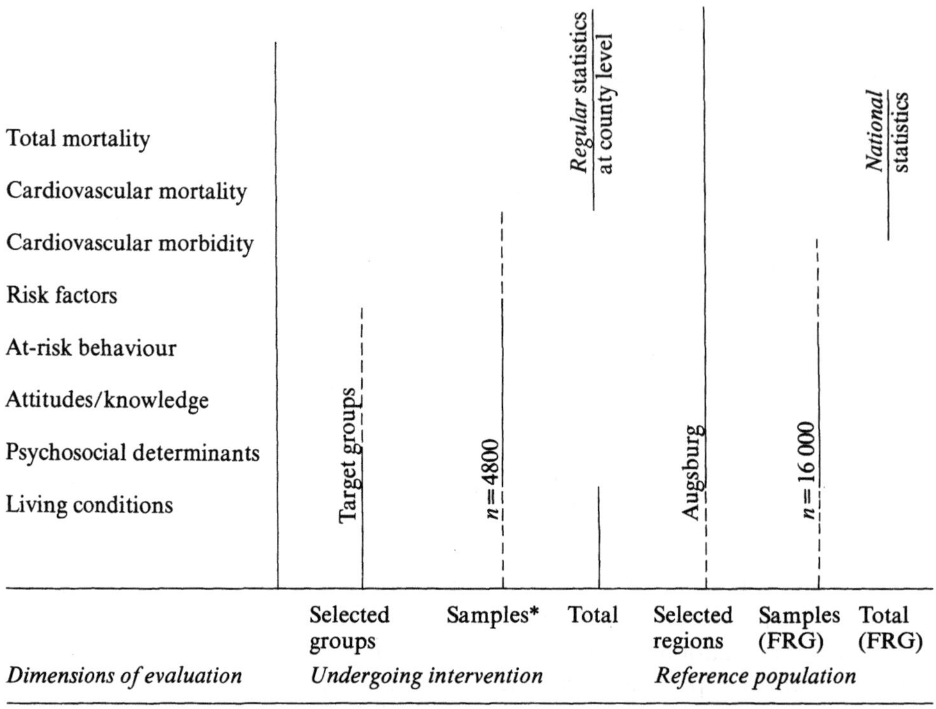

Fig. 6. Monitoring system for the Rhein-Neckar Community Study (in Mannheim and Weinheim, mid-study stable population aged 30–64 85 000 and 12 000 respectively) as part of the DHP study; —— evaluation definite, --- evaluation intended, * cross-sectional and prospective random samples

and hospital statistics, survey samples for risk factors and questionaire information) and process variables (living conditions, psychosocial determinants and at-risk modes of behaviour), the latter data being collected by formal (samples) and informal (action research) methods. Comparison will be made with the other three DHP intervention areas and with the Federal Republic as a whole (by means of the National Health Survey, using identical methodology and national mortality statistics). The analysis of cardiovascular morbidity for the determination of case fatality and survival times (required for the separation of preventive and curative influences) can be made only in comparison to the WHO-Monitoring System for Cardiovascular Disease (MONICA) in Augsburg (U. Keil, personal communication) and possibly elsewhere. Statistical calculation of required sample sizes shows [21] that quasi-significance can be expected for a comparison between Mannheim and Augsburg with regard to the 8-year mortality of cardiovascular disease (ICD 410–414 and 430–438) at standard levels of error I and II if a 10% differential reduction can be achieved. Linked together through detailed process evaluation it would be the first time that community action work in the health field could be shown to be effective at the outcome level. A summary of the monitoring concept of the GRN is shown in Fig. 6.

Conclusion

The "Rhein-Neckar Community Study" provides an advanced integrated approach to the community-based prevention of chronic and, specifically, cardiovascular disease, implementing participatory structures in the communities in order to enhance the development of life-styles conducive to health. The pilot phase 1982/83 has shown the feasibility of this approach.

References

1. Townsend P, Davidson N (1982) Inequalities in health. The Black report. Pelican, London
2. The Board of the German Cardiovascular Prevention Study (1983) DHP-study manual. Bonn
3. World Health Organization (1981) Community control of cardiovascular diseases: The North Karelia Project. Copenhagen
4. World Health Organization European Collaborative Group (1983) Multifactorial trial in the prevention of coronary heart disease. 3. Incidence and mortality results. Eur Heart J 4:141–147
5. Multiple Risk Factor Intervention Trial Research Group (1982) Multiple Risk Factor Intervention Trial: Risk factor changes and mortality results. JAMA 248:1465
6. Committee of Principal Investigators (1980) WHO cooperative trial on primary prevention of ischaemic heart disease using Clofibrate to lower serum cholesterol: Mortality follow-up. Lancet 2:76
7. World Health Organization (EURO) (1983) Lifestyles and their impact on health (fourth draft). 33rd session, Madrid, technical discussions. WHO EUR/RC33/TD, p 3
8. Trojan A (1982) Zur aktuellen Diskussion um die Förderung von Selbsthilfezusammenschlüssen, begriffliche Vorklärungen und Empfehlungen. In: Ergänzung zum 3. Zwischenbericht des Forschungsverbundes Laienpotential, Patientenaktivierung und Gesundheitsselbsthilfe. Düsseldorf, p 75
9. Bundesministerium für Forschung und Technologie (1983) Forschung und Entwicklung im Dienste der Gesundheit, Programm der Bundesregierung 1983–1986. Bonn
10. McEwen J, Martini CJM, Wilkins N (1983) Participation in health. London, Croom Helm, p 151
11. Sutherland I (1979) History and background. In: Sutherland I (ed) Health education, perspectives and choices. London, Allen and Unwin
12. Orth-Gomer K, Perski A, Theorell T (1983) Psychosocial factors and cardiovascular disease – a review of the current state of knowledge. The National Institute for Psychosocial Factors and Health, Stockholm
13. Siegrist J, Dittmann K, Rittner K, Weber I (1980) Soziale Belastungen und Herzinfarkt. Enke, Stuttgart
14. Karasek RA, Russel RS, Theorell T (1982) Physiology of stress and regeneration in job related cardiovascular illness. J Human Stress 8:29
15. Karasek RA (1979) Job demands, job decision latitude and mental strain: Implications for job redesign. Adm Sci Q 24:285
16. Karasek RA, Baker D, Marxer F, Ahlbom A, Theorell T (1981) Job decision latitude, job demands and cardiovascular disease: A prospective study of Swedish men. Am J Public Health 71:694
17. Berkman LF, Syme SL (1979) Social networks, host resistance, and mortality: A nine-year follow-up study of Alameda county residents. Am J Epidemiol 109:186
18. Medalie JH, Kahn HA, Neufeld HN, Riss E, Goldbourt M (1973) Five-year myocardial infarction incidence. J Chronic Dis 26:329

19. Marmot G, Syme SL, Kagan A, Kato H, Cohen JB, Belsky J (1975) Epidemiologic studies of coronary heart disease and stroke in Japanese men living in Japan, Hawaii and California: Prevalence of coronary and hypertensive heart disease and associated risk factors. Am J Epidemiol 102:514
20. Laaser U (1981) Epidemiologie: Wissenschaft, Methode oder Aufgabe? Med Klin 76:407
21. Schumann V, Laaser U (1983) Auswertung von Mortalitätsdaten mit Regressionsmethoden zur Beurteilung von Interventionseffekten bei Herz-Kreislauf-Studien. DIBHB, Heidelberg

Appendix

Results Obtained with Risk Display and Prevalence Display for Selected Social and Biological Determinants *

The 11 selected panels (Figs. 3 – 13) are very briefly described with the "co-control variable" as heading (Fig. 2).

Parity (Figs. 3 – 7)

The number of previous live births (parity) is a biologic determinant of the outcome of delivery for both mother and infant. Both primiparity (no previous live births) and grand-multiparity (4+ or 5+ previous live births) are generally associated with higher risk of death than intermediate parity (1 – 3 previous live births). While retaining the parity control, one can also introduce a second control, as shown in Fig. 2 and discussed below.

Registration Status (Fig. 3)

The peak risks of death coincide with grand-multiparous women admitted in emergency (44.8/1000 and 482.3/1000); the lowest; with women recorded as booked primiparous (0.40/1000 and 15.0/1000). Relative to intermediate-parity women (1 – 3 previous live births), grand-multiparous women have a 2.11-fold risk of maternal death and a 1.28-fold risk of perinatal death. Grand-multiparity thus has a more harmful effect on the life of the mother than on the life of the infant, with excess risks of death of 111% and 28%, respectively. Finally, the peak-to-base relative risk of maternal death is 112 (44.81/0.40), the largest bivariate control variation in risk noted so far in this control system. In future studies, emergency admissions and referrals will need particular attention since they carry the highest risks of death and thus merit priority attention even in each center's catchment area.

Maternal Health Status (Fig. 4)

The base risks refer to perfectly healthy women (HW) of moderate parity (0.88/1000 and 19.7/1000). By contrast, the peak risks exhibit dichotomized specificity: for maternal death it pertains to primiparas with hypertensive disorders of pregnancy (HDP; 18.00/1000); for perinatal death it pertains to grand-multiparas with hemorrhage per vaginam (HPV; 421.1/1000). Also, a concerted effort was made to fight the consequences of hemorrhage with blood transfusions with an apparent reduction of the maternal death rate. This documents by MCM the sequence "morbidity – intervention – outcome." Finally, deficiency anemia (AW) carries a 2.52-fold risk of perinatal death, and hemorrhage, a 19.6-fold risk of perinatal death compared with

* This note has been added in proof to supplement the chapter by Bernard and Sastrawinata (Sect. B, pp. 335 – 351) with a discussion of the results

Primary Health Care in the Making
Ed. by U. Laaser, R. Senault, H. Viefhues

risks calculated for healthy women of moderate parity. In other words, the risk of perinatal death with obstetric hemorrhage is 8 times that with deficiendy anemia.

Maternal Blood Hemoglobin (Fig. 5)

The peak risks are dramatic and apply to grand-multiparous women with less than 6 g hemoglobin per 100 ml on admission for delivery (81.6/1000 and 602.0/1000). An important cutoff point for survival of both the mother and the infant is between 7 and 8 g Hb/100 ml. Hence, less than 8 g Hb/100 ml is an extremely high risk factor for survival of both mother and infant. Prompt intervention will save life.

Complications of Labor/Delivery (Fig. 6)

The peak risks are carried by grand-multiparous women with placenta abruptio (33.1/1000 and 768.2/1000); the base risks by moderate-parity with no complications of labor and/or delivery (0.50/1000 and 38.6/1000). A significant problem emerges with prolonged/obstructed labor, since both involve very high risks for grand-multiparous women (25.5/1000 and 258.2/1000) and 10% of all deliveries were affected by this high-risk complication (3624/36, 321). A major priority is recognized in this sector for a national program to be launched.

Duration of Labor (Fig. 7)

Documentation of the previous problem is possible. For grand-multiparous women the risk of maternal death with more than 18 h duration of labor is 10 times that with labor lasting 7 – 12 h (31.9/3.1), the corresponding relative risk of perinatal death being 3.57 (263.7/73.9). Obviously, cases of difficult labor often arrive at the top referral level too late, leading to unacceptable mortality levels for both mother and infant. The whole referral system is currently in need of reassessment from top to bottom.

The 76-panel risk atlas contains several panels pertaining to the management of current deliveries. We have selected one as an example.

Type of Presentation and Type of Delivery (Fig. 8)

Analysis of risk patterns by type of presentation during labor and type of delivery exhibit important "end point differentiation." Among vertex occiput anterior presentations, a steep gradient of risk of maternal death extends from 0.99/1000 for spontaneous deliveries up to 21.30/1000 for cesarean sections – a relative risk of 21.5; while the corresponding relative risk for perinatal death is only 4.04 (158.8/39.3). Obviously, infant life was saved with cesarean section, but the 21-fold ratio for maternal death points to the "too-late-arrival-for-survival" syndrome that plagues the national referral system. Breech presentation with delivery by cesarean section instead of vaginal extraction carries a 37% lower risk of perinatal death (1 – 145.2/230.1), a documented example of intervention success. Breech presentation followed by spontaneous delivery carries a high risk of perinatal death of 244.9/1000, probably because of its frequent association with low birth weight. The same reason may be suspected to be operative with transverse presentation, which involves a risk of perinatal death of 818.2/ 1000. Finally, vertex occiput transverse/posterior presentation involves a serious degree of risk for both mother and infant. In 992 women this presentation led to cesarean section, and this was found to carry a maternal death risk of 14.1/1000 and a perinatal death risk of 193.5/1000. Obviously, prolonged/obstructed labor is one of the main factors behind this dual high risk.

The 76-panel risk atlas contains 18 panels of risks of maternal and perinatal death, with a specific co-control and the "counterpart mortality end point" used as the other control. In other words, across 18 variables the mother-infant death relationship is documented quantitatively. Two panels have been selected.

Counterpart Outcomes and Duration of Labor (Fig. 9)

For both control combinations (maternal death by infant outcome; perinatal death by maternal outcome, both across duration of labor), dramatic *risk fronts of mother-infant death* emerge across duration of labor. In addition, a serious "excess duration effect" on both single and dual loss is noted. For instance, among women with 7–12 h duration of labor, the risk of maternal death is 12.6 times higher when perinatal death occurs than when the infants survive (12.60/1.00). But that high risk increases 4.6-fold if the duration of labor extends to more than 18 h (57.88/12.60). It increases 5.76-fold if the duration of labor exceeds 24 h (72.63/12.60). This last risk affected 358 women, or 0.97% of all deliveries. Protracted labor thus emerges as a major perinatal killer for both mother and infant: in fact; 25.6% (34/133) of all maternal deaths were characterized both by "25+ h duration of labor" and by "infant death". Conversely, 12.8% (358/2797) of all infant deaths during the perinatal period were characterized both by "25+ h duration of labor" and by "maternal death." Clearly, *excessive duration of labor* is pernicious in its effect on the life of both mother and infant. Beyond 18 h duration of labor both risks rise dramatically, the base risks coinciding with a duration of 7–12 h.

Counterpart Outcomes and Maternal Age (Fig. 10)

For both control combinations (MAMO by INFOUT; PD by MATOUT, both across maternal age at current delivery), impressive *risk fronts of mother-infant death* emerge across maternal age. In addition, pernicious effects of "teenage" and "advanced reproductive age" become apparent on both maternal death combinations (without or with infant death). The risk of maternal death for *teenage deliveries* is 90% above base risk with infant death (29.15/15.33), and 113% above base risk with infant survival (2.22/1.04); the base risks are those associated with childbirth at age 20–24 years. Relative to these base risks, the risk of maternal death for *advanced age deliveries* is in excess by 191% with infant death (44.67/15.33) and by 263% with infant survival (3.78/1.04). Teenage and advanced reproductive age thus emerge as major perinatal killers for both mother and infant, and more for the mother than the infant: in fact, 31.7% (44/139) of all maternal deaths carried the dual characteristics: "35+ years of age" and "infant death"; conversely, 20.8% (582/2801) of all infant deaths during the perinatal period carried the dual characteristics: "35+ years of age" and "maternal death." At the lower age extreme, 12.9% (18/139) of all maternal deaths carried the dual characteristics: "teenage" and "infant death"; conversely, 12.2% (343/2801) of all infant deaths during the perinatal period carried the dual characteristics: "teenage" and "maternal death." In other words, *one eighth* of all maternal and perinatal deaths are associated with teenage delivery. Furthermore, since teenage and advanced reproductive age emerge as major biologic risk factors for the survival of both mother and infant for a given reproductive step (index delivery), the harm sustained should be quantitated routinely. Of all maternal deaths, 44.6% occurred in women aged either below 20 years or 35 or more years (62/139); the corresponding proportion of all infant deaths is 33% (925/2801). In other words, the absence of deliveries at the two extremes of maternal age would have reduced maternal deaths to 55.4% and perinatal deaths to 67.0% of the empirical occurrence in the top referral/teaching system. The J-shaped patterns of risks of maternal and perinatal deaths across maternal age can be viewed as a "biologic warning" that human reproduction should occur at intermediate ages only if high excess risks of a biologic nature are to be avoided for both mother and offspring. The *biologic argument* for limiting human reproduction to intermediate ages for health reasons constitutes a credible alternative to limiting human reproduction for demographic reasons. Also, the force of mobilization at the family level for biologically oriented optimization of reproduction patterns supports the health argument. Benefits of this approach are enhanced reproductive health, lower mortalities (all end points), and lower total fertility. The *biologically optimal period* for human reproduction can be ascertained by each nation with the aid of MCM.

Maternal morbidity and complications of labor and/or delivery appear to be key determinants of an unfavorable birth outcome for both mother and infant. Hence the need to study their prevalence in hospital and to control for maternal age and parity, two "biologic controls" which are, in addition, the twin variables defining fertility in general demography (all live births ever to women of a given maternal age). It is crucial that this *interdisciplinary methodologic understanding* be perceived by the health care professions, since it may provide a common base for discussing problems of fertility in developing countries and there may be a future significant input by the professions engaged in reproductive health care provision. In essence, the *risk approach* may start to generate information as important as that the *World*

Fertility Survey was able to publicize in the 1970s. Above all, by controlling for fertility, the *excess morbidities and mortalities* for unbiologic fertility combinations may give the demographic argument for "spacing and stopping" a more appealing "direct interest" connotation at the *microlevel* (the family) than it has so far been able to give it in the general population. Family health may emerge as a far more convincing argument for *behavioral change* in human reproduction than the high population growth rate has been at the macrolevel.

Hypertensive Disorders by Fertility (Fig. 11.1)

Age- and parity-controlled hypertensive disorders of pregnancy have a marked prevalence concentration among primiparas and women with advanced reproductive age, peaking at 18.5% in elderly primiparas. At all parities, advanced maternal age at index birth carries an excess prevalence of hypertensive disorders.

Hemorrhage per Vaginam by Fertility (Fig. 11.2)

Age- and parity-controlled hemorrhage per vagina increases at all ages with parity. Beside this parity effect, a teenage effect is noted at low parity and an advanced age effect at high parity, the latter culminating in an incidence of 6.83% for elderly grand-multiparous women with vaginal hemorrhage. The base prevalence of 1.26% applies to women aged 20–24 years with no previous live births. Had reproduction been confined to the "optimal biological window" of 20–34 years with 0–2 previous live births, this would have reduced hemorrhage per vaginam to 40.4%, i. e., to two-fifths of the current empirical occurrence. Overall, the prevalence rate of 3.19% would be reduced to 2.37% merely be confinement of reproduction to the optimal biologic window alone, – an improvement of 25.7%. The implications would be significant, since hemorrhage per vaginam carries a 10.27-fold risk of maternal death (8.63/0.84) and an 18.15-fold risk of perinatal death (401.2/22.1) compared with the corresponding base risks in perfectly healthy women (Fig. 4).

Prolonged and/or Obstructed Labor by Fertility (Fig. 12.1)

Age- and parity-controlled difficult labor shows a prevalence concentration among primiparas and women with advanced reproductive age, culminating for elderly primiparas at 25.4%. The dramatic drop in prevalence across all ages with increasing parity indicates that the first birth creates the greatest problems pertaining to pathologic features of labor. Since labor is difficult in exactly 10.0% of all deliveries, the *referral system* for cases of difficult labor must be reexamined. Difficult labor carries a 21.0-fold risk of maternal death (15.73/0.75) and a 4.6-fold risk of perinatal death (185.7/40.7) compared with the corresponding base risks carried by women with no complications (Fig. 6). Any decline in hospital prevalence of difficult labor as a result of reorganizing the referral system would lead to an important decline in the overall risks of maternal and perinatal death.

Placenta Previa by Fertility (Fig. 12.2)

Age- and parity-controlled placenta previa increases in incidence more with parity than with age. Nevertheless, beside this important parity effect a teenage effect is noted at low parity and an advanced age effect at high parity, peaking at 6.42% in "elderly grand-multiparous women." The base prevalence of 1.23% applies to women aged 20–24 with no previous live births. The data suggest an increasing likelihood of low implantation of a fertilized egg with increasing parity. This could be compatible with a parity-operated "biologic tiring effect." The hypothesis of "descending implantation" as a consequence of excess reproduction has thus been formulated empirically. Of all cases of placenta previa, 60.6% occurred in women below 20 years of age and those having a third or subsequent baby and/or aged 35+ years (717/1184). In other words, reproduction confined to the optimal biological window of 20–34 years of age with 0–2 previous live births would have reduced this condition to 39.4%, that is to two-fifths, of the current empirical hospital occurrence. Overall, the prevalence rate of 3.26% for placenta previa would drop to 2.44%, an improvement by 25.2%. The implications are significant, since placenta previa carries a 16.9-fold risk of maternal death (12.67/0.75) and a 7.8-fold risk of perinatal death (316.7/40.7) compared with the corresponding base risks for women with no complications (Fig. 6). The empirical hypothesis of descending implantation with increasing parity should be further investigated.

Moderately Low Birth Weight (MODLBW) by Fertility (Fig. 13.1)

Age- and parity-controlled women show the highest concentrations of moderately low birth weight (2000–2499 g) infants among primiparas, with important increases at both age extremes and significant decreases with increasing parity. Thus the first live-born child appears to be lighter than subsequent ones, but extremes of age increase this "reproduction start" effect on birth weight. Since hypertensive disorders show a somewhat similar pattern (Fig. 11.1) the latter may be causally related to moderate low birth weight. This suggests a new pathway of analysis for the near future.

Severely Low Birth Weight (SEVLBW) by Fertility (Fig. 13.2)

Age- and parity-controlled women exhibit a totally different prevalence pattern of severely low birth weight (< 2000 g) than of moderately low birth weight (2000–2499 g). The reproduction start effect has vanished, suggesting that moderate low birth weight among primiparas borders on biologic normality. By contrast, women with severely low birth weight infants are concentrated in the *teenage group* and that of *women with high parity in their early twenties.* This empirical observation amounts to a biologic warning against both teenage pregnancy and too-narrowly spaced pregnancies during the early twenties (there is thus an interesting parallel with the demographers' quest for later marriage and delay and spacing of low-order births). Obviously, this biologic warning is far more convincing than the demographers' quest, since it addresses the health status of the new offspring directly, with its links to morbidity and mortality at the family level. As shown in Fig. 13.2, there is a clearcut delineation of two contrasting levels of prevalence of women with severely low birth weight infants: (a) *Teens and high parity in the early twenties* (the 6 cells have a combined proportion of 8.21% of severely low birth weight infants); and (b) *the complementing age/parity fields* (the 14 cells have a combined proportion of only 4.44% of severely low birth weight infants). The implications of this 84.9% excess prevalence of severely low birth weight infants among births to teenagers and women of high parity in their early twenties are easy to perceive, since severely low birth weight involves a 16.5-fold risk of perinatal death compared with infants with optimal birth weight of 3000–3499 g (572.8/34.7, calculated from panel 44 of the risk atlas, which is not included).

Summary of Methodology

This paper reports selected findings from the first *dual risk of death at birth* analysis carried out with aggregated MCM data collected by the departments of obstetrics and gynecology in Indonesia from 1978 to 1980. Dual-control risk and prevalence tables derived from standard computer outputs (SCOs) are presented in 3D display for continuous documentation and broad access by various disciplines concerned with human reproduction.

A system of *basic information modules* has been created: self-contained single-page *Panels* that can be assembled ad libitum into *analytic pathways* with specific epidemiological focus. The panel is an epidemiologic building block that exists independently as an unalterable document referred to time and place. The focus in this report is on maternal age and parity (demography's "fertility") as *controls* and on maternal and perinatal deaths as *outcomes* (epidemiology's "mortalities"), by constructing an analytic pathway (Fig. 2) from 11 of 76 panels of a forthcoming Risk Atlas for the use of the professions concerned with reproductive health care provision in Indonesia.

The *maternal health status (ICD-9)* and *complications of labor and/or delivery* emerge as important determinants of delivery outcome for both mother and infant. This observation "directs" the analytic pathway to display various conditions of *morbidity and complications* as a function of *reproductive attainment* (age and parity = fertility). The study of institutional prevalence of "fertility-controlled" hypertensive disorders of pregnancy (Fig. 11.1), hemorrhage per vaginam (Fig. 11.2), prolonged/obstructed labor (Fig. 12.1), placenta previa (Fig. 12.2), moderate low birth weight (Fig. 13.1), and severe low birth weight (Fig. 13.2) then leads on to a battery of important findings and "empirical hypotheses," all pointing towards the same overriding behavioral necessity. The prevention/reduction of pathologic conditions linked with human reproduction and the prevention/reduction of the risks of maternal and perinatal death would make a leap forward if procreation were restricted in time and frequency to a relatively narrow "age/parity window" with optimal outcomes for mother and infant. The *optimal biological window in time and amount* for this data set collected from 11 university departments is 20 – 34 years of maternal age and 0 – 2 or 0 – 3 previous live births.

Any "expansion" to lower or higher ages (TEENS and ARA) and/or higher parities (GDMP) is associated with a sharp increase in morbidity and with complications leading to dramatic increases in the risks of maternal and perinatal death. Furthermore, initiation of childbearing in the early twenties and spacing between pregnancies is an "empirical dictate" derived from the low birth weight analysis (Fig. 13.2).

The findings of this epidemiological analysis are promising, since they make the *biological need for moderate human reproduction* a parade issue of preventive medicine at the microlevel (the family), as against a developmental need for the reduction of the population growth rate at the macrolevel (the society). Apparently, a shift in perception is currently emerging on the primary reason for moderate human reproduction: from demography to reproductive health. The "health argument" for moderate fertility is documentable by MCM. Similar systems studies are now needed in nations other than Indonesia.

Acknowledgements. The authors and the heads of departments of obstetrics and gynecology in Indonesian medical faculties express gratitude to His Excellency Dr. Suwardjono, Minister of Health, for his personal and continued encouragement and interest in the professional deployment of Maternity Care Monitoring. The first author is grateful for the many discussions and for general encouragement to engage in experimental methodology development with this empirical material. Prof. F. Kubli, Heidelberg, is thanked for encouraging the standardization of the 3D display technique in spring 1982 on the occasion of a Workshop on Monitoring and Reporting Perinatal Mortality and Morbidity held by the FIGO Standing Commitee on Perinatal Mortality and Morbidity. Prof. O. Käser, Basel, is thanked for a stimulating consultation about the risk atlas on maternal and perinatal mortality in summer 1983. For moral and material support the first author is indebted to Prof. H. de Watteville, Dr. E. Kessel, M. R. and Mme. N. Keller, Mme. L. Rothenbühler, and last but not least, Mme. A. Bernard. The second author is grateful to all colleagues and staff for their commitment to this intercenter project sponsored by BKS PENFIN. Comprehensive recording and experimentation with analytic epidemiology are now paying dividends beyond any participants' expectations. Finally, initial help from IFRP and the transfer of appropriate technology is gratefully acknowledged.

Subject Index

achievement motive 391
adaptive behaviour of patients 266
adiposity 416
adolescents 135
adolescents' life-style 162
adopted children from tropical (subtropical) countries 296
aftercare pattern 261
air pollutants 215
– pollution 222
alcohol 205
– prevention 207
allied health professions 42
ambulatory care 80
anti-adiposity training 416
antidepressants 140
arterial blood pressure 150
authority 241
autoprotective efforts 273

back problems 274
basic disorders 268, 269
– health service 386
– needs concept 386
behaviour 326
behavioural therapy 506
benign course 188
biographical perspective 285
birth weight 122
blue collar, white collar workers 179
– –, worker 175
body and health workshop model 165
bone and joint disorders 238
burns 307

cardiovascular 495
– disease 132, 274, 524
– mortality 454
– risk 135
causal model 127
childhood 285
child-psychiatry 125
cholesterol 495
chronic disease 227, 241, 274
– – of the respiratory organs 215, 238
– mental illness 256
– vascular disease 249
cigarette smoking 398
cigarettes with natural untreated tobacco 407
classification systems 88
cleaning personnel 295
clonidine 429
cluster analysis 141
coeliac disease 296
COHb Level 398
communication problems 305
community 132, 421, 500
– development 386
– diagnosis 387
– health councils 323
– involvement 378, 386
– nurses 505
– participation 11, 388, 516, 531
– prevention 510
– sector 378
– work 501
community-based 533
community-orientated care 261
compensation phenomenon 418
compensatory efforts 269
complex diagnosis 87
compliance 115, 240
comprehensive care 180
conditional, multinomial, distributions 276
confounding 216
consumer participation 501
context of gratification 177
– of performance 177
co-operating 31
coordination 500
coping 241
– behaviour 190

coronary heart disease 170, 181, 464, 495
– prone behaviour 170
– surgery 179
cosmic rays 252
cost and benefit 328
cost-effectiveness 483
costs 106
cultural background 287
– traditions 282
curative 418
cure 505
curriculum 47

dayas 379
decentralization 389
delivery 308
demand 329
demedicalisation 320
deprofessionalisation 320
desorientation 285
determinants, psychosocial 528
diabetes mellitus 238
diabetic diet 408
diagnostic vocabulary 274
dialysis 229
– patients 296
diet counseling 408
dietary therapy 418
digitalis 109
dihydralazine 429
discontinuity 285
discriminant analysis 276
disease-prevention 509
diseases, circulatory system 238
dissatisfaction 96
division of tasks 39
doctor-patient relationship 241
drug counselling 47
drugs 105
dual-career marriage 227

ecological concept 156
economics 106
education 502
– of Turkish infants 297
educational commission for foreign medical graduates 26
– level 217
– program 68, 434
educators 327
effectiveness 477
efforts to compensate basic disorders 268
electrocardiographic findings 109
emotional reactions 230
environmental factors 513

epidemiological 326
– project 125
– research 215
– studies 109, 138
episodes of schizophrenic disorders 267
equity 100
ethical 326
evaluation 325
exercise 144
experts 241

family confrontation 230
–, counselling 60
–, medicine 15, 49
–, physicians 505
–, rehabilitation 229
–, therapy 233
feasibility study 68
Federal Republic of Germany 75
feelt needs 388
follow-up 135, 154
foreign children 300
– families 294
Fourier analysis 255

gastro-intestinal ailments 304
general practitioner 96, 101
– practitioners 80
– prevention 528
geographic latitude 252
geomagnetic latitude 252
geophysical factors 252
government 321
graduate medical training 25
grammatical constructions 86
group medical practice 34
guest workers 294
gynaecologist 101

habits 132
Hadon's strategies 142
handicaps 307
health advisory 418
– centres 39, 322
– committee 502
– counselling 67
– disorders 513
– education 148, 150, 207
– – programmes 295
– effects research 215
– information 502
– insurance 274, 512
– – status 81
– needs 12

– planning 387
– policy 402
– promotion 163, 326, 503, 516, 521
– risk appraisal 23
– security 505
– status measures 101
– work 516
health-promoting functions 418
high blood pressure 421
– – –, education 464
– – –, trials 451
holistic approach 38
– health 158
home-blood pressure 428
hospital setting 231
hospitalized foreigners 295
– patients 265
human ecology approach 164
hypertension 183, 238, 428, 477
hypertensives 456

identification of patterns 274
illness and health 288
immigrant families 300
immigration 284
incidence 329
–, rate 263
indepent terms 88
industrial accidents 306
infant mortality 307
infections 307
informal sector 378
in-patient phase 506
insecurity 285
interaction between variables 278
interdisciplinary teamwork 42
internist 74, 80, 96, 101
inter-professional co-operation 38
– group practices 38
interruption of pregnancy 296
intersectoral co-operation 379
intervention 150, 206
interviews of doctors 74
involvement 320
ischaemic heart disease 238

job characteristics 175

knowledge 132

labour migration 304
lack of communicative rapport 232
lasting success 416
latent period 277
lay competence 158
– involvement 516, 524
– persons 503
lay-helper 505
"leaving one out" method 276
leisure-time activities 506
length of employment 277, 279
levels of aftercare 262
lifelong therapeutic strategy 505
life-style 157, 162, 237, 326, 506
light smoking 403
living conditions 297
long-stay patients 265
long-term trends 432
loss of weight 418

magnetic activity 253
malignant 188
– tumours 238
marital status 218
maternal 122
– perinatal death 335
medical care utilization 456
– education 11, 14
– knowledge 88
– pedagogy 3
– problems 294
– secondary prevention 530
– sociologist 280
– treatment 32, 287
medicalization 241
mental health problems 82
methods of suicide 139
migrant family 284
migration 25, 281, 304
minimal brain dysfunction 125
missing data 432
mortality 307
motivations 327
multi-dimensional nomenclature 87
multiple regression analysis 96
– sclerosis 188, 252
– – death rate 255
multivariate dependency analysis 153
myocardial infarction 244, 429
myocardinal infarction 179

natural course 261
neurophysiological abnormalities 126
non-compliance 242
non-compliers 262
non-smokers 216
nurses 381
nursing professions 43
nutritional intake 128

obese children 128
occupational careers 177
– diseases 306
– health services 181
– performance 188
– perspectives 40
– stress 170
oral contraceptives 136, 244
out-patient phase 507
overall diagnosis 230

parasitic infections 294
parent-child interactions 127
participation 320
participatory evaluation 386
patient education 408
patient-oriented local group 418
– teamwork 31
patient-physician contacts 82
patients 321
pattern of illness behaviour 280
– of support 391
people's medical society 510
perceived needs 387
periodicities 432
personal life narratives 288
– training 418
pharmacist 322
physical exercise 418
– fitness 128, 398
poisonings 307
policy of primary preventive health care 514
pollution abatement 222
polyclinic services 381
popular medicine 283
population intervention studies 531
positive auto-suggestion 418
practitioner's surgery 231
prazosin 429
prenatal 308
prescription patterns 112
prevalence 252
– of chronic bronchitis 215
prevention 132
– programmes 421
preventive 418
– care programme 308
– counselling 67
– measures 282
– medicine 11, 22, 402, 495
primary care 82
– – doctors 74
– – morbidity 79
– health 274
– – care 11, 60, 378, 386
– – – professions 43
– prevention 150, 512, 524
private practices 74
pro familia 47
problem solving 329
professional 321
– attitudes 8
– profile 9
– roles 39
programme 132, 464
prospective 266
psychiatric syndromes 300
psychological stress 433
psychosocial 326
– counselling 47
– situation 188
psychosomatic and psychosocial problems 79
psychotic patients 264
public health services 505

quality control 57

random-zero sphygmomanometer 155
receptionists 40
rehabilitation 179, 190, 249
– measures 306, 477
– professions 43
– services 32
renal diseases 115, 183
reproductive behaviour 305
rheumatic diseases 238
risk behaviour 163
–, display 335
– factor 67, 150, 170

sanitation 295
scalds 307
schizophrenia 267
schizophrenic patients 261
secondary schools 147
self blood pressure measurement 434
self-assurance 151
self-help 320, 505, 527
– groups 40, 323, 505
self-medication 321
self-monitoring 428
self-organization 501
self-reported health 456
self-responsibility 241
self-stabilisation 267, 269
semantic model 87
– patterns 89
separation of the family 285

services 83
severity 82
– rating 477
silent, impassive husband 232
simple diagnosis 87
slovenia 148
smokers 216
smoking 151, 391
– cessation 394
social and biological determinants 335
– change 388
– coping 528
– – strategies 514
– and environmental factors 215
– factors 122
– medicine 14
– network 285
– problem 281
– rights 285
– support 95
– workers 505
social-class 151, 229
socioeconomic status 100, 152
solar cycle 253
sotalol 429
sources of care 102
specific skills 126
status of residence 287
stepwise logistic regression analysis 479
– return to work 180
stigmatization 127
stillborn 307
strategies for prevention 138
strokes 464
subjective strain 175
suicide 264
– by firearms 137
– prevention 142
– rate 137
support of daily activities 32
surgery 249
survey 80
symptoms 280

team-work 13
technical health professions 43
telephone medicine 49
text processing 86
tracking 150
traditional customs 295
– family 227
traffic accident 307
training 49, 57
transplants 229
treating hypertensives 483
treatment demand 264
tuberculosis 307
turkish citizens 288

ulcers 304
uncertainties 328
unemployment 229
university curriculum 3
utilization 100, 261, 514

validity of medical diagnoses 274
vietnamese refugees 294
village health workers 386
visa qualifying examination 26
visiting nurse 308
vocational rehabilitation 183
– status 189
– training 45

well-being 326
work incapacity 274
working conditions 306, 513
– potential 189

yaws eradication 370
youth culture 161
– organization 156

MIX
Papier aus verantwortungsvollen Quellen
Paper from responsible sources
FSC® C105338

If you have any concerns about our products,
you can contact us on
ProductSafety@springernature.com

In case Publisher is established outside the EU,
the EU authorized representative is:
Springer Nature Customer Service Center GmbH
Europaplatz 3, 69115 Heidelberg, Germany

Printed by Libri Plureos GmbH
in Hamburg, Germany